EDITED BY

BRUCE J.CRISPIN

CONTEMPORARY ESTHETIC DENTISTRY: PRACTICE FUNDAMENTALS

9-25-95

Printing and Binding: Sun Art Printing Co, Ltd, Osaka
Printed in Japan
ISBN 4-87417-450-7 C 3047

CONTEMPORARY ESTHETIC DENTISTRY: PRACTICE FUNDAMENTALS

BRUCE J. CRISPIN, DDS, MS (EDITOR)
Director, UCLA Center for Esthetic Dentistry
Professor of Fixed Prosthodontics

EDMOND R. HEWLETT, DDS
Assistant Professor, UCLA Section of Operative Dentistry
Instructor, UCLA Center for Esthetic Dentistry

YOUNG HWAN JO, DDS, MSD, PhD
Director, Seoul Dental Institute, Seoul
Visiting Scholar, UCLA Center for Esthetic Dentistry

SUMIYA HOBO, DDS, MS, PhD
Director, International Dental Academy, Tokyo
Visiting Professor, UCLA Center for Esthetic Dentistry

DAVID S. HORNBROOK, DDS
Private Practice, La Mesa, CA
Visiting Lecturer, UCLA Center for Esthetic Dentistry

QUINTESSENCE PUBLISHING CO.,LTD. 1994
Tokyo, Chicago, Berlin, London, São Paulo, Moscow

PREFACE

This book is designed to provide an easy-to-access source of information on contemporary esthetic dental techniques and materials. Each chapter is divided into the following components for easy reference: (1) Historical and/or Scientific Background Information, (2) Clinical Techniques and (3) Related Materials. Materials used are described in a generic way due to the multitude of materials available and the amount of change that is constantly occurring.* Finally, (4) Laboratory Procedures are presented. The intention is to provide the restorative dentist with a basic review of laboratory procedures, which should enhance understanding and laboratory communication. It is the goal of the authors to make the process of learning easier and more organized in the everchanging and sometimes controversial area of contemporary esthetic dentistry.

The focus of the book is on esthetic approaches that are relatively new, minimally invasive, and within the ability range of the average practicing dentist. The exciting thing about contemporary approaches to esthetic dentistry is that no longer are highly esthetic results only achievable by a few elite dentists. The average dentist with a desire to learn and the commitment to pay attention to technique details can also achieve conservative, long-lasting and highly esthetic results.

* A Materials Reference Supplement containing up-dated information on specific materials is available from the author for a nominal postage/handling fee ($5.00 US, $10.00 outside US). Send original coupon on the back flap, including check or money order, to: Dr. Bruce J. Crispin, CHS, Room 33-009-A, 10833 Le Conte Avenue, Los Angeles, CA 90024-1668.

CONTENTS

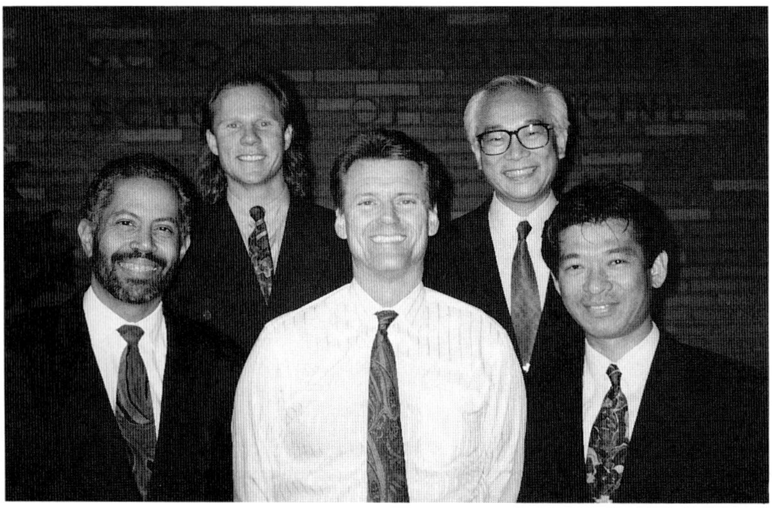

Top left Dr. HORNBROOK
Top right Dr. HOBO
Bottom left Dr. HEWLETT
Bottom center Dr. CRISPIN
Bottom right Dr. JO

ACKNOWLEDGMENTS

The authors wish to thank the following for their exceptional contributions in making this text a reality:

PUBLICATION ASSISTANT: Vicky A. Crispin

ILLUSTRATIONS: Irene Petravicius

EDITING: Dr. Jay Watson

PHOTOGRAPHY: Richard Friske

WORD PROCESSING: Mickey Stern
Larry Clarke

CERAMISTS: Dan Ortiz
UCLA Faculty Practice
da Vinci Studios
Katsumi Tamura, CDT
International Dental Academy

DEDICATION

This book is dedicated to all the dental professionals that have shared with us their clinical and research expertise for the advancement of esthetic dentistry. Secondly, this book is dedicated to the families that have supported us and allowed enough freedom to make this text possible.

INTRODUCTION

In the past 30 years, esthetic approaches to restorative dentistry have gone through an incredible transition, from esthetic partial coverage preparation designs and denture tooth pontics, to acrylic and later porcelain veneering of metal. The development of tooth colored restorative materials and finally the avalanche of techniques ushered in by the ability to "bond" different substrates together have led to the establishment of esthetic dentistry as a subspecialty.

As our ability to provide esthetic dentistry has improved, patient awareness and demands for esthetic excellence have increased. Consequently, the scope of esthetic dentistry has greatly expanded. Currently, the restorative dentist is a member of a team that works together to solve esthetically related problems. The dental specialists, related medical specialists, cosmetologists, the patient and the restorative dentist and staff work together to provide solutions to the esthetic problem in the orofacial region.

The demand for esthetically related services is immense and growing. The esthetic component of the average dental practices is currently significant and will continue to become more significant as dentists and patients become more aware and familiar with what is available to them. This book is designed to aid the restorative dentist in that developmental process.

CHAPTER 1

COMMUNICATION TECHNIQUES: THE FOUNDATION UPON WHICH TO BUILD AN ESTHETIC PRACTICE

INTRODUCTION TO PATIENT COMMUNICATION

Whether you are starting a new practice, converting the emphasis in an existing practice or expanding the esthetic component of a practice, one common denominator exists. The practice of dentistry is no longer involved exclusively with the prevention and elimination of disease. Today's contemporary esthetic practice also deals with elective procedures that may improve upon an already existing healthy situation. The primary reason that many of these elective esthetic procedures are being accepted by our patients is that these treatments do not require the same amount of tooth destruction once necessary to achieve an esthetic result.

The average patient wants to look as good as possible. Educating patients about contemporary esthetic dental techniques is the basis of their understanding and acceptance of treatment that will improve their appearance. Because in many instances esthetic procedures are elective and more expensive than other procedures, our ability to communicate and visualize the potential results of an esthetic procedure is essential. Buying esthetic dentistry often involves spending discretionary dollars that might be used for other items a patient feels are more important. Maximizing one's communication skills and techniques will significantly improve upon the ability to educate patients. Through understanding, a significant level of acceptance can be achieved. In addition, comprehensive diagnostic and communication techniques build confidence between the patient and the dental team. This is critical for optimizing patient satisfaction and minimizing dissatisfaction resulting from unrecognized unrealistic expectations.

Identifying Esthetic Concerns

The average patient goes to the dentist to fix a problem, prevent a problem or have his or her teeth cleaned. Almost every patient has esthetic conditions that could be improved upon. The emphasis in an esthetic practice must be to develop a patient focus that has previously not existed towards esthetic problems and to allow for easy access to information regarding possible solutions. All patients should be given an Esthetic Analysis Form as part of their new patient information packet (Fig. 1-1). This analysis must be given in an environment that will allow self-visualization when the patient answers the questions. A hand mirror or wall mirror is essential. A live video camera and monitor would be optimal. Patients could view themselves as others see them and not the usual mirror image they are accustomed to seeing. Some practices like to have the patient fill out all forms before the initial appointment. This may be helpful because it

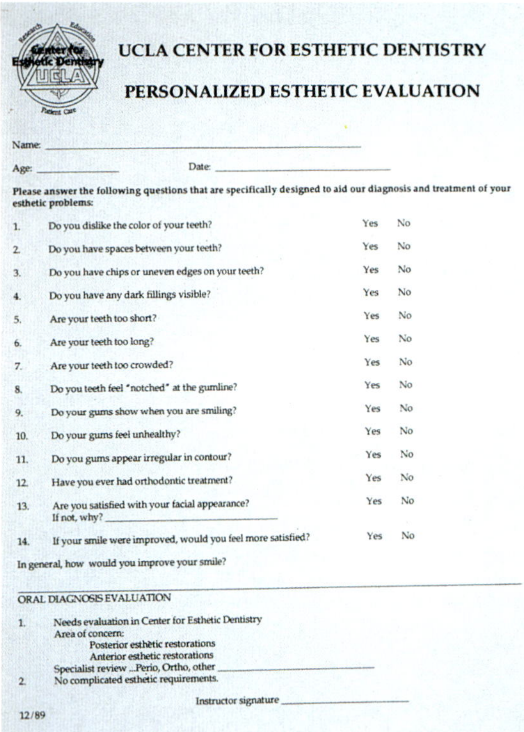

UCLA CENTER FOR ESTHETIC DENTISTRY

PERSONALIZED ESTHETIC EVALUATION

Name: ____________________

Age: __________ Date: __________

Please answer the following questions that are specifically designed to aid our diagnosis and treatment of your esthetic problems:

1.	Do you dislike the color of your teeth?	Yes	No
2.	Do you have spaces between your teeth?	Yes	No
3.	Do you have chips or uneven edges on your teeth?	Yes	No
4.	Do you have any dark fillings visible?	Yes	No
5.	Are your teeth too short?	Yes	No
6.	Are your teeth too long?	Yes	No
7.	Are your teeth too crowded?	Yes	No
8.	Do you teeth feel "notched" at the gumline?	Yes	No
9.	Do your gums show when you are smiling?	Yes	No
10.	Do your gums feel unhealthy?	Yes	No
11.	Do you gums appear irregular in contour?	Yes	No
12.	Have you ever had orthodontic treatment?	Yes	No
13.	Are you satisfied with your facial appearance? If not, why? __________	Yes	No
14.	If your smile were improved, would you feel more satisfied?	Yes	No

In general, how would you improve your smile?

ORAL DIAGNOSIS EVALUATION

1. Needs evaluation in Center for Esthetic Dentistry
   Area of concern:
   Posterior esthètic restorations
   Anterior esthetic restorations
   Specialist review ...Perio, Ortho, other __________
2. No complicated esthètic requirements.

Instructor signature __________

12/89

Fig. 1-1 Esthetic questionnaire.

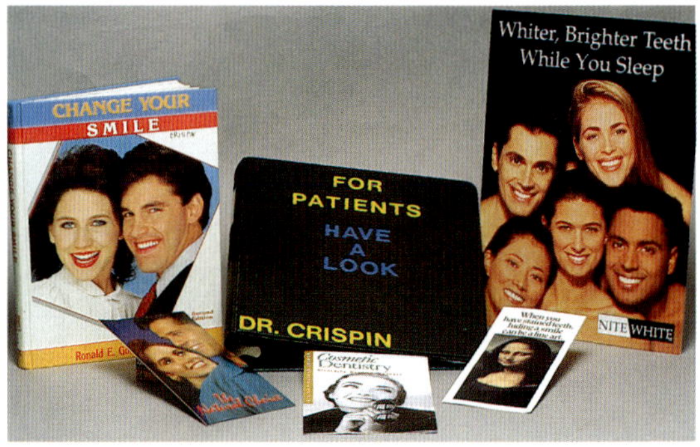

Fig. 1-2 Examples of reception room reading materials.

allows for a less rushed environment at home. Scheduling a time and area to complete certain forms just prior to an initial exam may be more useful in that the focus is more current. Photographs of "ideal" smiles should be positioned close by to allow patients a basis of comparison.

The written esthetic evaluation is the basis for identifying patient's esthetic concerns. It has been suggested that the esthetic questions should be placed in with the other questions in a new patient questionnaire. Many esthetic techniques are new, conservative and an improvement over traditional techniques. Keeping them separate underscores the fact that contemporary dentistry has many new and unique solutions to old dental problems that patients should be made aware of. For example, many individuals have lived for many years with sound but discolored teeth because they did not want crowns ("caps"), which require extensive removal of tooth structure—the only solution in the past. Design questions to have responses that make it easy to identify an esthetic concern. Auxiliaries interacting with the patient must be trained in observing this form and conversant in supporting the educational process about esthetic concerns.

The Reception Room

The reception room must be pleasant and comfortable but preferably in the taste of the dentist. This will set the style of the practice. Generic reception rooms might be interpreted as too complacent by patients looking for an excellent and confident professional. In the reception room, visual and educational aids must be present to focus attention on potential problems and suggest solutions a contemporary dentist has to offer.

Preprinted pamphlets or books are availa-

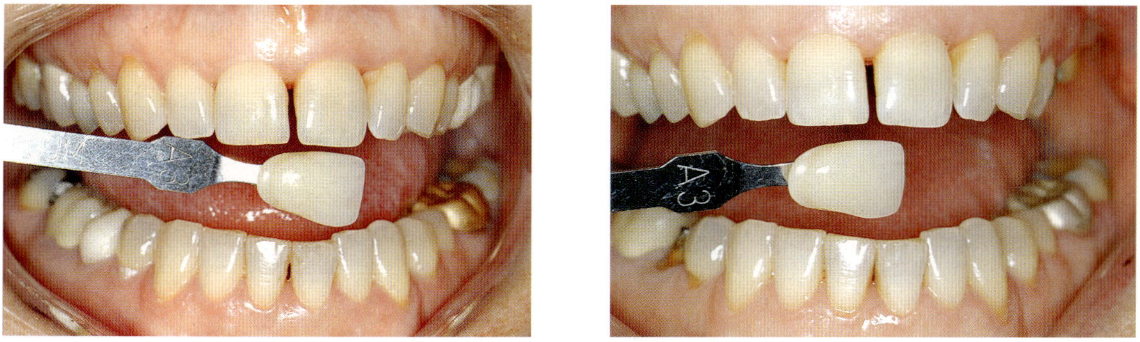

Figs. 1-3a and b Examples for patient book (bleaching preoperative and postoperative).

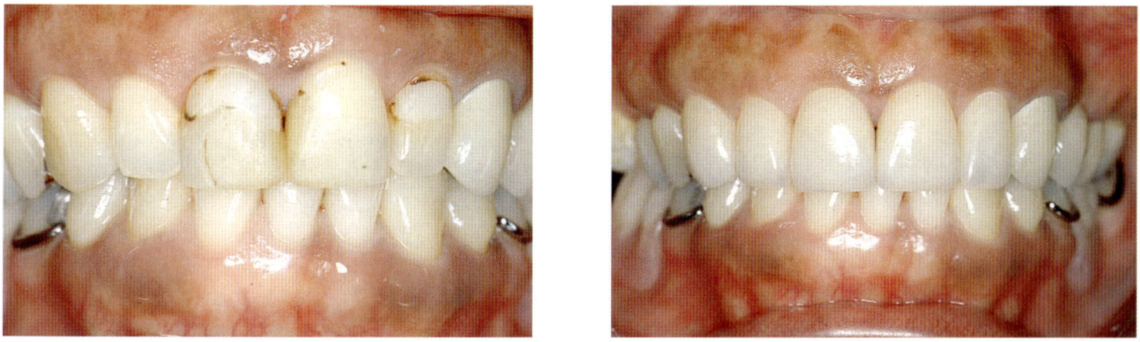

Figs. 1-4a and b Examples for patient book (porcelain veneers preoperative and postoperative).

ble from several sources (Fig. 1-2). A more customized approach is to develop your own patient-oriented books for your reception room. It will require more work but informative books can be designed to emphasize strengths of the practice and specific messages and can be modified as new techniques or better examples of treatment become available. These books require good computer developed text as well as before and after photographs. The novice or inexperienced dentist might have to buy patient education booklets. Obtaining a good quality camera for the documentation of treatment results is a must for any esthetic practice. Eventually, actual before and after pictures from the practice should replace those from outside sources (Figs. 1-3 and 1-4). Unfortunately these books may or may not be picked up by the patient and should be placed in a highly visible location.

A more sophisticated approach is to have a video monitor in the waiting room. Many sources for video tapes exist that will present a message on a specific topic. A more effective approach is to develop your own custom presentations. Some of the more sophisticated computer imaging systems provide the software that allows for the preparation of custom patient presentations. The key is to design presentations that heighten patient awareness of esthetic procedures that are available in the practice. The presentation should be only 5 to 10 minutes in length and prompt patients to ask questions on how these esthetic procedures apply to them. Video presentations require a larger capital outlay but attract more patient attention and acceptance (Fig. 1-5). These continuous loop video presentations repeat every few minutes.

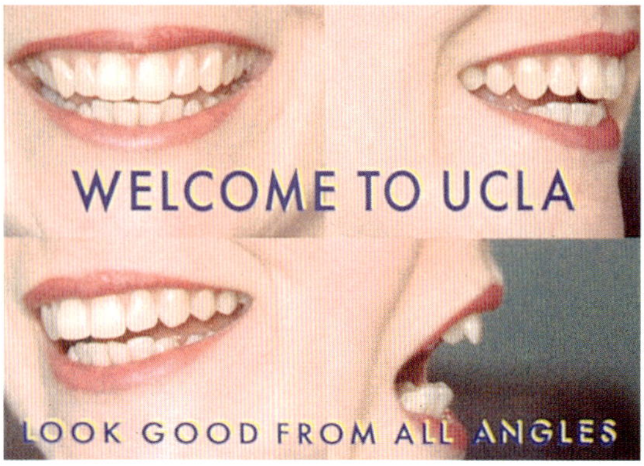

Fig. 1-5 Image from computer presentation.

One of the features of a computer imaging system should be a graphics and presentation software to develop short educational programs. These presentations are easy to program and modify, and different ones can be run as desired. In addition, computer imaging equipment can now be used 100% of the time.

Initial Examination

The initial examination time with the dentist should be relatively short. At this point little or no diagnostic information other than the patient questionnaires exist. In addition, the desires and dental needs of each patient are highly variable and a long appointment might be unnecessary. At the initial examination a review of written information is possible, and patient questions and concerns can be answered to a point, but the first appointment should be focused upon prescribing the diagnostic procedures that must be completed prior to the final diagnosis and treatment planning appointment. In a referral practice where patients are referred for specific treatment, first appointment procedures might be more predictable and easily scheduled. In the average general practice, new patients present with a variety of problems, desires and abilities to pay for services. A short initial appointment is a more efficient utilization of time. Depending upon patient needs, various diagnostic procedures and additional communication techniques can be prescribed or completed as time and staffing permit.

Depending upon the complexity of the case and diagnostic materials to review, an appropriate second treatment planning and consultation appointment should be made when all diagnostic materials are available. For patients that need procedures started as soon as possible, combination treatment–treatment planning appointments may be made. For very simple cases, all treatment planning procedures may be completed at the initial exam and confirmed when final diagnostic information such as radiographs are completed. In more complex cases, outside specialist consultations from the periodontist, orthodontist, oral surgeon, prosthodontist, endodontist or others may be necessary before a final treatment plan can be developed.

Referrals and traditional diagnostic procedures such as radiographs, study models and diagnostic wax-ups are well covered in most academic dental programs. Certain less routine techniques are valuable aids to patient communication, patient education and treatment plan acceptance. These techniques involve visualization using photography, computer imaging and intraoral video and will be discussed later in this chapter.

VISUAL DOCUMENTATION (WHY?)

A high quality camera(s) is a must for the contemporary esthetic practice. Photography or more sophisticated means of capturing, storing and reproducing images should be a standard procedure in every esthetic practice. There are many uses of such visual data.

Medical Records

Photographic documentation has many advantages. Visual documentation can improve insurance claim acceptance and will assist in any medical-legal action. Treatment planning using records with visual documentation allows for an exact recall of the patient's conditions and leads to a plan that is more complete and accurate.

Patient Motivation

Visualization is one of the best patient motivators. It clearly demonstrates a more comprehensive approach to diagnosis. Along with study models and radiographs, visual images clearly demonstrate the problems to the patient, which leads to a higher acceptance of treatment plans.

Patient Treatment Books

Before and after photographs of various esthetic cases are an excellent way to communicate esthetic dentistry to patients (Figs. 1-6 and 1-7). They show the esthetic results of various procedures and substantiate your experience. Brief educational components such as a photograph of a porcelain veneer prior to cementing or a bleaching stent in and out of the mouth all add to patient understanding and acceptance.

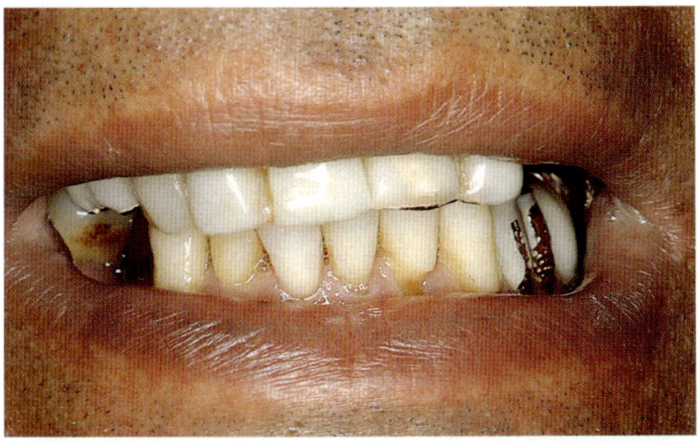
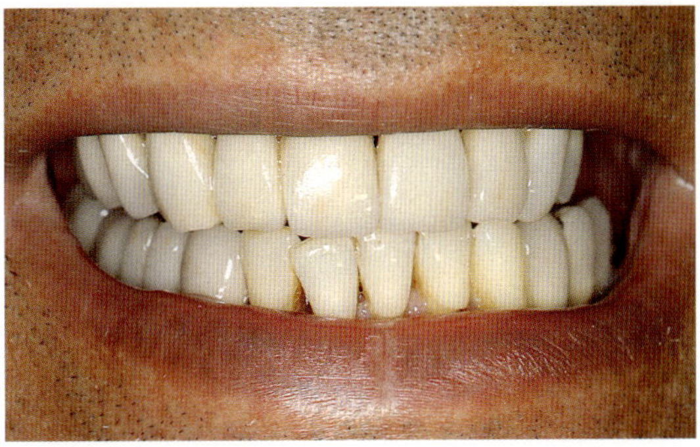

Figs. 1-6a and b Before and after photographs.

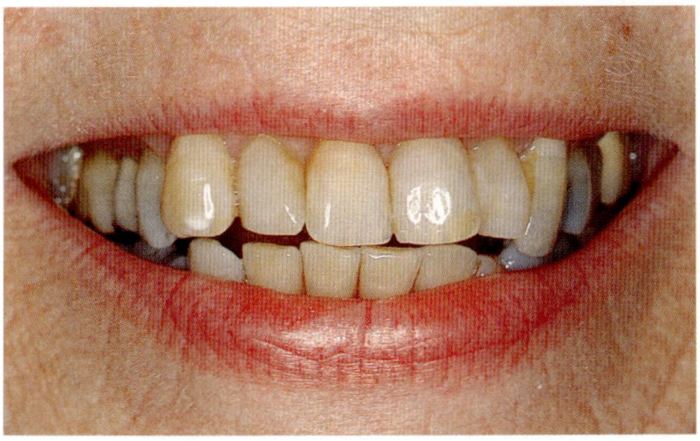
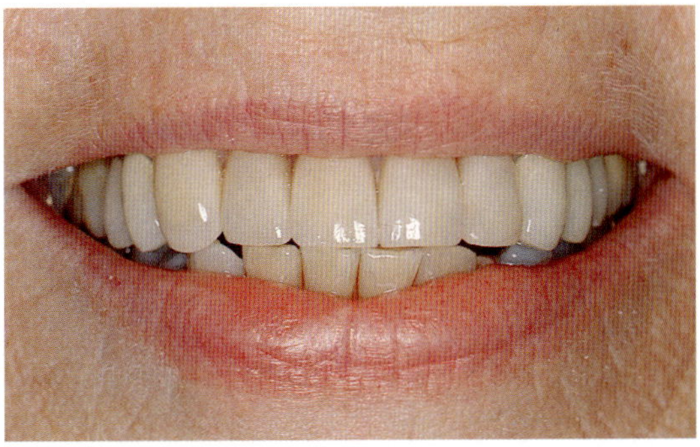

Figs. 1-7a and b Before and after photographs.

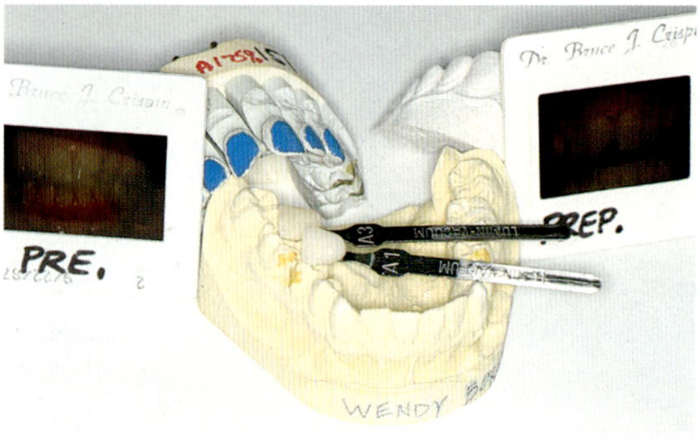

Fig. 1-8 Photographs included with study models, shade tabs and work models.

Books placed in the reception room must be readily available and easily understood. Books used for treatment planning can be more comprehensive and detailed. These will be used by the dental team when visualization techniques are required and provide an effective method of explanation during the consultation appointment.

Photo Walls

Many manufacturers of esthetic products are providing patient motivational materials. Such materials may also be developed internally to meet the specific needs and desires of the individual practices. Before and after photographs can be framed and posted on an appropriate wall along with photographs of smiling satisfied patients. Ultimately these techniques enhance your patients' ability to visualize esthetic results and divert their focus towards esthetic procedures. A tastefully done photo wall can be decorative and add a personal and highly professional touch to an esthetic practice. Photographs of staff members along with their names and positions also adds a more personal touch to the practice.

Self-evaluation

One of the best ways to self-evaluate esthetic results completed on patients is to project before and after slides on a wall or screen. Subtleties not seen when you look at a finished case intraorally become apparent when you look at magnified slides on the screen. Progressing in one's abilities is critical to longitudinal success. Evaluation of the results of dental treatment by the dental team will identify areas of strength and weakness in the practice.

Laboratory Communications

Preoperative photographs or computer produced before and after simulations of the desired results provide an excellent adjunct to communication (Fig. 1-8). Visual communication techniques provide an excellent way to demonstrate esthetic characteristics that are difficult to draw or verbalize. For example, how an incisal edge is developed by blending various translucencies and colors can be shown. While colors must be defined using various shade guides, the subtleties of how to blend various porcelains to achieve color variations mimicking an underlying tooth can be easily shown using visualization techniques. Visual documentation can be used in many ways and should be a standard part of any diagnostic sequence.

Education

Almost every aspect of a successful esthetic practice involves an educational process, educating patients, staff, laboratories or even yourself and other dentists. Visual documentation provides essential materials for many educational purposes. More formal dental educational lectures can be developed for lay audiences or for dental groups. This is a very positive form of public relations and may provide the critical component to practice success.

Patient referrals, whether from patients or other dentists, are critical for a successful esthetic practice. Providing awareness of what your dental team provides can be a very effective way to develop the kind of practice desired.

Newsletters

A practice newsletter is an excellent way to reach inactive as well as active patients with what's new and what's different in the practice and to keep communications open. Newsletters are a tasteful and personal method of public relations. Advertising is often viewed negatively as too aggressive but newsletters are considered an acceptable way to reach patients and expand the practice's referrals through education. A camera to provide visual images is essential for an effective newsletter produced in the office. General newsletters can be purchased with the practice name printed on it but lack the personal practice identity of a newsletter produced in the office. A timely informative newsletter sent out once or twice a year is a great way to enhance any esthetic practice by educating patients and their friends.

PHOTOGRAPHY

35-mm Photography

The least expensive way to develop visual materials is by using a camera designed for dental photography. A multitude of camera systems exist and can be designed for dental utilization. The 35-mm single lens reflex camera (S.L.R.) is the standard of quality and versatility. Instant type cameras provide the advantage of quick images but generally are limited in quality of image reproduction.

The basic components of a 35-mm camera system are the body, the lens and the flash or light source. The 35-mm format camera body is recommended because it can be used with a variety of macro lenses and lighting systems (Fig. 1-9). These systems are also portable, simple to operate and provide excellent results with a minimum of photographic experience. Film is readily available and processing is inexpensive. The standard of the Biological Photographers Association is based on the use of the 35-mm format when clinical photographs must be standardized. Standardization is necessary to allow for comparison of before and after images.

The 35-mm camera body is synchronized with a flash system. A simple camera body can be used, which saves more money for the more important lens and flash components. In nonautomatic systems, the camera body holds the film and is kept at a shutter speed that is determined by the flash. The lens is adjusted for each view to control the amount of light entering the body. Thus the extra features many camera bodies have may be unused unless the camera is used for purposes other than clinical photography. While this may be necessary when starting a practice, ultimately a camera should be dedicated for practice utilization.

Automatic systems have been developed

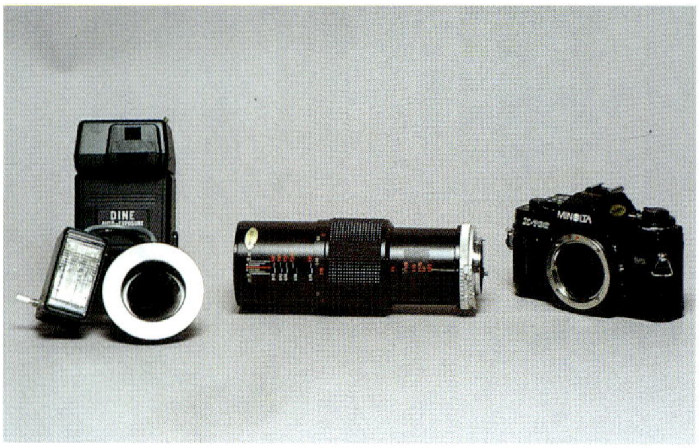

Fig. 1-9

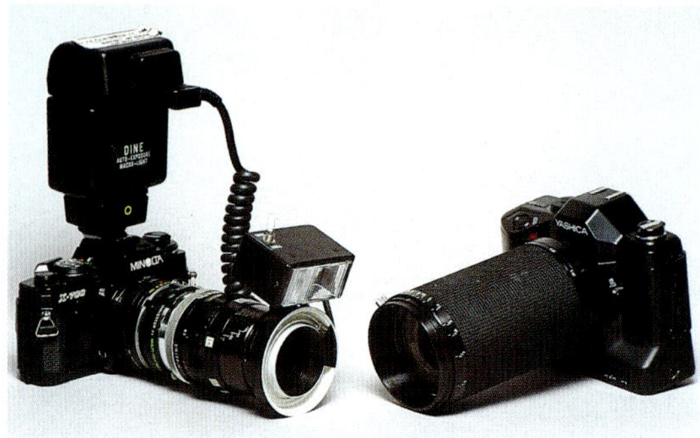

Fig. 1-10

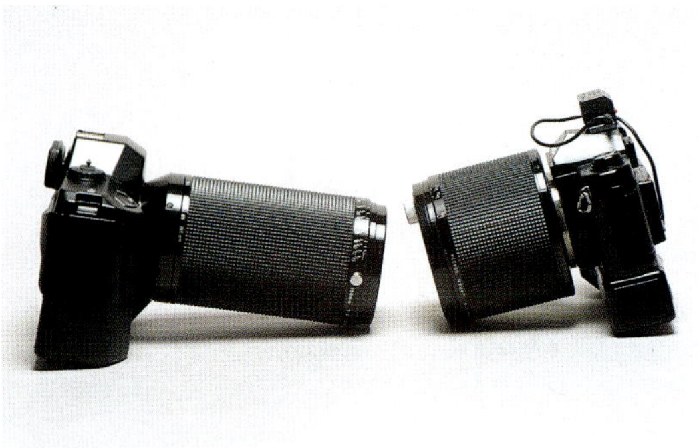

Fig. 1-11

Fig. 1-9 Camera system components: **(left to right)** flash, lens and body.

Fig. 1-10 Automatic camera systems.

Fig. 1-11 Camera lenses: **(left)** 100-mm; **(right)** 50-mm.

Fig. 1-12a Focal length of 50-mm lens (1:1).

Fig. 1-12b Focal length of 100-mm lens (1:1); note not as close to subject.

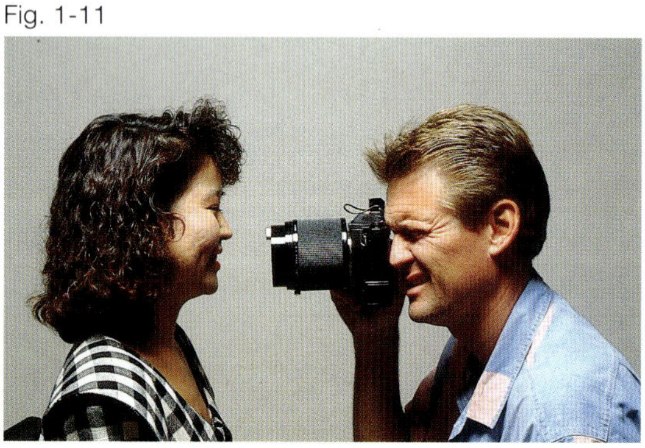

Fig. 1-12a

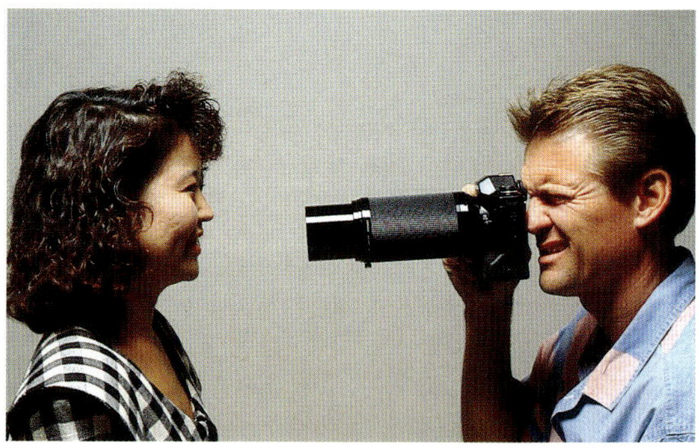

Fig. 1-12b

that require a more sophisticated camera body. These cameras have "through the lens" (TTL) metering, which uses computerized connections between the camera, lens and lighting source to optimize the results automatically (Fig. 1-10). Automatic systems generally are more convenient and results are more predictable, especially if several staff members use the system. These systems are usually more costly and may be less versatile but overall results are excellent.

A macro or close up lens is designed to provide the specialized optics required for close-up photography. The factors of peripheral image distortion, working distance, required apertures and focal length are taken into consideration and built into the lens to provide optimal image quality. The "magnification ratio" of subject to image is imprinted on the lens. A 1:1 ratio means that the actual size of the object is equal to the actual size of the image on the film. This allows for ease of adjustment. This is the lens of choice for dental photography. A focal length in the 90-

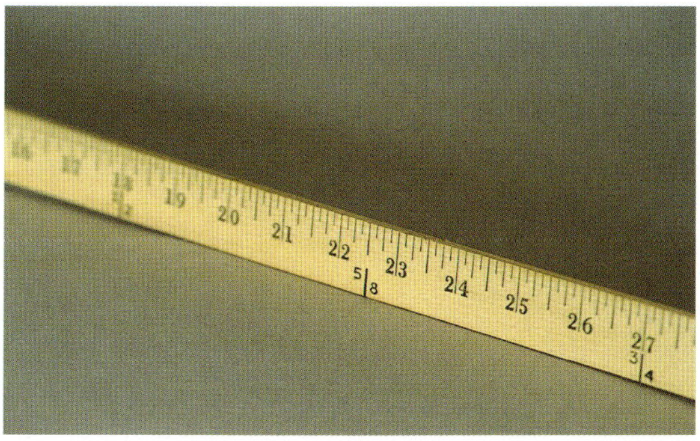

Fig. 1-13a

Fig. 1-13a Depth of field example; note out of focus portions.

Fig. 1-13b Depth of field example with higher f-stop; note greater depth of ruler in focus.

Fig. 1-14 (**left to right**) Ring light, combination and point source.

Fig. 1-15 Shadows from using point source.

Fig. 1-16 No shadows using ring light.

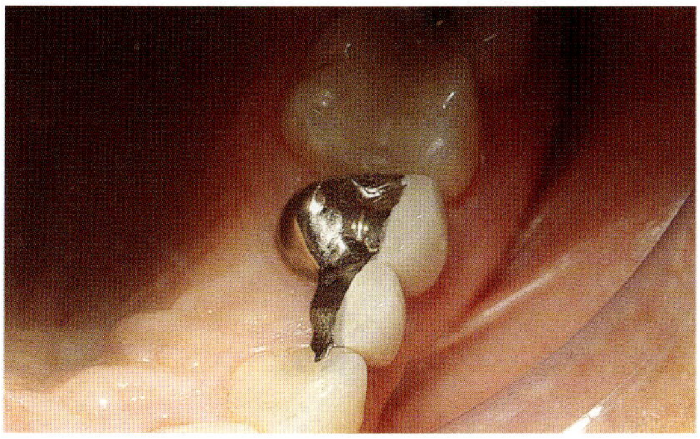

Fig. 1-15

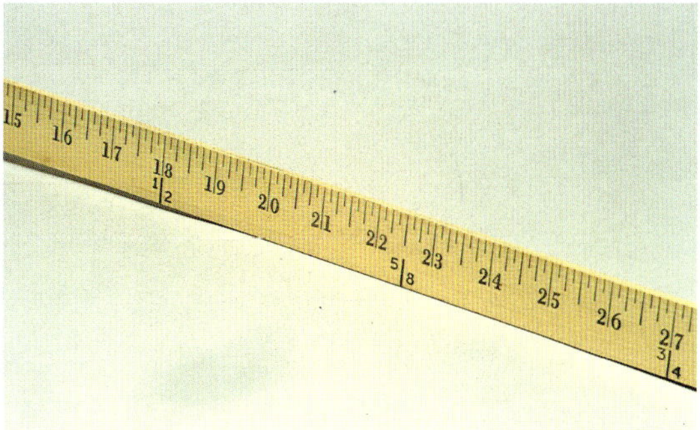

Fig. 1-13b

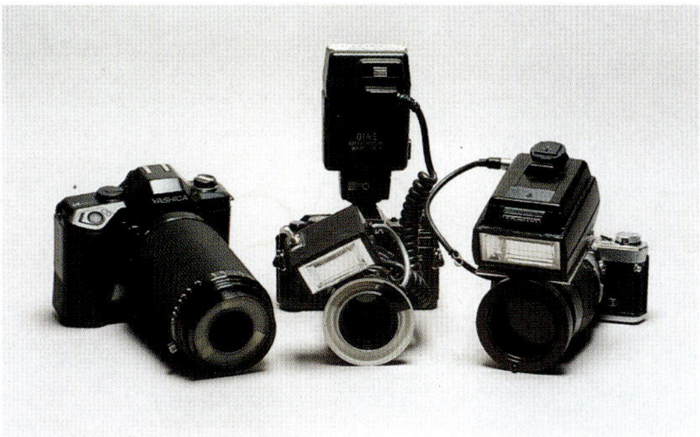

Fig. 1-14

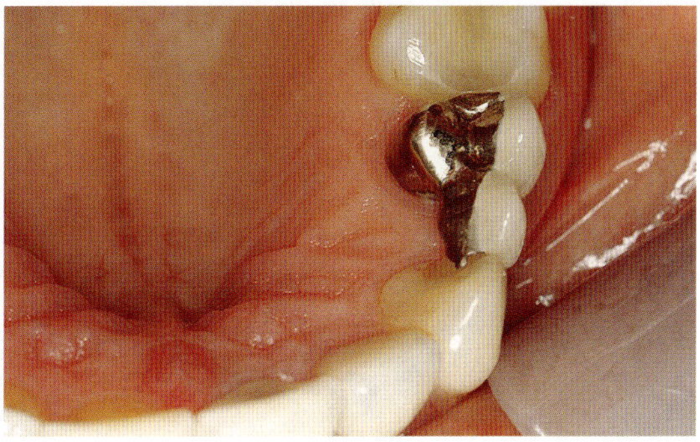

Fig. 1-16

to 105-m range is recommended (Fig. 1-11). This will allow for close-up photography without having to position the lens so close to the subject (Fig. 1-12). The macro lens should also have a high f-stop rating (minimum aperture). A setting of f:32 is ideal with f:22 being the absolute minimum. The smaller the aperture setting (higher f-stop rating) the greater the depth of field. With close-up photography the depth of field is much smaller and maximizing this depth is necessary or portions of the photograph may be out of focus (Fig. 1-13).

The last component of the camera system is the light source. The flash component must be mounted at the end of the lens to minimize shadows. It must have enough intensity to allow for a f:32 (minimum aperture) setting using films in the 25 to 100 ASA/ISO film speed range. This will produce quality results and a maximum depth of field for close-up shots.

The light source comes in three configurations. The point source which is a small flash

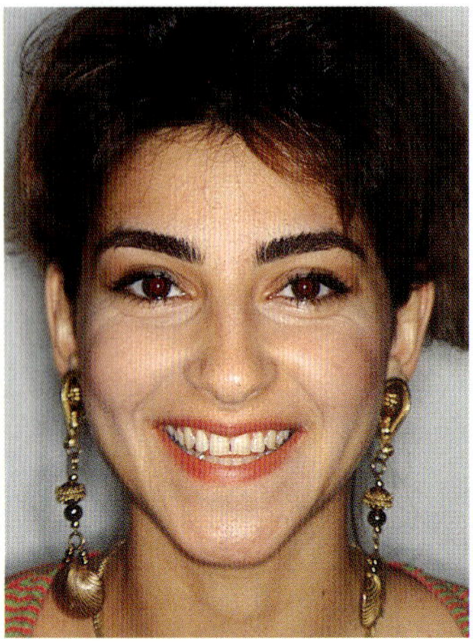

Fig. 1-17a

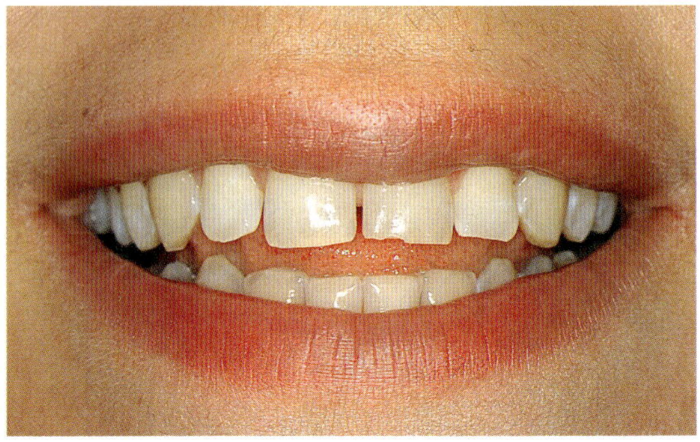

Fig. 1-17b

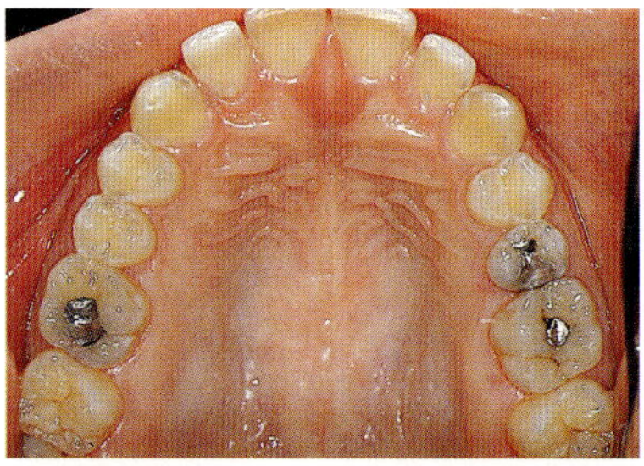

Fig. 1-17c

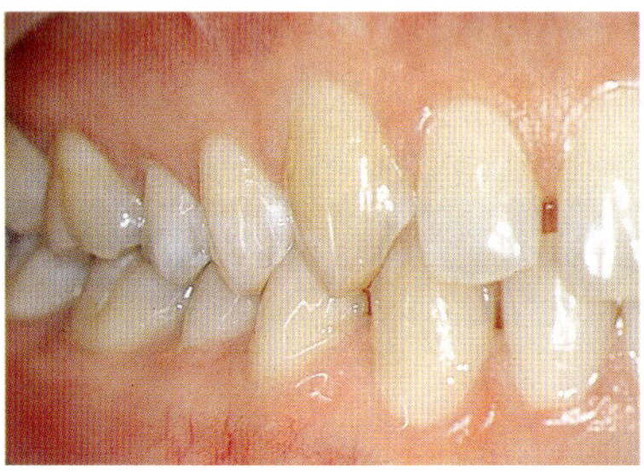

Fig. 1-17d

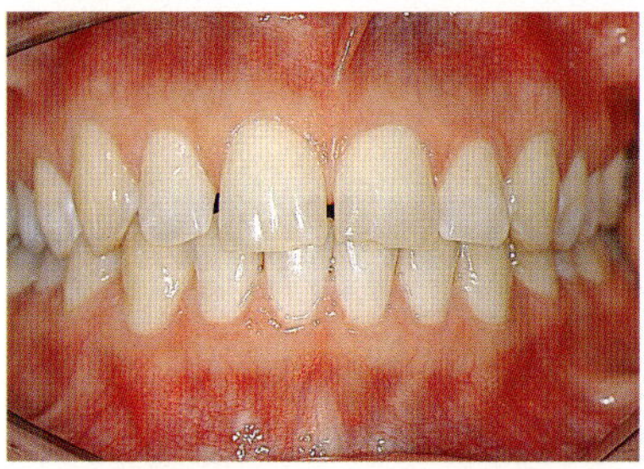

Fig. 1-17e

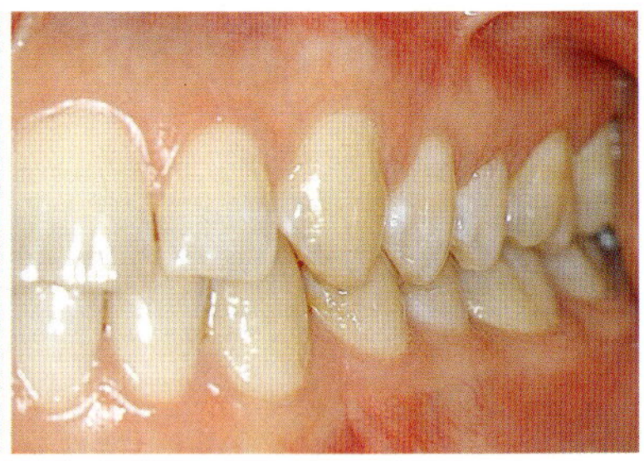

Fig. 1-17f

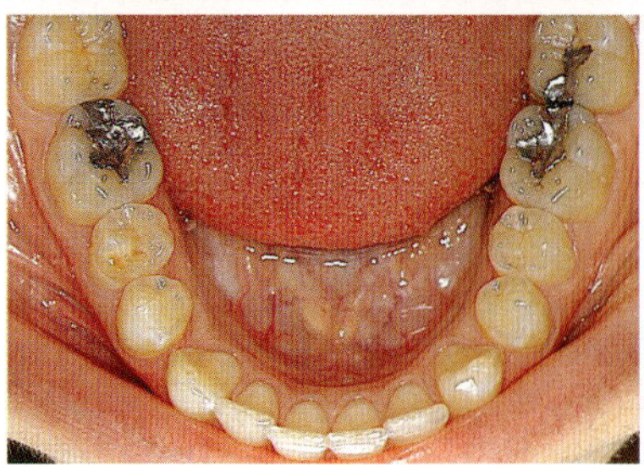

Fig. 1-17g

Figs. 1-17a to g Example of a standard photographic series.

tube that is mounted on a rotating bracket, the ring light which is circular flash tube that surrounds the end of the lens and a combination point source–ring light (Fig. 1-14). For close-up work the ring light may be the best illuminator with less chance of unwanted shadows. The point source may be used for a larger more accessible view like a full smile or larger. One advantage of using the ring light is not having to reposition the flash for various views to control shadows as is necessary with a single point source (Fig.

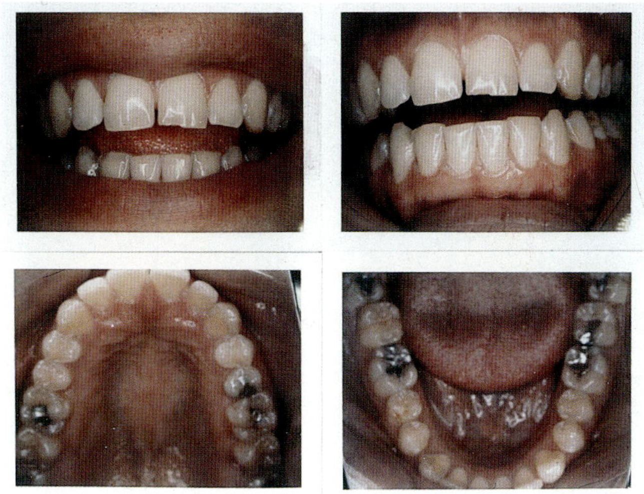

Fig. 1-18 Instant photographic print series.

Fig. 1-19a Instant print showing smile line.

Fig. 1-19b Instant print showing close-up detail of teeth.

Figs. 1-20a and b Comparison of instant (a) and 35-mm (b) picture quality.

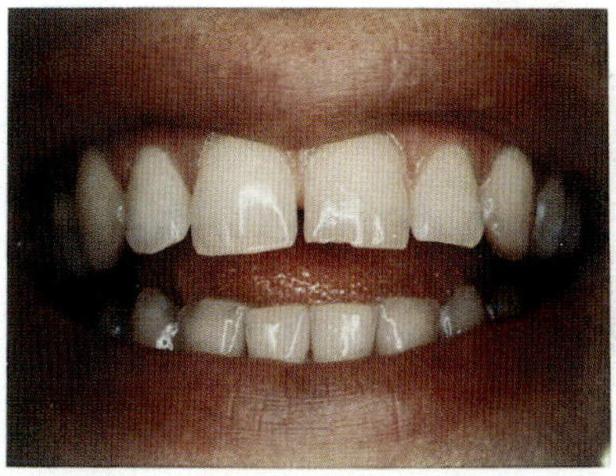

Fig. 1-19a

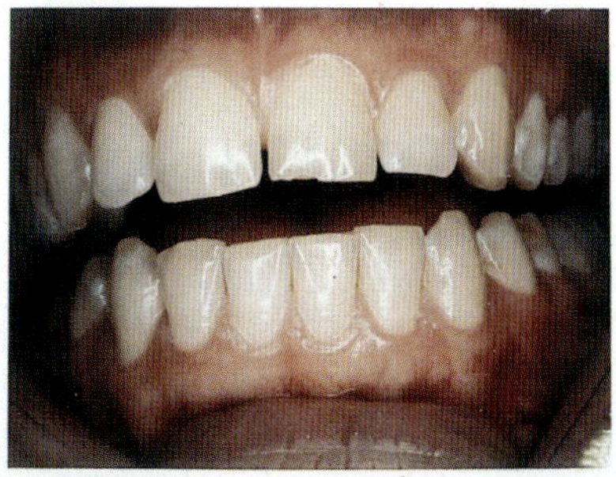

Fig. 1-19b

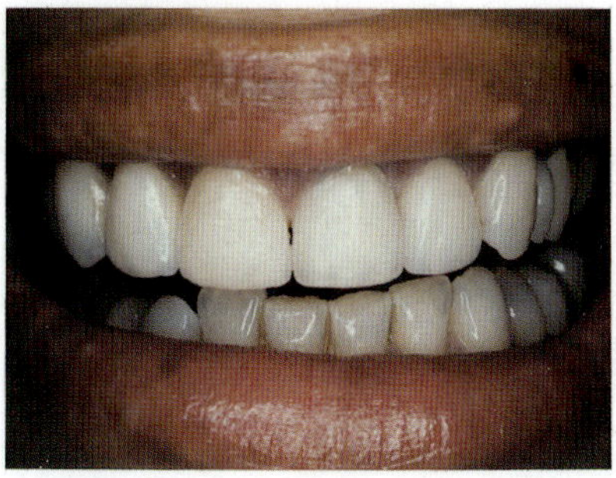

Fig. 1-20a

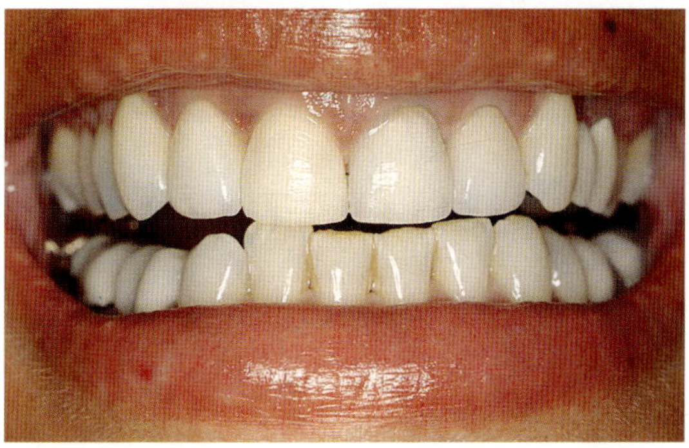

Fig. 1-20b

1-15). A dual point source will minimize this problem. The ring light will flood the areas more completely (Fig. 1-16). Shooting a trial series prior to the purchase of a camera system is recommended. Compare different systems for results, ease of utilization and certainly cost. More comprehensive publications on dental photography should be reviewed by the novice (see references).

The key to photographic documentation is to standardize the photographic technique. Each subject should have a series of photos taken that consist of the same views using the same magnification ratios and techniques. This will allow for direct comparison over time and between subjects. A standard series is shown in Fig. 1-17. While individuals may develop their own series of photography, standardizing whatever series is selected is necessary for optimal comparison.

Instant Photography

Polaroid® or instant-type photographic

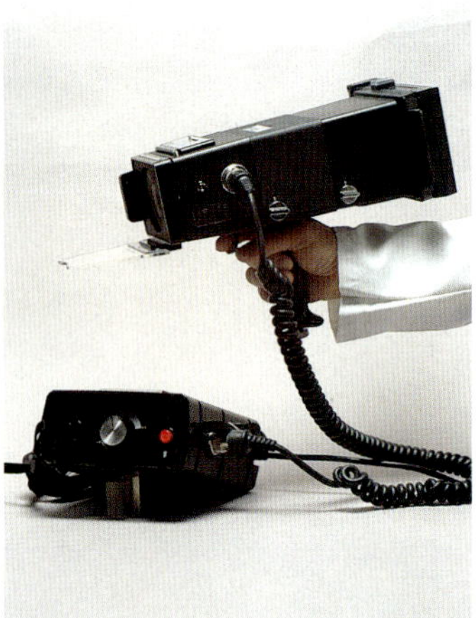

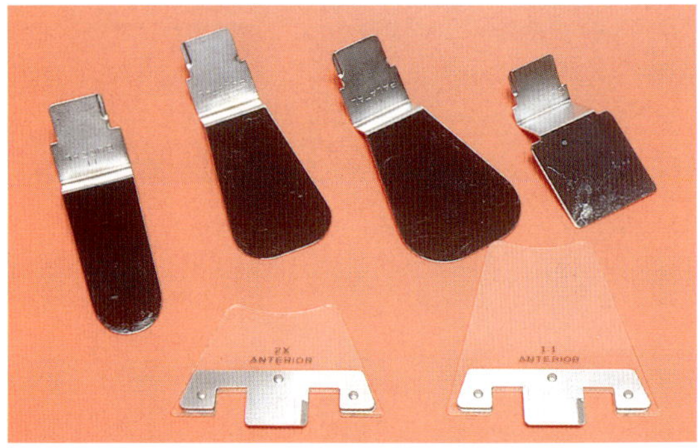

Fig. 1-22 Instant camera accessories.

Fig. 1-21 Instant camera with power pack.

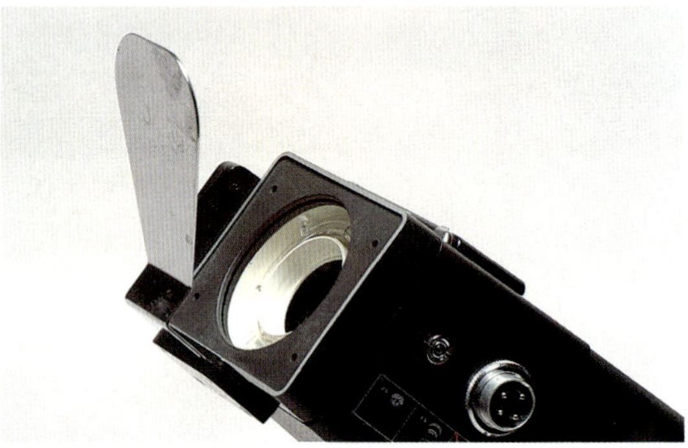

Fig. 1-23 Intraoral mirror attached to camera.

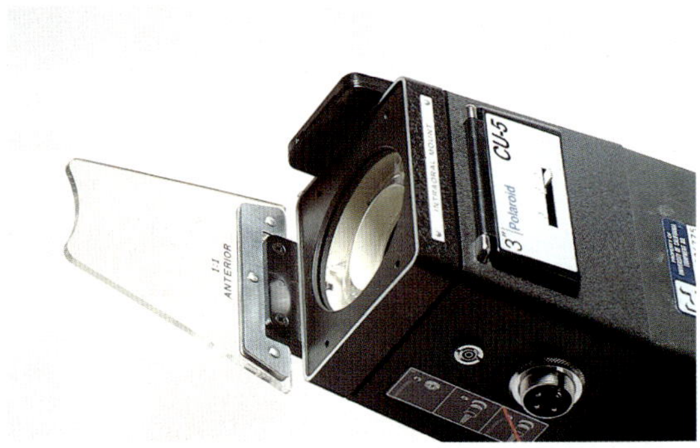

Fig. 1-24 Focal length chin guide for positioning camera.

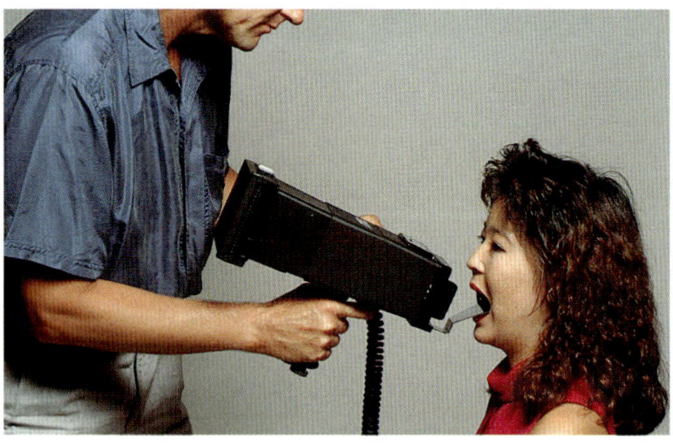

Fig. 1-25a Visual orientation of camera position for mirror shot.

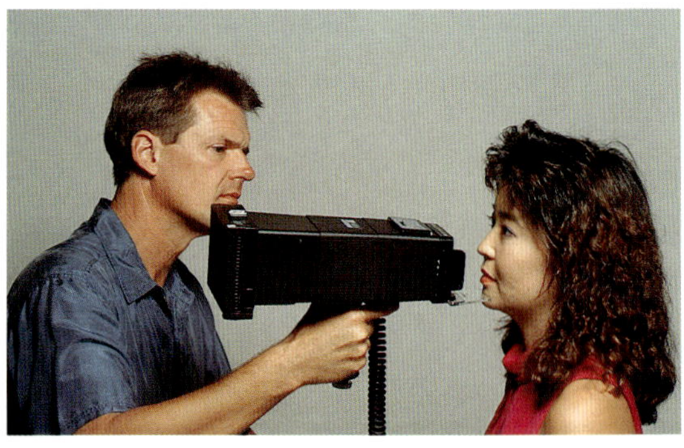

Fig. 1-25b Visual orientation of camera position for direct shot.

systems offer some unique advantages for improved visual communications in dentistry. An instant print can show a patient how others see them and can be used immediately as a focal point for dialogue. A routine series of views should be placed in the chart (Fig. 1-18). It is an extremely helpful reference for treatment planning after the patient has left, and provides improved case documentation. A full face view on the chart cover can

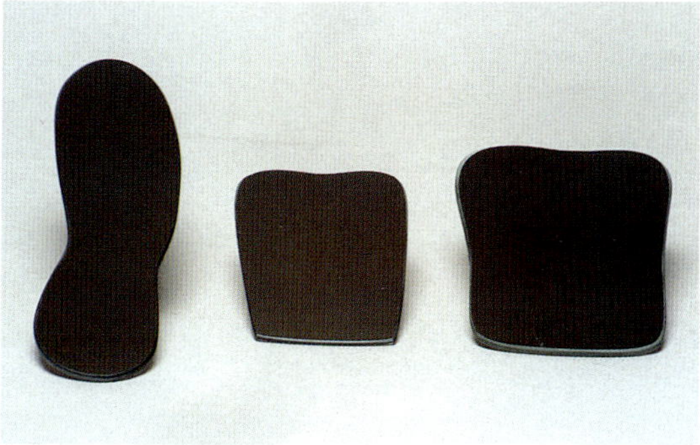

Fig. 1-26 Basic mirrors required.

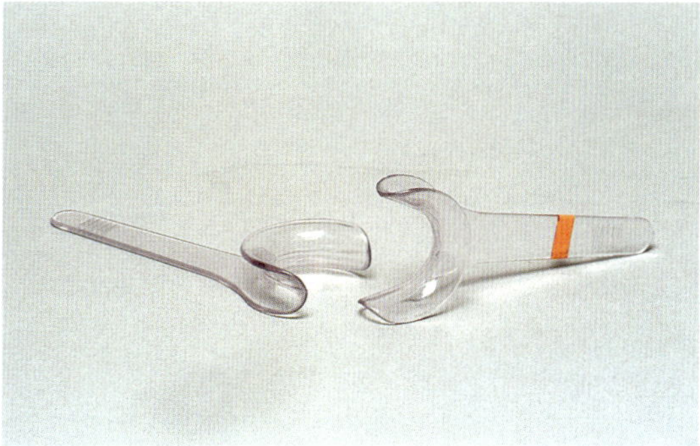

Fig. 1-27 Clear plastic check retractors.

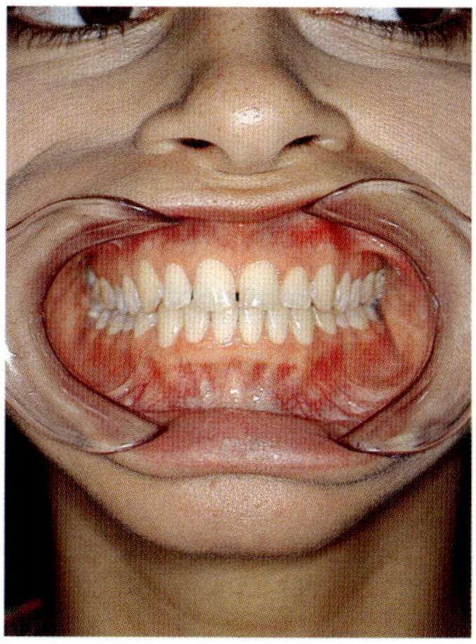

Fig. 1-28 Clear plastic check retractors positioned intraorally.

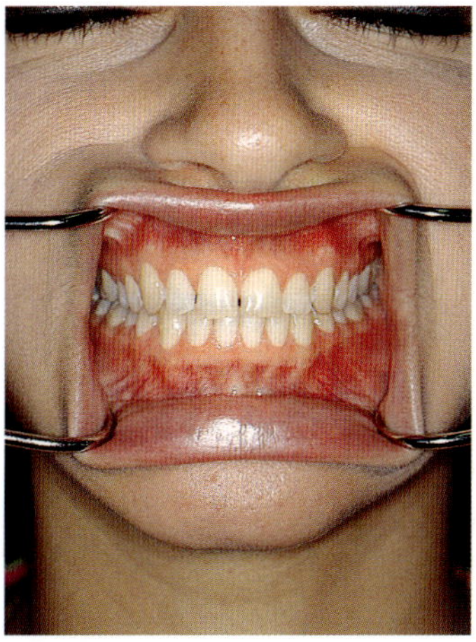

Fig. 1-29 Metal retractors positioned; note the more limited retraction.

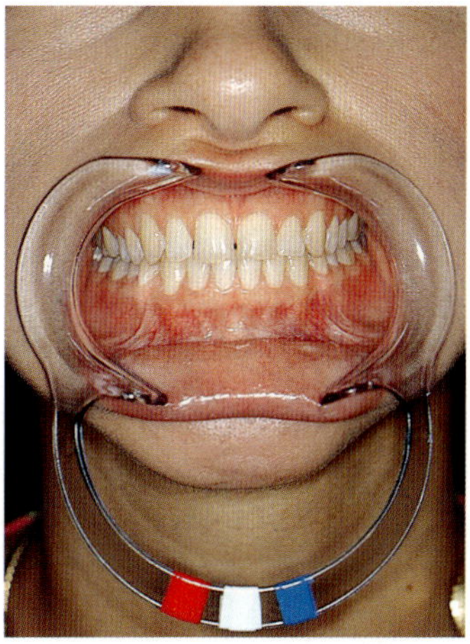

Fig. 1-30 One piece retractor positioned intraorally.

be a public relations builder allowing patients to be recognized and treated more personally. Instant prints are also useful for improved laboratory communications by allowing visualization of the total patient showing esthetic subtleties that are difficult to describe on the written prescription (Fig. 1-19). Enhancement of communications to insurance companies using instant prints will reduce written documentation and improve authorization percentages.

Unfortunately, instant photography is not without disadvantages. The quality of the picture is only just acceptable when compared to that of 35-mm prints (Fig. 1-20). The quality of instant prints is not suitable for professional publication. Another limitation is the fact that these camera systems have fixed focal lengths. With the addition of different lens components this focal length and the resultant magnification ratios change, but instant cameras are far less versatile than a 35-mm camera (Fig. 1-21). In addition, they do not conform to the standard magnification ratios established by the Biological Photographers Association. By using various mirrors and chin rest accessories, an adequate series of views can be attained (Figs. 1-22 to 1-24). Instant photographs are more difficult to orient properly because there is no TTL focusing (Fig. 1-25).

Instant camera systems require a minimum

of photographic experience to use and, when an immediate print is desirable, provide a useful adjunct to an esthetic practice.

Photographic Accessories

Intraoral mirrors are an essential component of any dental photographic system. Occlusal and buccal front surfaced glass mirrors will provide the quality of image reflection and the sizes necessary for most indirect views (Fig. 1-26). Polaroid systems use special mirrors that must be attached to the camera lenses.

Clear cheek retractors are also necessary to achieve adequate visualization for intraoral photography (Figs. 1-27 and 1-28). Double ended or assorted sizes are required. Metal retractors generally do not provide adequate retraction (Fig. 1-29). Colored retractors may be distracting, and one piece attached retractors lack the versatility necessary for a complete series of views but are useful for prolonged retraction during selective restorative procedures such as porcelain veneer cementation (Fig. 1-30).

COMPUTER IMAGING

Introduction

Utilization of "hi tech" is becoming a routine part of doing business in many industries. While the cost of "hi tech" in dentistry seems at first high, the benefits of computer imaging systems and intraoral video cameras, if used properly, will more than compensate for the cost. The keys are understanding how they should be applied, utilization techniques and a dedication to application.

The basic components of a computer imaging system are a computer, a video camera, a monitor and a cart (Fig. 1-31). A thermal printer is recommended so an instant print of results can be produced and a copy given to the patient and another placed in the chart (Fig. 1-32). The computer should have ample capacity to efficiently run the imaging software and sufficient flexibility to handle additional software and expansion capabilities to include other computer driven dental items, such as radiographic or periodontal programs. A properly designed system will minimize the need for additional computers.

The camera and lens should be of high quality and capable of producing full face to close-up images that have excellent resolution and color using a simple lighting source.

The monitor should also be of high quality. The size of the monitor may vary from 13 inches to larger depending upon space availability and personal preference.

A thermal printer will provide an instant print. The type of printer used should be dictated by applications. The size of the print produced and the number of views possible on each print will vary with different printers. A cart may be used for portability or the system may be built into a diagnostic suite.

As with any item of dental equipment, cost should not be the only determining factor in selecting an imaging system. One of the primary determining factors is software. Imaging software must produce a desired result. It must be fast, clear and accurate but more important it must be easy to use. Any software that is difficult to learn will probably be underutilized. Computer imaging is often a delegated procedure and, when staff changes occur, the training of a new staff member should be quick and easy. The dentist must also be competent at using the equipment and easy to understand software will reduce frustration and encourage utilization.

Visual Communications

The primary application of computer imag-

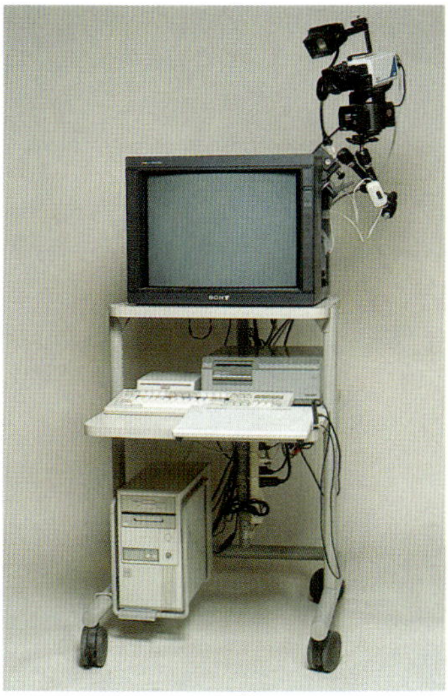

Fig. 1-31 Computer imaging system.

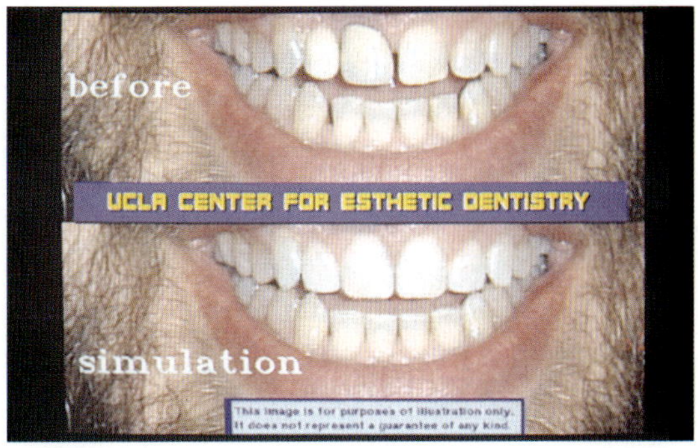

Fig. 1-32 Computer imaged print.

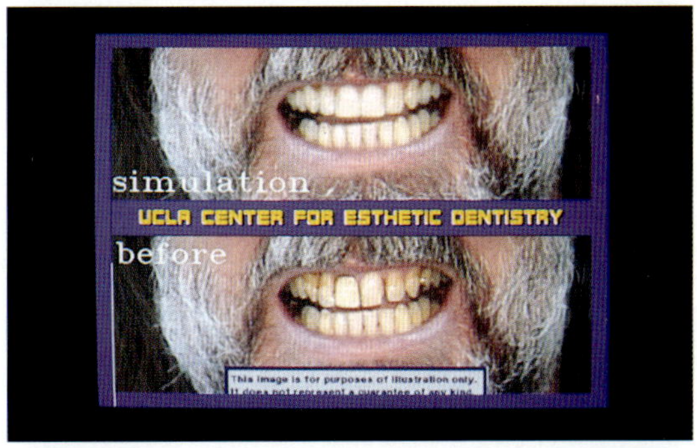

Fig. 1-33a Pretreatment print of computer imaged simulation.

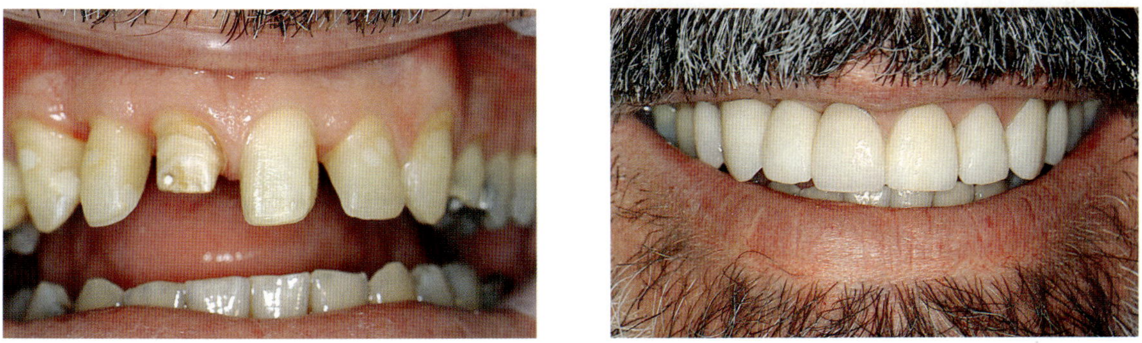

Figs. 1-33b and c Pretreatment and posttreatment views of the imaged patient, who was treated by a third year student.

ing is to enhance communications through visualization. The patients can see themselves as others see them and not the mirror image that they are accustomed to seeing. Patients are used to seeing themselves in a mirror and they subconsciously block out areas they do not like. Asymmetries and chipped or missing teeth are blocked out through a process known as "subliminal esthetic mapping." Areas are mapped out and subconsciously overlooked. When patients see themselves on a video camera, it is the reverse of the mirror image and mapped out areas become immediately obvious to them. Now they are seeing themselves as others see and perceive them and they can make a more objective analysis of their appearance.

Areas of concern can quickly be changed on the computer imaging system. Hard and soft tissues can be modified; color, contour, size and position of teeth are changed and the patient can visualize the benefits of the proposed changes. A communication process begins between the patient and the dental team. Because all parties are visualizing the same image, there is little possibility of misunderstanding. The patient becomes involved in the treatment planning process and often will want more treatment than he or she was originally seeking.

Accuracy of Communication

A perceived problem with imaging is the possibility of demonstrating results that are unachievable by the dentist. Any knowledgeable dentist should easily be able to match imaged simulations (Fig. 1-33). The real problem is often a lack of patient understanding. Misunderstanding is a critical component of patient dissatisfaction with the results of esthetic procedures. For instance, a patient requests longer teeth so the dentist increases length incisally. In reality the patient wanted them longer gingivally. This is an example of two people independently imagining a final result and verbalizing the problem, which each appears to understand, but with totally different results. This could have been avoided through imaging. Imaging is a key to treatment plan acceptance through enhanced patient understanding.

Tasteful Marketing

Almost every item sold is marketed to individuals using visualization techniques in order to compete for discretionary dollars. Computer imaging is the dentist's modality to visualize, communicate and compete with other items of value to the patient. The print produced should have the practice name and logo on it so it is easily identified. Patients will show this to their friends thus exposing the practice to others and a clear practice emphasis on excellence in esthetic dentistry is evident. Computer imaging offers a broad range of marketing possibilities.

Laboratory Communications

Communicating with a laboratory about desired esthetic changes or needs is difficult. Computers allow for images to be transmitted directly to the laboratory through a modem or copies of the simulated changes can be included with the laboratory prescription. These visual images can show subtle features not shown on models, such as lip line, asymmetries relative to the face or lips as well as the more obvious changes in color and contour. As with the patient, visual communication with the laboratory will minimize misunderstandings and improve results.

Reception Room Presentations

One feature of a complete imaging system should be the ability to produce visual presentations that can be shown in the reception room. Visual images stored in the computer memory can be combined with written graphics to present a practice message to everyone in the reception room. These presentations are easy to make and easy to change. They run on a continuous repeating loop and should last around 5 to 10 minutes. The imaging system may be positioned in the waiting room or a separate monitor may be installed. This monitor can be connected to other input sources when the imaging system is being used.

This presentation software will allow for continuous utilization of the imaging equipment, which significantly enhances its value and application.

Utilization

Imaging systems only benefit the practice if utilized. Utilization of this technology is important but will be variable from practice to practice.

A dentist with the aptitude and desire may be the primary imaging system user during the consultation and treatment planning appointments. As outlined in the next section the dentist may want to delegate this responsibility to the appropriate staff member, such as the dental hygienist. When delegated, the dentist must prescribe desired changes. The imaging results and patient's opinions must be placed in the dental record and returned to the dentist along with a print to be used during the final consultation.

Flexibility of the imaging system is the key to proper utilization and the dentist or a properly trained staff member may utilize the imaging system. Each practice can decide on the most effective use of the equipment. Underutilization of the equipment will occur if the practice does not have a commitment to implement the system effectively.

The individual practice will decide which patients are appropriate for imaging. All patients in the practice or selected patients may be scheduled for imaging. The latter is generally more practical for the average general practice and care must be given to include imaging into the list of diagnostic services prescribed, along with study models and radiographs. A fee should also be charged for this service but the fee may be returned if treatment is provided. If a fee is a deterrent to utilization, the service may be provided free. But remember, "a service provided for nothing has no perceived value."

Clinical Procedures

At the initial imaging session, the patient should first be allowed to see themselves on the monitor in motion. Have them count to 10, smile, show as much of their teeth as possible, or use other exercises that allow them to observe themselves under different circumstances.

Next, the actual imaging procedures are completed. They include the following steps:

- Freeze images as desired.
  - Full face.
  - Close up of smile.
  - Lateral views.
- Make changes as desired.
- Make prints of the pretreatment condition and simulated changes.
- Record highlights of the patient's input and procedures performed in the simulated image for future treatment plan reference.

Subsequent imaging sessions may be used during try-in procedures or for evaluation of possible final adjustments prior to making changes intraorally.

Computer imaging is a very effective visualization tool that can be used to increase treatment plan acceptance and minimize esthetic problems due to poor communications. The many utilizations and advantages of computer imaging clearly make this a necessary component of any contemporary esthetic practice that is committed to proper application.

INTRAORAL VIDEO

Intraoral video utilizes a small camera that can be placed in the mouth to transmit a view of oral structures to a TV monitor. Patients can now see inside their mouths along with the dentist. Intraoral video has many diagnostic and patient education uses which involve both esthetic and nonesthetic functions. Intraoral video is often used in the posterior part of the mouth, which is generally less esthetically demanding than anterior regions. It clearly shows the need to replace existing restorations or restore broken down teeth. Esthetic bonded restorations are often the treatment of choice (Fig. 1-34). When

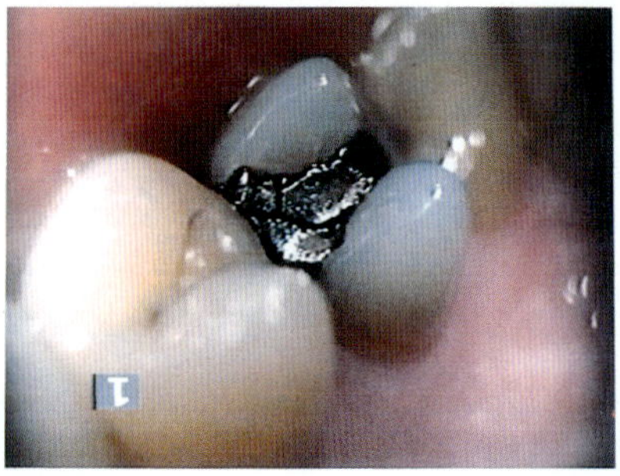

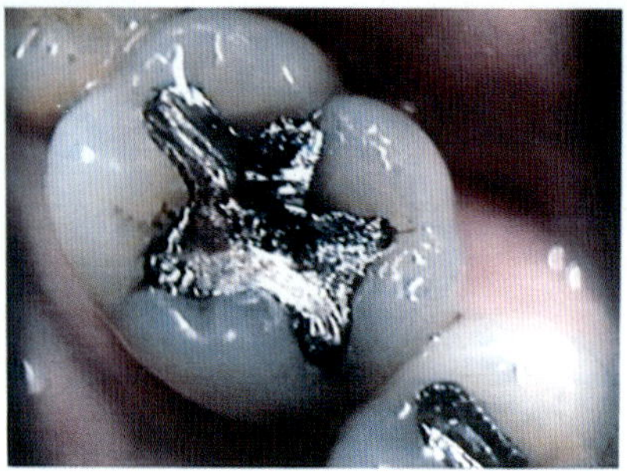

Figs. 1-34 and 1-35 Color prints taken with a dental intraoral video (taken with a Pro-Dentec system, compliments of Joy Moeller).

patients can actually see the problems, the acceptance of treatment is enhanced.

Prints made from the intraoral video recording are useful in communicating with dental insurance companies to improve acceptance of treatment plans. Traditional radiographs often do not show the extent of oral disease as clearly as an occlusal print (Fig. 1-35).

Intraoral prints can also be used to enhance laboratory communications for difficult cases by giving the laboratory technician a clear picture of the oral condition.

Intraoral video is very different from computer imaging in both use and application. Both are essential tools for today's demanding practices but imaging has far greater esthetic applications while intraoral video has more general practice applications.

TEAM APPROACH

A dental practice that wants to expand and improve its esthetic treatment component must utilize the entire staff. All staff members must be educated in the esthetic procedures provided and the benefits resulting from such procedures. It is the dentist's responsibility to educate the staff and develop this understanding. Dentists should have their staff members attend continuing education courses, have weekly staff meetings, review videotapes, read dental literature and have demonstrations to educate everyone with patient contact. Treating the esthetic problems of staff members at no cost provides living examples. This will also develop a real enthusiasm for the benefits of the esthetic treatment you are providing. This enthusiasm will be very contagious. In many instances patients will discuss issues and ask questions of the staff that they hesitate to ask the dentist. An informed, enthusiastic and experienced staff is a key to directing focus towards esthetic procedures provided by the practice.

The Receptionist

The receptionist is the first person a patient contacts for each appointment. Scheduling a little extra time before appointments and using waiting periods for patient education can be effective. The receptionist can show video presentations, or hand out patient books and brochures that describe the services provided in the practice. This will focus the patient's attention on treatment options, reduce anxiety by presenting information during waiting periods or present specific information that may apply to that patient. It will also educate an existing patient that might discuss the unique procedures you perform with a nonpatient. Reception room time can be very productive if used in an organized way. The receptionist is the key and this should not be an entry level position but demanding of a knowledgeable personable, an enthusiastic individual who can motivate and communicate to patients and others.

The Hygienist

The hygienist is a critical and important member of the esthetic dental team. New patients will see the hygienist early in the treatment process and existing patients will return on a regular recall basis. An informed, motivated, and enthusiastic hygienist will talk to and direct patient focus to possible problems. During the hygiene appointment, there is time for the hygienist to talk to and educate patients. Many existing patients may not be aware of new esthetic procedures available. The emphasis for existing and new patients should be to communicate and educate. Many esthetic procedures are elective and compete with discretionary funds that might be spent elsewhere. A well educated patient will accept treatment more readily.

Another key function that can be delegated to the hygienist is that of "computer imaging." The hygienist is the ideal staff member to image patients, with techniques ranging from simple video visualization techniques to more sophisticated computer imaging. Imaging can be scheduled in the approximate time frame as a normal hygiene appointment. The fee should be similar to the hygiene fee and if procedures are performed as a result of visualization, the fee may be absorbed by the dentist. Imaging appointments provide a wonderful change of pace from the redundancy of a typical hygiene schedule, which is a motivation for the hygienist to promote such procedures. This is a very important staff position and will require an energetic, positive, enthusiastic and motivated individual.

Finally, maintenance of many esthetic services will require special knowledge, skills, and instrumentation by the hygienist. Minimally, the hygienist must be trained in the appropriate techniques used to maintain and enhance esthetic restorations and services. Otherwise deterioration will be accelerated. Many of the same techniques used by the dentist to finalize esthetic procedures must also be taught to the hygienist for effective long term maintenance.

Financial Consultant

The staff member discussing fees and payment must also be well educated and capable of discussing advantages of the proposed esthetic treatments. Discussing financial arrangements or collecting money is always a difficult task. Payment procedures to be followed must be made clear to the patient prior to starting treatment. Positive reinforcement and encouragement by an informed staff consultant will increase patient acceptance of the treatment plan.

Dental Assistant

The dental assistant will usually work with the dentist and may often take a secondary or supportive role. In practices where the dental assistant independently performs selected procedures, their significance level may be enhanced. When multiple assistants are utilized, delegation of independently performed procedures such as making bleaching stents without direct dentist supervision is routine. During these periods the assistant assumes the same staff role and priorities discussed above. Patient education and creating a strong patient awareness of the benefits of esthetic dentistry must be a consistent focus by the dental assistant as part of the esthetic dental team. The dental assistant may also direct patients' attention to viewing educational video tapes or other related written and visual materials.

The Dentist

The dentist is the team captain and coach. The amount and level of team aggressiveness must be clearly established by the dentist and along with it the responsibility for staff training, enforcing policy and ensuring that the team is a functional unit. Nonfunctional members of the team must be educated or removed from patient contact. Practices will differ in their approaches but those approaches must be established as a team under the direct supervision and guidance of the responsible dentist. Weekly meetings to discuss, modify and reinforce the team policies and duties are mandatory to maintain effectiveness. Communication is also the key for a successful dental team!

TREATMENT PLAN VS. PLAN OF TREATMENT

Treatment Plan

The final step before treatment begins is establishing a "treatment plan." The "treatment plan" is a listing of services to be performed or referral services necessary (Fig. 1-36). With minimal "treatment plans," this may be all that is necessary. With more extensive treatment plans timing of procedures become more critical; a simple list of procedures is inadequate for efficient and synchronized treatment and may lead to compromised final results.

Plan of Treatment

A "plan of treatment" is an exact listing of procedures to be performed at each appointment (Fig. 1-37). For example, time required for each procedure, specialist procedures to be performed, laboratory materials or special

"TREATMENT PLAN"

PROCEDURES	COST
Computer imaging	$
Study models	$
Diagnostic mounting and waxup	$
Refer to periodontist (Dr. UCLA)	$
Tooth #3° composite	$
Tooth #4^{mod} ceramic inlay	$
Tooth #7^{m} composite	$
Tooth #9^{d} composite	$
Tooth #5-12 porcelain veneers	$
Tooth #14 porcelain fused to metal (PFM) crown	$
Tooth #19^{mod} ceramic inlay	$
Tooth #21° composite	$
Tooth #29do ceramic inlay	$
Tooth #30 PFM crown	$
Tooth #30 composite build-up	$
Bleaching (mandibular)	$
TOTAL	

Fig. 1-36 Example.

"PLAN OF TREATMENT"

I. DIAGNOSTIC AND STABILIZATION PHASE

A. Referral to Periodontist (Dr. UCLA)

Appointment #1 (1 1/2 hours)
- caries control #14, #30 (temporize and evaluate for Endo)
- study models and facebow (Lab: stents and diagnostic waxup) Fee due $_______

Appointment #2 (1 1/2 hours)
- deliver bleaching stent
- computer image Fee due $_______

Appointment #3 (1/2 hour)
- check bleaching
- review imaging and diagnostic waxups
- final consultation to establish priorities — (review perio)
- (8 weeks delay #5-12 due to esthetic perio) Fee due $_______

II. FIRST TREATMENT PHASE

Appointment #4 (1 1/4 hours)
- #3, 7, 9, 21 composites Fee due $_______

Appointment #5 (1 1/4 hours)
- #14 prep, temp. impression, shade (2 weeks to next appointment) Fee due $_______

Appointment #6 (3/4 hour)
- #14 deliver crown Fee due $_______

Appointment #7 (1 1/2 hours)
- #30 build-up, prep, temp, impression, shade (2 weeks to next appointment) Fee due $_______

Appointment #8 (3/4 hour)
- #30 deliver crown
- evaluate periodontal status #5-12 Fee due $_______

Appointment #9 (1 1/2 hours)
- #5-12 prep, impression, shade, photos (one week to next appointment) Fee due $_______

Appointment #10 (3 hours)
- #5-12 seat veneers (3 weeks to next appointment) Fee due $_______

Appointment #11 (time variable)
- #5-12 final contour and polish (ceramic inlays wait 3 months) No fee

III. SECOND TREATMENT PHASE

Appointment #12 (1 hour)
- #19 inlay prep, temp, impression (2 weeks to next appointment) Fee due $_______

Appointment #13 (1 hour)
- #19 deliver inlay (wait three months)
  Note: may prefer composite on remaining teeth. Fee out $ _______

IV. THIRD TREATMENT PHASE

Appointment #14 (1 hour)
- #4 inlay prep, temp, impression (2 weeks to next appointment) Fee due $_______

Appointment #15 (1 hour)
- #4 deliver inlay (wait three months) Fee due $_______

V. FOURTH TREATMENT PHASE

Appointment #16 (1 hour)
- #29 inlay, prep, temp, impression (2 weeks to next appointment) Fee due $_______

Appointment #17
- #29 deliver inlay Fee due $_______

NOTE: This sequence should take about 12 months. Extension beyond that period may be subject to fee increases.

The above should be condensed and abbreviated per individual desires. The basic ideas should be used as an effective "plan of treatment."

Fig. 1-37 Example.

equipment needed, time required between appointments, possible detour points if decisions need to be made, payments due, etc. are critical components of a "plan of treatment." For the organized practice, a "plan of treatment" is a critical component to efficient utilization of practice time and leads to maximum efficiency in patient treatment. A more optimal result is also achieved with greater consistency, fewer mistakes, compromises, or setbacks. This is especially true in the less experienced practice.

A critical component of a "plan of treatment" is patient involvement. By this time the patient knows what procedures can or should be done from the "treatment plan." A patient who has been adequately educated about the proposed procedures is necessary in assisting the dentist in finalizing the "plan of treatment." Certain factors such as desire, priorities, ability to pay, etc. are only answered by the patient and may modify the sequencing of treatment. Patient desires should not modify sequencing that ensures health or an optimum prognosis but is used when treatment order is flexible and patient input is helpful in sequencing.

A plan of treatment will provide an easy reference that allows the entire dental team to know exactly what is going on and when. Appointments can be made correctly even if circumstances interrupt an appointment sequence. Assistants know what supplies and equipment to prepare for each appointment, financial agreements are not a surprise or overlooked and communication and proper sequencing with laboratories and other specialists is ensured. The plan of treatment is the blueprint for treatment. Imagine building a sophisticated structure without a blueprint. The "plan of treatment" provides the master plan that leads to successful esthetic practices with satisfied patients.

REFERENCES

Albers, H.F.: Intraoral Photography. (1992). Adept. Report, Vol. 1: 2, 3.

Joseph Clayton, Personal Communications.

Dzierzak, J.: Computer Imaging: Its Practical Application. (1991). J.A.D.A., Vol. 122, March, p. 41.

Freghe, C.: Dental Photography. (1983). Dent. Clin. N.A., January.

Ganz, G.H.: Computer Video Imaging: Computerization, Communication, and Creation. (1989). QTD Yearbook, p. 64.

Goodlin, R.M.: The Complete Guide to Dental Photography. (1987). Montreal: Michael Publishing Co., Inc.

Goldstein, R.E. and Lancaster, J.S.: Survey of Patient Attitudes Towards Current Esthetic Procedures. (1984). J. Prosthet. Dent. Vol. 52 (6), p. 775.

Hanks, C.T., Fat, J.C., Wataha, J.D., and Corcoran, J.F.: Cytotoxicity and Dentin Permeability of Carbamide Peroxide and Hydrogen Peroxide Vital Bleaching Materials, in vitro. (1993). J. Dent. Res. Vol. 72 (5), p. 931.

Nathanson, D.: Dental Imaging by Computer: A Look at the Future. (1991). J.A.D.A., March, p. 45.

Neuman, K.A.: Cosmetic Imaging in Private Practice. (1990). Esth. Dent. Update. June, Vol. 1 (2), p. 30.

Reality: (1992) Vol. 7 (2). Houston: Reality Publishing Co.

Singer, B.: Special Report: A Buyer's Guide to 35mm Intraoral Photographic Accessories. (1992). J. Am. Acad. Cosmetic Dent. Spring, Vol. 7 (3).

Singer, B.: Marketing your Cosmetic Practice Through Photography. (1991). J. Am. Acad. Cosmetic Dent. Vol. 6 (7), p. 6.

Singer, B.: All you Need for Intraoral Photography: The Sullivan System. (1991). J. Am. Acad. Cosmetic Dent. Vol. 7 (1), p. 6.

Singer, B.: Special Report: 35mm Intraoral Camera Systems. (1992). J. Am. Acad. Cosmetic Dent. Vol .7 (2), p. 1.

Walk, E.B.: Buying a "Budget 35mm Camera System." (1992). J. Am. Acad. Cosmetic Dent. Vol. 7 (2), p. 2

Wander, P.A. and Gordon, P.D.: Dental Photography. (1987). London: British Dental Association.

CHAPTER 2

NONRESTORATIVE ESTHETIC PROCEDURES

COLOR MODIFICATION

Introduction

Often the only complaint a patient has about his or her teeth is that of unacceptable color or irregularities in color. In the absence of other problems that would require restorative procedures, such as shape or size deficiencies, color modification should be considered as a possibility first. This chapter will analyze and discuss the currently available color modification procedures.

Most color modification procedures utilize hydrogen peroxide or a stabilized form, carbamide peroxide, to bleach the teeth. Another technique called microabrasion uses hydrochloric acid and actually dissolves away surface enamel stains.

Bleaching procedures may be divided into two main categories. They are office bleaching, which is dentist and staff administered, and home bleaching, which is patient administered, or a combination of the two. Finally a distinction is sometimes made between external and internal bleaching. External bleaching is the application of the bleach to the outside of the teeth and internal bleaching requires a nonvital tooth or a calcified pulp so the bleach can be placed inside the tooth.

The actual mechanism of tooth bleaching is not fully understood. Bleaches contain unstable peroxides that produce highly unstable free radicals of oxygen that chemically break down larger and highly pigmented organic carbon ring compounds, contained in the enamel matrix, into less pigmented smaller chain molecules. This process is known as oxidation. If continued for long periods beyond the point of continuous lightening, the oxidation process could break down organic materials into carbon dioxide and water. This could result in a loss of the enamel matrix. It is important that bleaching procedures be supervised by a professional that understands these potential hazards to avoid the possibility of unnecessary enamel porosity or brittleness. Remineralization in vivo may minimize these potential problems.

Office Applied External Bleaching (Historical Background)

Attempts to lighten teeth date back to the late 19th century. They evolved into two basic approaches. The first is the use of hydrochloric acid, which is a microabrasion process. The second is the use of hydrogen peroxide; this constitutes the majority of the actual bleaching techniques used in dentistry today.

Westlake in 1895 used parazone (hydrogen peroxide and ether) with an electric current to lighten teeth. Abbot in 1918 and Prinz in 1924 reported success using a stabilized peroxide in water (30% superoxol).

Ames in 1937 reported the first alternative to hydrochloric acid for removing fluorosis stain: five parts 100% hydrogen peroxide and one part ether. Saturated cotton rolls that covered the teeth were heated with a hand instrument for 30 minutes. The number of treatments ranged from five to 25 with the most noticeable results in the first few. Younger in 1939 condemned the use of hydrochloric acid to remove fluorosis stains because of the amount of enamel decalcification that occurred. He advocated his own bleaching solution consisting of five parts 30% hydrogen peroxide and one part anesthetic ether which was applied to the teeth and heated. He reported acceptable fluorosis removal with five to 15 treatments. Hydrogen peroxide remained the treatment of choice until the mid 1960s when enamel etching with phosphoric acid for bonding made hydrochloric etching more acceptable to the dental community.

In 1970, Cohen and Parkins reported the use of 30% superoxol and the rheostatically controlled application of heat for bleaching the teeth of cystic fibrosis patients, which had been stained due to the use of tetracycline. Each patient received eight treatments and the heat was adjusted to be just below each patient's threshold for pain. Improvements were noted in five of six patients; no reversals in tooth color were reported at monthly recalls and no side effects were noted.

In spite of the potentially irritating effect hydrogen peroxide and heat might have on the dental pulp, interest flourished. In 1972, Arens reported results with tetracycline stained teeth using a modified technique of Cohen and Parkins. Arens reduced treatment time to three weekly treatments of 20 minutes each using 30% to 35% superoxol and a thermostatically controlled heating device developed with the Union Broach Company. Of the five patients treated, one did not have permanent results. Arens reported that yellow and brown stains were more easily removed than grey. In 1974, Corcoran and Zillich, using the techniques of Cohen and Parkins at a higher temperature, reported significant lightening in all six cases treated. They also noted that light yellow and brown stain responded more favorably to bleaching than dark brown or grey.

Walton et al, in a 1982 dog study, reported poor long term improvement in tetracycline stained teeth bleached with hydrogen peroxide, with and without phosphoric acid etching. Their findings contributed to the growing clinical evidence that bleaching of tetracycline stained teeth may be temporary and possibly only a surface phenomenon.

In 1984, Jordan and Boksman described three major categories of tetracycline staining and offered a rationale for treatment with hydrogen peroxide and heat. "First-degree" stain is a light yellow, brown or grey stain that is uniform throughout the crown without color bands "Second-degree" stain is dark yellow, brown or grey without color bands. Both of these satisfactorily bleach with hydrogen peroxide. "Third-degree" stain is characterized by dark grey or blue-grey stain with marked banding in the crown (Figs. 2-1 to 2-3). These respond to bleaching but the bands persist even after repeated treatment. Third-degree staining requires combination treatment including esthetic restorative therapy to achieve satisfactory results.

In 1987, Feinman, Goldstein and Garber expanded the indications and advanced the techniques for the utilization of hydrogen peroxide bleaching with various dental stains. They advocated the use of a 20-second pre-etch with 37% phosphoric acid and the use of a heating light to temperatures of 115°F to 140°F with 35% hydrogen peroxide. The pre-etch removes some stains and may facilitate hydrogen peroxide absorption. The light allows for more teeth to be treated at one time and activation of the bleaching solution.

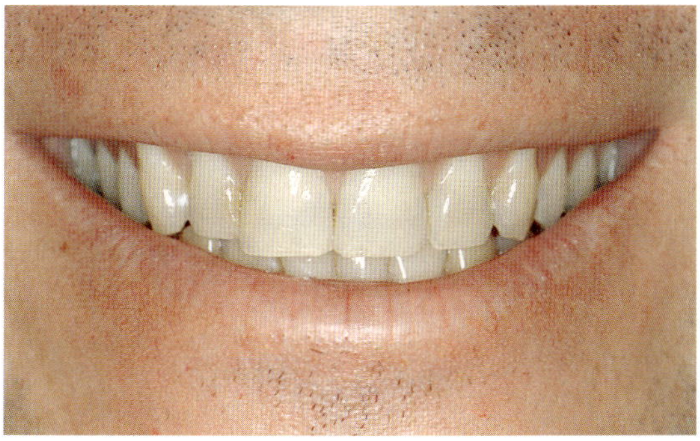

Fig. 2-1

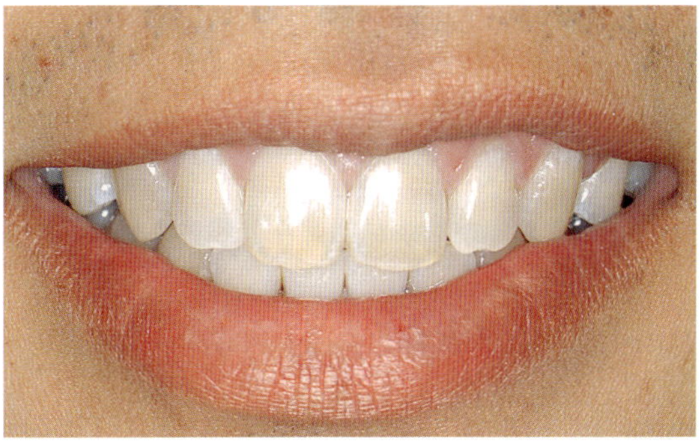

Fig. 2-2

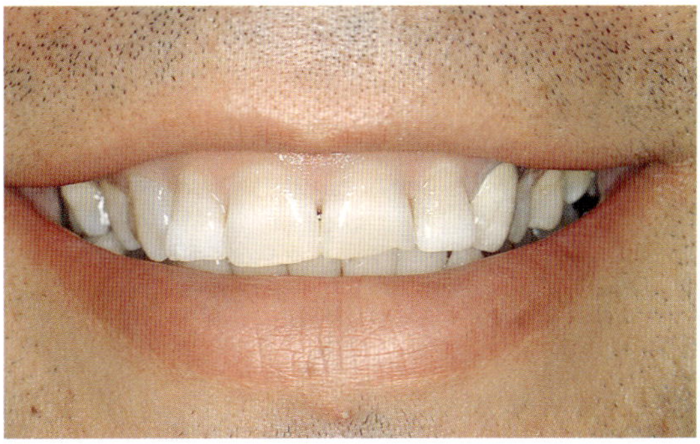

Fig. 2-3

Fig. 2-1 Minimally tetracycline stained teeth.

Fig. 2-2 Darker tetracycline stained teeth.

Fig. 2-3 Third-degree tetracycline stained teeth.

Three to 10 treatments may be necessary at 2- to 4-week intervals. They also described the use of a combination of hydrogen peroxide and hydrochloric acid along with diethyl ether (McInnes' solution) for the removal of fluorosis stains.

In 1988, Haynie and Emett introduced an unheated hydrogen peroxide technique. By mixing 35% hydrogen peroxide with silica dioxide, an inert powder, a gel is formed. Because of the higher viscosity of the gel mixture, it stays in place on the teeth thus minimizing the need to ligate the rubber dam, use protective gingival gels under the dam or use additional dam sealing procedures. The elimination of heat allows for a large simultaneous bleaching area and no need for heating equipment. Other manufacturers have recommended alternatives to rubber dam placement. A fatty acid mucoprotectant, based on sodium stearate, is recommended as a protective layer on intact epithelium against hydrogen peroxide bleaching. A liquid light cured paint on rubber dam material was also developed to protect the tissues from the in-office application of 35% carbamide peroxide. Trends, innovations and new and improved materials will continue to be developed in a search for the yet to be discovered ideal bleaching system.

In conclusion, the use of hydrogen peroxide for in-office bleaching techniques has been well accepted as an effective treatment for many discoloration problems. While hydrochloric acid microabrasion techniques may work faster for superficial stains, hydrogen peroxide is the bleaching material of choice for intrinsic discolorations. Unfortunately, there is still a lack of complete understanding about the exact mechanisms of tooth bleaching. Clearly, different stains respond differently to bleaching and, in some instances, extensive time and money may be spent for what may be considered "limited success" that falls short of patient expectations. Careful treatment planning and patient consultation must precede treatment. An understanding of bleaching potential and techniques is essential. Patients should read and sign an informed consent form prior to starting bleaching.

Heat Application Office Bleaching Technique

Note that this section is based upon the recommendations of Albers (1991), Feinman et al (1987), and Union Broach (1987).

Preoperative Procedures

Prior to starting any bleaching procedures, patients must be informed of potential results and possible limitations. Lighter yellow, orange or brown stains in the incisal two thirds bleach best while darker stains, such as blue or grey and especially banded teeth, bleach less effectively. Stains in the gingival one third often bleach slower. Bleaching may have to be repeated every 1 or 2 years and some postoperative sensitivity may be expected.

Questionable teeth should be tested for vitality and any leaking restorations should be sealed prior to bleaching. Temporary margin sealing can be accomplished using light cured unfilled resin applied to acid etched marginal deficiencies.

Patients' habits such as smoking or coffee and tea drinking may affect the long-term prognosis of the bleaching procedures and patients should be advised accordingly. Finally a preoperative photograph with a shade guide for a reference is helpful to document bleaching progress (Fig. 2-4). If a ceramic crown exists the shade guide may not be necessary. At a minimum, record the prebleaching shade in the chart. It is often advisable to bleach only one arch to provide the patient with an easy reference for improvement and provide additional motivation.

Treatment Procedures and Materials

- Do not use anesthesia. Any discomfort or adverse symptoms should be identified immediately to avoid unnecessary hard or soft tissue irritation.
- Polish the teeth with pumice.
- Apply a plain oral protective paste (petroleum jelly or Orabase™) to protect the soft tissues labially, lingually and interproximally. Do not use topical anesthetic. Hydrogen peroxide bleaching solution is very irritating to the tissues and detecting any leakage is essential.
- Place a well fitting rubber dam. Holes should be as small as possible in a heavy dam material. Invert the dam and ligate with waxed floss around all the teeth (Fig. 2-5). Place rubber strips interproximally at the distal of the isolation area to hold the dam in place.
- Reapply an oral protective paste to seal

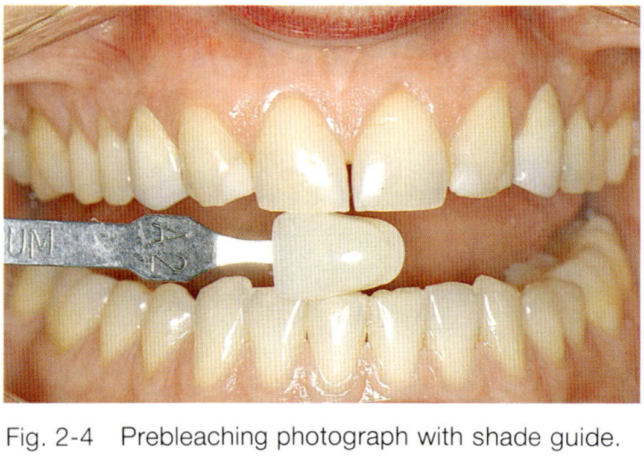

Fig. 2-4 Prebleaching photograph with shade guide.

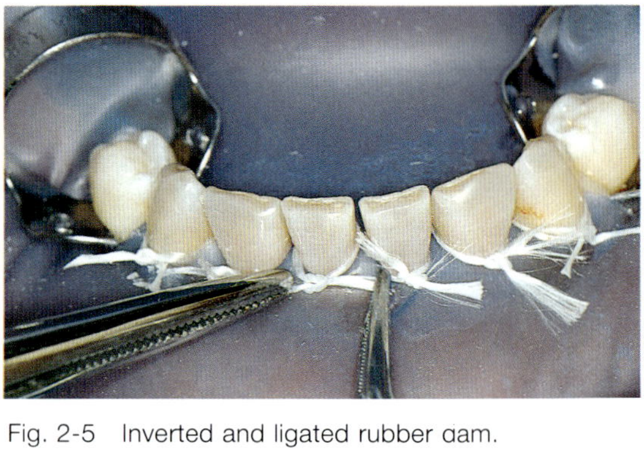

Fig. 2-5 Inverted and ligated rubber dam.

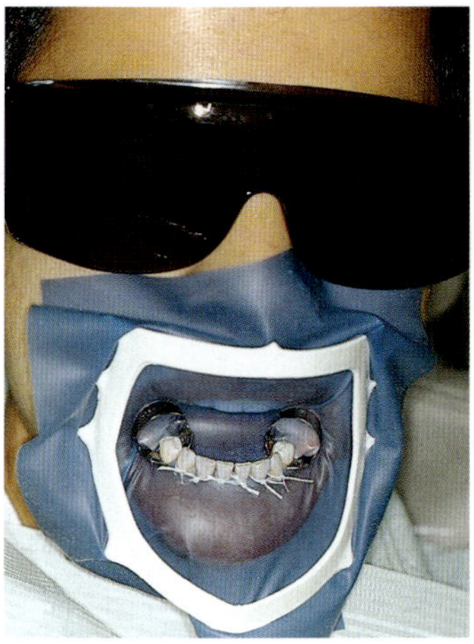

Fig. 2-6

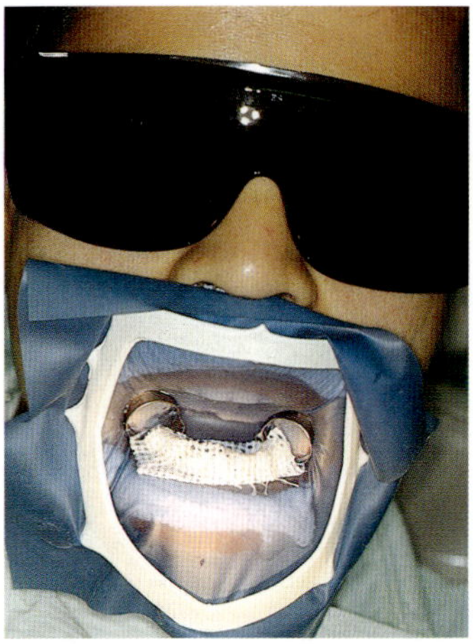

Fig. 2-7

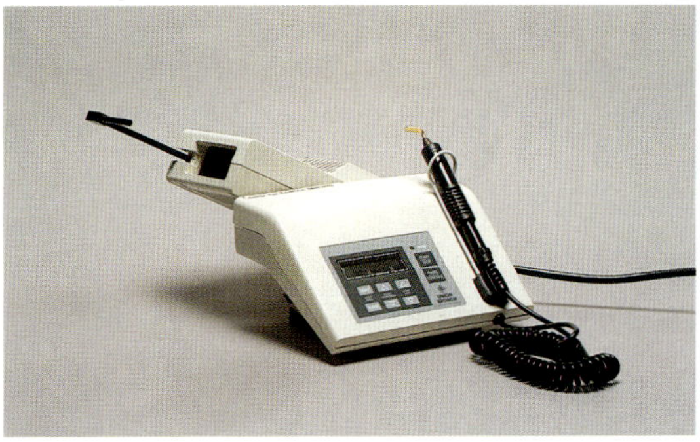

Fig. 2-8

Fig. 2-6 Bleaching patient with protective eyewear.

Fig. 2-7 Bleaching in progress; note light illuminated area, wet gauze over lower lip to cool and H_2O_2 saturated gauze over the teeth.

Fig. 2-8 Example of a bleaching light as part of a total bleaching system. Note guide arm (**left**) to determine the appropriate light distance from the subject (Union Broach®).

against leakage. Place the rubber dam frame in such a way as to form collection areas that prevent bleach from dripping on the patient. A 2×2-inch gauze pad may also be placed in a run off area to absorb excess bleaching solution. Also place cold wet gauze under the dam and over the lips to cool the area. Cold wet gauze may also be placed over the dam and clamp areas to cool them.

- Safety glasses should be worn by the dental staff and patient. Drape the patient with a heavy plastic cover. Gloves are mandatory for staff (Fig. 2-6).
- Polish the teeth again with pumice to remove any protective paste.
- Pre-etching the teeth with 37% phosphoric acid for 15 to 60 seconds will enhance porosity of the enamel. It may be advisable with banded or selectively stained teeth to limit this etching to the darker areas. Routine etching may not be necessary in all instances. Rinse thoroughly with water.
- Cut a piece of gauze to match the size of area to be bleached. Saturate it with the 35% hydrogen peroxide bleaching solution and place it over the exposed teeth. Note that both the buccal and lingual areas are bleached simultaneously (Fig. 2-7).
- This gauze should be blotted with dry gauze every 5 to 10 minutes and new solution applied.
- Apply heat with a bleaching light according to manufacturer's instructions. Place the light on a stable base and adjust the temperature so the patient feels the heat but is not uncomfortable (Fig. 2-8). Monitor this as time goes on for temperatures will vary and the light intensity may need to be reduced. The patient can control this with

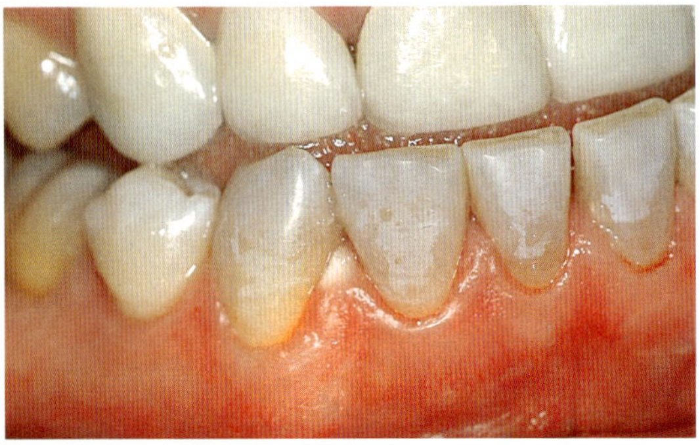

Fig. 2-9 White papillae due to exposure to hydrogen peroxide.

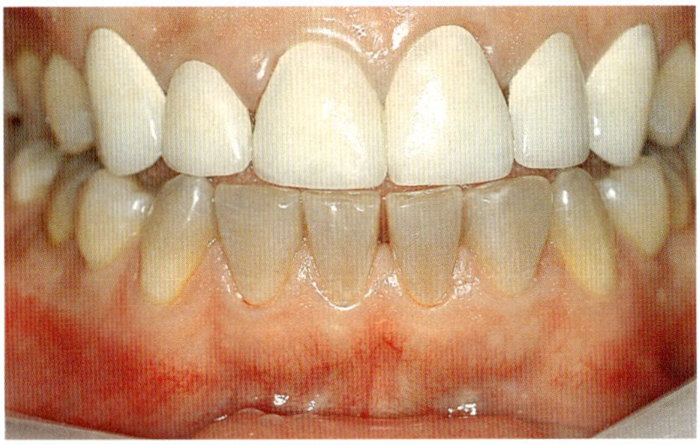

Fig. 2-10a (**left**) Prebleaching.

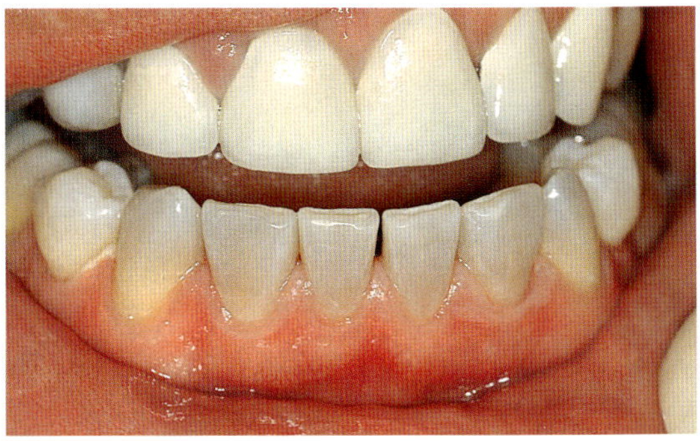

Fig. 2-10b (**right**) After two bleaching sessions.

some bleaching lights. Note that any discomfort must be checked and the cause diagnosed and corrected. Leaks or an uncomfortably high temperature setting must be corrected immediately.

- Continue the bleaching process for 30 to 45 minutes. Record bleaching time and temperature in the patient's chart.
- Remove the heat source and let the teeth cool for 5 minutes. Remove the saturated gauze and rinse thoroughly with water.
- Postbleaching the etched surfaces should be polished with fine rubber porcelain polishing cups and a clear neutral sodium fluoride gel should be placed for 2 minutes.
- Remove the rubber dam and any remaining oral protectant. Any white tissues should be rinsed with water for at least 2 minutes (Fig. 2-9).
- The patient should be advised that postoperative cold sensitivity is common, especially in the first 48 hours. Pain generally subsides in 24 hours. Neutral fluoride rinse may be provided to restore the fluoride rich enamel layer and to reduce sensitivity. If sensitivity increases, advise the use of a desensitizing toothpaste.
- Check results in 2 weeks after rehydration and repeat (Fig. 2-10). Five to 10 bleaching sessions may be necessary, depending upon the nature and severity of the discoloration. If painful postoperative symptoms occur, heating temperature and duration of the session should be reduced.

No-Heat Office Bleaching Techniques

The use of heating equipment in conjunction with liquid bleaching solutions requires meticulous isolation and has been a deterrent for many dentists. It is time consuming, technique sensitive, and often costly to patients. The trend in office bleaching is to simplify. The main modification that has taken place is to increase the viscosity of the bleaching solutions using silica dioxide or other additives. This allows the bleach to be placed on the teeth with minimal flow. Due to this increased viscosity, the need to meticulously ligate each tooth for maximum isolation is minimized. To simplify the process further, paint on light cured rubber dam materials may be substituted for traditional rubber dams depending upon individual preference. For extensive isolation areas, a traditional rubber dam may be easier. For localized areas with irregular tissue heights and random root exposure, the control of the light cured dam material may be advisable. Both systems should be used as necessary.

Treatment Procedures

- The paint on rubber dam material should be painted on to cover soft and hard tissues where exposure to bleaching solutions is to be avoided. Excess material can easily be cut away with a scalpel (Fig. 2-11). A heavy rubber dam may also be placed and inverted. Ligation is not necessary for every tooth.
- Selectively etching darker areas may be advisable to enhance bleach penetration.
- The viscous bleach should be applied to the area to be bleached according to the manufacturer's instructions (Fig. 2-12). Some new systems actually change color when the bleach is exhausted (Fig. 2-13).
- Repeat the bleach application as needed or time allows.
- Rinse thoroughly; remove the rubber dam. Topical fluoride may also be applied (Fig. 2-14).

The newer office bleaching systems are

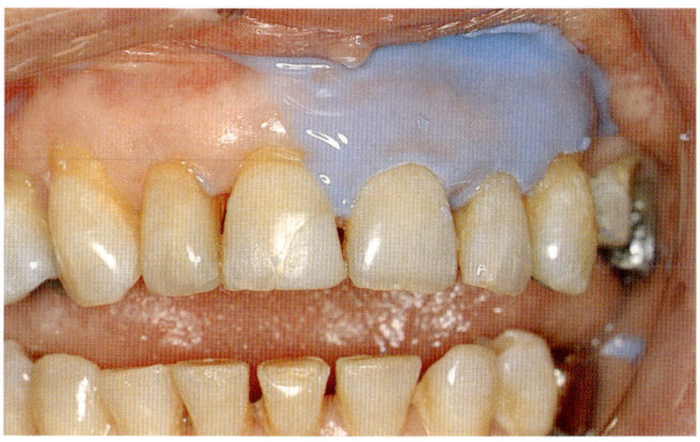

Fig. 2-11a Application of paint on rubber dam material.

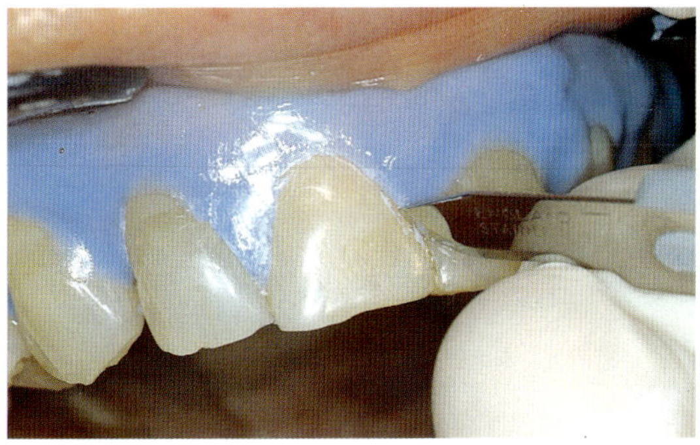

Fig. 2-11b Use scalpel to cut away excess.

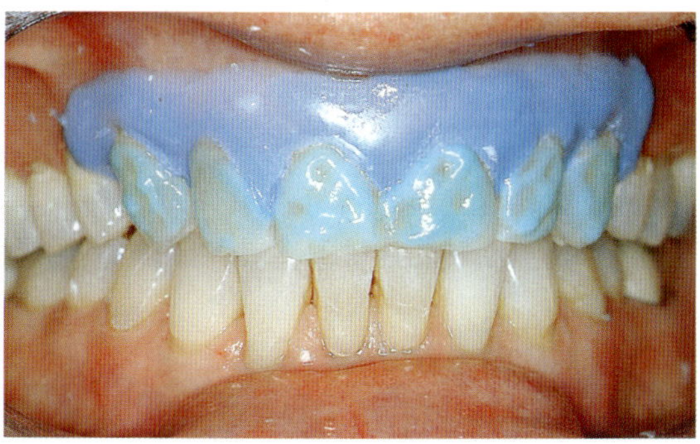

Fig. 2-12 Viscous bleach applied to teeth.

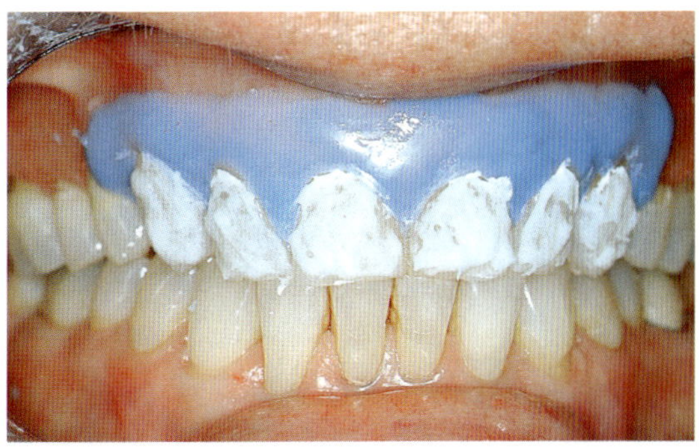

Fig. 2-13 Note color change of bleaching material (Shofu®).

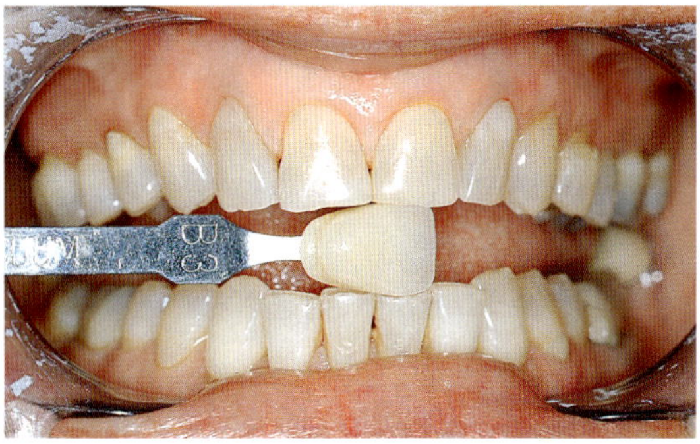

Fig. 2-14a Pretreatment.

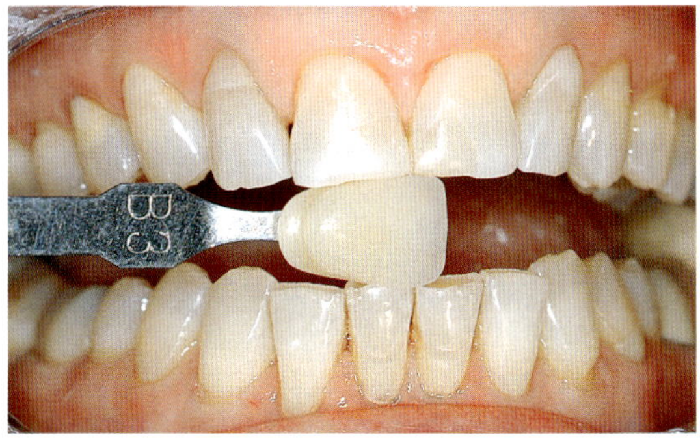

Fig. 2-14b After one bleaching session.

certainly easier to use and less costly to the patient. Whether or not they are as effective as heat application systems is questionable. This approach has greater appeal to most dentists and may be attempted first before more aggressive approaches are used. They may also be used in conjunction with home bleaching approaches to accelerate the total bleaching process and minimize the total time necessary to attain acceptable results.

One of the main failures of home bleaching systems, to be discussed later, is patient compliance. These newer office applied techniques offer an attractive alternative for patients who are willing to pay more for eliminating the inconvenience of home bleaching.

Single Tooth Bleaching

A single intact vital tooth may occasionally be different from the remaining dentition and present an esthetic problem (Fig. 2-15). This may be the result of trauma and resultant internal hemorrhaging or premature internal calcification. It may also be normal as in the case of canine teeth naturally being darker than incisors. Single tooth vital bleaching uses the same office techniques already presented. Heat applied techniques are useful here and a spatula shaped heating instrument may be used to localize heat application (Fig. 2-16). No-heat techniques may also be used by simply applying the viscous bleach to the localized area to be bleached (Fig. 2-17).

Discolored nonvital teeth are a more com-

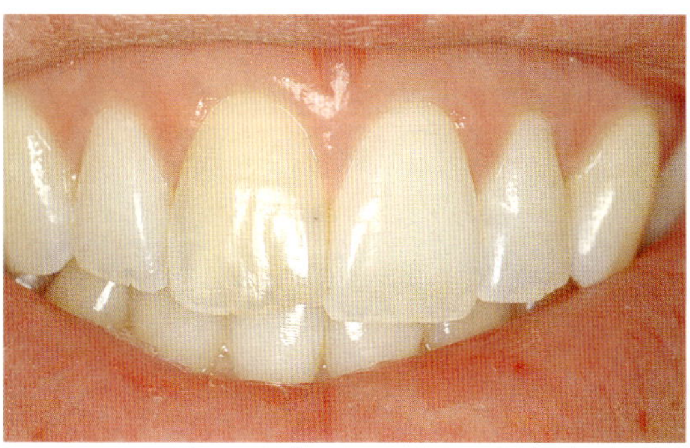

Fig. 2-15 Single discolored right central incisor.

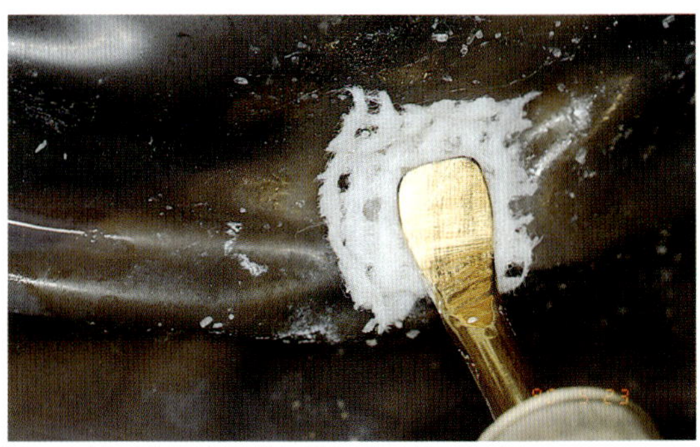

Fig. 2-16a Heat applied with heating wand to singe isolated central incisor.

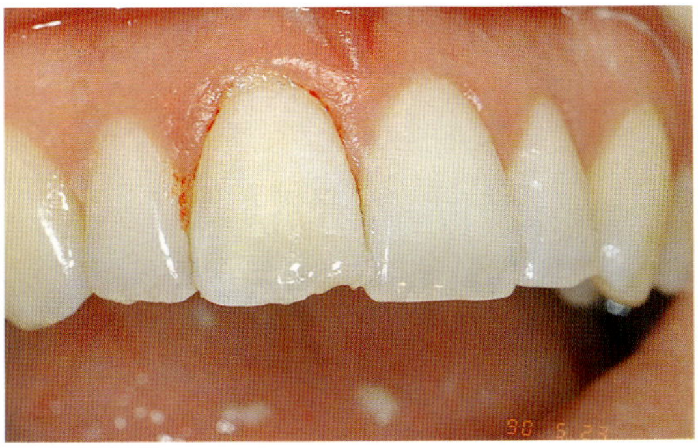

Fig. 2-16b Central incisor after one session.

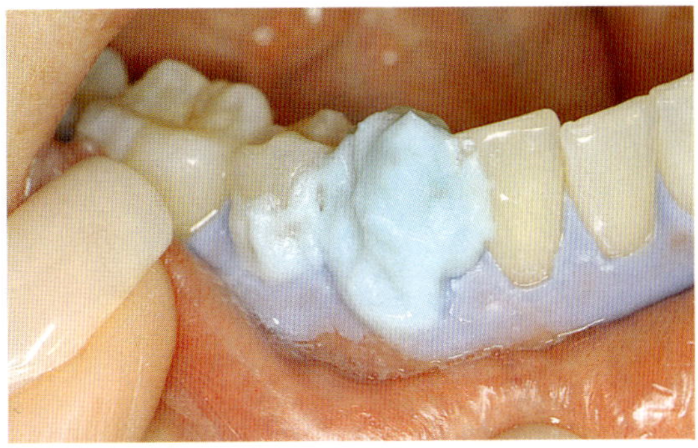

Fig. 2-17 Viscous bleach applied to one tooth only.

mon problem and bleaching may provide an acceptable solution. The two major concerns include (1) lack of color stability over time and (2) more importantly the possibility of external root resorption several years postoperatively and possible tooth loss. The patient must be advised of these potential problems during the consultation appointment and an informed consent signed. For teeth with large restorations or heavily stained from lingual amalgam restorations, a restorative procedure may be a more appropriate and predictable solution.

Historically, nonvital bleaching was first successfully documented by Spasser in 1961. Sodium perborate was used as a "walking bleach." Nutting and Poe combined superoxol with the sodium perborate to create a very popular walking bleach. Techniques for meticulously cleaning the pulp chamber and increasing bleach penetration using phosphoric acid were advocated along with the addition of heat to accelerate the process. Finally, internal bleaching techniques were combined with external bleaching techniques to enhance the result as described by Boksman in 1983.

Technique

- The tooth should be evaluated for an adequate root canal filling. Retreatment may precede bleaching if the root canal filling is clinically unacceptable.
- Bleaching materials used, as in vital office bleaching, are very caustic. The tooth to be bleached must be meticulously isolated with a rubber dam, ligated and a protective gel placed under the rubber dam. Safety glasses should be worn by the patient and the dental team.
- Remove all root canal filling material and debris from the pulp chamber to a depth of 1 to 2 mm below the gingival crest but short of the periodontal ligament attachment (Fig. 2-18). Measure with a periodontal probe to verify this depth. Reseal this apical area with a 1- to 2-mm thick layer of base cement or a light cured glass ionomer base if access permits (Fig. 2-19). Depth of the apical seal should be no deeper than 0.5 mm below the gingival crest. It may be placed further coronally in nonesthetic lingual and proximal areas.

CAUTION: NEVER DO INTERNAL BLEACHING UNLESS THE APICAL SEAL IS COMPLETED.

- Acetone may be used to dissolve any fatty debris left in the tooth. Extremely discolored teeth should be etched internally with 37% phosphoric acid for 60 seconds to facilitate bleach penetration.
- Place a cotton pellet into the chamber and carefully saturate it with 30% to 35% hydrogen peroxide using a small syringe.

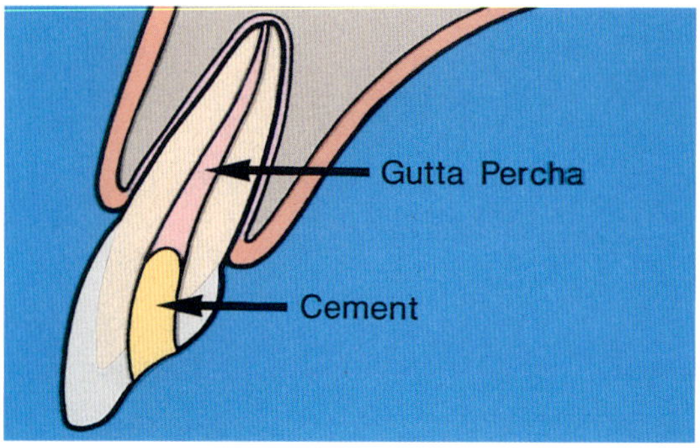

Fig. 2-18a Preoperative.

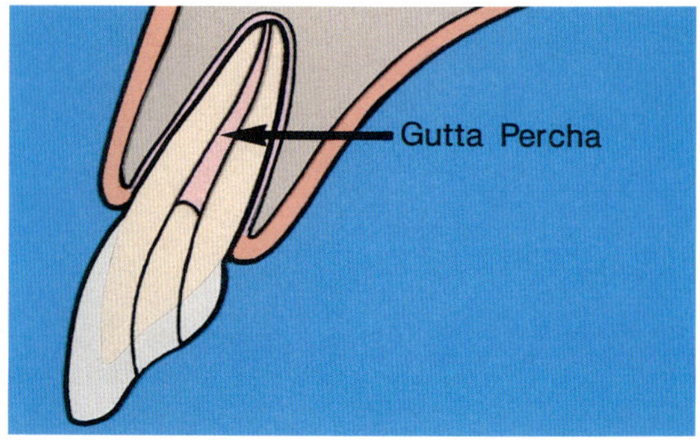

Fig. 2-18b Gutta percha removal just short of periodontal ligament attachment.

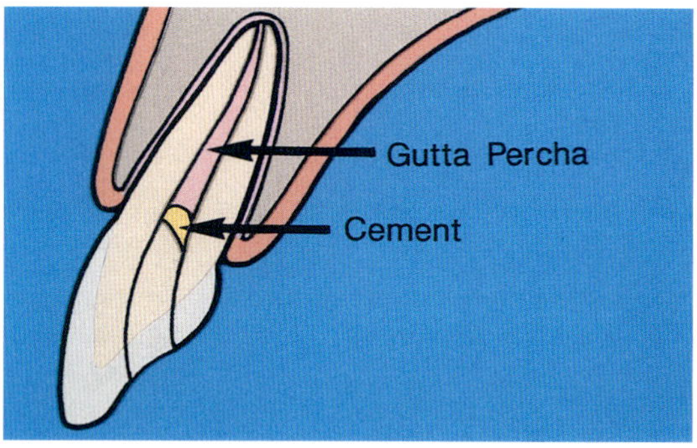

Fig. 2-19 Cement layer to seal gutta percha.

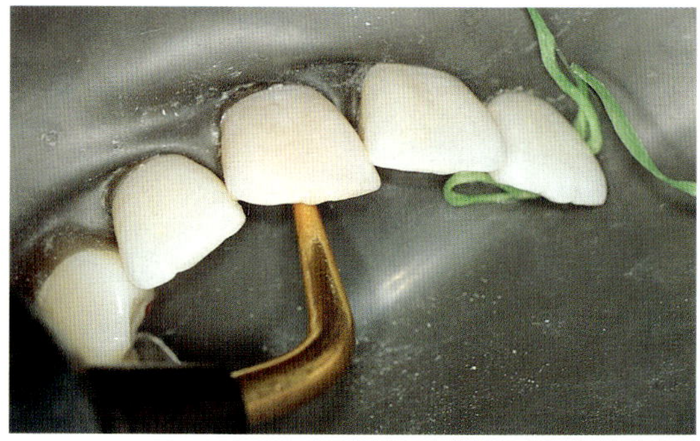

Fig. 2-20 Pointed heating instrument used to heat bleach in tooth.

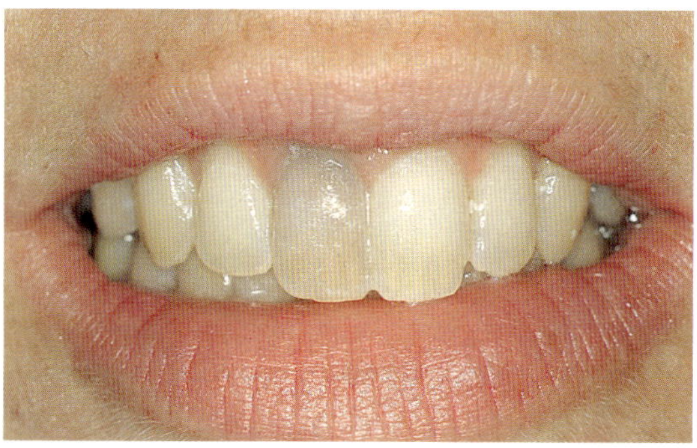

Fig. 2-21a Preoperative.

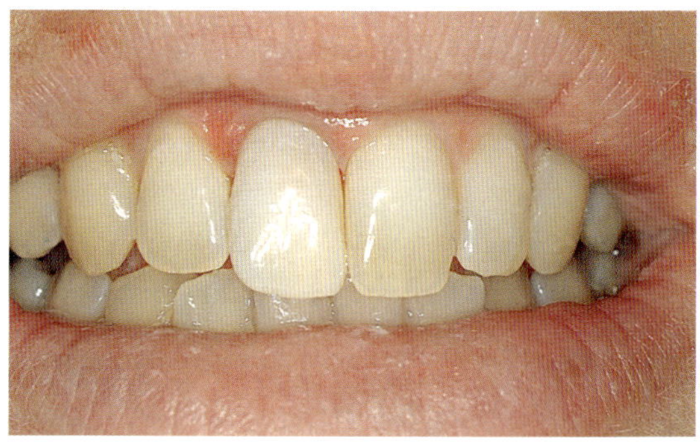

Fig. 2-21b After one bleaching session.

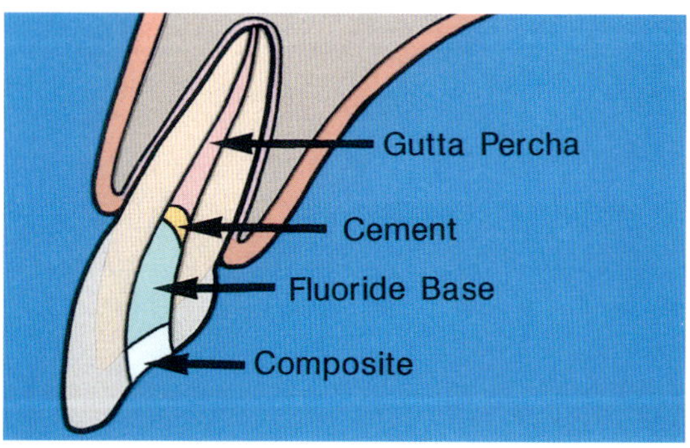

Fig. 2-22 Pulp chamber is filled with a fluoride releasing base and sealed (if necessary) with a tooth colored restorative material (composite).

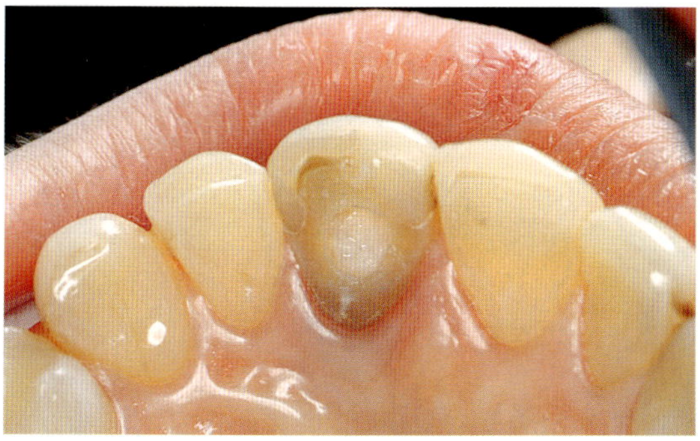

Fig. 2-23a Bleaching solution in tooth.

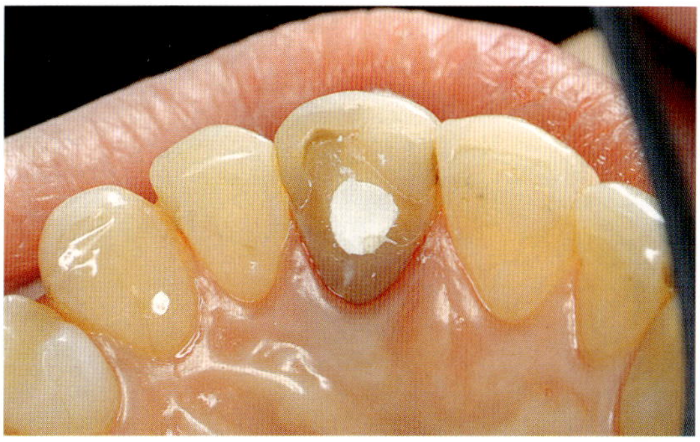

Fig. 2-23b Tooth sealed with temporary cement.

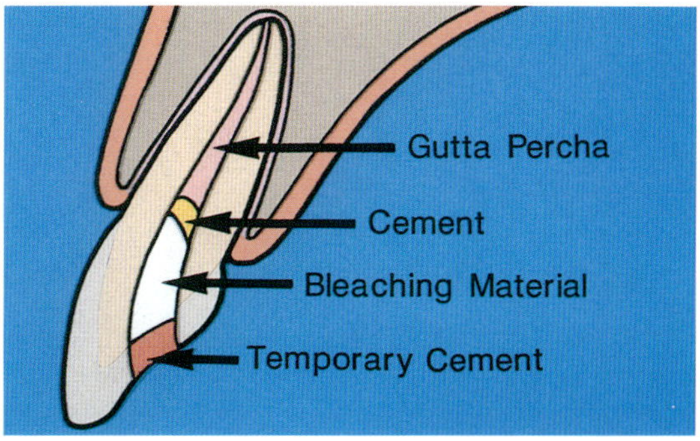

Fig. 2-24 Diagram of tooth prepared for "walking" bleach.

Care must be taken to avoid excess. A piece of gauze may also be placed over the facial surface and saturated with the bleaching solution. Using a pointed heating instrument set at 165°F (73°C), apply heat to the internal portion of the tooth for 5 minutes (Fig. 2-20). This procedure is repeated three to six times with new solution. Heat may be applied externally as described in vital single tooth bleaching (Fig. 2-16a). Heat may be reduced if uncomfortable to the patient. Repeat these procedures for 30 minutes or until desired results are achieved (Fig. 2-21). A slight overbleaching is recommended. If inadequate bleaching is achieved, the process may be repeated at a future date.

- If the bleaching is adequate, fill the pulp chamber with a mixture of calcium hydroxide and water. Calcium hydroxide will reduce the acidity and return the tooth and surrounding structures to a neutral pH. It also induces the formation of a calcified matrix when multiple bleaching visits have denatured the organic matrix. The tooth is thus strengthened and the possibility of external resorption minimized. The calcium hydroxide is left in place for a minimum of 2 days.
- When results are stable and acceptable, the pulp chamber can be filled with a tooth colored fluoride releasing restorative and sealed externally with a composite resin restoration (Fig. 2-22).

Another technique that may be combined with office nonvital bleaching or used by itself is called "walking bleach." In this technique the first four steps are the same. A thick mixture of 30% to 35% hydrogen peroxide and sodium perborate is condensed into the pulp chamber. This is sealed in place with a 1- to 2-mm thick layer of a temporary cement (Figs. 2-23 and 2-24). The bleach is left for 7 days and the process repeated a maximum of two times. If adverse symptoms arise, the patient should return immediately. Once complete, the tooth should be stabilized with calcium hydroxide and restored as above.

Office Monitored Home Bleaching

Historical Background

In the mid to late 1960s, an orthodontist in Arkansas, Dr. Bill Klusmier, began advising patients who were using postorthodontic positioners (a mouthguardlike appliance) and who developed inflammation to use Gly-oxide™ (Marion Merrell Dow, Inc.). This carbamide peroxide oral antiseptic, when placed in the positioner, would reduce inflammation, but in addition he noticed that the teeth were also lighter. He started to use this technique to lighten teeth on family and friends and presented the technique at two Arkansas State Dental Association meetings and the Southwestern Orthodontic Society meeting. In 1972 he switched to Proxigel™ (Reed & Carnrick's Pharm.) because its increased viscosity aided in longer retention. He also started to use this technique in custom fitted trays.

In the early 1970s, Dr. Jerry Wagner, a pedodontist from Arkansas, used Proxigel in positioning appliances to reduce inflammation in older patients he was treating for minor orthodontics. Upon recall he noticed improved soft tissue health and tooth lightening. Both dentists noticed that it took longer to bleach the mandibular arch. Dr. Wagner and Dr. Klusmier both participated in the same dental society in Arkansas. Dr. Wagner went on to promote the treatment as a practice builder.

In 1984, Dr. Tom Austin, a general dentist from North Carolina, learned the technique from Dr. Wagner. He shared the technique with Dr. David Freshwater, a general dentist also from North Carolina, who treated his daughter and shared the technique with the Coastal Dental Study Club. In 1988, the technique was shared with Dr. Van Haywood as he lectured to the Study Club. In conjunction with Dr. Harald Heymann, clinical and laboratory testing of the technique began at the University of North Carolina. In 1989 the first article on nightguard bleaching was published.

Parallel to this professional introduction, in 1986, Dr. John Munro, a general dentist from Tennessee, used 10% carbamide peroxide to control bacterial growth after root planing. In selective cases, a vacuum formed plastic splint was used to hold this neutralized Glyoxide solution that was refilled two or three times a day for 3 to 7 days or until a normal pink appearance returned to the tissues. He noticed that as a side effect the teeth were whiter and in 1988 he presented his findings to a manufacturer who in 1989 developed the first commercial product specifically used for this technique (White & Bright™, Omni International). Commercial promotion began and thus the massive exposure to the dental profession and public sector began. The "Home Bleaching Revolution" was started and with it a vast increase in bleaching popularity and acceptance and a large variety of bleaching solutions, accessories and techniques.

The revolution in bleaching has largely been initiated by the Office Monitored Home Bleaching (OMHB) techniques. The significant reduction in office time and equipment needed and consequent reduction in cost has made these techniques attractive to both the patient and dentist. In addition, they are simple procedures that appear relatively safe and reasonably effective.

Office monitored home bleaching works best on yellow, orange or light brown stains and is less effective on dark grey, dark blue and tetracycline banding as with office bleaching. Some improvement in brown fluorosis has been noted.

This technique is inexpensive and conservative. The current trend is to try this approach first and only use more costly and aggressive techniques as required.

Materials

This OMHB technique requires the use of an intraoral stent or mouthguard-type appliance. Generally this is fabricated by a vacuum molding technique on a stone model of the dental arch. A clear soft vinyl material, .02 to .035 inches thick, is advised. Thicker .08-inch material may be used but is often less comfortable and less esthetic. Stiffer materials often crack and reduce the longevity of the appliance (Fig. 2-25).

The stent is now trimmed. For lower viscosity to medium viscosity bleaching materials, extend the stent 2 or 3 mm beyond the free gingival margins (Fig. 2-26). If high viscosity bleaching materials are used, it is advised to cut the stent 0.5 mm short of the free gingival margins (Fig. 2-27). This will minimize potential tissue irritation. It has also been recommended that a reservoir be placed over the facial surfaces of the teeth to be bleached. This is accomplished by placing wax or a light cured block-out resin on the facial surfaces of the study model prior to vacuum molding the bleaching stent (Fig. 2-28). Thus a larger space is created in this area under the stent, which will hold a larger volume of bleaching solution. Creating this extra space is not mandatory for OMHB to work but may extend the time required before additional bleaching material needs to be added due to washout. A potential disadvantage of a reservoir may be a loose stent due to decreased frictional retention.

A vacuum forming device is necessary for the above stent fabrication techniques (Fig. 2-29). These devices have many utilizations in restorative dentistry and quickly pay for themselves in reduced laboratory costs and convenience. Use of quick setting stone at

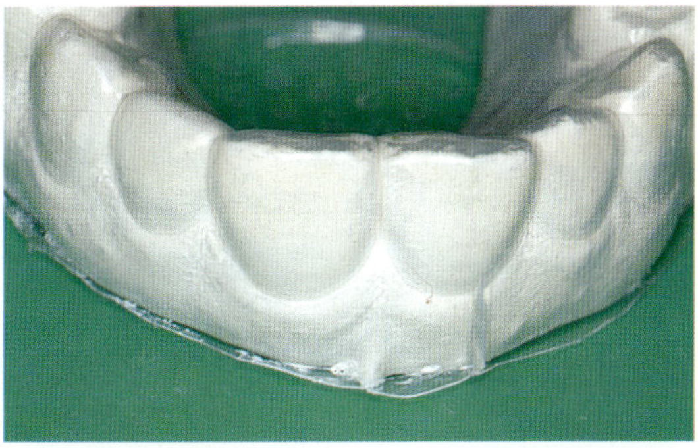

Fig. 2-25 Note wrinkle in stiff vinyl matrix.

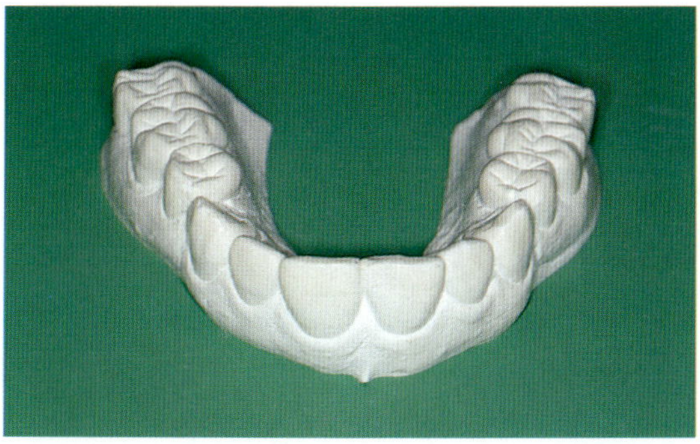

Fig. 2-26a Quick set stone model trimmed to extend 3 to 4 mm beyond free gingival margin.

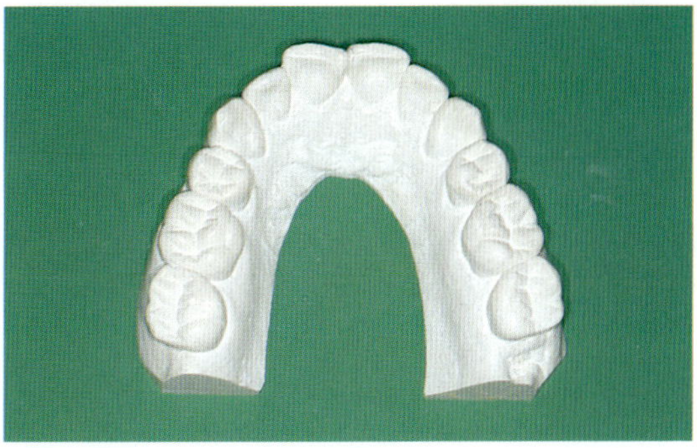

Fig. 2-26b Open palate to aid in vacuum forming.

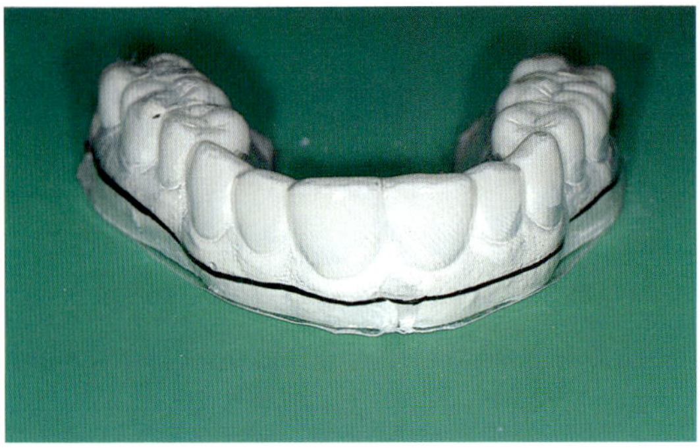

Fig. 2-26c Vinyl material formed and marked for trimming.

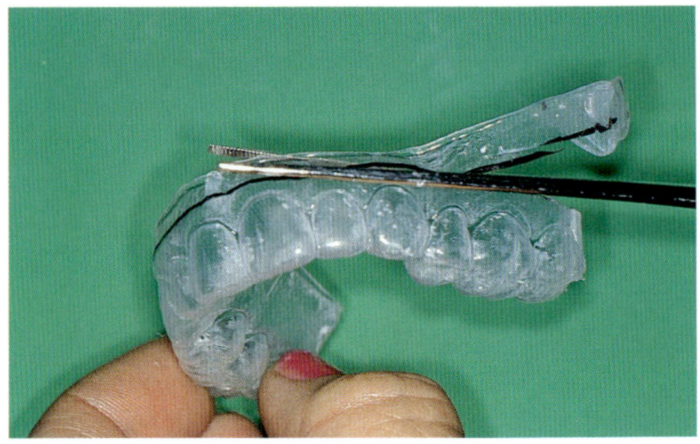

Fig. 2-26d Use scissors to cut matrix material.

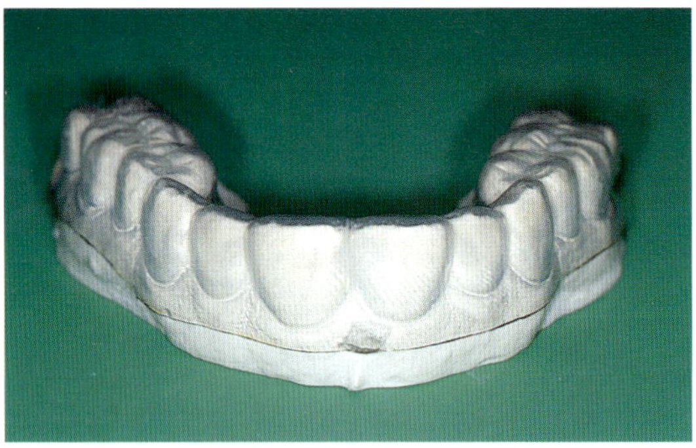

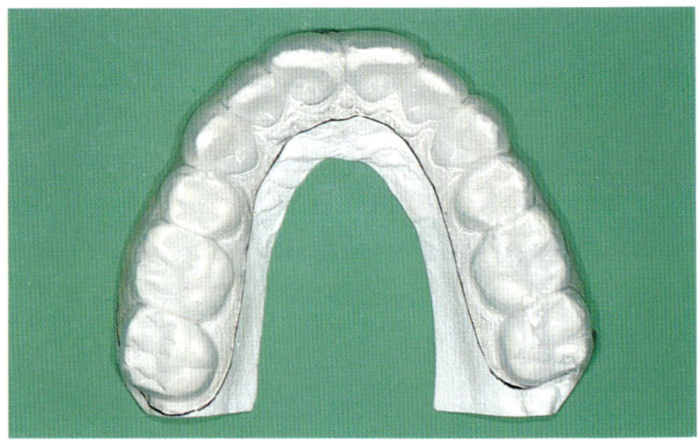

Figs. 2-26e and f Completed medium viscosity stent extending 2 to 3 mm beyond free gingival margins.

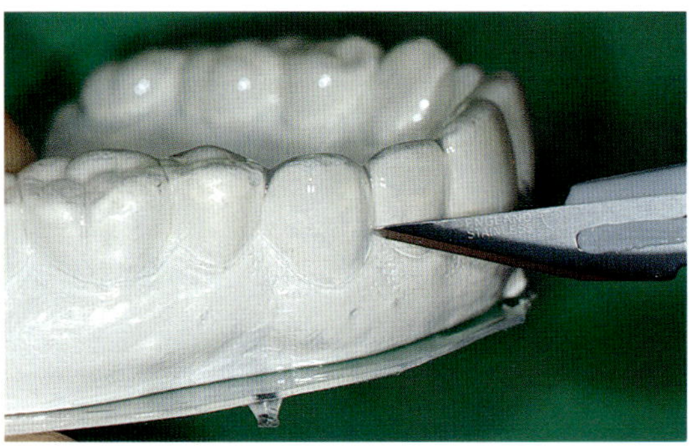

Fig. 2-27a Using a scalpel or scissors to cut the bleaching stent on the model.

Figs. 2-27b and c Completed high viscosity bleaching stent extending 0.5 mm short of the free gingival margin.

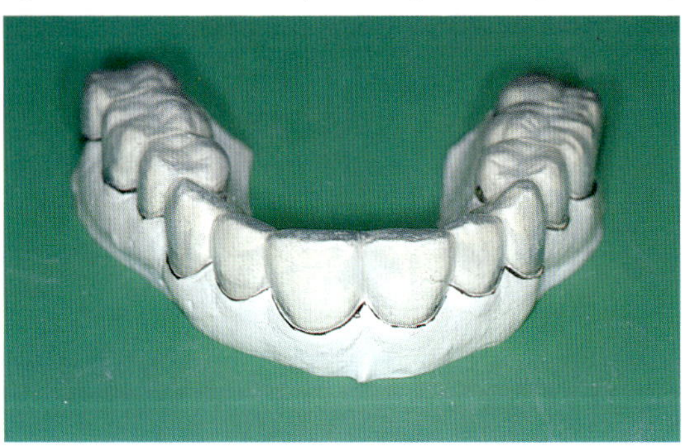

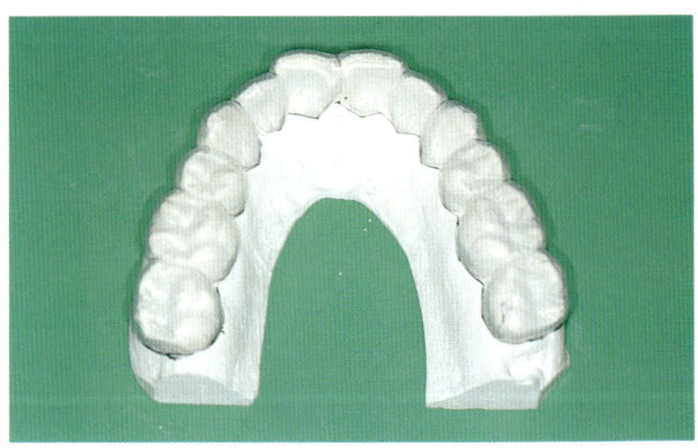

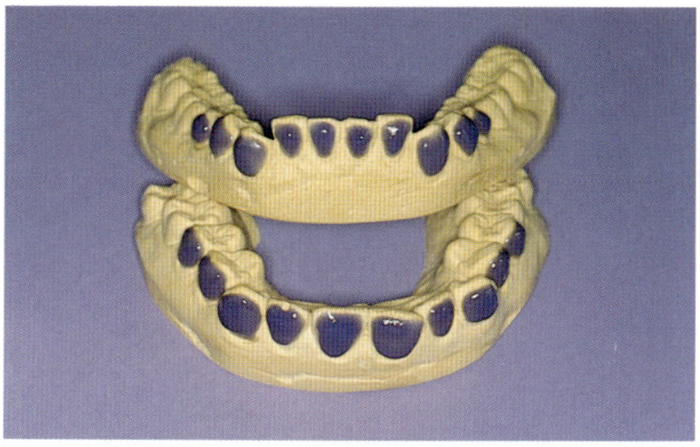

Fig. 2-28 Light cured block-out resin on model to form bleach reservoir.

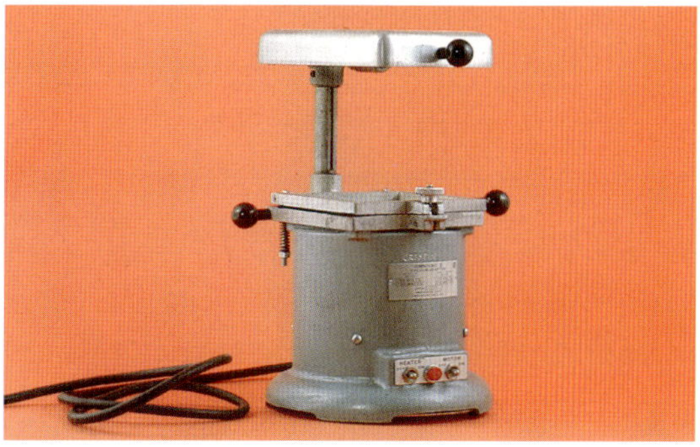

Fig. 2-29 Vacuum forming device.

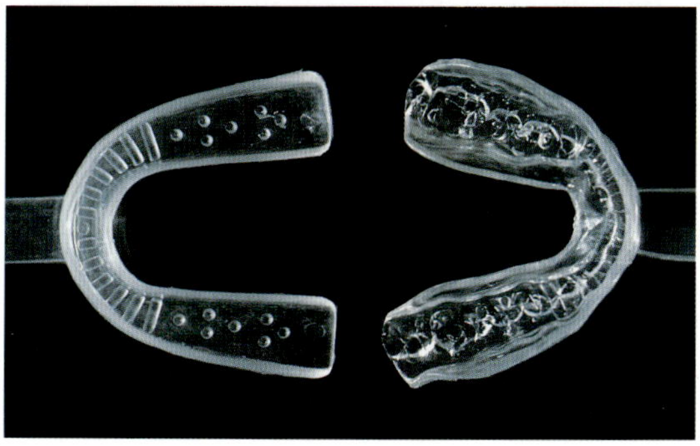

Fig. 2-30 Stent material is boiled (**left**) and formed directly in the mouth (**right**).

the initial bleaching appointment means that the model can be easily fabricated and a vacuum bleaching stent made, saving the patient a return delivery appointment.

One system uses a thermal plastic material that can be put in hot water and molded directly in the mouth (Fig. 2-30).

The bleaching solutions used are primarily 10% to 15% carbamide peroxides (Fig. 2-31). The remaining components are 85% or more glycerin or propylene glycol, sodium stannate, and flavors. Carbamide peroxides have been classified by the FDA since 1979 as an oral antiseptic. One of the only side effects is a laxative effect from ingesting large amounts of glycerin. Ingestation of these materials from OMHB is generally only about 2 ounces over 3 to 5 weeks. In addition, small amounts of acid may be added to reduce the pH to between 5.0 to 6.5 which greatly increases the shelf life. This lower pH has been questioned as a possible etchant for enamel or dentin. The critical pH for etching enamel is 5.2 to 5.8 and for dentin is 6.0 to 6.8. Preliminary SEM studies have not demonstrated any significant etching of the enamel. A slight reduction in surface fracture toughness has been demonstrated in vitro.

An additive to many carbamide peroxide bleaching solutions is carbopol. Carbopol is an extremely large molecular weight (4 to 5 million) polyacrylic acid polymer. This water soluble resin, when used with carbamide peroxide, increases the shelf life and binds with carbamide peroxide and increases the active peroxide release by 3 or 4 times. In addition, carbopol greatly increases the viscosity of the bleaching solution. Thus by increasing the carbopol content of the bleaching solution, the material will stay in place and remain active for longer periods of time. Noncarbopol containing materials are less acidic but must be replenished more frequently.

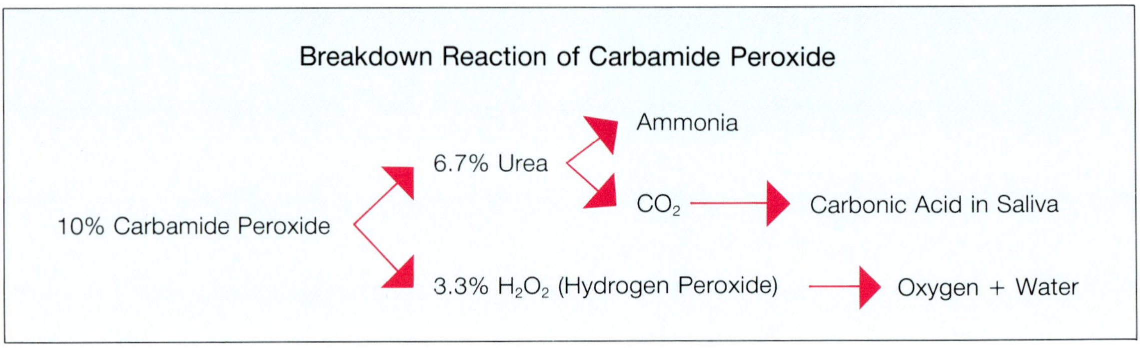

Fig. 2-31

Hydrogen peroxide OMHB materials are also available. It is claimed that hydrogen peroxide works two to three times faster than the same concentration of carbamide peroxide and at a neutral pH. In both materials it is the hydrogen peroxide that is the active bleaching ingredient.

One hydrogen peroxide OMHB starts with a 35% hydrogen peroxide solution that is diluted to 2%, 5%, or 10% by adding it to a gel solution containing a hydroxyl ethyl cellulose gel, 0.5% fluoride, a fatty acid mucoprotectant (based on sodium stearate), and water.

This material offers the flexibility to control the active hydrogen peroxide concentrations but has only a limited shelf life (4 to 6 days). This may be desirable, because it requires the patient to return more frequently for new material and ensures more patient control and contact. The mucoprotectant requires intact epithelium and should not be used on lacerated tissues. When this material is used, a low concentration is used at first and the concentration is increased as needed and tolerated. Whether this material works faster has yet to be determined, but the higher hydrogen peroxide concentration potential may prove to be a significant factor for more demanding situations.

Treatment Procedures

- A consent form must be read and signed by the patient.
- Polish the teeth. A complete prophylaxis is recommended.
- Take preoperative photographs with a shade guide placed horizontally between the teeth (Fig. 2-32a). When only one arch is to be bleached, or if an existing ceramic restoration is present, the shade guide may be omitted. Minimally the prebleaching shade should be recorded in the chart.
- Alginate impressions are made and vacuum formed stents are fabricated, trimmed and tried in. Retention is checked and any areas of tissue blanching modified. Patient comfort and a passive fit should be verified.
- The patient is shown how to load the stent with bleaching material. Enough material should be used to fill the voids between the stent and teeth with minimal excess being forced out. Excess can be wiped out or expectorated.
- Patient instructions:
  1. Use a minimum of 3 hours per day.
  2. Use more if time and lack of symptoms allow.
  3. Overnight utilization is advisable.
  4. During waking hours, medium viscosity materials should be replenished every 1.0 to 1.5 hours. High viscosity materials may need to be replenished less frequently.
  5. Some minor tooth symptoms are normal. If it is very uncomfortable, reduce

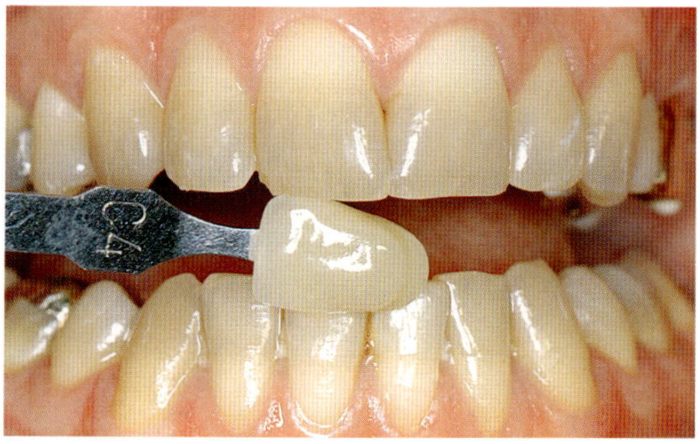

Fig. 2-32a Prebleaching photograph.

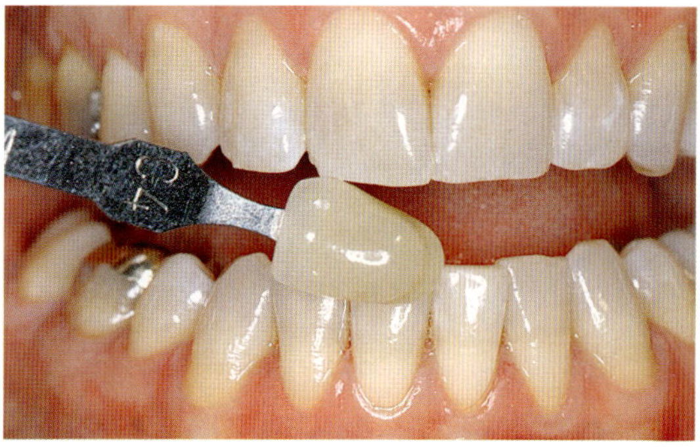

Fig. 2-32b Postbleaching photograph.

utilization time. If intolerable, discontinue use and return to the office immediately for evaluation of the problem.

6. If tissues become irritated, reduce utilization time. If continuous irritation persists, discontinue use and return immediately.

- Recall at 1 week and 1 month. Additional utilization time is determined at the 1-month recall. Any adverse hard or soft tissue changes must be monitored. Progress of the bleaching should also be checked and verified using shade tabs for comparison.
- When using hydrogen peroxide bleaching solution, weekly recalls to replenish the material will be necessary.
- When improvement is no longer seen, bleaching should be discontinued and postoperative photographs and shade determinations made (Fig. 2-32b). If results are not satisfactory, office bleaching procedures may be necessary or restorative procedures initiated.

NOTE: Proceeding with acrylic resin bonding techniques immediately after bleaching is contraindicated. Residual oxygen in the tooth tissues may inhibit polymerization and result in a significant decrease in bond strength. A 2-week period of time is recommended to minimize this potential and to allow for any remineralization and color stabilization to occur prior to esthetic restorative therapy.

Enamel Microabrasion

Historical Background

Enamel microabrasion is not a bleaching technique but a selective erosion process that removes stained enamel. Chemical erosion has its roots in a technique used in 1916 by Dr. Walter Kane, a Colorado Springs dentist, who used 18% hydrochloric acid to remove endemic fluoride stains. While effective, the use of hydrochloric acid went out of favor when it was shown by Younger in 1939 that it decalcifies enamel and may increase caries susceptibility. The use of hydrogen peroxide was the most popular technique until 1966 when McInnes revived a technique that combined five parts 30% hydrochloric acid with five parts 30% hydrogen peroxide and one part ethyl ether to remove fluorosis stains. The solution was placed on the affected areas for 15 to 30 minutes, neutralized with sodium bicarbonate and then polished. No postoperative pain was noted with this technique. This technique was modified by Bailey and Christen in 1970 and stain removal was accelerated by using fine cuttle discs to apply the bleaching mixture. In 1983 Murrin and Barkmeier used a combination bleaching technique for fluorosis stain removal. Flour of pumice and 36% hydrochloric acid was applied to the teeth for 5 to 10 seconds using a prophy cup. This was neutralized with Clorox and water and then treated with hydrogen peroxide soaked in cotton and heated (120°F) for 5 to 10 minutes. McCloskey in 1984 updated Kane's technique of applying 18% hydrochloric acid by using pumice abrasion for better enamel penetration. This technique was advanced again in 1986 by Croll and Cavanaugh. They mixed 18% hydrochloric acid and fine flour of pumice into a thick paste and burnished it into the enamel with a modified tongue blade for 5 seconds. This material was rinsed off with water and reapplied at 5-second intervals until desired results were achieved. This technique is advocated for all types of superficial stains. Electron microscopic studies show that each 5-second treatment removes an average of 10 μm (range 7 μm to 22 μm) of enamel.

Currently microabrasion is recommended for the removal of stains that are superficial and localized in enamel. It is the primary treatment of choice for superficial fluorosis stain removal, small white stains and some multicolored stains.

The generic use of 18% hydrochloric acid and pumice can be used for enamel microabrasion. Only one commercially developed system currently exists for enamel microabrasion. The PREMA™ system (Premier Enamel Microabrasion) compound contains an abrasive mixed with hydrochloric acid of approximately 10%. This system offers a unique, easy and safe approach to enamel microabrasion and will be described in the technique section. The alternative is the use of rotary instrumentation, which is faster but potentially more destructive and less discriminating in selective tissue removal.

Procedures

- Patients with superficial fluorosis or white stains are excellent candidates for enamel microabrasion. Deeper internal stains are not (Fig. 2-33a).
- Preoperative photographic documentation is recommended (Fig. 2-33b).
- View the teeth to be treated from the incisal direction to estimate enamel thickness. Thicker teeth may be treated more aggressively (Fig. 2-33c).
- Safety precautions should be used to avoid unwanted hydrochloric acid exposure. Safety glasses should be worn by the patient and the treating dental team. Protective gloves are mandatory and high speed suction and a water rinse should be available should contamination occur.
- Rubber dam isolation is mandatory. Margins of the dam should be sealed with copal varnish or as recommended for office administered bleaching (Fig. 2-33d).
- The microabrasion compound should only be applied with a 10:1 gear reduction contra-angle or a hand instrument to avoid

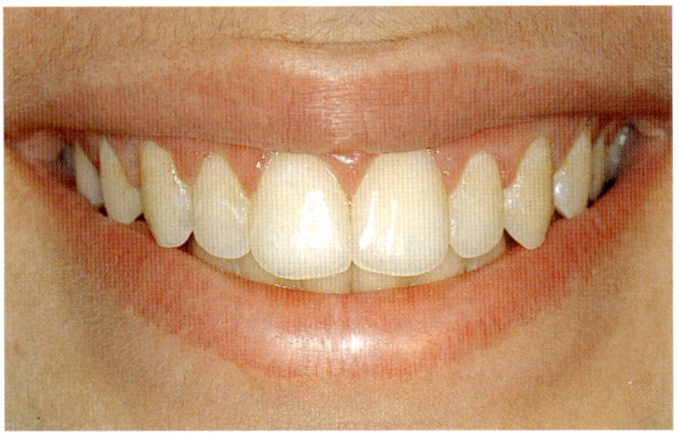

Fig. 2-33a Upper right lateral with line of hypocalcification.

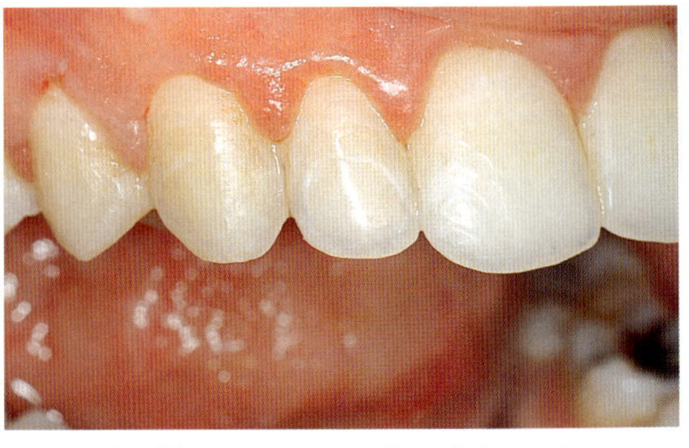

Fig. 2-33b Close-up preoperative photograph.

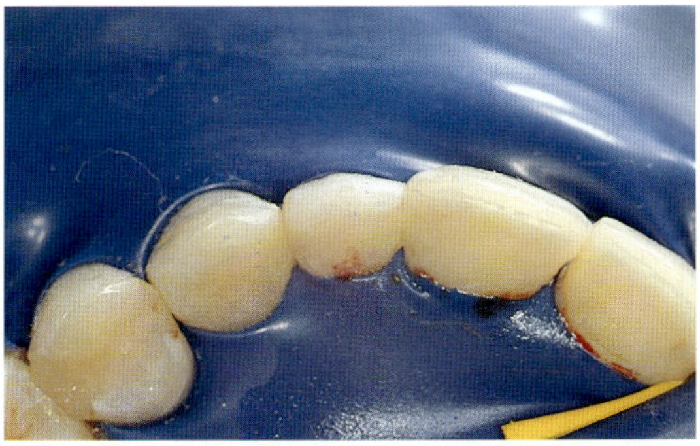

Fig. 2-33c Incisal view to note facial-lingual tooth thickness.

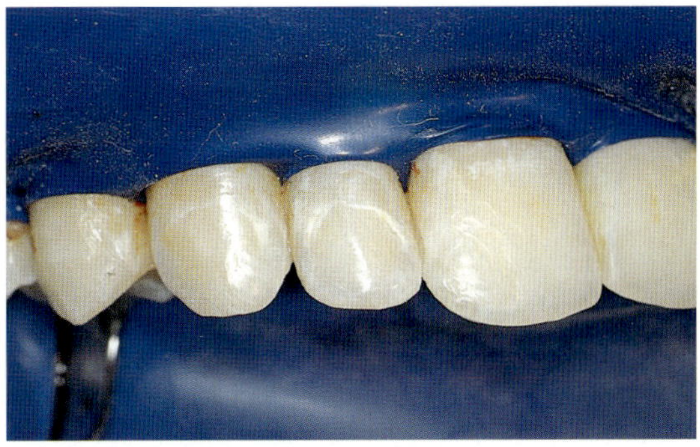

Fig. 2-33d Tooth isolated with a rubber dam.

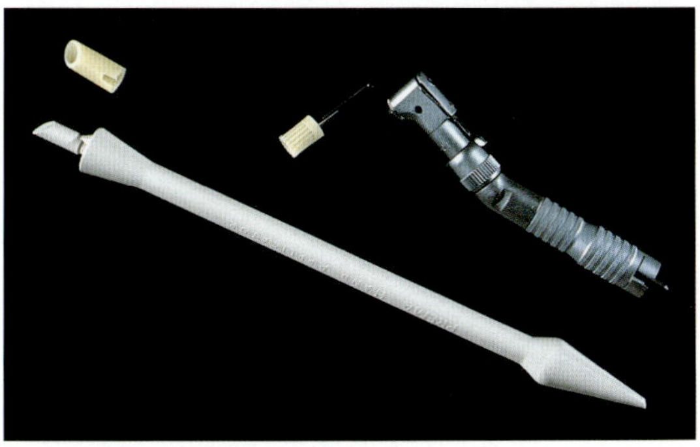

Fig. 2-33e Microabrasion instrumentation.

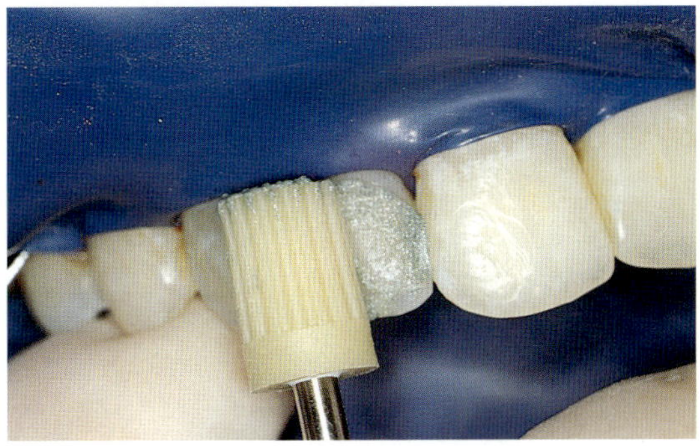

Fig. 2-33f Rotary handpiece application.

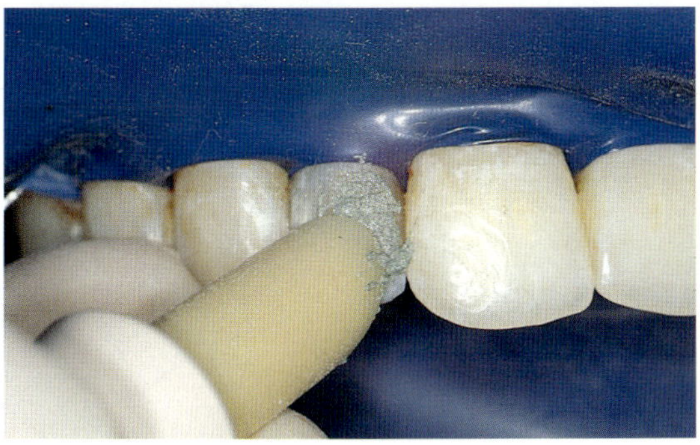

Fig. 2-33g Hand instrument application.

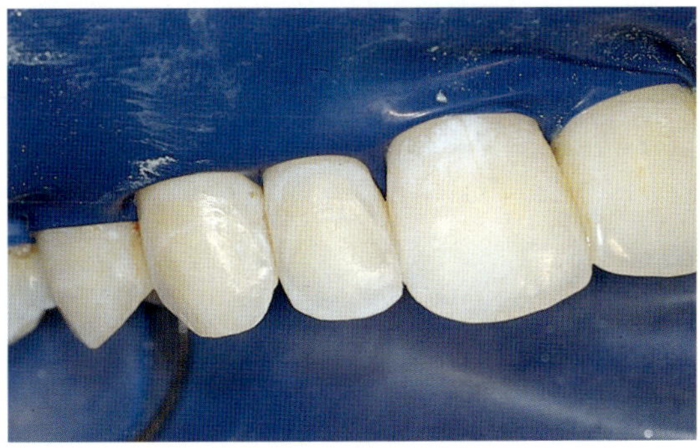

Fig. 2-33h Dry surface after microabrasion.

spattering (Fig. 2-33e).

- Rotary application is done by placing a small amount of the PREMA™ compound on the disposable PREMA™ mandrel tip and using rotary abrasion over the stained area of the tooth for 20 to 30 seconds (Fig. 2-33f). The compound is rinsed off and the stain and enamel thickness are evaluated.
- Manual application, for small isolated stains, can be accomplished using the PREMA™ hand applicator. Small concentrated stains are best removed with manual application and 20- to 30-second treatment cycles (Fig. 2-33g).
- Microabrasion treatment cycles are continued until the stain is removed. Should the enamel begin to appear slightly concave and the stain remains, alternative

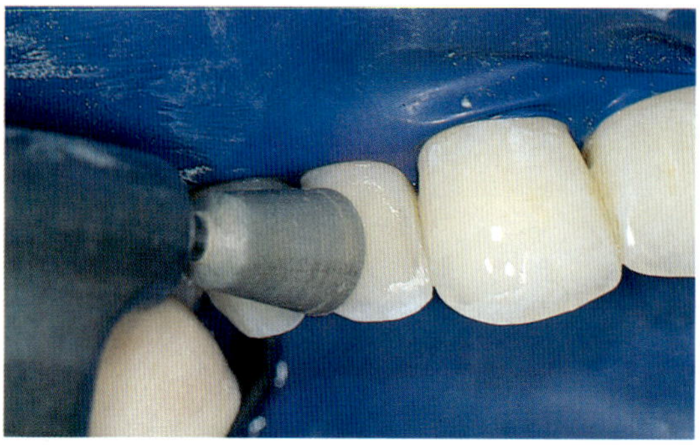

Fig. 2-33i Polish surface with fine fluoridated prophy paste.

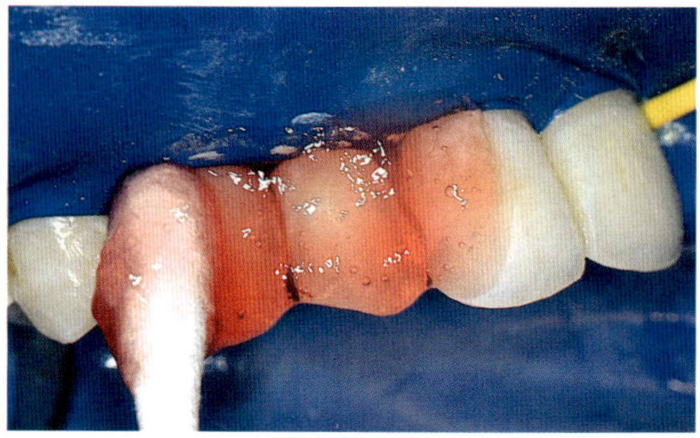

Fig. 2-33j Apply neutral sodium fluoride gel.

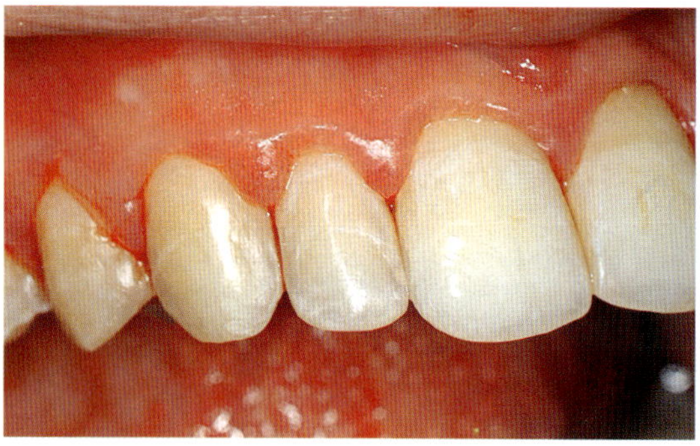

Fig. 2-33k Immediately after treatment.

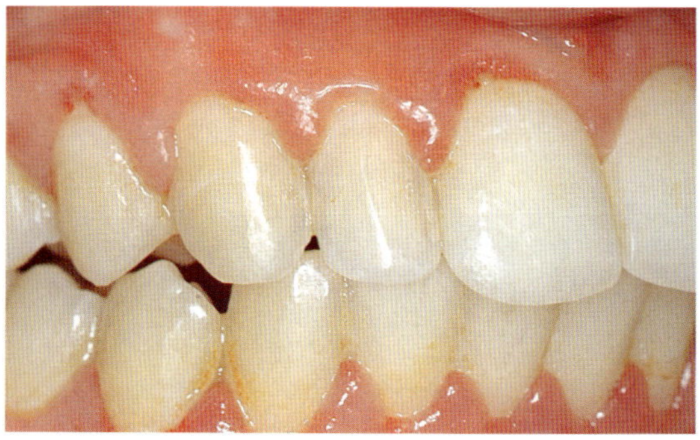

Fig. 2-33l View 3 months later (good results, poor hygiene in an adolescent).

treatment approaches may be pursued. If the stain is not superficial, enamel microabrasion alone is not indicated.

- When evaluating the results of enamel microabrasion, wet the enamel surface since dry enamel surfaces may exaggerate the discoloration (Fig. 2-33h).
- Upon completion, the treated enamel should be polished with a fine grit fluoridated prophy paste and a rubber cup (Fig. 2-33i).
- A 4-minute application of a neutral sodium fluoride gel is recommended (Fig. 2-33j).
- Patients should be recalled in several weeks. Some additional treatment may occasionally be necessary once the enamel has rehydrated. Postoperative photographs can be taken at this recall appointment (Figs. 2-33k and l).

ESTHETIC TOOTH CONTOURING

Esthetic modification of an existing dentition by enameloplasty is often simple and quick but frequently overlooked as a component of conservative esthetic treatment. Dramatic results can often be attained from this procedure (Fig. 2-34). Esthetic enhancement of restorative procedures may also be accomplished through appropriate preoperative tooth contouring (see Porcelain Veneer Preparation in chapter 6). These techniques are not new to esthetic dentistry and will be described primarily as a reminder of their value as part of the total esthetic treatments.

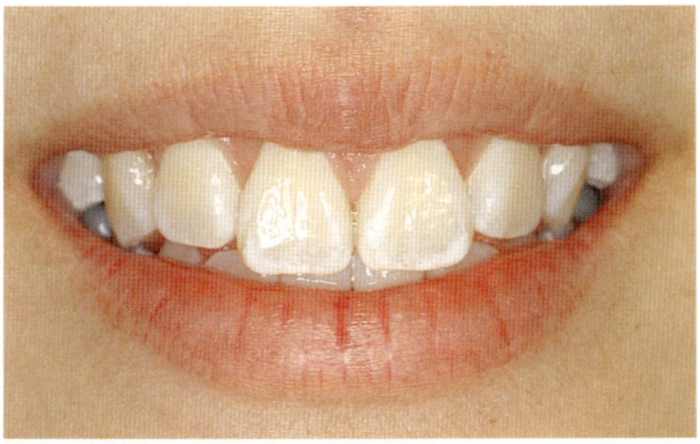
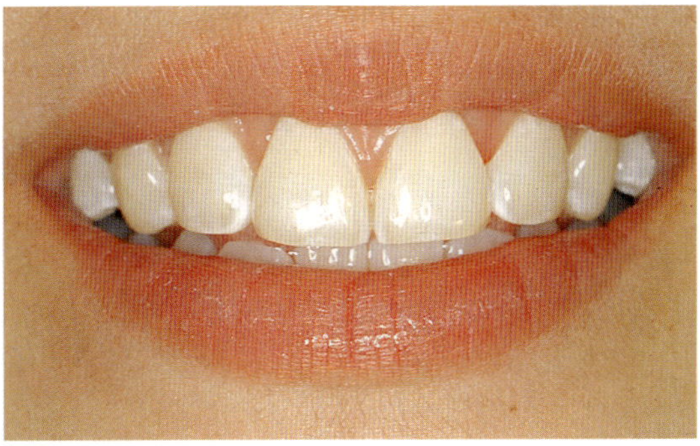

Figs. 2-34a and b Precontouring and postcontouring photographs of young female with very large teeth (smile).

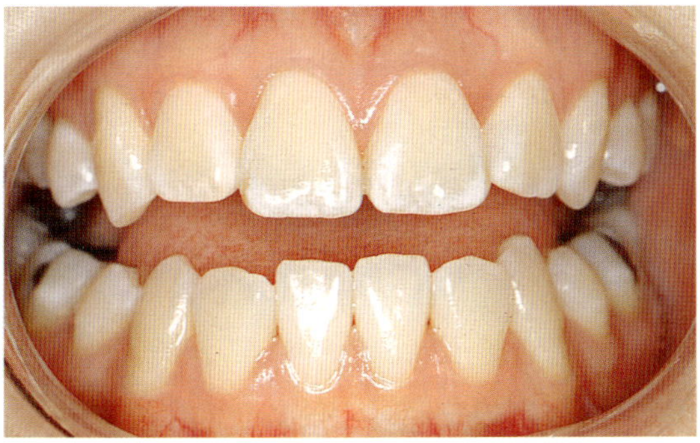
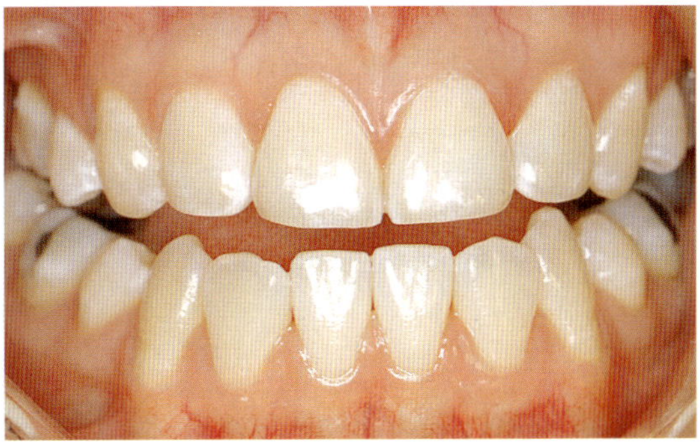

Figs. 2-34c and d Precontouring and postcontouring photographs of the same young female (close up).

Procedures

- Determine the need for possible esthetic tooth contouring through the normal diagnostic process and patient consultation.
- The use of diagnostic models or other means for visual communication is mandatory to show the patient the problem and proposed solution preoperatively.
- Very simple contour modifications may be communicated to the patient by simply drawing over the tooth structure to be removed with a fine black felt tip pen (Figs. 2-35a and b). This will show the patient the illusion of tooth removal prior to the actual procedure. Adequate communication of the proposed changes preoperatively is essential to avoid any misunderstanding. Study models can also be marked or modified with the patient observing to illustrate proposed changes (Figs. 2-35c and d). Computer imaging is one of the most effective means to communicate changes. Always make sure the patient has a hand mirror available to observe their teeth and the sequential modifications as performed.
- Always document the preoperative dentition with photographs or unaltered models.
- Once the patient agrees to the proposed modifications, begin with a 12-fluted carbide bur using water and no anesthesia (Fig. 2-35e).
- Always be conservative with tooth reduction and have the patient frequently check the progress. Remember, a simple contour change can make a significant esthetic change. Some individuals will respond to change negatively at first, even if it is an improvement.
- If teeth become sensitive, stop. Tooth con-

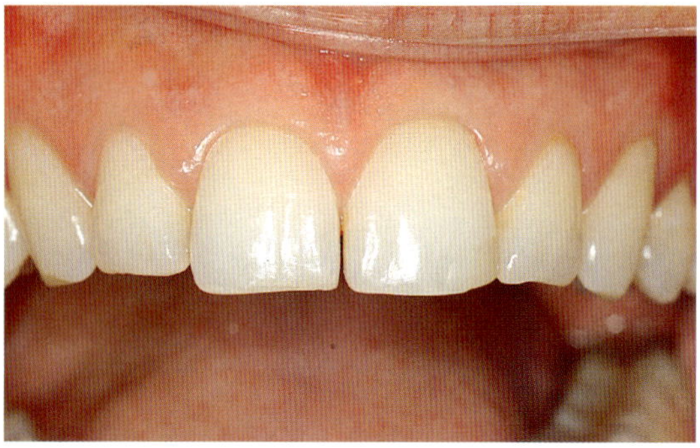

Fig. 2-35a Precontouring photograph.

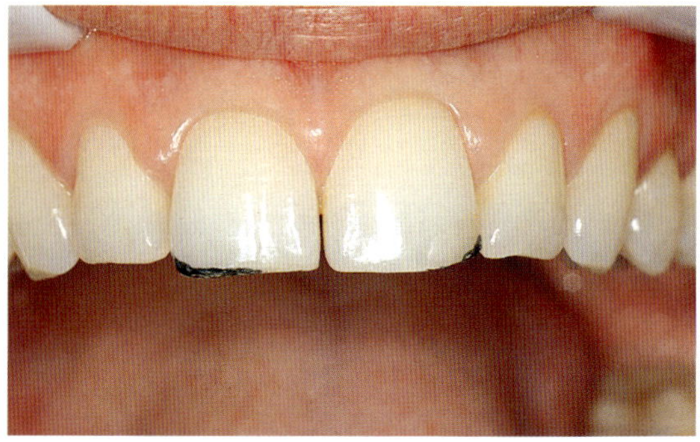

Fig. 2-35b Black ink on proposed areas to be contoured.

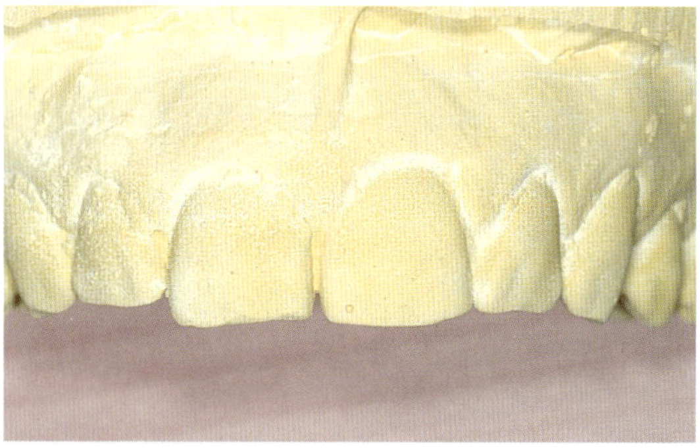

Fig. 2-35c Precontouring models.

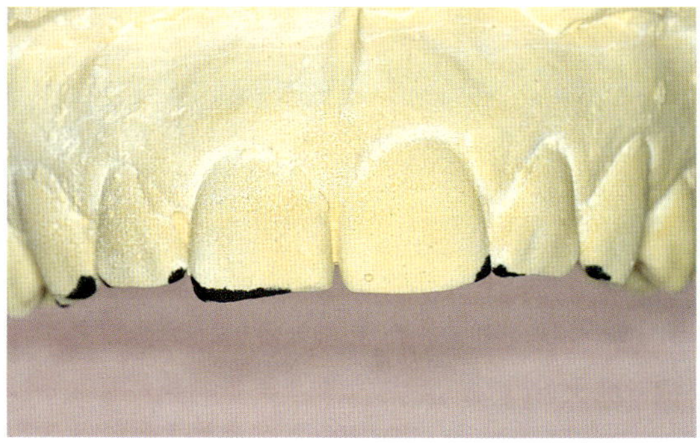

Fig. 2-35d Black ink on preposed areas to be contoured.

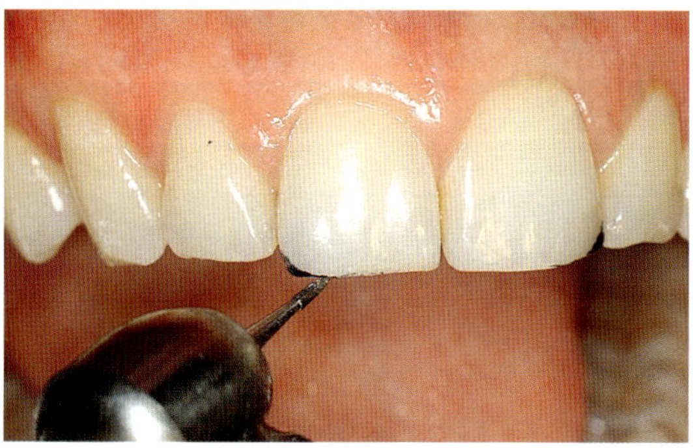

Fig. 2-35e Use a 12-fluted carbide bur to contour teeth.

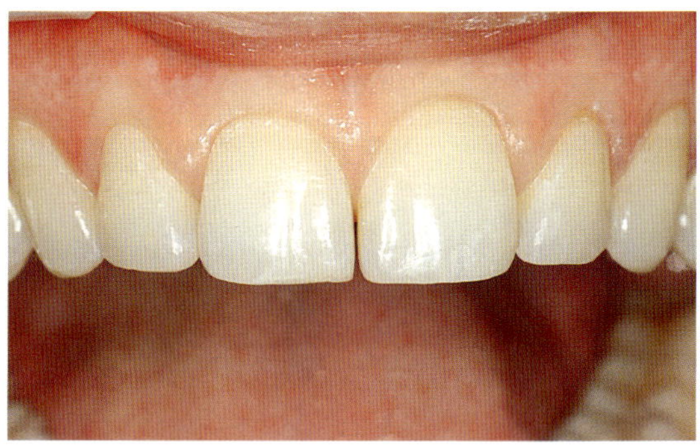

Fig. 2-35f Postcontouring photograph.

touring may have to be accomplished over multiple appointments. Apply topical fluoride and continue in 1 or 2 weeks.

- The basic rules of esthetic contouring are well established in other texts and will not be covered (Fig. 2-35f).
- Once the desired result is achieved, the teeth should be polished with porcelain polishing cups and points and returned to their original luster and surface texture (Figs. 2-35g and h). Reapplication of topical fluoride is recommended.
- Postoperative photographs should be taken and/or models made to document results.
- A fee for esthetic contouring should always be assessed no matter how simple. Services performed for no charge may be

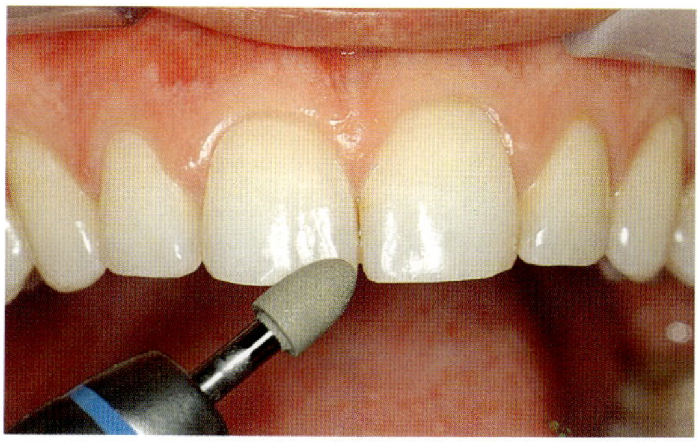

Fig. 2-35g Porcelain polishing point used to polish the roughened enamel.

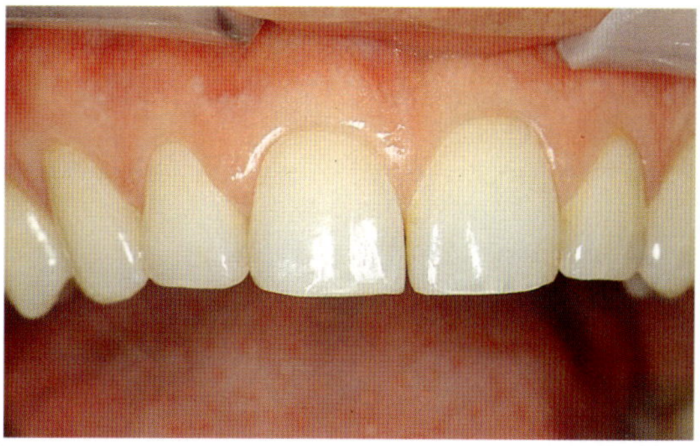

Fig. 2-35h Postcontouring photograph 1 month later.

perceived as having little or no value. Esthetic contouring requires time, expertise and a thorough understanding of esthetic and functional parameters.

REFERENCES

Adams, T.C.: Enamel Color Modifications by Controlled Hydrochloric Acid Pumice Abrasion: A Review of Case Summaries. (1987). Ind. Dent. Assn. J. Vol. 66, p. 23.

Albers, H.F.: Lightening Natural Teeth (1991). Adept. Report, Vol. 2 (1), Winter.

Ames, J.W.: Removing Stains from Mottled Enamel. (1937). J.A.D.A., Vol. 24, p. 1674.

Anderson, M.H.: Dental Bleaching. (1991). Current Opinion in Dentistry. Vol. 1, p. 185.

Appleby, D.C. and Craig, C.: Subtleties of Contour. A System for Recognition and Correction. (1986). Comp. Cont. Ed. Vol. 7 (2), p. 108.

Arens, D.E., Rich, J.J., and Healey, H.J.: A Practical Method of Bleaching Tetracycline-Stained Teeth. (1972). Oral Surg. Vol. 34, p. 812.

Bailey, R.W. and Christen, A.C.: Bleaching of Vital Teeth Stained with Endemic Dental Fluorosis. (1976). J. Dent. Res. Vol. 49, p. 168.

Bartelstone, H.J.: Radioiodine Penetration Through Intact Enamel with Uptake by Blood Stream and Thyroid Gland. (1951). J. Dent. Res. Vol. 30, p. 728.

Baumgarther, J.C., Reid, D.E., and Pickett: Human Pulpal Reaction to the Modified McInnes Bleaching Technique. (1983). J. Endodont. Vol. 9, p 527.

Berry, J.H.: What About Whiteners? Safety Concerns Explored. (1990). J.A.D.A., Vol. 121, p. 223.

Bowles, W.H. and Thompson, L.R.: Vital Bleaching: The Effects of Heat and Hydrogen Peroxide on Pulpal Enzymes. (1986). J. Endodont. Vol. 108, p. 112.

Cohen, S.C. and Chase, C.: Human Pulpal Response to Bleaching Procedures on Vital Teeth. (1976). J. Endodont. Vol. 5, p. 134.

Cohen, S., Parkins, F.M.: Bleaching Tetracycline-Stained Vital Teeth. (1970). Oral Surg. Vol. 29, p. 465.

Cooley, R.C. and Burger, K.M.: Effect of Carbamide Peroxide on Composite Resins. (1991). Quint. Int. Vol. 22 (10), p. 817.

Clinical Research Associates Newsletter (1989). Vol. 13 (12), Provo, Utah, USA.

Croll, T.P. and Cavanaugh, R.R.: Enamel Color Modification by Controlled Hydrochloric Acid-Pumice Abrasion. I. Technique and Examples. (1986). Quint. Int. Vol. 17, p 81.

Croll, T.P. and Cavanaugh, R.R.: Enamel Color Modification by Controlled Hydrochloric Acid-Pumice Abrasion. II. Further Examples. (1986). Quint. Int. Vol. 17, p 157.

Croll, T.P.: Enamel Microabrasion for Removal of Superficial Dysmineralization and Decalcification Defects. (1990). J.A.D.A., Vol. 120, p. 411.

Croll, T.P. and Cavanaugh, R.R.: Hydrochloric Acid-Pumice Enamel Surface Abrasion for Color Modification: Results After Six Months. (1986). Quint. Int. Vol. (17), p. 335.

Croll, T.P.: A Case Report of Enamel Color Modification: 60 Year Results. (1987). Quint. Int. Vol. 18, p. 493.

Davies, A.K., Cundall, R.B., Dandiker, Y., and Slifkin, M.A.: Photo-Oxidation of Tetracycline Absorbed on Hydroxyapatite in Relation to the Light-Induced Staining of Teeth. (1985). J. Dent. Res. Vol. 64 (6), p. 936.

Dietz, E.: Many Practices Offer Dentist-Monitored Bleaching. (1990). Dental Economics, May, p. 72.

Faunce, F.: Management of Discolored Teeth. (1983). D. Clin. N.A. Vol. 27 (4), p. 657.

Feiglin, B.: A 6-year Recall Study of Clinically Chemically Bleached Teeth. (1987). Oral Surg. Oral Med. Oral Pathol. Vol. 63 (5), p. 610.

Feinman, R.A.: Matix Vital Bleaching: A Review. (1991). Esth. Dent. Update. Vol. 2 (2), p. 42.

Feinman, R.A., Goldstein R.A., and Garber, D.A.: Bleaching Teeth. (1987). Chicago: Quintessence.

Garber, D.A., Goldstein, R.A., Goldstein, C.E., and Schwartz, C.G.: Dentist Monitored Bleaching: A Combined Approach. (1991). Pract. Perio. Esth. Dent. Vol. 3 (2), p. 22

Haywood, V.B.: Nightguard Vital Bleaching, A History and Products Update: Part I. (1991). Quint. Int. Vol. 22, p. 515.

Haywood, V.B.: Nightguard Vital Bleaching, A History and Products Update: Part 2. (1991). Esth. Dent. Update Vol. 2 (5), p. 82.

Haywood, V.B. and Heymann, H.O.: Nightguard Vital Bleaching, How Safe Is It? (1991). Quint. Int. Vol. 22, p. 515.

Howard, W.H.: Patient-Applied Tooth Whiteners: Are They Safe, Effective with Supervision. (1992). J.A.D.A. Vol. 123, p. 57.

Jordan, R.E. and Bohsman, L.: Conservative Vital Bleaching Treatment of Discolored Dentition. (1984). Comp. Cont. Educ. Dent. Vol. 5, p. 803.

Jordan, R.E.: Esthetic Composite Bonding Techniques and Materials. (1986). Toronto and Philadelphia: B.C. Decker, Inc.

Lado, E.A., Stanley, H.R., and Weisman, M.I.: Cervical Resorption in Bleached Teeth. (1983). Oral Surg. Oral Med. Oral Pathol. Vol. 55, p. 78.

Ledoux, W.R., Malloy, R.B., Hurst, R.V.V., McInnes-Ledoux, P., and Weinberg, R.: Structural Effects of Bleaching on Tetracycline-Stained Vital Rat Teeth. (1985). J. Prosth. Dent. Vol. 54, p. 55.

Lemieux, J.J. and Todd, M.J.: Simplified Bleaching of Discolored Pulpless Teeth. (1981). J. Canad. Dent. Assoc. No. 11, p. 729.

Lisanti, V.F. and Zander, H.A.: Thermal Injury to Normal Dog Teeth: Measurements of Pulp Temperature Increase and Their Effect on the Pulp Tissue. (1952). J. Dent. Res. Vol. 31, p. 548.

McClosky, R.J.: A Technique for Removal of Fluorosis Stains. (1984). J.A.D.A. Vol. 109, p. 63.

McEvoy, S.A.: Chemical Agents for Removing Intrinsic Stains from Vital Teeth. I. Technique Development. (1989). Quint. Int. Vol. 20 (5), p. 323.

McLaughlin, G. and Freedman, G.A.: Color Atlas of Tooth Whitening. (1991). St. Louis: Ishyiaky Euroamerica, Inc.

Montgomery, S.: External Cervical Resorption After Bleaching a Pulpless Tooth. (1984). Oral Surg. Oral Med. Oral Pathol. Vol. 57 (2), p. 203.

Nyborg, H. and Brannstrom, M.: Pulp Reaction to Heat. (1968). J. Prosthet. Dent. Vol. 19 (6), p. 605.

Pearson, H.H.: Bleaching of the Discolored Pulpless Tooth. (1958). J.A.D.A. Vol. 56, p. 64.

Prinz, H.: Recent Improvements in Tooth Bleaching. (1924). Dent. Cosmos. Vol. 66, p. 558.

Richardson, S.E.: Home Bleaching: Effectiveness, History, Technique, Bleaches, Cost and Safety. (1989). J. Greater Huston D.S., Nov., p. 22.

Robertson, W.D. and Melfi, R.C.: Pulpal Response to Vital Bleaching Procedures. (1980). J. Endodont. Vol. 6 (7), p. 645.

Rotstein, I., Lehr, Z., and Gedalia, I.: Effect of Bleaching Agents on Inorganic Components of Human Dentin and Cementum (1992). J. Endodont. Vol. 18 (6), p. 290.

Scherer, W., Cooper, H., Ziegler, B., and Vijayaraghavan, T.V.: At-Home Bleaching System: Effects on Enamel and Cementum. (1991). J. Esthet. Dent. Vol. 3 (2), p. 54.

Seale, M.S., McIntosh J.E., and Taylor, A. N.: Pulpal Reaction to Bleaching of Teeth in Dogs. (1981). J. Dent. Res. Vol. 60 (5), p. 948.

Seale, M.S. and Thrash, W.J.: Systemic Assessment of Color Removal Following Vital Bleaching of Intrinsically Stained Teeth. (1985). J. Dent. Res. Vol. 64 (3), p. 4547.

Seghi, R.R.: Personal Communication.

Simons, J.F., Allen, H., Woodson, R.G., and Eilers, A.S.: Efficacy of Vital Home Bleaching. (1993). Cal. Dent. J.

Titley. K.D., Torneck, C.D., and Ruse, N.D.: The Effect of Carbamide-Peroxide on the Shear Bond Strength of a Microfil Resin to Bovine Enamel. (1991). J. Dent. Res., Vol. 71 (1), p. 20.

Tong, L.S.M., Pang, M.K.M., Mok, N.Y.C., and Wei, S.H.Y.: The Effects of Etching, Micro-Abrasion and Bleaching on Surface Enamel. (1993). J. Dent. Res. Vol. 72 (1), p. 67.

Union Broch: Bleaching Procedure Manual: Illuminator. (1987).

Wahl, M.J.: At-Home Bleaching of a Single Tooth. (1992). J. Prosthet. Dent. Vol. 67 (2), p. 281.

Yarborough, D.K.: Tooth Bleaching Safety and Efficacy: A Review of the Literature, 1988-1990. Brite-Smile, Inc. Technical Paper, Birmingham,. AL, USA.

CHAPTER 3

ESTHETIC RESTORATIVE MATERIALS

EARLY DEVELOPMENT

INTRODUCTION

The desire by patients and practitioners alike for practical and reliable esthetic dental restorative materials is certainly not new to dentistry. The demand, however, for techniques and materials that can be used to conservatively and esthetically restore teeth has never been greater, and continues to grow. Many factors are responsible for this phenomenon. The acid etch technique and composite resin resulted in restorations with markedly improved durability and longevity as compared to silicates. Introduction of visible light polymerization dramatically expanded the applications for composites, giving rise to the wide range of procedures collectively known as "esthetic bonding." Increased patient awareness of such procedures produced increased demand, with patients commonly seeking elective dental treatment to improve esthetics. Additionally, the business of dental private practice has grown more competitive, especially in larger metropolitan areas, as fluoridation and other preventive strategies continue to reduce the caries rate in the general population. The marketing of "esthetic dentistry" by dentists has become commonplace as elective procedures comprise an increasing percentage of the mix of services provided in general practice. Catch-phrases such as "painless," "no drilling" and "in one appointment" have piqued the curiosity of many a prospective patient.

As physical properties of direct esthetic materials improve, dentists are increasingly confident in offering these materials to patients as alternatives to the traditional metallic restoratives for posterior teeth. The adhesive characteristics of these materials reduce or eliminate the need for removal of sound tooth structure to obtain adequate retention and resistance forms. In vitro studies also indicate that teeth restored intracoronally with adhesive materials are rendered more resistant to cusp fracture than those restored with amalgams or gold inlays. Many Class I and II cases, particularly initial carious lesions, can thus potentially be treated more conservatively, and with a stronger tooth as the result.

The increased use of adhesive esthetic materials has additionally been driven by concerns over the safety of dental amalgam. While the level of risk, if any, associated with exposure to mercury from amalgam restorations has yet to be definitively determined, many patients now request amalgam alternatives or choose such materials when informed of available options. The disposal of amalgam-containing waste from dental offices has also emerged as a controversial issue due to the potential for environmental mercury contamination from this source. These issues will continue to raise questions regarding the propriety of using dental amalgam as a dental restorative. Practitioners must accordingly be prepared to discuss and offer appropriate alternatives to amalgam when these questions arise.

Virtually all restorative dental procedures currently include or can be adapted to include the use of adhesive materials. This trend will potentially improve the esthetics and longevity of restorations, but is accompanied by a significant increase in technique sensitivity as compared to the more traditional procedures. As the adhesive materials increasingly occupy such a fundamental position in the restorative armamentarium, it is incumbent upon the practitioner to develop an understanding of their basic chemical and physical characteristics and their modes of interaction with enamel and dentin. Only then can optimal results be consistently obtained with these useful but complex materials.

This chapter describes the composition and mechanisms of action of materials used for direct esthetic and adhesive restorations, and provides a brief history of their development.

SILICATES

Silicate cement, the first translucent dental restorative material, was introduced by Thomas Fletcher of England in 1878 as "Translucent Cement." Improvements on the original formula in Germany in 1904 (by chemist Paul Steenbock and dentist Hugo Ascher) led to wide acceptance around the world for the material as an anterior restorative in the early 1900s. This powder-liquid system consists of acid-soluble glass particles and a liquid solution of 35% to 50% phosphoric acid. The mixture of these components produces a material with good initial esthetic appearance. The high fluoride content of the glass also imparts a caries-retarding quality to the restoration. Additionally, silicate cements have a coefficient of thermal expansion similar to that of tooth structure. The correspondingly similar expansion and contraction when exposed to temperature extremes reduces stress at the marginal interface between tooth and silicate.

The disadvantages of silicates, though, rendered it far less than ideal as a dental restorative. The chemical reaction of the powder and liquid produces a gel-like matrix that matures to a hard cement, binding together any unreacted glass particles. Sensitivity of the material to both dehydration and moisture contamination in this early setting phase necessitated the use of a protective layer of cocoa butter or cavity varnish during setting. Such agents were only partially effective in protecting the surface, though, resulting in increased solubility in the set restoration. Opacity and staining would thus soon develop, as well as loss of material due to its poor resistance to wear. The acidity of the liquid has been implicated in the occasional pulpal damage or death of teeth following placement of silicate cement onto freshly cut dentin. Silicates, at best, produced a highly soluble and potentially irritating restoration with a short clinical life span.

Subsequent efforts to produce an improved esthetic restorative were to be centered around organic resins. However the chemical principles, as well as the glasses, used to produce silicates would later be applied to the production of glass ionomers (see page 72).

ACRYLIC RESIN

Developed in Germany in the 1930s and becoming widely used following World War II, acrylic resins were an attempt at producing a tooth colored restorative with a longer clinical life span than silicate cement. These systems, usually supplied in powder-liquid form, utilize the organic molecule methyl methacrylate (Fig. 3-1), as do resins for dentures and crown and bridge provisionalization. The powder (methyl methacrylate polymer particles) and liquid (methyl methacrylate monomer and chemical initiators) react chemically when mixed to polymerize at room temperature. Once placed into the cavity and allowed to set, the resin can be polished to a smooth luster. Pigments added to the powder also made it possible to achieve a good color match with the surrounding enamel.

Like silicates, however, the physical properties of acrylic resin severely limited its clinical performance as a direct restorative. High polymerization shrinkage (7%) led to poor marginal adaptation at initial placement. A high coefficient of thermal expansion (compared to that of tooth structure) produced excessive microleakage, leading to secondary caries and unsightly staining at these poorly adapted margins. Abrasion resistance was low, and water absorption caused further softening as well as poor color stability. Improvements in the material and in placement techniques reduced these problems slightly, but acrylic resins proved to be only slightly better than silicate cement with respect to clinical longevity. Thus silicates and acrylic resin both remained in use as efforts to develop improved direct esthetic restoratives continued.

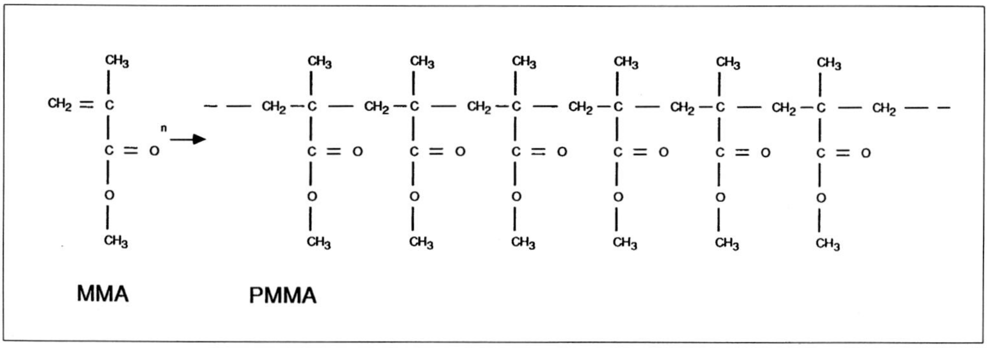

Fig. 3-1 Polymerization of methyl methacrylate (MMA) to poly(methyl methacrylate) (PMMA).

COMPOSITE RESINS

DESCRIPTION

Composite resins, introduced in 1962, are the result of the work of Ray Bowen at the National Bureau of Standards. The term "composite" refers to the combination of two distinctly different component phases to produce the final material. One phase consists of a soft organic resin polymer (Bisphenol-glycidyl methacrylate, or Bis-GMA). Dispersed throughout this resin matrix is the second phase, consisting of ground particles of an inorganic ceramic (originally quartz). The resin phase is both continuous and reactive in nature, while the inorganic "filler" phase is discontinuous (interrupted), and inert.

The resin phase of the composite would perform very poorly as a stand-alone restorative; i.e. resin is the weak link in the composite system with respect to physical properties. In general, as the resin (organic) component of the composite is decreased, and the filler (inorganic) component is increased, problems related to the properties of the resin are reduced. The remaining resin is said to be "reinforced" by the filler particles. The addition of the inorganic filler particles, then, produces a material with substantially improved physical properties over both unfilled resin (including acrylic) and silicate cement. Polymerization shrinkage is reduced by 75%, and coefficient of thermal expansion by approximately 60% of the unfilled resin values. Water sorption is also reduced, while compressive and tensile strength, fracture toughness, hardness and stiffness are all increased. Correspondingly improved cavity margin adaptation and reduced microleakage, as well as improvements in wear resistance and color stability, are seen clinically. Newer composite formulations can even be used, albeit judiciously, to restore selected stress-bearing areas. While composites still suffer from many of the problems seen with silicates and acrylic, it is to a far lesser degree.

A more detailed discussion of each of the composite resin components follows.

COMPONENTS

Resin Matrix

Bowen's original resin, Bis-GMA, is produced by combining bisphenol-A with glycidyl methacrylate. Its chemical structure imparts qualities that are more favorable than those of methylmethacrylate. The larger molecular size and aromatic structure increase stiffness and compressive strength, and reduce polymerization shrinkage and water sorption. When combined with a diluent (e.g. triethylene glycol dimethacrylate, or TEG-DMA) to control its high viscosity, Bis-GMA was found to exhibit suitable handling characteristics for use as a direct restorative. Bis-GMA and a newer, lower viscosity resin introduced by Foster and Walker in 1974 (urethane dimethacrylate, or UDMA) comprise the resin matrix of virtually all composites currently in use. Figure 3-2 illustrates the chemical structure of resins commonly used in composites.

Fillers and Classification

The inorganic filler component of composite resin is responsible for its improved physical properties as compared to the older unfilled silicates and acrylics. Composed of quartz, silica or glass, composite fillers tend to be hard, inert and similar to tooth struc-

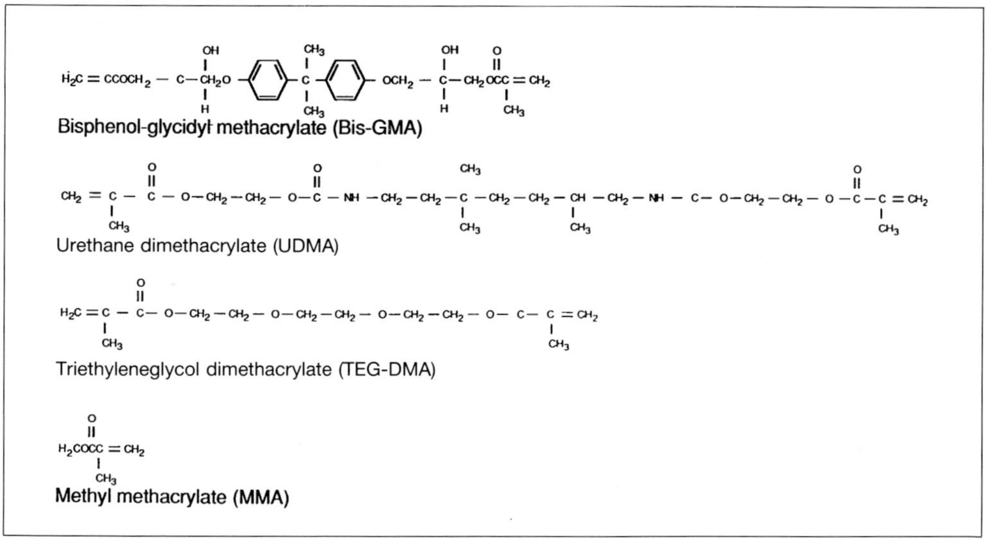

Fig. 3-2 Resins commonly used in dental composites. Methyl methacrylate is shown for comparison.

ture with respect to translucency and refractive index. Many physical properties, notably fracture and wear resistance and polymerization shrinkage, improve as the amount of filler in the composite material increases. It is important to know the level of filler content, or "loading," which is reported both as percentage by weight and percentage by volume. Weight percentage is used more commonly as it is easier to measure. Filler particle size is also significant. The ability to polish and resistance to wear increase as particle size decreases. Since composites that differ with respect to size (as well as composition and amount) of filler particles will also differ in clinical behavior, composites are classified based on their filler type: macrofilled, microfilled and hybrid.

Macrofilled Composites (or Conventional, Traditional, Large Particle, Small Particle)

Early composite resins were of the macrofilled type, utilizing fillers of ground quartz. The radiolucency of quartz made radiographic detection of secondary caries under these restorations difficult at best. Filler particle sizes averaged 15 to 30 μm ("large particle"), but ranged as high as 100 μm (Fig. 3-3). These large sizes allowed 75% to 80% loading by weight of inorganic filler. Producing a smooth surface on these materials was difficult, as polishing procedures exposed portions of the large, irregular particles by selectively removing the softer surrounding resin (Fig. 3-4). Continued clinical wear of the resin matrix leading to further exposure and eventual "plucking" of filler particles from the surface (Fig. 3-5) would increase roughness over time. Difference in the coefficients of thermal expansion between the resin matrix and filler also contributed to loosening of surface filler particles when subjected to thermal changes. Rough surfaces promote staining and plaque accumulation, rendering these restorations esthetically compromised and irritating to adjacent gingiva. These materials also exhibited low resistance to abrasion, producing a loss of contour for restorations exposed to functional stresses. Frequent replacement of macrofills was necessary to correct these problems.

More recently introduced macrofills utilize particle sizes in the 1- to 5-μm range ("small particle"), with similar levels of inorganic load-

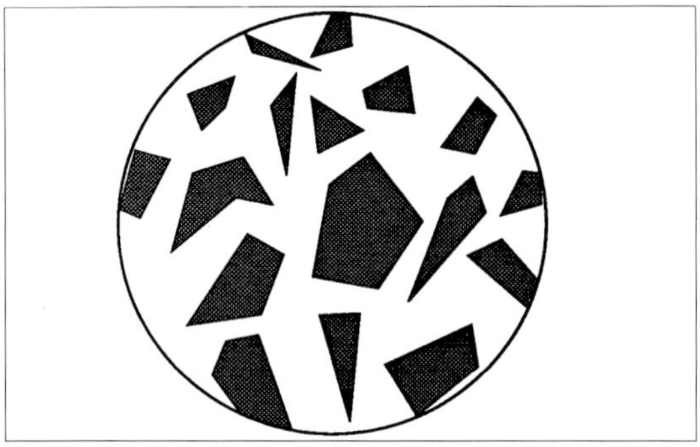

Fig. 3-3 Macrofilled composite consisting of large, irregular filler particles surrounded by resin matrix.

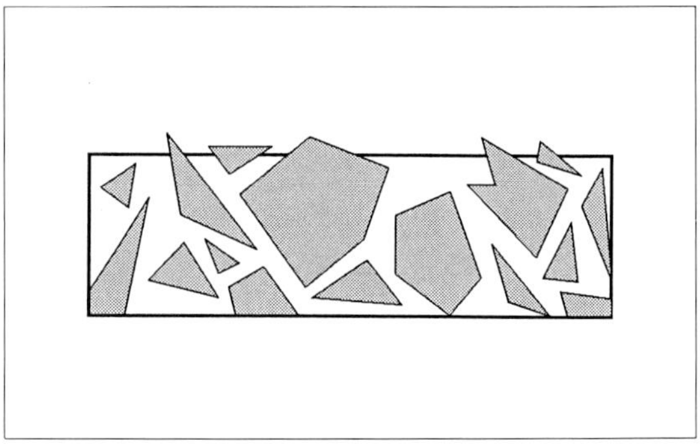

Fig. 3-4 Initial placement of macrofilled composite. Polishing selectively removes softer resin matrix, exposing filler particles, and producing a rough surface.

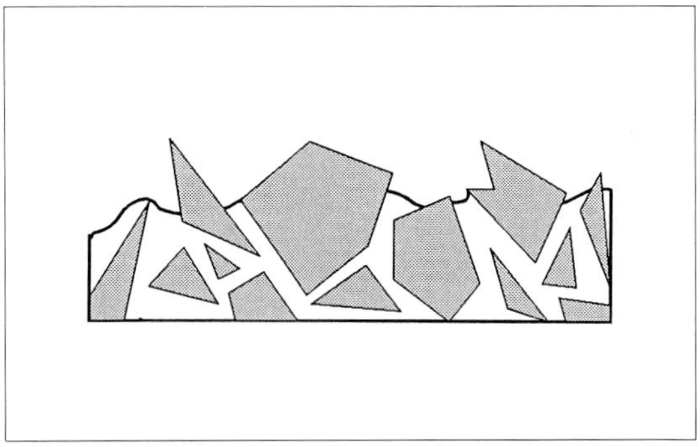

Fig. 3-5 Surface wear of a macrofilled composite continues as resin matrix erosion leads to loss of filler.

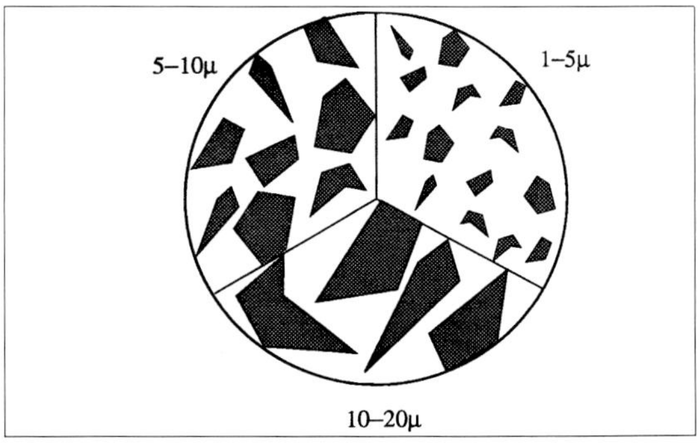

Fig. 3-6 Comparison of early macrofilled composites (10- to 20-μm filler particles) with later, more polishable formulations.

ing (Fig. 3-6). The smaller, as well as softer, fillers (barium and strontium glasses) improved polishability and slowed the development of roughness and staining. The newer glass fillers also imparted the distinct advantage of being radiopaque. All macrofills currently in production are of the small particle variety.

Microfilled Composites

Developed in the late 1970s, microfills were designed to eliminate the problem of polishability common to macrofill composites. Rather than ground quartz or glass, microfills contain submicron-sized (0.04 μm) particles of silica as an inorganic filler. Such minute particles enable polishing to a surface texture that approaches the smoothness of enamel.

The silica ash (pyrolithic silica) used in microfills has been used in industry as a thickening agent for products such as paints and cosmetics. Addition of a small amount of microfiller to a liquid will dramatically increase its viscosity, due to the substantial surface area of the microfiller. Thus only low levels of filler loading (<35% by weight) can be achieved by direct mixing of resin and microfiller in order to maintain suitable handling characteristics. Such materials (homogenous microfills) have exhibited correspondingly poor physical properties and clinical performance.

Microfills in current use are of the heterogenous variety, produced using one or two methods of increasing filler loading. The first

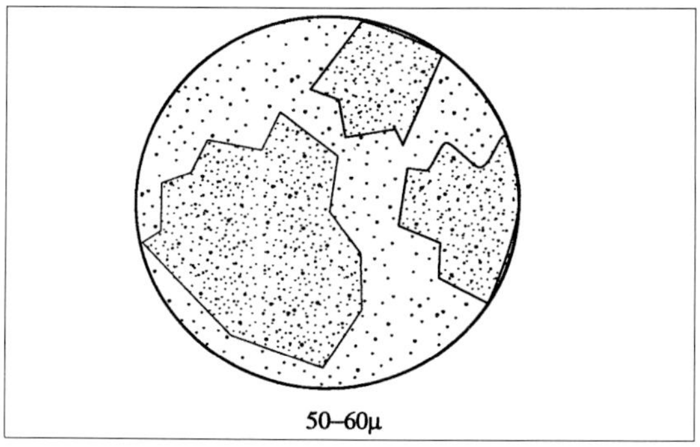

Fig. 3-7 Microfill composite containing prepolymerized particles (50 to 60 μm) to increase filler loading.

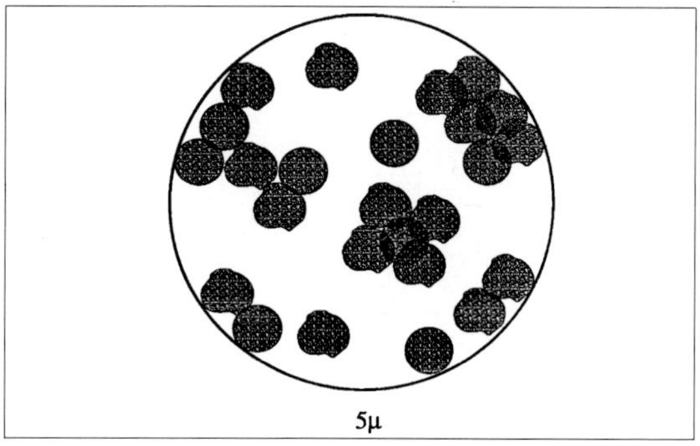

Fig. 3-8 Microfiller (0.04 μm) particles condensed into agglomerates, then added to resin to increase filler loading.

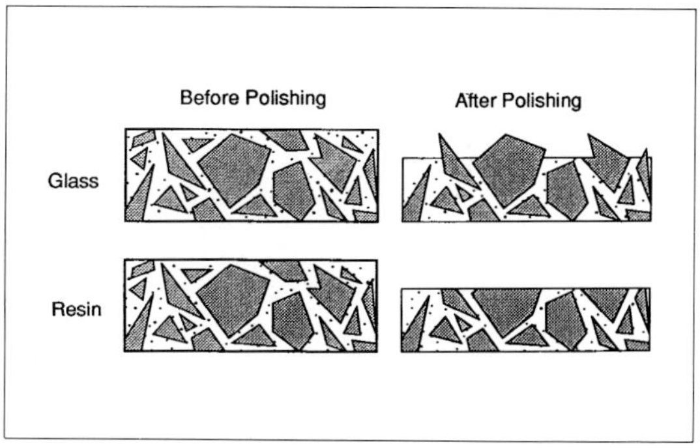

Fig. 3-9 **(top)** Glass fillers become exposed during polishing and wear due to the hardness differential between filler and resin matrix. **(bottom)** Prepolymerized resin fillers in microfilled composites polish and wear at a similar rate as the matrix, producing a smooth surface.

employs mixing microfiller and resin under heat (to increase the capacity of the resin to accept the filler), polymerizing the mixture, and grinding or splintering the hardened mixture into particles 1 to 200 μm in size. These splintered prepolymerized particles are then added to a similar nonpolymerized resin (Fig. 3-7). The second method uses sintering to agglomerate (combine) the microfiller into pellets (0.07 to 0.2 μm) or larger complexes (3 to 5 μm), which are then added to nonpolymerized resin (Fig. 3-8). Microfill composites currently in production use one or both of these methods to produce final products with filler loading of slightly greater than 50% by weight.

While the finishing qualities of microfills far exceed those of macrofill composites (Fig. 3-9), their higher resin content gives rise to less favorable physical properties. Specifically, microfills exhibit a higher coefficient of thermal expansion, polymerization shrinkage and water sorption, and lower strength than their macrofilled counterparts.

Hybrid Composites

Hybrids offer the best combination of the advantages of macrofills and microfills, and as a class represent the closest approximation yet to an "all-purpose" direct tooth colored restorative. Hybrids can generally be described as small particle (0.6 to 5 μm) macrofill composites with 0.04-μm microfiller added to the resin matrix (Fig. 3-10). The microfiller has the effect of reinforcing the resin matrix, theoretically increasing the resin's stress-bearing capability and reducing microcrack propagation. The microfilled matrix also has a coefficient of thermal expansion that is more compatible with that of the macrofiller particles, reducing particle loosening during thermal changes. Filler

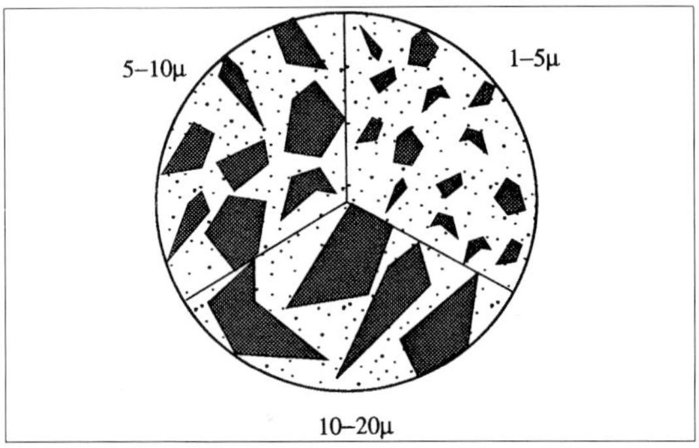

Fig. 3-10 Hybrid composite consisting of macrofiller particles in a microfilled resin matrix.

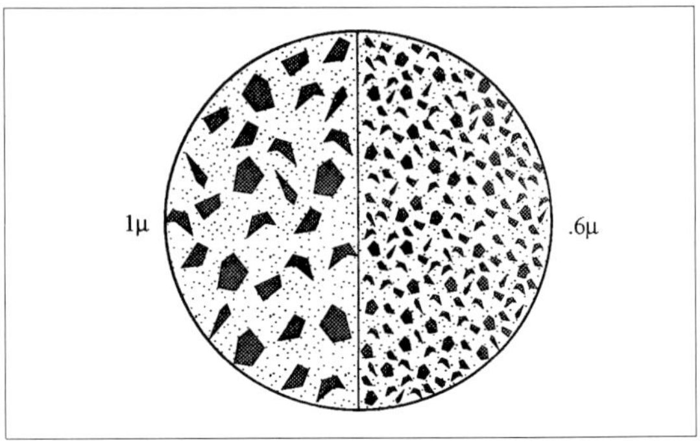

Fig. 3-11 "Micron" and "submicron" hybrid composite classes, based on average size of macrofiller particles.

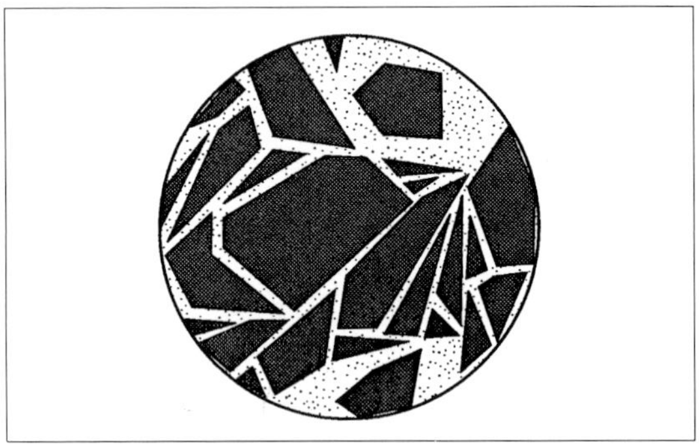

Fig. 3-12 A "heavily filled" hybrid composite. Note the large macrofiller size and close packing of filler particles.

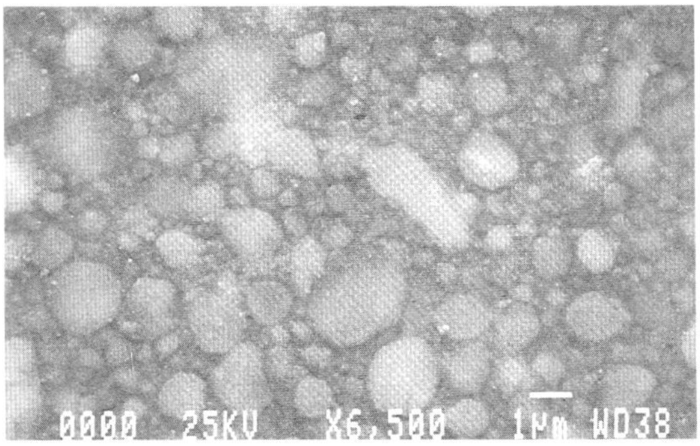

Fig. 3-13 Scanning electron micrograph of Restorative Z100 (3M). Note the size distribution and rounded shape of filler, allowing high filler loading (From 3M Dental Products Division, St. Paul, Minn., USA, with permission).

loading of up to 80% by weight imparts physical properties on a par with those of macrofills. The interspersion of microfiller in the matrix allows a smooth surface to be attained and maintained. Utilization in newer systems of 0.1-μm agglomerated microfiller pellets, in combination with 0.04-μm microfiller and small particle macrofiller, produces further improvements in reinforcement and hardening of the resin matrix via increased filler loading. Hybrid composites possess superior physical properties and exhibit improved clinical performance over macrofills and, with the exception of polishability, microfills.

The class of hybrid composites can be further subdivided, based on the size of the macrofiller used. "Submicron" hybrids contain macrofiller of an average particle size of less than 1 μm (usually 0.6 μm to 0.7 μm), while the macrofiller in "small particle" hybrids averages 1 μm to 5 μm (Fig. 3-11). The combination of the submicron-sized particles (consisting of the newer, softer glasses) with 0.04-μm and agglomerated microfiller provides for high loading and good polishability. Additionally, current polishing systems contain abrasive points, disks, and pastes that are specifically formulated to produce an optimal surface on hybrids. Thus, the polishability of submicron hybrids approaches that of microfills, making these hybrids the material of choice for a single, general-purpose composite restorative.

A third group of hybrids, the "heavily filled"

variety, possesses the highest filler loading (>80%) yet to be attained in a composite resin. These materials are produced using specific size distributions of filler particles to achieve close packing, minimizing the amount of microfill-reinforced resin between the particles (Fig. 3-12). This method of production increases stiffness and resistance to fracture. While very durable and well suited to stress-bearing areas, filler particle size (as high as 10 to 25 μm) makes hybrids of this type less polishable than either the small particle or submicron hybrids. They are thus best applied to posterior areas of occlusal or proximal contact, and as a reinforcing lingual or core layer (under a submicron or microfill) in large anterior restorations.

The most recently introduced composite restoratives are characterized by their manufacturers' efforts to exercise greater control over filler particle size distribution. These materials have average particle sizes of less than 1 μm, with maximums of 2 or 4 μm, depending on specific brand. Earlier submicron hybrids, however, typically display a bimodal distribution of particle sizes, i.e. the sizes tend to be clustered around two values (usually 1 μm and 0.05 μm) with a lack of some sizes in between these extremes. Newer materials, utilizing improved milling techniques, contain a more continuous particle size distribution, allowing closer packing and an increased number of filler particles per unit volume of material (Fig. 3-13). Initial in vitro tests indicate physical properties as good or better than previous composite restoratives. High translucency and excellent polishability allow use in esthetically critical areas.

Initiator Systems

Acrylates such as Bis-GMA are polymerized by addition polymerization. Each monomer molecule of Bis-GMA contains an unsaturated carbon double bond. If this bond is opened, the resultant free electron renders the molecule highly reactive. It will now

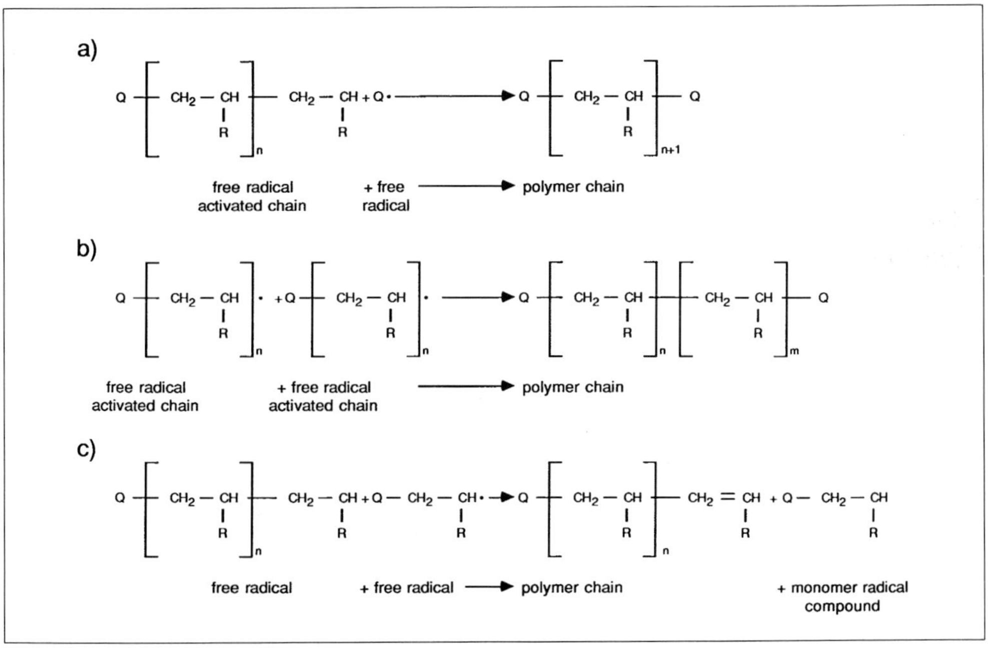

Fig. 3-14 Polymerization reaction of dental restorative resin.

induce a double bond on a neighboring molecule to split, will bond to that molecule and leave yet another reactive electron at the end of this newly formed bimolecular chain. This chain reaction continues, linking and cross-linking the resin molecules together until most of the monomer. becomes polymerized (Fig. 3-14).

In order to initiate the reaction, i.e. to initially split the monomer's double bond, composite systems utilize chemical initiators. Initiators, when activated, are converted to free radicals, compounds that have a highly reactive unpaired electron but that are electrically neutral. The free radical reacts with the monomer's carbon double bond, binds to the molecule and transfers the free electron, initiating the reaction described above.

Activation of the initiator to produce free radicals can be produced by heat, chemical reaction, or photochemical reaction. As direct restorative composites must polymerize at room temperature, only the latter two modes of activation are used with these materials. Thus composite resins can be classified according to activation mode: chemically activated (or, more commonly, chemically cured) and light activated (light cured). Light activated resins can be further classified according the wavelength of light used for activation: ultraviolet (UV) or visible light.

It is important to point out that initiation and polymerization of composite resins is inhibited by exposure of the material to air. This is true for both chemically and light activated systems. This "air-inhibited layer" occurs only at the superficial outer surface of the resin, and is rich in unreacted double bonds. This makes it feasible, then, to apply composite restoratives in multiple increments, as good chemical bonding occurs between each increment via the air-inhibited layer. Incremental placement can facilitate control of contours in large restorations, and is critically important with light activated materials, as will be discussed below. Unpolymerized resin at the surface of the final increment is removed by normal finishing and polishing procedures.

Chemical Activation

Chemical activation was the mode utilized by Bowen in the first composite restorative, and it remains in use in a few products today. Chemically activated systems are usually supplied as two pastes, commonly referred to as "base" and "catalyst." The base contains an initiator (benzoyl peroxide), the catalyst an activator (a tertiary aromatic amine). Upon mixing the two pastes, the amine, acting as an electron donor, reacts with the benzoyl peroxide to form the free radical.

The two paste chemically activated composite replaced silicates and acrylics as the dominant tooth colored restorative. These composites, in turn, have largely been replaced by light activated systems. Chemically activated composites do remain useful in selected situations such as core buildups, where bulk is required and access of all preparation areas to light curing units may be compromised. Incremental buildup, required for light activated resins, may also be impractical in such situations. Combined use of light and chemically activated composites has been proposed for the restoration of Class II cavities in the "Directed Polymerization Shrinkage" technique (see chapter 4). Routine use of chemically activated composites does remain common in many parts of the world.

Ultraviolet Light Activation

Light activated composite was first reported by Michael Buonocore in 1970, and was introduced in 1971 by the L.D. Caulk Company. It contained a photoinitiator (benzoin methyl ether), which reacts with UV light with a wavelength of 365 nm. The reaction converts benzoin methyl ether into free radicals without the need for chemical initiators.

Ultraviolet-activated systems were initially well received, due to the unlimited working time as compared to the chemically activated materials. Concern regarding the safety of these systems arose, however, particularly with respect to potential corneal and soft tissue damage from direct exposure to UV radiation. Additionally, UV curing units require a warm-up period of several minutes, efficiency of output decreases over time, and output level cannot be discerned visually. Even at 100% efficiency, a minimum of 60 seconds of exposure is required for a depth of cure of only 1.5 mm. Placement and curing of the material in individual 1.5-mm increments is thus necessary to assure thorough polymerization throughout medium and large restorations. Ultraviolet light also has very limited ability to penetrate enamel. Because of these disadvantages as compared to visible light activated systems, UV-activated composites are no longer manufactured.

Visible Light Activation

Visible light activated systems improved on many of the problems inherent in UV systems, and represent the preferred composite restorative materials available at this time. Depth of cure is greater (up to 3 mm), and less exposure time is required (a minimum of 30 to 40 seconds per increment is generally recommended). Although significantly attenuated by enamel, visible light can polymerize composite in preparation undercuts. The units do not require warm-up, and the halogen bulbs used in visible light units maintain efficiency at a much more constant level than do UV sources.

Diketone photoinitiators (e.g. camphoroquinone) produce free radicals when exposed to visible light in the blue (420- to 450-nm) range. While these substances are capable of curing the resin, small amounts (as compared to chemically activated resins) of tertiary amines are also added to accelerate the initial reaction and markedly decrease curing time. As these amines, as well as the chemical initiator benzoyl peroxide, are implicated as causative agents in postcure color shifts, visible light activated composites exhibit improved color stability over their chemically activated counterparts.

Counter-top curing units consist of a box containing all functional components (light bulb, cooling fan or heat sink, on/off and timer switches), and utilize a fiber optic cord to transmit light from the unit to the curing tip. Care must be taken with these units not to bend the cord, which can cause breakage of individual optical fibers. Gun-type units (Fig. 3-15) place functional components in a compact unit used at the operative site, eliminating the need for the fiber optic cord. Interchangeable tips of varying diameter and curvature add versatility to these units.

Visible light curing units are considered to be less hazardous than UV units; however, precautions must be taken against retinal

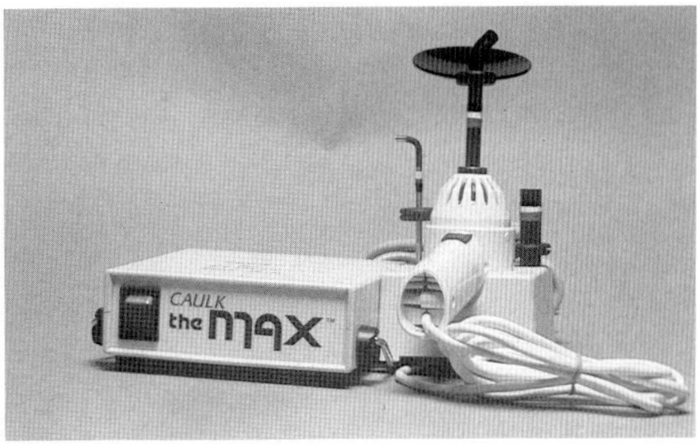

Fig. 3-15 Typical "gun-type" light curing units. Note interchangeable tips and protective shields.

damage from both direct and reflected visible light output. Exposure to intense blue light can severely damage photoreceptors in the eye, with the effect being cumulative. Transparent hand-held shields or protective eyewear designed to absorb blue light provide effective protection. Most curing units are supplied with attached shields, which can be removed and used in a hand-held manner (Fig. 3-15).

Effect of Initiation System on Physical Properties

While conversion of a monomer to a polymer is the end result of all initiation systems, the amount of conversion, i.e. the conversion rate, will vary with the initiation system used. As conversion rate increases, residual uncured monomer in the resin is reduced, and physical properties correspondingly improve.

Chemical activation results in the least complete cure of any of the systems discussed. Unreacted double bonds of 25% to 70% have been reported for chemically activated composites. Physical mixing of the two pastes by the user produces variable and inconsistent levels of homogeneity in the final resin. Oxygen inhibition of polymerization, via air incorporation during mixing, also reduces conversion rates significantly. These factors give rise to the high levels of water sorption and polymerization shrinkage, poor coefficient of thermal expansion and low resistance to fracture exhibited by these composites. Clinical consequences are increased discoloration and margin breakdown, and decreased resistance to wear, as compared to more completely polymerized resins.

Light activation, especially using visible light, produces high conversion rates in composite resins. The higher efficiency of light activated systems results in materials that exhibit physical properties superior to those of their chemically activated counterparts. Incomplete polymerization can occur, however, if several factors affecting light activation are not considered and controlled:

Curing unit output. Visible light curing units were initially not thought to suffer from the gradual and undetectable decrease in output intensity seen in their UV predecessors. It has been shown, however, that output can decrease as the halogen bulbs in these units age, resulting in incomplete polymerization, especially at the deepest aspect of the increment being cured. The bulb's reflective surface blackens with use, reducing intensity of light emitted. Excessive bending of fiber optic cords can produce breakage of individual fibers, resulting in decreased output intensity. Radiometers (Fig. 3-16) that measure the amount of blue light being emitted from a curing unit are very useful for monitoring individual units for loss in output intensity.

Curing time. As previously stated, composite must be exposed to the curing light for a minimum of 30 to 40 seconds to effect optimum polymerization. Prolonged curing times have not been shown to adversely affect resin or tooth structure; i.e. it is not possible to "overcure" a composite. The polymerization reaction, however, continues after exposure to the light ends. Composites have thus been shown to not achieve maximum hardness until more than 24 hours after polymerization is initiated (Fig. 3-17). Since the improvement in surface hardness increases exponentially during the period immediately following exposure to the curing light, and in consideration of practicality, a waiting period of 10 minutes after the last curing cycle before finishing of a composite has been recommended.

Distance between light source and composite. Intensity of light reaching a surface will decrease as a function of the square of the distance to the surface. A curing unit tip must be as close as possible (1 mm) to the composite for optimum curing efficiency. As light-to-resin distance increases, curing time

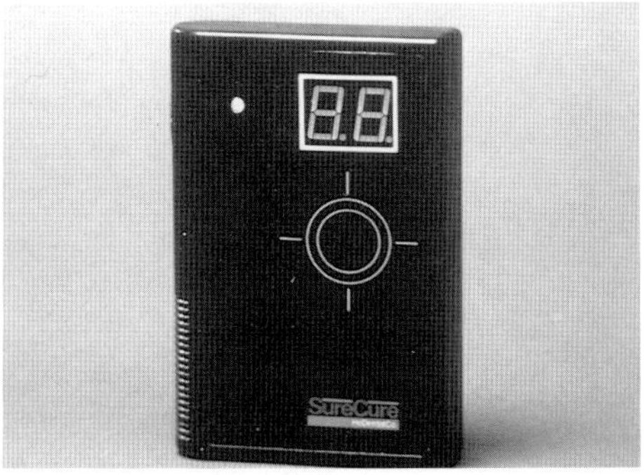

Fig. 3-16 A radiometer (Sure Cure Meter, HO Dental), used to monitor curing light output.

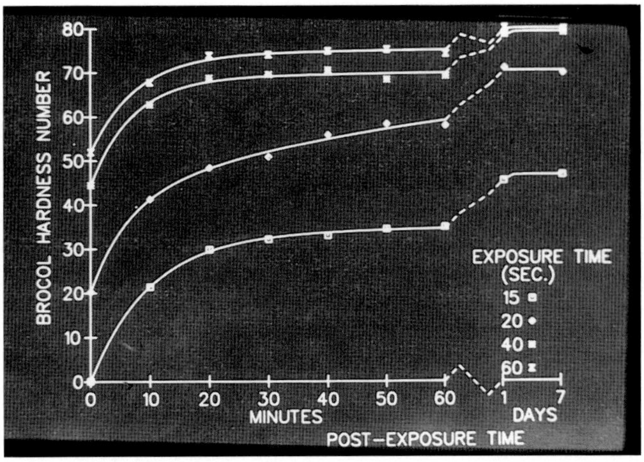

Fig. 3-17 This graph illustrates the degree of polymerization of a composite resin, as measured by hardness, achieved with different durations of exposure to the curing light. Note the continued increase in hardness following light curing, and the low early and final values for 15 and 20 second exposures. (From R. Leung, J. Dent. Res., 62 (3): 363-365, March 1983, with permission.)

must be increased accordingly.

Incremental thickness of composite. Hardness of cured composite has been shown to decrease as distance from the composite surface increases. Restorations should therefore ideally be built up in individually cured increments of 1 mm thickness (and should not exceed 2 mm) to assure thorough polymerization.

Composite shade. Light is transmitted more easily through lighter shades of resin than through darker shades. Increment thickness should then be reduced, and curing time increased, when darker shades are used.

Filler type. Glass filler particles transmit more (and absorb less) light than either microfillers or the organic resin matrix. A given amount of light, then, will generally cure a macrofilled or heavily filled hybrid more thoroughly than a microfilled composite.

Tooth undercuts. Blue light does penetrate both enamel and dentin, but with markedly reduced intensity. Curing time must be increased two to three times to ensure adequate polymerization in preparation areas that cannot receive direct light exposure.

Heat activation produces the highest conversion rate, and the correspondingly best physical properties in the resin, of any activation method. Though not practical for direct-placement composites, indirectly fabricated heat cured composite restorations are used for a variety of applications (see chapter 5).

Other Components

1. Coupling Agents. Properties of a composite will improve as the affinity of the filler for the resin matrix increases. Adhesion between resin and filler facilitates transfer of stresses between these components, and resists loss of filler from the restoration surface. Coupling agents have resulted, then, from efforts to bond filler to resin. Silanes (bipolar organic molecules) are commonly used for this purpose in dental composite resins, as well with indirect resin-bonded ceramic restorations (see chapter 6).

Glass surfaces, including those used for inorganic fillers, readily pick up a layer of water when exposed to the atmosphere. Silanes

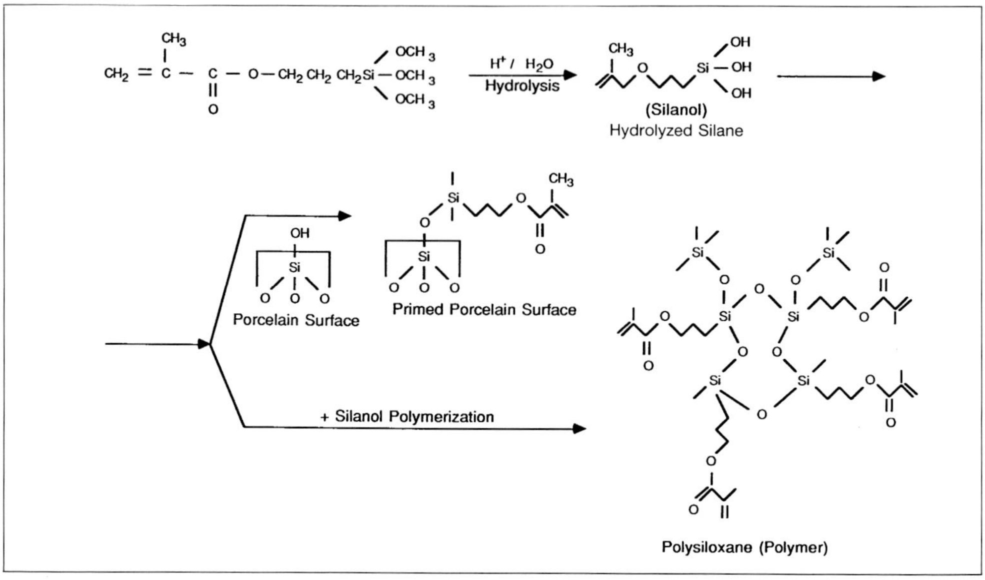

Fig. 3-18 Activation (hydrolysis) of silane coupling agent and subsequent attachment to porcelain surface.

are bifunctional molecules composed of a hydrolyzable silicone group at one end, and an organofunctional group (usually methacryl) at the other. Once hydrolyzed, the silicon group theoretically bonds ionically to water at the glass surface, leaving the organic end free to covalently bond to the resin matrix (Fig. 3-18).

Most microfillers and macrofillers currently in use are treated with silane prior to incorporation into resin. As the silane bond to filler is easily hydrolyzed, water sorption is thought to decrease composite longevity by accelerating loss of exposed filler at the restoration surface. Silanation of filler has been shown, however, to result in overall improved physical properties of composite.

2. Diluents. The high viscosity of Bis-GMA requires the addition of lower viscosity organic monomers to facilitate the clinical handling characteristics of composite resins. The most commonly used diluent is TEG-DMA, which produces a more flexible and less brittle material.

3. Inhibitors. Small amounts of compounds that inhibit polymerization are added to composites to increase shelf life. Both 4-methoxyphenol (PMP) and 2,4,6-tritertiary-butyl phenol (BHT) are commonly used.

RESIN CEMENTS

Cements composed of composite resin and other resin formulations are used for cementation and bonding of a variety of indirect restorations. Resin cements have been available since 1952, with the first composite resin cement being introduced in 1970. With the dramatic increase in conservative and esthetic techniques such as resin-bonded bridges and esthetic restorations (crowns, veneers, inlays and onlays composed entirely of ceramic or composite), resin cements have become very popular in recent years.

Resin cements typically consist of low-viscosity microfill or hybrid composite resins, formulated from Bis-GMA or UDMA resins, and the other components described in chapter 3. Degree of inorganic filler loading ranges from 20% to 75% by weight. An additional type of formulation utilizes 4-methacryloxyethyl trimellitic anhydride (4-META) in polymethyl methacrylate (PMMA).

Adhesion to tooth structure and restorative materials is enhanced by using resin cements in conjunction with the current generation of dental adhesives (see chapter 3). Various treatments designed to increase mechanical and chemical adhesion to restoration surfaces are also required to produce optimal bond strengths to these materials. These treatments include acid etching and silanation of ceramic, chemical softening of indirect (post-cured) composite and microabrasion (sandblasting) of metals, ceramics, composites and (for intraoral repairs) surfaces of existing restorations. Some resin cements and adhesives also require tin-plating of precious metals to obtain maximum adhesion. Resin bond strengths to materials treated with these techniques can exceed 20 MPa.

The adhesive properties of resin cements allow restorations to be bonded to tooth structure, allowing more conservative preparation designs than those traditionally recommended for indirect techniques. While conventional protocols dictate the removal of weakened areas of tooth structure, bonded restorations are capable of strengthening and supporting these areas. Other advantageous properties include compressive strength (100 to 340 MPa) and film thickness (13 to 20 μm).

Resin cements vary in both mode of polymerization and opacity, depending on the application for which they are designed. Chemical cure versions are used for conventional fixed prostheses and resin-bonded bridges, where visible light curing is not possible. These materials also tend to be opaque, facilitating removal of excess, and a reduction of potential "graying" of anterior teeth by resin-bonded retainers. Dual-cure resin cements polymerize via both chemical and light activation. They are used for ceramic and composite inlays, onlays and crowns, where the restoration thickness may hamper complete polymerization by light activation alone. Dual-cure cements are typically translucent, allowing the restoration to blend into and reflect the color of surrounding or underlying tooth structure ("chameleon" effect). Chemical and dual-cure cements are supplied in either a two-paste or powder-liquid form. Light-cure cements are used for ceramic veneers, where access and restoration thickness do not impede the penetration of visible light. Lack of a chemical activator also increases working time, enabling verification of veneer seating and removal of excess cement. A wide range of shades and opacities, as well available color modifiers, enables the user to esthetically customize restorations. Many light-cured cement systems also include a dual-cure catalyst, allowing the cement to also be used for posterior restorations. Similar dual-cure options are also included for the adhesive resin component of some dental adhesive systems, to assure thorough polymerization when used in indirect techniques.

GLASS IONOMERS

Glass ionomers are similar to silicates in that they too are formed by the reaction of ion-leachable, fluoride-containing glasses and an acid solution. They bear no resemblance to silicates, however, with respect to clinical performance and versatility. They also differ significantly from resin-based systems in chemistry and handling characteristics. Initially marketed as a direct restorative for cervical erosion and abrasion lesions, glass ionomer materials are used for several different restorative applications. Glass ionomers are classified as dental cements, hence the common use of the term "glass ionomer cement" in reference to all variations of the material.

GLASS IONOMER RESTORATIVES

Composition

Introduced in 1974 by Alan D. Wilson and Brian E. Kent, glass ionomers combine components from silicates and zinc polyacrylate materials to gain the favorable qualities of both. The ionomer systems are generally chemical cured in nature and consist of powder and liquid. Originally aqueous solutions of polyacrylic acid, glass ionomer liquids presently consist of acrylic/itaconic or acrylic/maleic copolymers, as these are more stable. These high molecular weight polyacids have been shown to be biologically compatible and far less irritating to the pulp than the phosphoric acid used with silicates. Tartaric acid is also added to reduce what would otherwise be an impractically long setting time.

Glass ionomer powder consists of finely ground aluminosilicate glass which is approximately 20% fluoride by weight. Particle size for restoratives averages 40 μm. Fluorides incorporated into the glass improve the working characteristics of the powder/liquid mixture and increase the strength of the set cement. Fluoride release via ion exchange also has the therapeutic effect of providing caries resistance to glass ionomer restorations.

Glass ionomer restoratives contain clear glasses which give rise to translucency to the set material. These glasses tend to have high silica/alumina ratios, resulting in a slow setting reaction (see below). Other glass ionomer materials contain opaque glass powders of finer grain size, reducing setting time and facilitating their handling.

Setting Reaction and Vulnerability to Water

An understanding of the glass ionomer setting reaction of glass is necessary to properly manipulate these materials and to obtain optimal clinical performance. The reaction is of the acid-base variety, and requires an aqueous medium for cement-forming ions leached from the glass to react with the polyacid. Water is additionally important as it hydrates the set material and becomes permanently incorporated into it. The reaction process can be divided into three distinct phases (Fig. 3-19).

Initial mixture of the liquid (acid) and powder (base) elicits release of soluble metal ions (Al^{3+} and Ca^{2+}) from the glass particles and migration of these ions into the surrounding aqueous solution. This leaching process depletes the outer layer of each glass particle of metal ions, degrading this layer to a silica gel.

Accumulation of sufficient metal ions in the

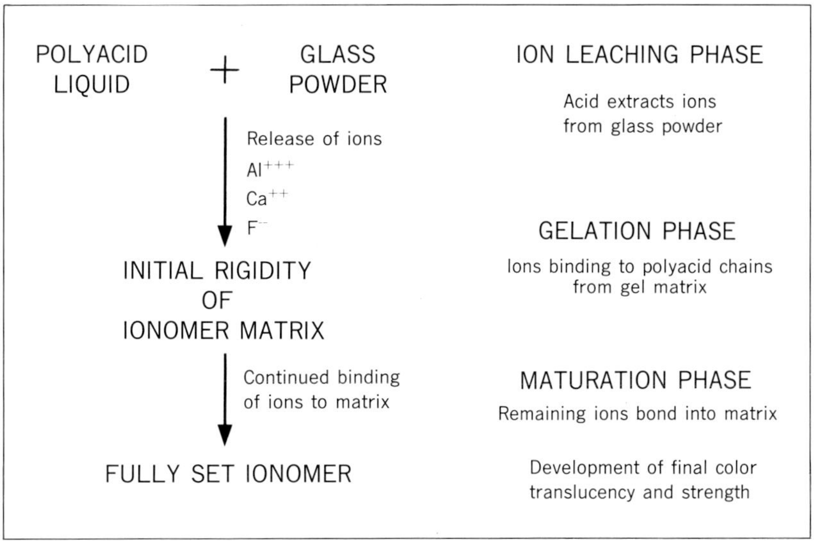

Fig. 3-19 Setting reaction of glass ionomer.

liquid initiates the gelation phase, during which these ions are bound to the polyacid chains, leading to development of metallic salt bridges between these chains. The resulting cross-linked hydrogel acts as a matrix to surround and bind together the unreacted glass particles. As ions are incorporated into the matrix, they are rendered insoluble, forming the final set material. The process, however, is gradual for restoratives, as the clear glasses used have a relatively low alumina content. Unbound ions remain soluble and highly vulnerable to leaching out by water. Thus, exposure to water permanently removes these yet-to-be-bound ions from the matrix, permanently weakening the set material, and leading to softening and opacity of the surface. The material is also adversely affected by dehydration during this phase, as water loss slows and prematurely halts the matrix-forming reactions. A weakened final material is again the result, manifested as crazing, loss of translucency or partial loss of the restoration. Isolation with rubber dam, matrix application during initial set and protection of the restoration surface with varnish or unfilled light polymerized Bis-GMA resin have proven effective in preventing these untoward occurrences (see chapter 4).

The final stage of hardening and maturation continues for about 24 hours. Remaining ions are bound into the hydrogel matrix during this period, rendering it hard and no longer vulnerable to attack by moisture. Translucency, as well as increasing strength and rigidity also develop at this time.

Mechanism of Adhesion

Adhesion to tooth structure has been described as the most important property of glass ionomer restoratives, as it reduces the need for mechanical undercuts in low-stress-bearing areas. While generally believed to be chemical in nature, the exact mechanism has yet to be elucidated.

Early speculation was that during the gelation stage of setting, the chelation of leached calcium ions by the polyacid was occurring with calcium in enamel and dentin. The process probably involves a more complex ionic exchange, displacing calcium and phosphate in hydroxyapatite. Hydrogen bonding to collagen has also been postulated, but not verified.

Figs. 3-20a and b (From E. Hewlett, et al., J. Prosthet. Dent., 66 (6): 767-772, December 1991.)

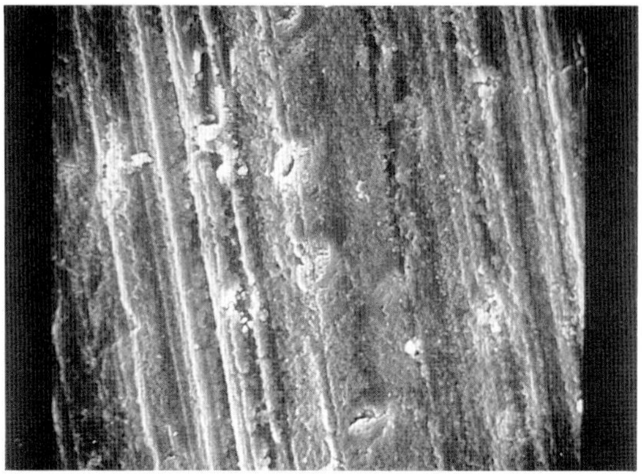

Fig. 3-20a Scanning electron micrograph showing intact smear layer.

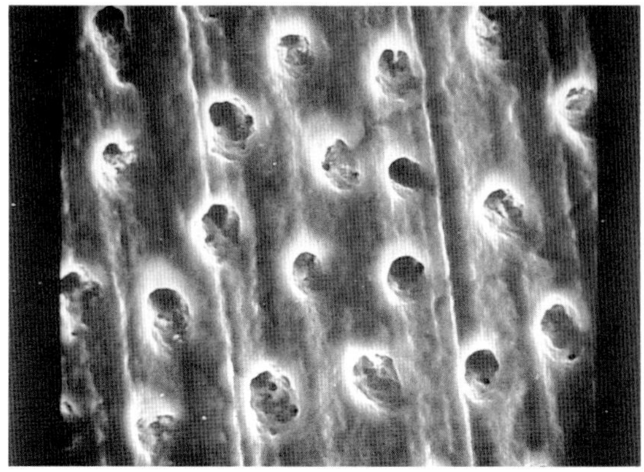

Fig. 3-20b Scanning electron micrograph showing dentin surface following removal of smear layer with 40% polyacrylic acid.

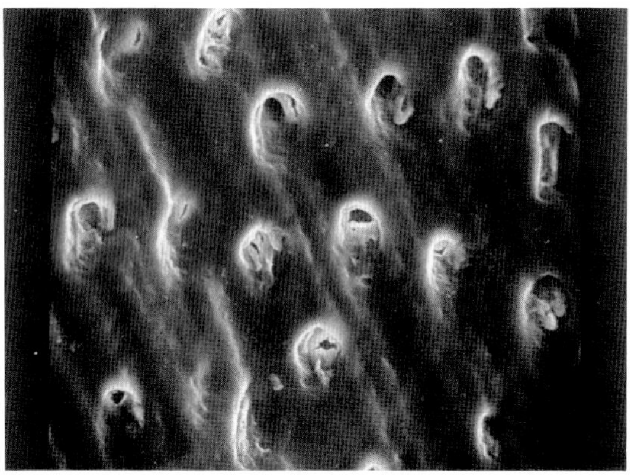

Fig. 3-21 Scanning electron micrograph of cut dentin surface following conditioning with 10% polyacrylic acid. Note partial smear layer removal, with smear remnants occluding tubular orifices. (From E. Hewlett, et al., J. Prosthet. Dent., 66 (6): 767-772, December 1991).

"Conditioning" of a cut dentin surface with a mild acid to remove the smear layer has been commonly recommended to improve the adhesion of glass ionomer to dentin. The initial use of citric acid for this purpose has given way to the use of aqueous solutions of polyacrylic acid polymer. Polyacrylic acid is chemically compatible with glass ionomer systems, nonirritating and effective in removing smear debris from dentin in 10 to 15 seconds (Fig. 3-20). Research results vary widely regarding the increase, if any, of glass ionomer bond strength to conditioned dentin. Since, however, the smear layer is highly variable in the tenacity of its attachment to dentin, smear removal and exposure of the dentin substrate with polyacrylic acid have been shown to produce more consistency in glass ionomer bond strength measurements. Lower concentrations (e.g. 10% vs. 40%) of polyacrylic acid are recommended as they ideally effect only a partial removal of the smear layer, leaving dentinal tubules plugged (Fig. 3-21). These plugs eliminate a direct pathway (via the tubules) to the pulp, preventing ingress of bacteria and other potential irritants.

The aqueous nature of the glass ionomer setting reaction requires a slightly moist dentin surface for optimal wetting and adhesion. Desiccation of the dentin surface immediately prior to placement of glass

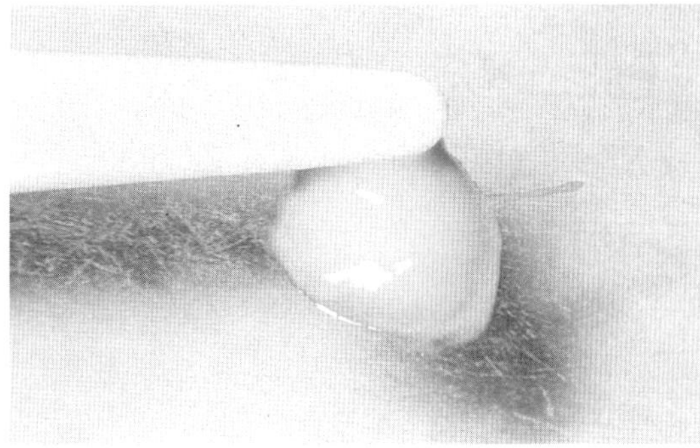

Fig. 3-22 Freshly mixed glass ionomer. Note shiny surface appearance, indicating that the gelation stage of the setting reaction has not yet begun.

Figs. 3-23a and b Encapsulated versions of glass ionomer materials.

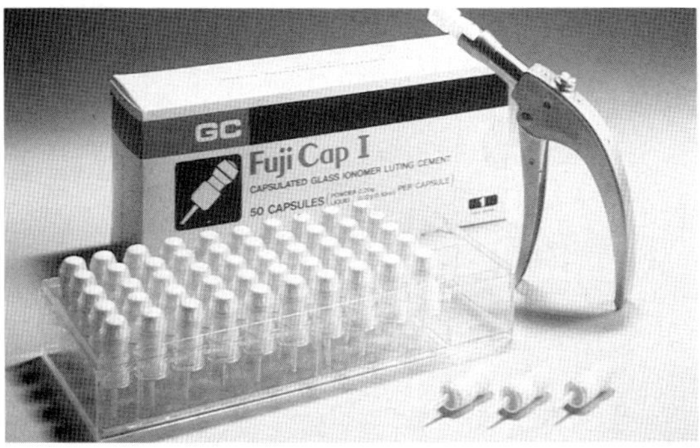

Fig. 3-23a Luting agent.

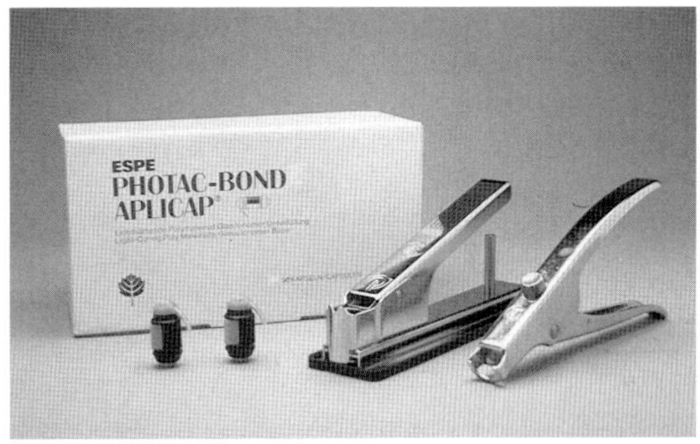

Fig. 3-23b Liner/base.

ionomer is thus contraindicated. Adequate moisture should be present to produce a glisten on the dentin surface without pooling in line angles.

Handling Considerations

Adhesion of glass ionomer to tooth structure (as well as to metal, in the case of luting agents) will only occur during the initial reaction phase immediately following mixture of powder and liquid. The mix has a characteristically shiny appearance during this phase (Fig. 3-22), and is able to optimally wet and adhere to a slightly moist dentin surface. As the gelation phase begins, the surface shine gives way to a dull, opaque appearance, indicating that the mix has progressed from a liquid to a rigid state. It is imperative, then, that all manipulation and placement be completed prior to the start of gelation, i.e. while the mix appears shiny.

Encapsulated systems eliminate measuring and hand mixing of powder and liquid components. In addition to easier handling, mechanical mixing can accommodate a higher powder-liquid ratio, improving physical properties. While these systems are more expensive, they produce optimal and more consistent results. Encapsulated versions are available for all types of glass ionomer materials (Fig. 3-23).

Physical Properties

Glass ionomer cements generally exhibit high compressive strength, but comparatively low flexural strength and toughness. Compressive strength increases as the cement ages for at least a year, due to continuation of both ion incorporation into the matrix and cross-linking of the matrix.

Resistance levels of glass ionomers to dissolution and erosion are highest of all dental cements, but lower than those of composite resin. Gain or loss of water offsets the low inherent setting shrinkage, and is thus responsible for dimensional stability. Water is absorbed by the cement in conditions of high relative humidity (>85%) or in the presence of water, which tends to make the cement expand. Shrinkage occurs if the cement is allowed to desiccate, which occurs in an environment of less than 80% relative humidity. The net result, then, is slight expansion, provided that proper techniques for maintaining water balance have been employed. Very low water sorption renders restorations highly color stable and stain resistant.

While not well suited to stress-bearing areas, glass ionomer restoratives perform well in cervical areas (especially root caries) due to dimensional stability (good marginal integrity), adhesion to tooth structure (low microleakage), and fluoride release (inhibition of secondary caries development).

OTHER GLASS IONOMER MATERIALS

With utilization of various formulations of glasses, glass ionomer materials can be produced that are applicable for uses other than direct restorations. Handling characteristics and physical properties accordingly vary among these different glass ionomer types, but they all share the same basic chemical reactions and cement formation processes described for the restoratives.

It should also be noted that the following terminology is frequently used with regard to the classes of glass ionomer materials: Type I (luting agents), Type II (restoratives) and Type III (bases and liners).

Luting Agents

Glass ionomer luting agents exhibit many desirable properties, notably low solubility, high compressive strength, adhesion to dentin, and anticariogenic activity. Use of finer particle-size glasses ($<20\ \mu m$) with a higher alumina/silica ratio than those used in the restoratives increases strength and reduces the setting time to practical levels, producing a set cement within 10 minutes. While these improvements are obtained at the expense of some translucency as compared to restoratives, translucency is not critical to the performance of luting agents in conventional cementation.

Classification of glass ionomer luting agents is based on the form in which the acid is supplied:

Hydrous. Hydrous glass ionomers contain all of the acid in the liquid component of the material. The first glass ionomer luting agents were of this type, utilizing a standard calcium fluoroaluminosilicate glass powder and an aqueous copolymer of acrylic and itaconic acids. This high viscosity liquid makes it difficult to judge consistency when mixing. The resultant tendency to develop a lower than optimal powder/liquid ratio produces a weaker cement. Film thickness is also substantial, and shelf life of the liquids limited.

Anhydrous. Anhydrous, or water-hardening, glass ionomers were developed to overcome the problems associated with the hydrous materials. In these systems, the polyacid is freeze-dried and incorporated into the glass powder. Barium glass is also added to improve radiopacity. The liquid component, a water solution containing tartaric acid, reconstitutes the acid upon mixing. The low viscosity makes it easier to achieve adequate powder/liquid ratios and improved physical properties (highest strength, lowest solubility). Low film thickness facilitates complete seating of restorations, and shelf life is greatly extended as it is now limited by the long term stability of the powder.

High initial acidity of anhydrous glass ionomers has been associated with a higher incidence of postoperative sensitivity as compared to other luting agents. Strict adherence to proper handling techniques should minimize these untoward reactions. Dentin must be adequately hydrated, and deep areas of dentin should be lined with calcium hydroxide. Proper powder/liquid ratio must be developed to reduce solubility. Isolation should be maintained during set to again minimize solubility of the set cement at the margins, preventing early microleakage. For prepared teeth that are extremely sensitive upon exposure to air, indicating large, open tubules or close proximity to the pulp, a milder cement (semihydrous glass ionomer or polycarboxylate) should be considered.

Semihydrous. This classification represents an intermediate step between the hydrous and anhydrous luting agents, in that the polyacid is contained both in the powder (freeze-dried) and in liquid solution. The levels of viscosity, film thickness and initial acidity correspondingly lie between those for hydrous and anhydrous materials. Physical properties, as for all glass ionomer luting agents, are good.

Liners and Bases

Glass ionomer liners and bases (Fig. 3-24) are useful for cavities requiring sealing of dentin, cariostatic action and replacement of dentin to provide thermal protection and to idealize cavity form. They are unique among liner and base materials in their ability to adhere to dentin. Formulations are designed to produce strength, radiopacity and rapid setting. Zinc oxide is occasionally added as a buffering agent and to increase radiopacity, albeit at the expense of slightly decreased strength.

Low viscosity glass ionomer liners have been recommended for pulpal protection under direct composite resin. Their use has also been shown to reduce microleakage at dentin margins of composite restorations. The so-called sandwich technique additionally calls for etching of the set liner surface with phosphoric acid to effect micromechanical bonding between the liner and the composite resin. The etching selectively removes areas of cement matrix, producing a roughened surface analogous to that of etched enamel. The rationale for the technique is that (1) the liner seals the dentin, provides a chemical barrier against the resin and releases fluoride, and (2) bonding occurs at each interface (dentin/liner and liner/resin), thereby increasing retention and resistance to microleakage.

This technique, initially thought to be advantageous, has several shortcomings. Studies conducted in vitro have indicated that while bonding does occur between the etched liner and the resin, polymerization

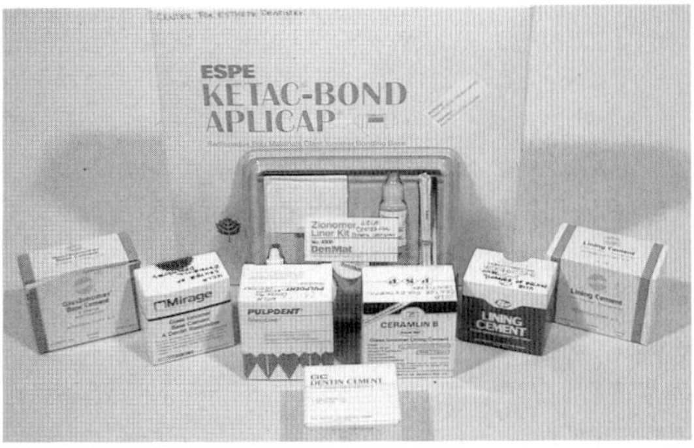

Fig. 3-24 Glass ionomer liners and bases.

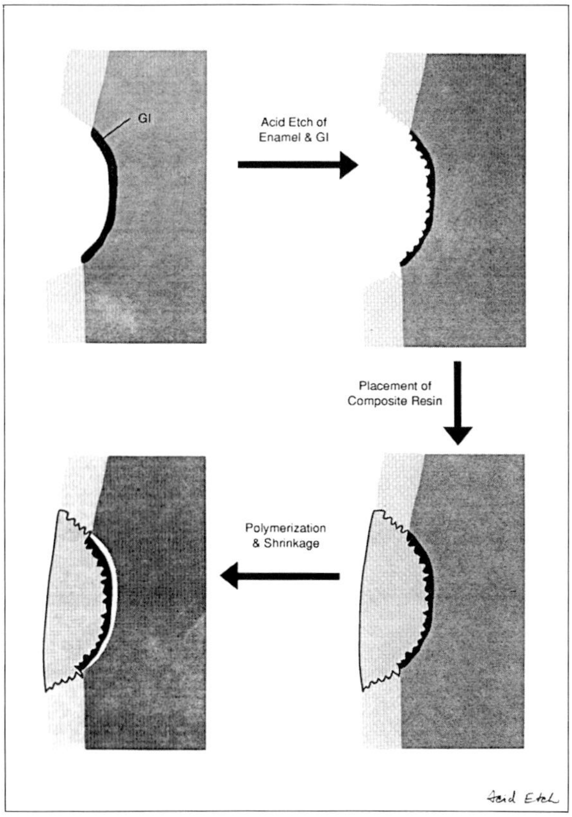

Fig. 3-25 Glass ionomer and composite "sandwich technique." Forces produced by composite polymerization shrinkage are sufficient to detach glass ionomer liner from dentin.

shrinkage of the resin is forceful enough to pull the liner away from the dentin (Fig. 3-25). The resultant void between liner and dentin has been implicated in postoperative sensitivity, especially related to chewing, in composite restored teeth. Excessive etching of the liner removes cement all the way down to the dentin surface, eliminating the seal the liner was to provide. These problems, combined with continued development of improved materials, have rendered the sandwich technique obsolete. Newer generations of resin bonding agents are capable of sealing the dentin surface and providing both a more chemically compatible and strongly attached substrate than that provided by liners. Deep areas (near pulp exposures) should still be protected, but products combining visible light cured resin and glass ionomer are increasingly being used for this purpose, as well as for any situation where a fluoride-releasing liner is desired.

Glass ionomer bases typically exhibit high compressive strength, and are applicable to any situation in which cement bases are traditionally used. Their adhesive quality also makes them useful for blocking out undercuts in preparations for indirect restorations. Fluoride release imparts an additional advantage over other cement bases.

Glass Ionomer and Metal Combinations

Inclusion of metallic components into glass ionomer cement has been attempted in efforts to improve strength and abrasion resistance, thereby making them applicable to the restoration of posterior stress-bearing areas. Addition of amalgam alloy to the glass

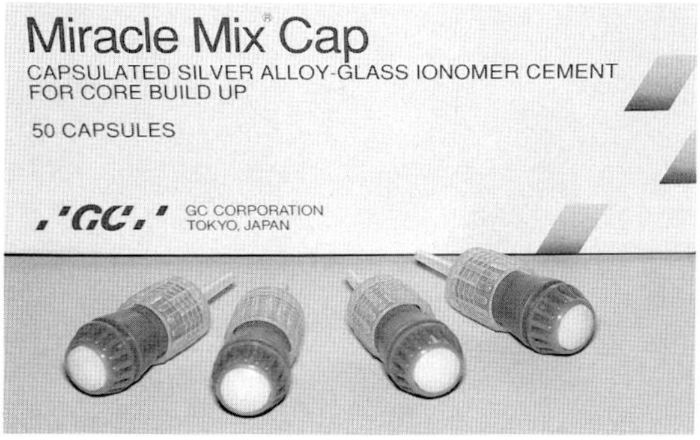

Fig. 3-26 Miracle Mix (GC), a combination of glass ionomer and silver amalgam alloy.

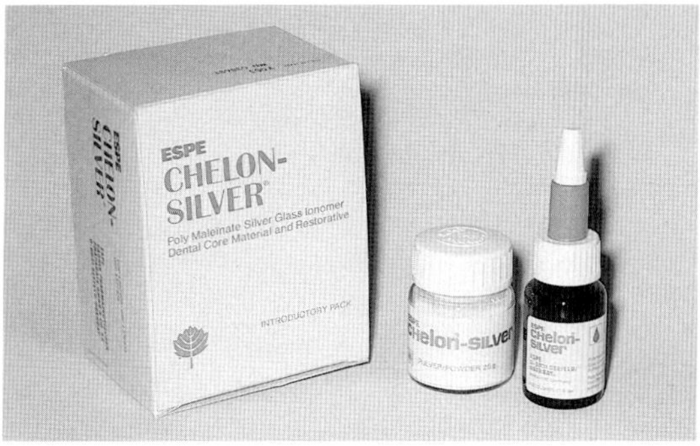

Fig. 3-27 Chelon Silver (ESPE Premier), a cermet-ionomer, produced by fusion of the ionomer's glass component with silver metal.

powder (e.g. Miracle Mix, Fig. 3-26) did increase flexural strength, but resulted in a material with less abrasion resistance than regular glass ionomer restoratives.

Cermet-ionomer cements (Fig. 3-27) are produced by fusing silver powder into the glass component under heat and pressure (sintering). While this process slightly improves physical properties as compared to regular glass ionomers, cermets are not suitable for use in stress-bearing restorations. These materials are commonly used, however, as core buildups due to qualities of strength, adhesion, fast set and fluoride release.

Glass Ionomer/Resin (Light Cured Glass Ionomers)

The combination of glass ionomer components with visible light cured resins has produced materials that have desirable qualities of both of these components. These "light cured glass ionomers" have improved handling characteristics over their chemical cured counterparts. Working time is increased, facilitating placement. Reduced setting time via photocuring decreases sensitivity to water loss/gain of the material in the early stages of the setting reaction. Shear bond strengths to dentin and enamel are increased and have been shown to approximate those of some dentin bonding agents. Base and liner versions chemically bond to composite resin restoratives and cements. The addition of a resin component increases toughness and compressive strength and decreases brittleness.

Glass ionomer/resin materials exhibit low solubility, but fluoride release, in some instances, approaches levels observed in conventional glass ionomers. Higher levels of fluoride release are exhibited by formulations that contain higher percentages, by weight, of glass ionomer (vs. resin). Products in this category thus vary with respect to amount and duration of fluoride release. The anticariogenic qualities and resistance to microleakage of these materials as compared to conventional glass ionomers continues to be evaluated.

The powder component of these systems is a traditional ion-leachable glass. The liquid consists of polyacrylic acid, visible light activated monomers such as hydroxyethyl methacrylate (HEMA), organic copolymers (e.g. polyalkenoic acid) and water. These materials, then, are true glass ionomers, as the glass and acid components react with each other in an aqueous environment in the manner described earlier. This reaction continues after polymerization of the resin, with

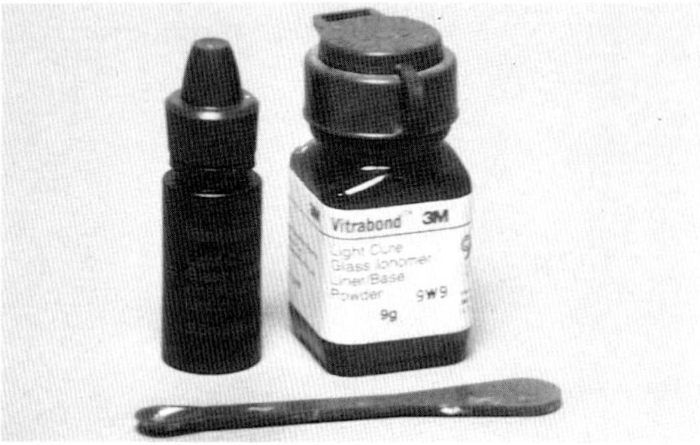

Fig. 3-28 Vitrabond (3M), a glass ionomer liner combined with light curable resin.

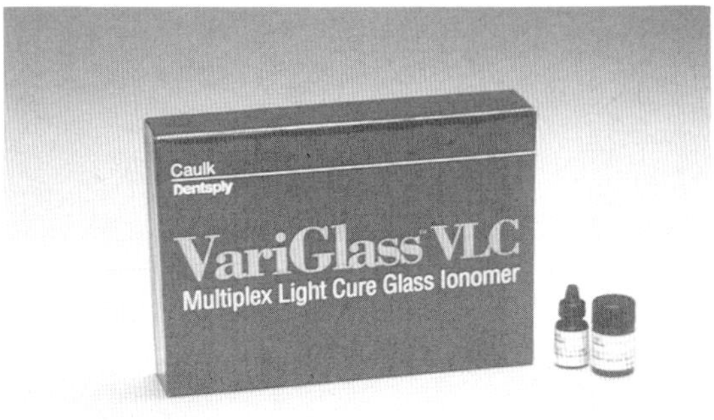

Fig. 3-29 Variglass (Caulk), a glass ionomer and resin combination designed for multiple uses, including direct restorations.

the resin imparting resistance to changes in water balance and becoming an integral part of the set material. The resins of some products in this category contain initiators for both chemical and visible light polymerization. Terms, then, such as "triple-cure" or "tri-cure," referring to the dual mode of resin curing plus the glass ionomer setting reaction, are used to describe these products. Incremental placement and curing is nevertheless recommended to assure thorough resin polymerization. Increment thickness should not exceed 2 mm.

A distinction should be made between true glass ionomer/resin materials and products that are essentially composite resins that contain fluoride and fluoridated fillers. While such composites exhibit handling and physical property characteristics generally associated with restorative resins, they tend to have significantly lower levels of fluoride release than glass ionomers.

The first glass ionomer/resins were formulated for use as cavity liners (Fig. 3-28), and remain useful and effective for this application. Subsequently introduced products allow variation of the powder/liquid ratio to expand the use to bases, core build-ups and non-stress-bearing restorations (Fig. 3-29). Encapsulated restoratives are available as well, further increasing ease of handling and consistency. A wide range of available shades, and ease of finishing, give these materials great potential for use in esthetically critical areas where fluoride release is desired.

RESIN ADHESION TO TOOTH STRUCTURE

BONDING RESIN TO ENAMEL

The discovery of a technique for producing an adhesive bond between tooth structure and a restorative material revolutionized restorative dentistry. Michael Buonocore in 1955 first reported a process in which enamel was modified to effect adhesion to acrylic resin. Specifically, the enamel was treated (etched) with an acid solution, rinsed with water and air dried, allowing attachment of a methyl methacrylate resin via penetration into microporosities created by the acid. This acid etch technique was combined with Bis-GMA composite resins in the early 1970s to produce what continues to be the standard for bonded restoration techniques.

Acid application acts to selectively dissolve the ends of enamel rods at the surface. An irregular, porous surface is produced, dramatically increasing the surface area of the treated enamel (Fig. 3-30). The acid additionally removes saliva pellicle, which would otherwise interfere with bonding, and renders the enamel surface more wettable by altering its surface energy. The effects of etching have been shown to be greater for permanent teeth than for deciduous teeth, due to the aprismatic structure of outer deciduous enamel. Removal of a small amount (0.1 mm) of this outer enamel prior to etching, however, appears to improve bond strength between enamel and resin for deciduous as well as permanent teeth, which may also contain aprismatic enamel. In a similar manner, etching effects are greater for prepared enamel at the cavosurface margin than for unprepared enamel.

The resins (referred to as bonding agents) applied to etched enamel are generally Bis-GMA materials in low viscosity liquid form. The bonding agent wets the irregular surface, flowing into the pores created by enamel rod dissolution. Polymerization of the resin then creates rigid tags interlocked into the etched enamel, producing a significant degree of micromechanical retention of the resin to the enamel. Composite restorative placed into the preparation then chemically bonds to the air inhibited layer at the outer surface of the bonding agent, effectively bonding the composite to the tooth. The bond provides retention for the restoration, and in many situations may eliminate the need for removal of sound tooth structure to create mechanically retentive undercuts in the preparation.

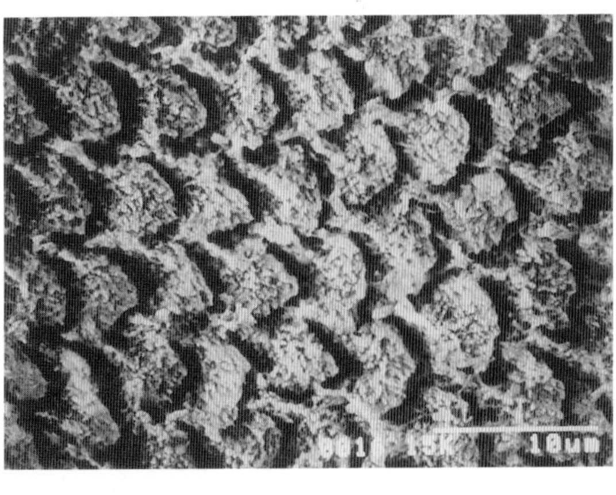

Fig. 3-30 Scanning electron micrograph of enamel etched with phosphoric acid.

Figs. 3-31a and b Phosphoric acid preparations for enamel etching.

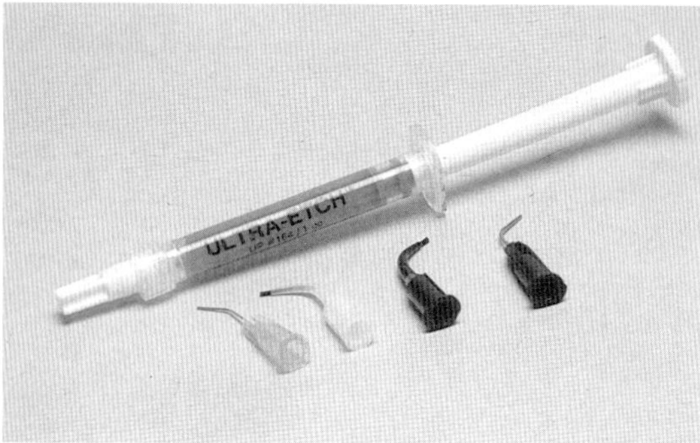

Fig. 3-31a Gel versions are designed to allow more precise placement than possible with low viscosity liquid.

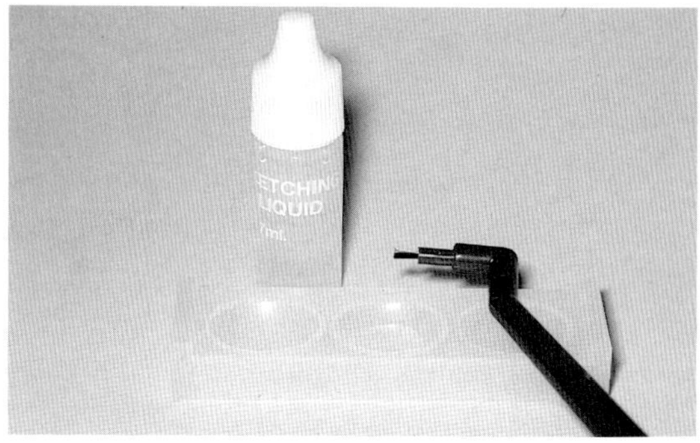

Fig. 3-31b Low viscosity liquids.

Figs. 3-32a and b Newer conditioning agents that use non–residue-forming polymers as thickening agents.

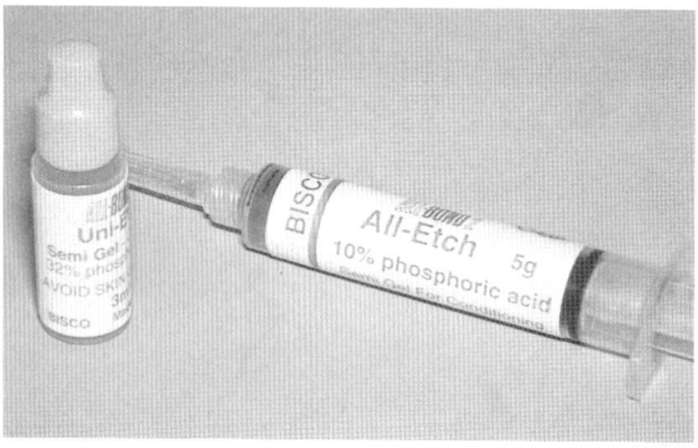

Fig. 3-32a Phosphoric acid, 37% and 10% (All-Bond, Bisco).

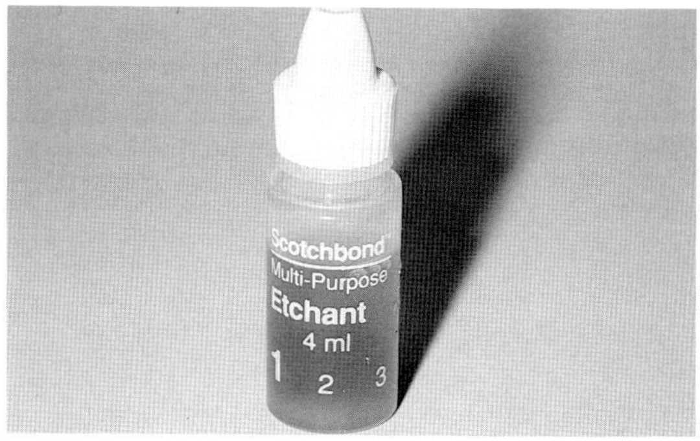

Fig. 3-32b Maleic acid, 10% (Scotchbond Multipurpose, 3M).

The bond also resists the tendency of the restorative material to pull away from the cavosurface margin as it undergoes polymerization shrinkage. The resultant restoration margin thus retains excellent adaptation and is highly resistant to microleakage.

Several acids have been used to etch enamel, but phosphoric acid (30% to 40%) has become the standard. Placement of the acid on enamel for 15 to 30 seconds produces an optimal etch pattern. Etching for longer periods tends to decrease the depth of the surface irregularities and should be avoided. A 20- to 30-second water rinse followed by air drying completes the etching procedure. Protection of the enamel from contamination (e.g. with saliva) is critical at this point. It has even been suggested that condensation of moisture from exhaled air can reduce adhesion to etched enamel, especially on posterior teeth. Rubber dam isolation is most effective in preventing contamination. In cases where rubber dam prevents adequate access or is otherwise impractical, cheek retractors, cotton rolls and gingival retraction cord may be useful. Warm air dryer units are also very effective and eliminate contamination by water or oil in air lines on some chairside units.

Liquid solutions of phosphoric acid were used initially and were effective, but placement was difficult to control, and contact with prepared dentin and uninvolved enamel surfaces was a concern. Liquids have largely

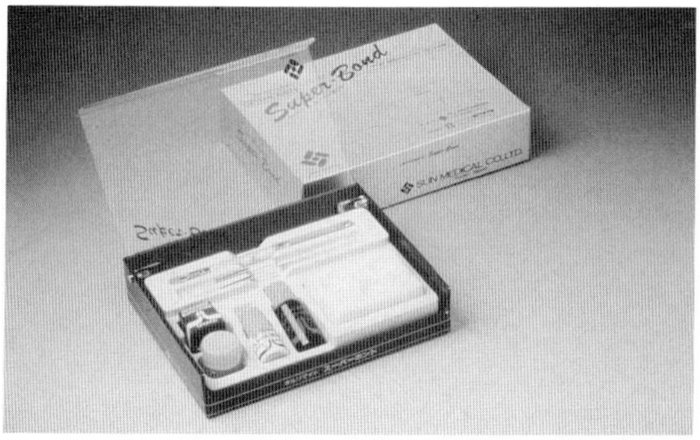

Fig. 3-33 Bonding kit for orthodontic brackets.

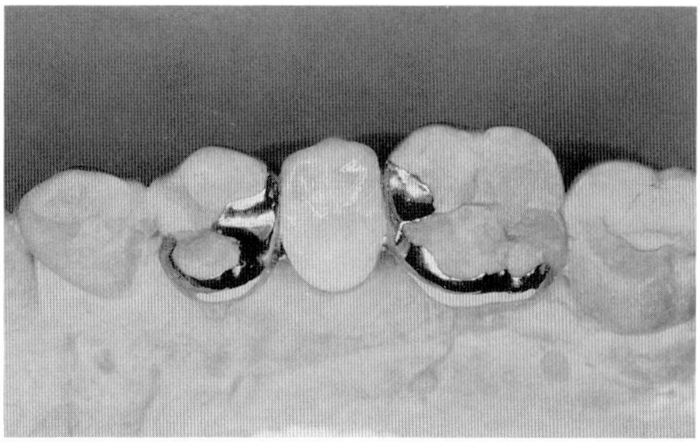

Fig. 3-34 Resin-bonded bridge.

given way to gels as their placement may be controlled much more precisely (Fig. 3-31). Some studies have indicated that longer rinsing may be required to remove debris and residue following use of a gel vs. a liquid etchant. It has also been suggested that silica thickening agents used in gels leave a residue on etched enamel even after thorough rinsing. Newer gel preparations (Fig. 3-32) use polymer thickening agents that rinse away more completely, leaving a cleaner etched surface. Liquids do remain useful, though, for placement of pit and fissure sealants, where penetration of the acid into occlusal grooves is desired. Liquids also allow quick application to multiple teeth, e.g. in the placement of ceramic labial veneers.

With the recognition that application of acidic conditioners to dentin is required for optimal performance of current adhesive resins, phosphoric acid has been replaced in some systems by single agents formulated for use on both enamel and dentin. Consisting primarily of maleic or citric acid, these agents are applied to enamel and dentin simultaneously, simplifying the conditioning or "etching" procedure. They also tend to be of liquid viscosity as the need to limit placement to enamel no longer exists. The development of dentin conditioning and adhesive resins is discussed further in the next section.

In addition to increasing the longevity of conventional composite restorations, the acid etch technique makes a wide array of other procedures not only possible but predictable. Fractured anterior teeth can be esthetically restored in a single appointment without the use of retentive pins. Incipient caries can be treated with maximum conservation of tooth structure. Orthodontic brackets are routinely attached directly to labial or lingual enamel, eliminating the need for full bands on all but molar teeth (Fig. 3-33). Resin-bonded bridges can be used to conservatively replace missing teeth (Fig. 3-34). Direct esthetic bonding can be applied to modify shape and color of anterior teeth. Bonded ceramic restorations, most notably ceramic labial veneers, can be reliably attached to teeth to make dramatic and long-lasting improvements in esthetics.

BONDING RESIN TO DENTIN

The acid etch technique for enamel bonding has remained essentially unchanged since its introduction, and its success is well documented. Development of a system to bond resin restoratives to dentin, however, is more aptly described as an evolution rather than a discovery. Attempts have varied widely in method and degree of success and have been the source of considerable controversy. Techniques have improved significantly during this evolution and should continue to improve, as this remains a most highly active area of research and development.

Dentin Composition and Structure

The difficulty in producing reliable adhesion between resins and dentin is a direct consequence of dentin physiology and structure. Any dentin bonding system that is to work effectively and consistently must take these characteristics of dentin into account. Unlike enamel, whose composition is largely inorganic (96% hydroxyapatite, 4% organic substance and water), dentin is a complex living tissue composed of 65% hydroxyapatite, 20% organic matter, and 15% water. The hydroxyapatite crystals of dentin are plate shaped and are much smaller than those of enamel. Dentin's organic component consists of collagen fibers and a mucopolysaccharide ground substance. These fibers form the dentinal matrix throughout which the hydroxyapatite crystals are deposited to form the final mineralized dentin tissue.

Dentin is permeated by a system of tubules that originate at the pulp and terminate in a branching network near the dentino-enamel and dentinocemental junctions. Odontoblast cells arranged along the pulpal surface of the dentin give rise to long cytoplasmic processes (one process per cell), each of which extends into a tubule through most of the tubule's length (Fig. 3-35). Intercellular fluid also fills each tubule, and can be visualized as it flows onto the surface of cut dentin in a cavity preparation. Diameter of the tubules is typically 3 to 4 μm near the pulp, becoming smaller at the ends near enamel (1 μm) (Fig. 3-36). The number of tubules per unit area is also higher in pulpal dentin than in outer dentin by a factor of four. Because of these differences, the clinical behavior of deep and outer dentin as substrates for

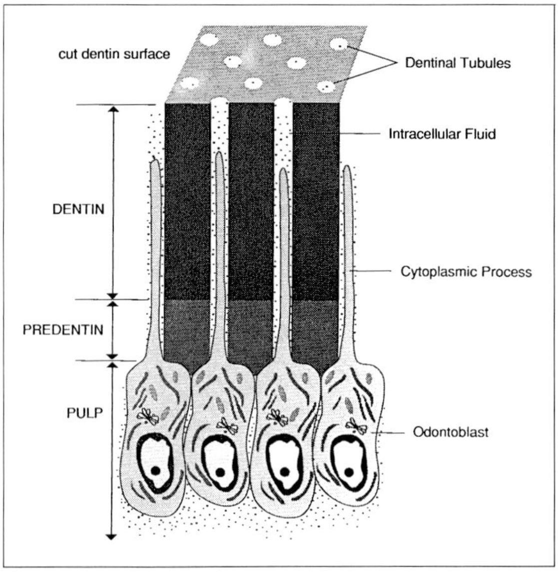

Fig. 3-35 Block section of dentin.

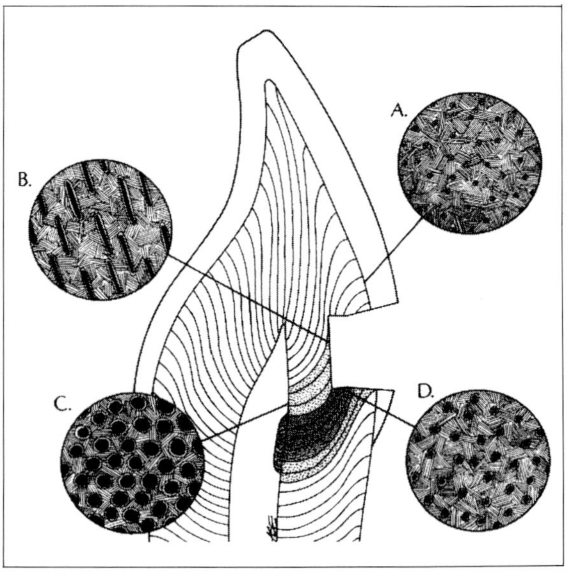

Fig. 3-36 Variations in dentinal tubule morphology at various depths. (From Bhaskar, S.N. (Editor), Orban's Oral Histology and Embryology, 11th Ed., St. Louis: Mosby-Year Book, Inc., 1991, with permission.)

Figs. 3-37a and b (From Bhaskar, S.N. (Editor), Orban's Oral Histology and Embryology, 11th Ed., St. Louis: Mosby-Year Book,Inc., 1991, with permission.)

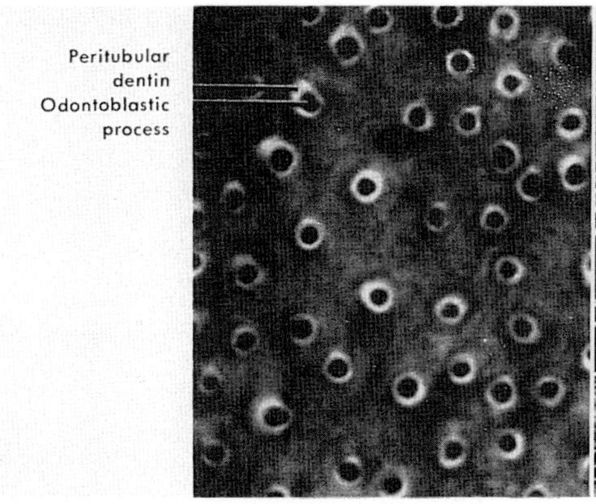

Fig. 3-37a Radiograph of an undemineralized ground section of peritubular dentin showing higher density in the peritubular zone (approx. X2000).

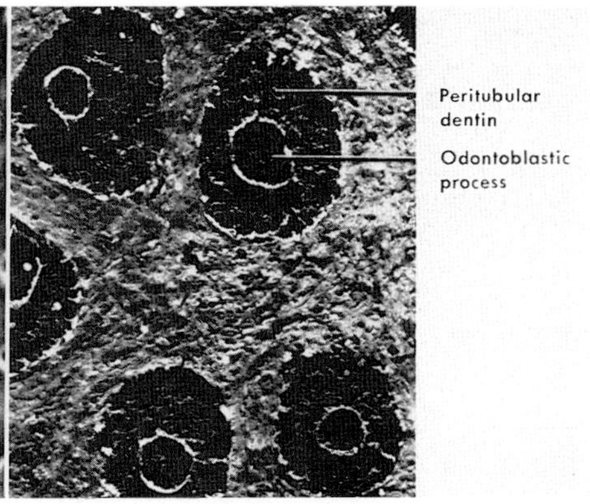

Fig. 3-37b Electron micrograph of demineralized dentin. Note loss of mineral in peritubular area (approx. X4000).

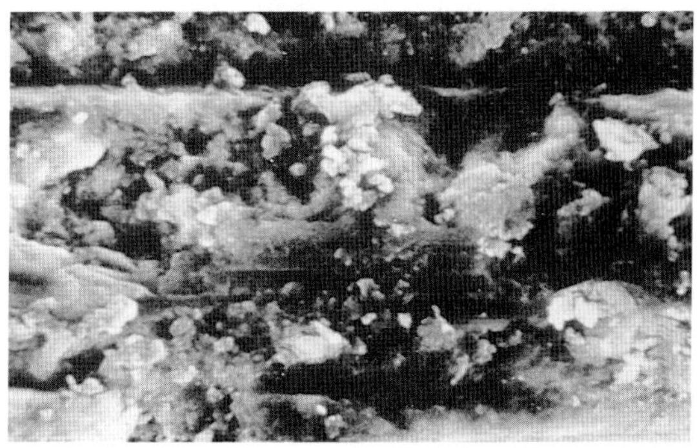

Fig. 3-38 Scanning electron micrograph of smear layer on cut dentin.

bonding can be expected to differ.

Dentin immediately surrounding the tubules and forming tubule walls is referred to as peritubular dentin, while the main body of dentin between the tubules is termed intertubular dentin. Of the two types, peritubular dentin is more highly mineralized (about 9%). It is thicker in outer dentin (approximately 0.75 μm) than in inner dentin (0.4 μm), thereby constricting tubular diameter to about 1 μm near the dentinoenamel junction. This has important clinical implications, as "etching" or conditioning of dentin walls in a cavity preparation with an acidic substance opens up the tubules, i.e. increases the tubular orifice diameter, by demineralizing the peritubular dentin (Fig. 3-37).

In addition to these factors, it is important to consider alterations to the surface of dentin that occur during cavity preparation procedures. Cutting of dentin with hand or rotary instruments produces a layer of debris on the cut surface referred to as the smear layer (Fig. 3-38). It is analogous to the surface debris produced by wet sanding of plaster. Consisting of very small particles of mineralized collagen matrix mixed with saliva and bacteria, the smear layer varies with respect to both thickness and tenacity of attachment to the underlying dentin surface. The attachment is such, however, that removal by simple rinsing and scrubbing is prevented. As it plugs orifices of dentinal tubules, removal of the smear layer is thought to create a wet bonding surface (effusion of dentinal fluid) and facilitate bacterial invasion of the dentin and pulp. In developing strategies for bonding to dentin, different approaches to handling the smear layer (maintenance, modification or removal), as well as the consequences of each approach, must be considered.

Second-Generation Bonding Agents

The term "second-generation" has been applied to resin bonding agents designed for enamel and dentin bonding, and consisting of modified versions of the unfilled Bis-GMA materials used successfully with enamel bonding. Specifically, these so-called dentin bonding agents were halophosphoesters of Bis-GMA, i.e. phosphate ester groups were substituted for hydroxyl groups. Designed to bond to dentin with the smear layer left intact, these agents were hypothesized to infiltrate and penetrate the smear layer (Fig. 3-39). Chemical adhesion was then thought to occur via ionic bonding between the resin's negatively charged phosphate groups and positively charged calcium ions in both the smear layer and the underlying dentin matrix (Asmussen, 1985; Asmussen and Munksgaard, 1988) (Fig. 3-40). Preservation of the smear layer was desired as it reduces dentin permeability and flow of fluid onto the dentin surface. Examples of these agents include Scotchbond (3M Dental Products), Bondlite (Sybron/Kerr), Prisma Universal

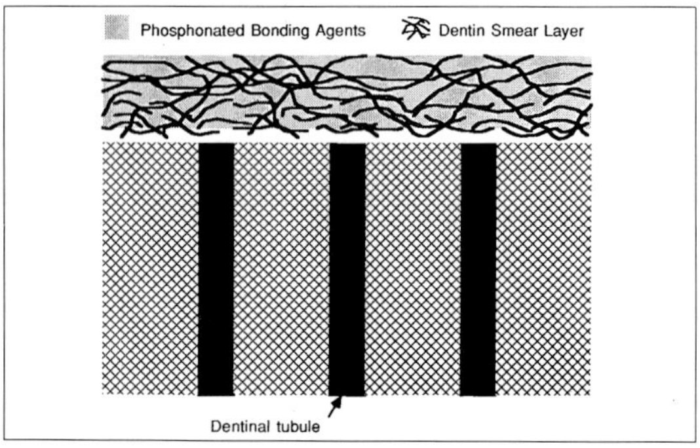

Fig. 3-39 Proposed absorption of a second-generation bonding agent into the dentinal smear layer.

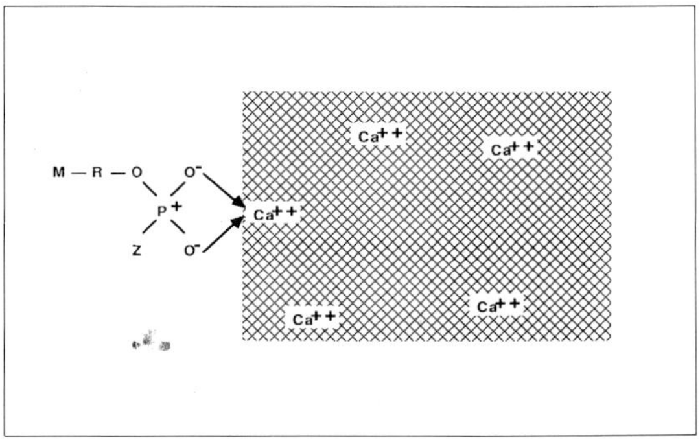

Fig. 3-40 Proposed adhesion mechanism of second-generation bonding agents, involving ionic bonding between phosphate groups and dentinal calcium.

Figs. 3-41a and b Examples of second-generation bonding agents, consisting of enamel etchant, and a two-component resin to be mixed and applied to enamel and dentin.

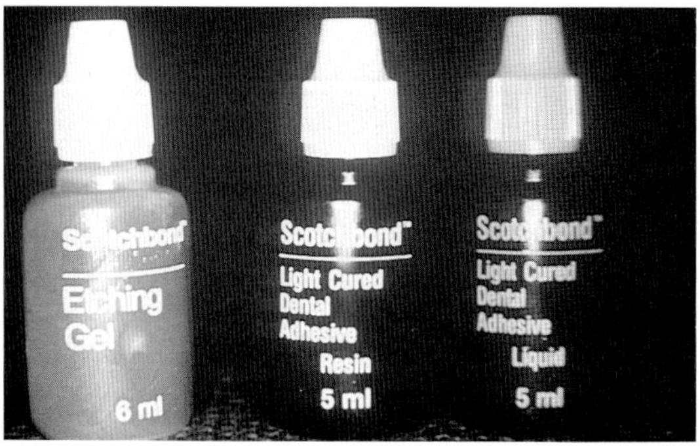

Fig. 3-41a Scotchbond (3M).

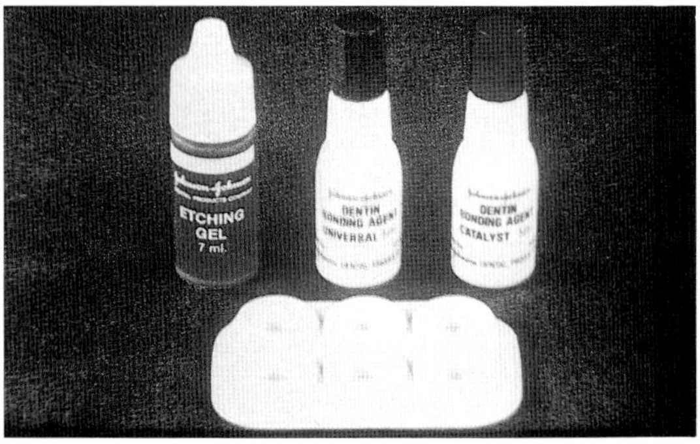

Fig. 3-41b Dentin Bonding Agent (Johnson & Johnson).

Bond (L.D. Caulk/Dentsply) and Dentin Bonding Agent (Johnson & Johnson) (Fig. 3-41).

Shear bond strengths to dentin obtained with these products (4 to 6 MPa) were significantly lower than those routinely observed with etched enamel (13 to 18 MPa). These dentin bond strengths are roughly equivalent to contraction forces in composite resin generated by polymerization shrinkage. The resultant pulling away of composite from dentin walls and margins resulted in poor adaptation of restoration to cavity. Marginal staining and microleakage around dentin margins, as well as poor retention of composite in cervical cavities lacking mechanical undercuts, were observed clinically.

Phosphate ester bonding agents were eventually shown to wet the dentin surface very poorly, largely due to their hydrophobic nature and the aqueous nature of the dentin and its smear layer. Dentin with a smear layer intact has also been shown to have a high surface tension (Benediktsson, 1991). Evidence of chemical bonding between resin and dentin has yet to be produced, and is thought by many researchers not to be significantly responsible for any adhesion that was observed. Tao, Pashley and Boyd (1988) demonstrated bond failure of these agents within the smear layer itself, indicating incomplete penetration of the smear layer, and that the measured bond strengths (5 to 7 MPa) probably represent the cohesive strength of the smear layer itself. Second-generation agents, then, probably achieved some degree of attachment to the smear layer only. The ultimate adhesion of the resin to the dentin substrate was thus limited by the inherent strength of the smear layer and by the tenacity of the layer's attachment to dentin.

Third-Generation Bonding Agents

The phosphate esters have been succeeded by what are accordingly referred to as the "third generation" of resin bonding agents. These systems are characterized by a multistep approach to producing bonding of resin to dentin. While specific methods vary between individual products, third-generation agents generally consist of three components, applied in succession: an acidic dentin conditioner, a hydrophilic resin primer, and an adhesive resin agent. Each of these components will be discussed separately.

Dentin Conditioner

Recognition of the presence of the smear layer and of its effects on resin-dentin bonding led to the use of dentin conditioners. Conditioning agents are acidic solutions designed to modify the cut dentin surface in such a way that a more favorable bonding substrate is produced. Pashley, et al. (1988) and other investigators have shown that such modification can even improve the bond strength of hydrophobic phosphate ester bonding agents, probably by facilitating wetting (reduced surface tension). Many specific agents with different modes of action have been and continue to be used in the various bonding systems currently available.

Much of the controversy related to dentin bonding agent development has its origins in the area of dentin conditioning, specifically with respect to the use of phosphoric acid (H_3PO_4). Upon initial consideration, phosphoric acid would appear to be a convenient choice of acidic conditioner as it could simultaneously be used to etch enamel. The prevailing body of evidence during the early stages of dentin bonding agent development, however, indicated that placement of phosphoric acid on dentin should be avoided. "Etching" of the dentin was shown to have deleterious effects on both the ability of the resin to bond and on the vitality of the pulp (Vojinović, Nyborg, and Bränström, 1973; Bränström and Vojinović, 1976; Macko, Rutberg, and Langland, 1978; Eriksen and

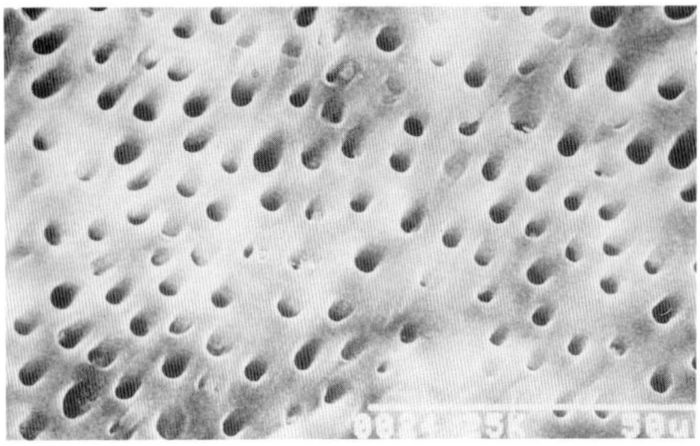

Fig. 3-42 Scanning electron micrograph of dentin treated with phosphoric acid.

Leidal, 1979). It should be noted that although the term "etch" is commonly used in this context, acid treatment of dentin does not produce a true etch pattern such as that resulting from the selective demineralization by acid of enamel. Scanning electron microscopy demonstrates that phosphoric acid is very effective in smear layer removal (Fig. 3-42). The permeability of dentin correspondingly increases following such treatment, allowing fluid to flow from the tubules and significantly wet the dentin surface (Bränström and Nordenvall, 1977). This phenomenon was thought to be responsible for decreased bond strengths in early attempts to bond phosphate ester agents to acid-etched dentin. Equally compelling were numerous reports of adverse pulpal reactions following dentin etching. Dentin treatment with phosphoric acids was thus contraindicated according to most experts, and conventional composite restoration protocol strictly prohibited placement of phosphoric acid on any tooth surface other than enamel.

Fusayama, et al. (1979) nonetheless reported the successful use of phosphoric acid to etch dentin prior to placement of composite resin. Enamel and dentin were treated simultaneously with a 37% solution of H_3PO_4 for 1 minute. Using a phenylphosphate derivative of dimethacrylate (Clearfil New Bond, Kuraray), numerous clinical trials were conducted in Japan in which this technique was applied. Hosoda and Fusayama (1984) reported that acid etching increased the bond strength of Clearfil New Bond to dentin. This, as well as reports of successful trials (Shintani, et al., 1989) were at odds with previously mentioned studies that concluded that phosphoric acid treatment of dentin was contraindicated. Referred to as "total etch," Fusayama's technique was adopted and taught by clinicians in other countries (Bertolotti, 1990, 1991a), but was slow to gain acceptance, especially in the United States.

It is important to note that chemically polymerized composites were used in the Japanese trials referred to here. Bertolotti (1991b) has suggested that these materials do not challenge bonding agent strength to the degree that light polymerized composites do upon polymerization shrinkage. This factor, as well as some unique characteristics of the bonding agent used, may be factors in the success reported by Fusayama and others.

Continued research into the interaction of dentin with phosphoric acid has been enlightening. Wang and Hume (1988) described the ability of dentin to significantly buffer acid solutions applied to its surface. This is in agreement with evidence that hydrogen ion exhibits very shallow penetration into dentin following brief exposure to acid (Chan and Jensen, 1986). Pashley, et al. (1992) suggested that the hypertonicity of phosphoric acid should draw dentinal fluid toward the surface, further restricting hydrogen ion diffusion. Perhaps most significant is the idea of Bränström (1982) that the level of pulpal response to restorative materials is directly related to the number of bacteria under the restoration. This was later confirmed in studies by Browne and Tobias (1986) and Cox, et al. (1987), where Class V cavities were restored and surface sealed with zinc oxide in eugenol to prevent bacterial penetration around restorative margins. Even silicate cements, used as positive controls, failed to elicit pulpal inflammation.

These findings support the widely accepted notion that bacterial infiltration into dentin via its increased permeability following phosphoric acid treatment is responsible for the adverse pulpal reactions seen in these cases. Restorative materials used in these studies failed to adequately seal the cavities at dentin margins (unless specifically surface sealed with an antibacterial agent). Bacterial ingress and penetration into dentin that had been stripped of its protective smear layer was thus allowed. This scenario can be applied to years of anecdotal and experimental observations of pulpal inflammation following exposure of dentin, both inadvertent and intentional, to phosphoric acid. Many clinicians now routinely use chlorhexidine soap solutions to disinfect preparations and surrounding tooth structure prior to placement of restorative materials.

Concomitant with these developments was the introduction of the "third-generation" bonding agents. Common to these systems is the use of a conditioning agent to modify or remove the smear layer. Combined with the use of hydrophilic resin "primers," conditioning has produced significant improvements in bond strengths over those obtained with phosphate esters. The fact that these conditioners are acids (nitric, maleic, citric, EDTA and others are used) makes the distinction between conventional techniques and dentin etching less clear. Evidence does exist, though, that over aggressive conditioning of dentin (e.g. with phosphoric acid concentrations of 37% or higher) may produce a zone of demineralized dentin that is too deep for the resin primers to completely infiltrate (Nakabayashi, et al., 1991). A weakened layer of softened dentin, susceptible to long term degradation, may thus potentially be left beneath a restoration. Several proponents of dentin etching have accordingly modified their recommendations to include the use of lower concentrations of phosphoric acid (10%) to treat dentin. Use of this agent produces a dentin surface that more closely approximates the results seen with many of the currently available conditioners. At least one manufacturer (Bisco) now provides a 10% H_3PO_4 gel for use as a dentin conditioner with its bonding system. It is clear, then, that the once wide philosophical gap between dentin etching and conventional methods is virtually nonexistent.

Dentin Primer

To effect resin adhesion to dentin, it has been necessary to overcome the poor reaction of the inherently hydrophobic resin and the moist dentin surface. This is accomplished by the application of priming agents to the conditioned dentin. Dentin primers are typically very low viscosity comonomers containing two distinctly different types of functional groups. Carboxyl groups, due to their affinity for water, impart a hydrophilic quality to the primers and allow excellent wetting of the dentin. Thus able to compete with water for positions in the dentin matrix, primers are able to penetrate and infiltrate the conditioned dentin surface. Hydrophobic methacryl groups remain oriented away from and exposed at the dentin surface, providing a favorable and polymerizable substrate for the adhesive resin agent applied in the final step (Fig. 3-43). Examples of hydrophilic resins commonly used as primers (also referred to as adhesion

Figs. 3-43a to c Adhesion of third-generation systems to dentin.

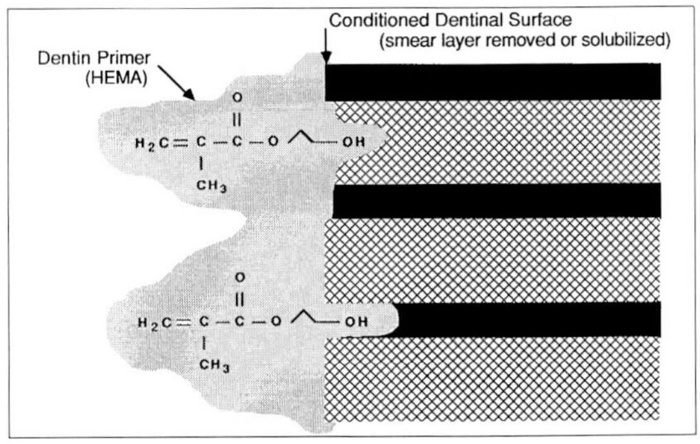

Fig. 3-43a Dentin primer, hydrophillic by virtue of a carboxyl group, is able to penetrate the conditioned dentin surface.

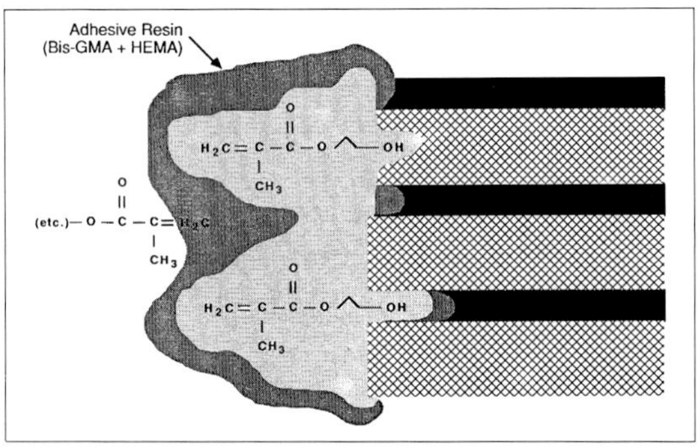

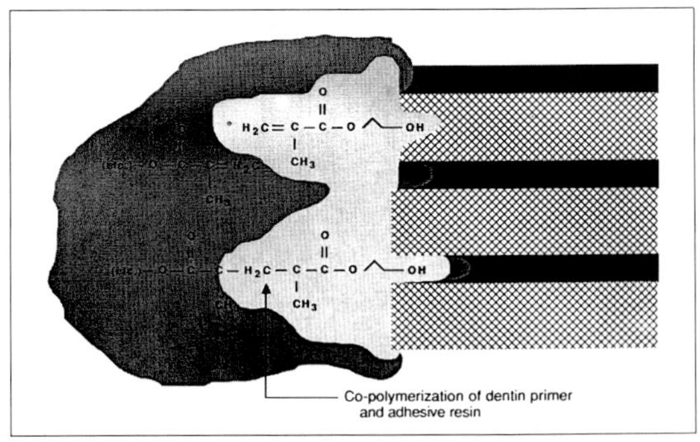

Figs. 3-43b and c Methacryl groups remain exposed at the surface, and bond chemically to the adhesive resin.

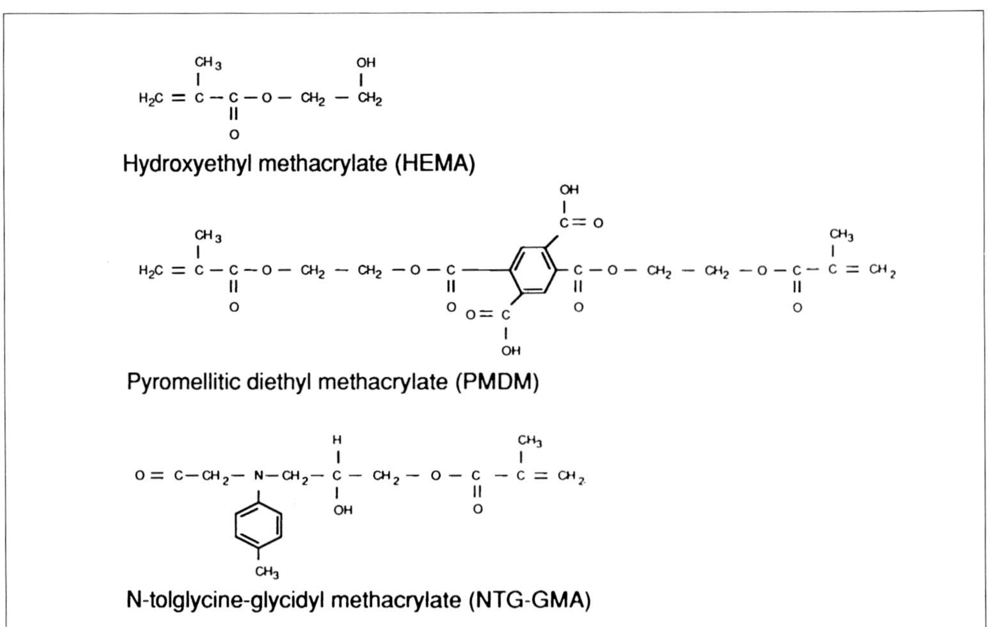

Fig. 3-44 Examples of hydrophillic resins used in the dentin primer components of current adhesive systems.

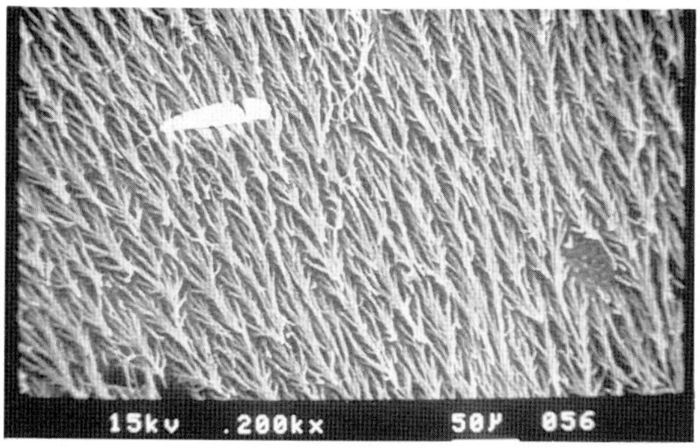

Fig. 3-45 In vitro resin tags formed by applying the All-Bond System (Bisco) to dentin. (From B.I. Suh, J. Esthet. Dent., 3 (4): 139-147, July-Aug. 1991, with permission.)

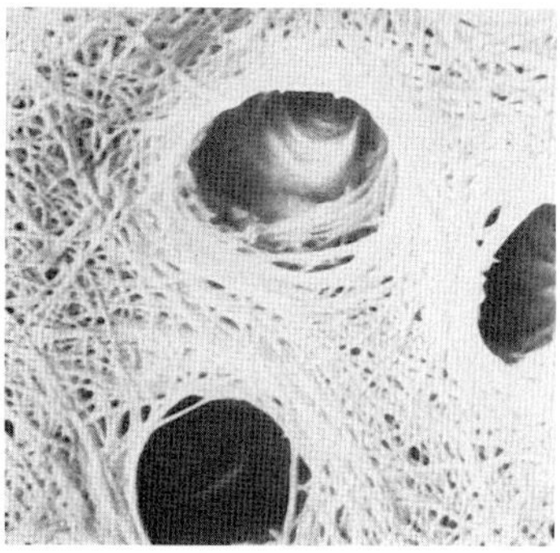

Fig. 3-46 Scanning electron micrograph of pulpal dentin showing calcifying collagen fiber surrounding tubules. (From Bhaskar, S.N. (Editor), Orban's Oral Histology and Embryology, 11th Ed., St. Louis: Mosby-Year Book,Inc., 1991, with permission)

Figs. 3-47a and b (From B.I. Suh, J. Esthet. Dent., 3 (4): 139-147, July-Aug. 1991, with permission.)

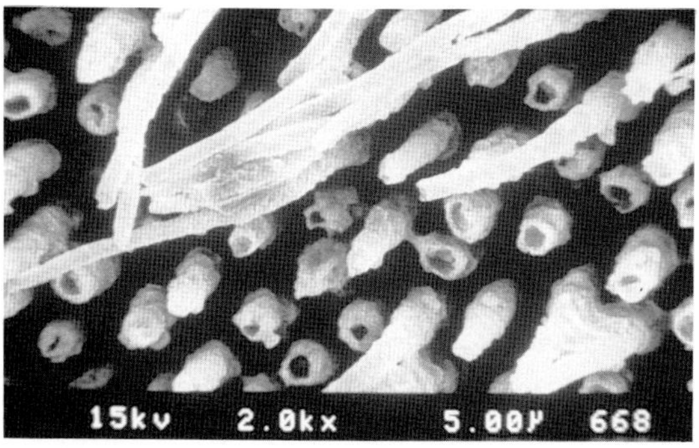

Fig. 3-47a In vitro resin tags extending into dentin tubules produced using the All Bond System (Bisco).

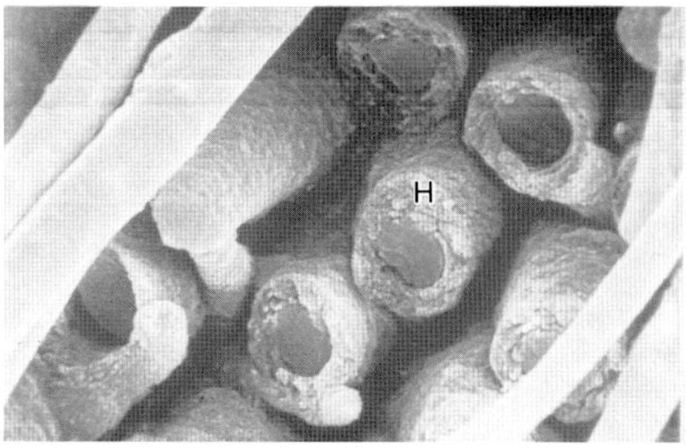

Fig. 3-47b Higher magnification shows a resin core surrounded by the dentin-resin hybrid layer (H).

promoters) include hydroxyethyl methacrylate (HEMA), pyromellitic diethylmethacrylate (PMDM), biphenyl dimethacrylate (BPDM), and N-tolglycine-glycidyl methacrylate (NTG-GMA) (Fig. 3-44).

Tags of primer resin (produced in vitro) extending into tubules can be visualized with scanning electron microscopy (Fig. 3-45). This appearance suggests that resin attachment to dentin is achieved through micromechanical interlocking similar to that seen in enamel-resin bonding (Nordenvall and Bränström, 1980). While such evidence indicates the degree of wetting in vitro, there exists some doubt as to the ability of resins to develop similar tags in vivo, where tubules are not empty. Nakabayashi (1982) first described a more plausible and now widely-accepted mechanism, referred to as the dentin-resin "hybrid layer." Conditioning of dentin removes apatite mineral, leaving a network of exposed collagen fibers (Fig. 3-46) and some remaining hydroxyapatite crystals. Hydrophilic resin primers diffuse into this network and entrap collagen and hydroxyapatite upon polymerization. A resin-reinforced layer of dentin, the hybrid layer, is thus produced. Observations of lower bond strengths in deeper dentin where intertubular dentin comprises a smaller fraction of the surface area lend support to this theory (Pashley, 1990). Nakabayashi has demonstrated this phenomenon with a single unique bonding agent system (4-META). Similar impregnation of conditioned intertubular dentin, however, has been demonstrated in many other third-generation systems (Erickson, 1989; Suh, 1991; Van Meerbeeck, et al., 1992, Inokoshi, et al., 1993) (Fig. 3-47).

Primers are supplied in a solvent, usually ethanol, acetone or water. Gentle but thorough air drying is necessary after primer application to eliminate all traces of solvent. Remaining solvent may interfere with bonding between primer and the subsequently applied adhesive resin.

In addition to effecting improved bonds to dentin, the primers described here have also been shown to improve the adhesion of composite resin to various restorative materials, including cast metal, porcelain and fresh or set amalgam. Dental adhesive systems are thus typically utilized in a wide variety of restorative techniques, including cementation and bonding of indirect restorations and repair of existing restorations. Accessory items such as porcelain etchants, silane and metal primers are often included with the basic system components. As a result, then, of the broadened range of applications for dental adhesives, current systems are commonly referred to as "multiple purpose adhesives."

Adhesive Resin

Unfilled methacrylate resins (Bis-GMA and urethane dimethacrylate, or UDMA) remain the agents of choice for application to conditioned/primed dentin and etched enamel. This component is commonly referred to as the "bonding agent" in many systems. Specific formulations vary from one system to the next. Variations are usually limited to addition of viscosity controllers such as TEG-DMA (triethylene glycol-dimethacrylate) and hydrophilic resins (e.g. HEMA) to improve wetting.

Copolymerization with the primer's exposed methacryl groups completes the sequential process of dentin-resin bonding. Adequate thickness of adhesive resin must be applied to prevent air inhibition of polymerization at the resin/primed dentin interface. Curing of the adhesive resin with visible light prior to placement of the restorative assures sufficient penetration of the light into the hybrid zone to produce thorough polymerization. This also renders the zone more resistant to possible disruption by polymerization shrinkage of the restorative resin. Optional agents containing chemical initiators can be mixed with the adhesive resin to convert it from light-cured to dual-cured. This additional mode of curing helps to insure complete polymerization beneath indirect restorations bonded with resin cement. Chemical adhesion between the adhesive resin and the composite restorative (or resin cement) occurs in the conventional manner described in "Bonding Resin to Enamel."

Some newer dental adhesive systems include an additional modification to the adhesive resin step. Specifically, a low-viscosity filled resin (40% to 50% by weight) is placed and cured prior to placement of the restorative material. This filled resin "liner" is either applied after the unfilled adhesive resin (as a fourth step in the bonding sequence) or is substituted for the adhesive resin, depending on the system being used. Use of a fluoride-containing filler in this component is thought to effect continued fluoride release after the restoration is completed. The filled liner may also act to reduce stresses at the tooth/restoration interface, as its modulus of elasticity value should lie between those of tooth and composite restorative. It should be noted, however, that these supposed benefits of a filled liner, as well as improvements in bond strength and microleakage, have yet to be demonstrated.

Classification of Systems

Considerable diversity exists among the current generation of adhesive systems, making classification difficult. Grouping according to the number of steps in the system (usually two or three) has been used. A more meaningful method groups systems according the dentin conditioning strategy employed. Van Meerbeek, et al. (1992) classified the available systems as follows: dentin adhesive systems that completely dissolve or remove the smear layer (most systems), those that partly dissolve the smear layer, and those that preserve or modify the smear layer. Systems in each classification will be described. It should be noted that tooth conditioning procedures in the technique descriptions usually refer to treatment of dentin only. Unless otherwise stated, separate etching of enamel with 37% to 40% H_3PO_4 is performed immediately prior to all dentin bonding sequences.

Results of *in vitro* tests measuring shear bond strengths to dentin are imported where available. It should be noted that currently such tests are not conducted using a standardized protocol. Experimental methods vary between investigators with respect to such aspects as freshness of and storage conditions for extracted teeth, storage time for bonded specimens and thermocycling procedure (if any). Such measurements nonetheless do provide a basis for comparison, provided that these factors are kept in mind. Additionally, *in vitro* test results do not fully reflect all factors (dentinal fluid, etc.) that affect bonding to teeth *in vivo*.

Dissolution or Removal of Smear Layer

Bowen, et al. (1982) described a system in which the smear layer is not only removed but also replaced. N-phenylglycine-glycidyl methacrylate (NPG-GMA), a hydrophilic resin, was thought to interact with the dentin surface via chelation. Acid conditioning, however, depleted the dentin surface of calcium ion needed for this interaction. Conditioning with a solution of dilute nitric acid (2.5%) and ferric oxalate removed the smear layer and replaced it with an insoluble precipitate. This "artificial smear layer" was more tightly bound to the dentin than the original, effectively sealed the tubules and was rich in metallic cations. Hydrophilic monomers NPG-GMA and PMDM were then mixed with acetone and applied separately. The system was subsequently modified, simplified and marketed as Tenure (DEN-MAT Corp.) (Fig. 3-48). Aluminum oxalate replaced ferric oxalate in the nitric acid conditioner due to marginal staining attributed to ferrous ions. Following rinsing off of the conditioner with water and air drying, acetone solutions of NTG-GMA (Tenure A) and PMDM (Tenure B) are mixed and applied to the conditioned dentin. Unfilled Bis-GMA resin is then placed and polymerized in the conventional manner.

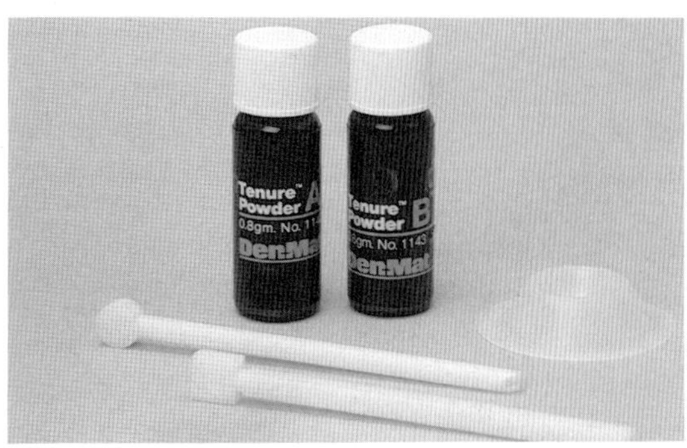

Fig. 3-48 Tenure (DEN-MAT), the first commercial adhesive based on Bowen's oxalate system.

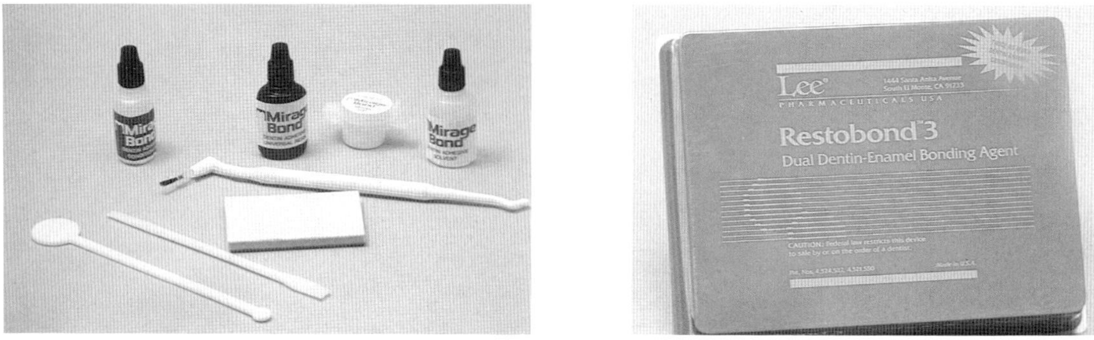

Figs. 3-49a and b Mirage Bond (Chameleon) and Restobond 3 (Lee) represent further modifications of Bowen's oxalate system.

Bond strengths to dentin of 18.1±5.4 MPa have been reported (Barkmeier, et al., 1990).

The chemistry of Mirage Bond (Chameleon) and Restobond 3 (Lee Pharmeceuticals) (Fig. 3-49) is derived from Bowen's oxalate system and represents a further modification of the system. No metallic oxalates are present in the conditioner, as it was found that oxalate elimination did not reduce bond strength. Additionally, N-phenylglycine (NPG) has been substituted for NTG-GMA and added to the conditioner (2.5% nitric acid and NPG). Solutions such as this, combining acidic conditioners and primer agents, are referred to as "self-etching primers." Conditioning, rinsing and drying is followed by application of 10% PMDM primer. Placement of Bis-GMA adhesive resin completes the process. Barkmeier and Cooley (1992) reported a bond strength to dentin of 15.5± 4.9 MPa using this system.

Adhesive By Choice (Chameleon) is the successor to Mirage Bond, and incorporates additional modifications designed to increase the system's versatility, and adapt it to the current trend of bonding to moist dentin. A nitric acid enamel/dentin conditioner (supplied) is applied with agitation and is not rinsed off, or 10% phosphoric acid etch of enamel and dentin may be employed as an option. With the dentin surface left moist, the two-component primer is mixed and applied in multiple coats. Primers A and B contain 5% NTG-GMA in acetone and 2% pyromellitic glycerol methacrylate (PM-GDM) in acetone, respectively. PM-GDM is an analog of PMDM, and is the reaction product of pyromellitic dianhydride and glycerol dimethacrylate. Venz and Dickens (1990) report a significant increase in bond strength with PM-GDM vs. PMDM. The adhesive resin base may then be applied alone and light-cured, or mixed with the catalyst to impart dual cure properties (for indirect restorations). Product literature indicates bond strength to dentin of 19.8 MPa (Knight, 1991).

Restobond 4 Multipurpose Bonding Agent (Lee Pharmeceuticals) represents a similar evolution of the Restobond 3 product. Enamel and dentin are conditioned simultaneously with a 2.5% solution of nitric acid, then rinsed and dried. The two-component primer now consists of PM-GDM ("Adhesive") and NTG-GMA ("Composite Activator"). The mixed primer is applied in multiple layers and dried. A light-cured unfilled resin is applied as a final step, and, according to manufacturer's instructions, may be cured simultaneously with the composite restorative material. The use of a dual cured resin is recommended for use in cementation of direct restorations, but is not supplied with the kit.

Scotchbond 2 (3M) (Fig. 3-50) is a two-

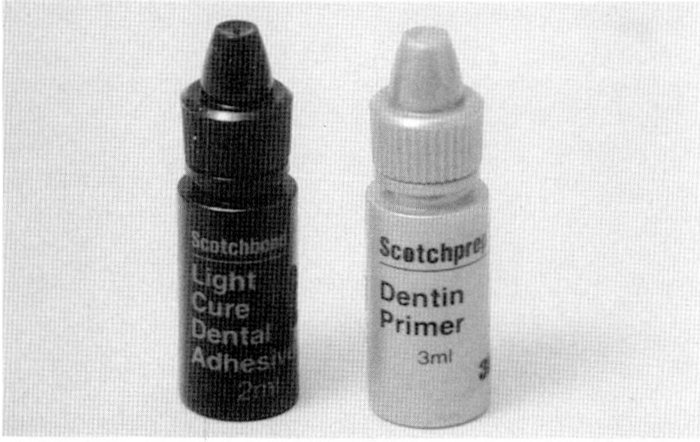

Fig. 3-50 Scotchbond 2 (3M) utilized a self-etching primer, eliminating a separate dentin conditioning step.

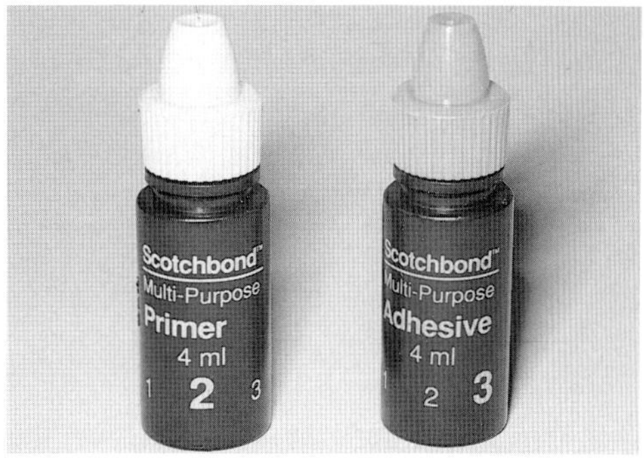

Fig. 3-51 The Scotchbond Multipurpose system (3M) contains a single component enamel-dentin conditioner. The manufacturer reports a lower film thickness than its predecessor, Scotchbond 2.

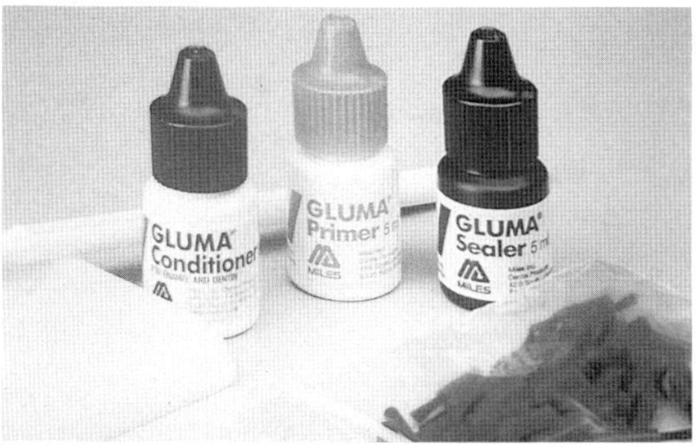

Fig. 3-52 Gluma (Bayer) is formulated with glutaraldehyde to chemically bond to tooth structure.

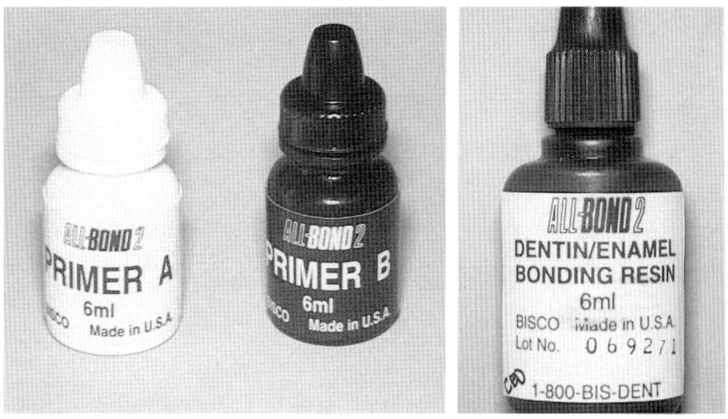

Fig. 3-53 All-Bond (Bisco) was the first system to include a phosphoric acid conditioner (10%) designed specifically for dentin.

step system, utilizing a self-etching primer composed of maleic acid and HEMA in an aqueous solution. Primer is placed on the dentin surface and air dried rather than rinsed off. It is designed to solubilize and dissolve the smear layer as well as to demineralize the dentin surface. Infiltration of HEMA into the dentin surface occurs simultaneously with these conditioning processes. A Bis-GMA/HEMA adhesive resin completes the technique. Barkmeier and Cooley (1992) reported a bond strength to dentin of 8.8 MPa using this system.

Scotchbond Multi-Purpose (3M) (Fig. 3-51) is the successor to Scotchbond 2. The first of three steps utilizes a aqueous 10% solution of maleic acid. It is described as a multipurpose etchant for use on both dentin and enamel, and contains a non silica thickener. The etchant has a liquid viscosity as the need for controlled placement, i.e. on enamel only, no longer exists. Recommended application time is 15 seconds, followed by rinsing and drying. Primer consists of aqueous solution of HEMA and the polyalkenoic copolymer used in Vitrabond. The copolymer is thought to reduce moisture sensitivity observed for other systems in conditions of high relative humidity. The adhesive resin again combines Bis-GMA and HEMA. A proprietary photoinitiator system is said by the manufacturer to reduce film thickness and cure time compared to the Scotchbond 2 resin. Bond strength to dentin of 24 MPa is reported in product literature.

Gluma (Miles/Bayer) (Fig. 3-52) was designed to adhere to dentin via chelation of calcium and chemical attachment to collagen. EDTA (ethylene diamine tetra acetic acid) is used as a conditioner and chelating agent. Glutaraldehyde is added to the hydrophilic resin primer HEMA to promote bonding to collagen. Resin bonding agent (Bis-GMA and triethylene glycol-glycidyl methacrylate, or TEG-GMA) completes this three-step process. Bonds to dentin of 10.0±4.2 MPa have been reported (Barkmeier and Cooley, 1989a).

Gluma 2000, consisting of only two solutions, is an updated and simplified version of the Gluma system. Solution 1 (1.6% oxalic acid, 2.6% aluminum nitrate and 2.7% glycine in water) is designed to simultaneously etch enamel and remove the dentinal smear layer. Application is followed by rinsing and drying. Solution 2 is a primer composed of mono and polyfunctional methacrylates in ethanol and water. After applying and drying, directions call for placement of composite, which then copolymerizes with the primer.

All-Bond 2 (Bisco, Inc.) (Fig. 3-53) is supplied with a choice of two dentin conditioners, and is thus classified twice according to the two respective modes of action. All-Bond 2 was the first system to provide 10% phosphoric acid gel for use as a dentin conditioner, rinsing and drying, a two-part silica thickening agents. After applying the conditioner, rinsing, and drying, a two-part dual-cure primer of NTG-GMA and biphenyl dimethacrylate (BPDM) is mixed and applied in multiple coats. Adhesive resin is composed of Bis-GMA, UDMA and HEMA. Bond strengths exceeding those commonly reported for enamel-resin (20 MPa) have been reported for this system. Barkmeier, et al. (1991) reported 14.7±4.3 MPa. Using a "wet bonding" technique, Kanca (1991) reported bond strengths of 29.34±4.09 MPa. In this technique, conditioned dentin is blot-dried rather than air-dried, leaving the surface visibly moist. Additional moisture is said to promote penetration of the hydrophilic primers into the conditioned dentin (Suh, 1991). Barkmeier, et al. (1991a) reported bond strengths exceeding 30 MPa when the wet technique was used. Samples in this study exhibited bond failure within the dentin itself (cohesive fracture of dentin). Van Meerbeek (1992), however, reported that a 7.5-μm zone of decalcified dentin was produced by 10% phosphoric acid that was impregnated with All-Bond 2 primer to a depth of 2.5 μm. While this level of resin penetration was the deepest of any system in the study, the longterm effect, if any, of the residual 5 μm of decalcified dentin on the integrity of dentin bond is unknown.

Powerbond (Cosmedent) bears some chemical similarity to All Bond 2; however, its two-component primer has no dual cure properties. It is supplied with both a light-cured and a dual cure adhesive resin, for use in direct and indirect restorations, respectively.

Nakabayashi's (1982) initial demonstration of the hybrid layer used the 4-META/MMA-TBB adhesive resin system. A substantially thick hybrid layer (5 μm) was observed. 4-META (5% 4-methacryloxyethyl trimellitate anhydride) is described as an adhesion promoter. Nakabayashi found that adding 4-META to methyl methacrylate (MMA) increases the diffusion of this resin into conditioned dentin. Tri-N-butyl borane (TBB) is an initiator that works in conjunction with water and oxygen. As both water and oxygen are abundant in dentin, TBB is said to effect a thorough polymerization of the infiltrated resin, with shrinkage in the direction of the dentin substrate. The conditioner in this system is 10% citric acid with 3% ferric chloride. The improvement in bond strength seen using this conditioner vs. citric acid alone is attributed to stabilization of collagen fibers with ferric ions. Collagen collapse following acid removal of supporting mineralization (Fig. 3-54) has been observed by other

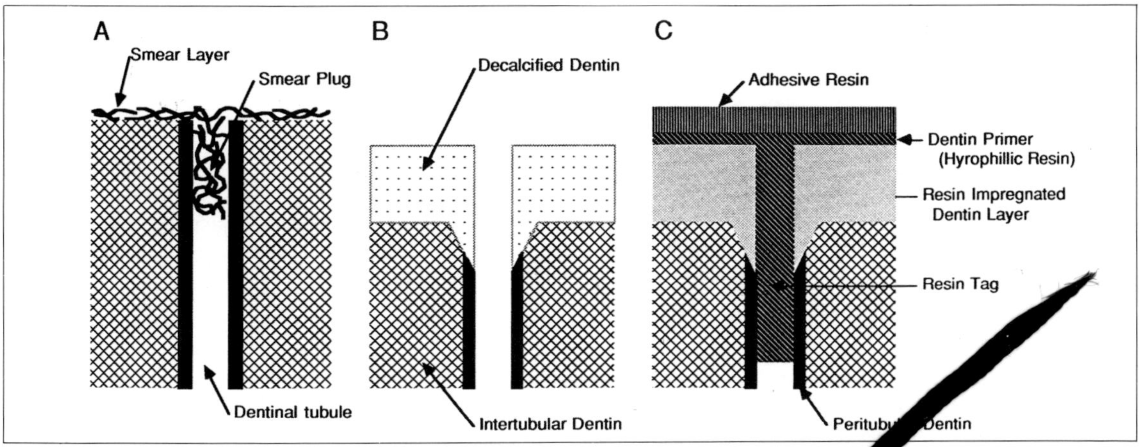

Fig. 3-54 The surface of cut dentin (A) has been observed in vitro to undergo shrinkage or collapse following demineralization produced by conditioning (B). The 4-META system theoretically minimizes collagen collapse, producing a wider layer of resin-impregnated dentin (hybrid layer) (C).

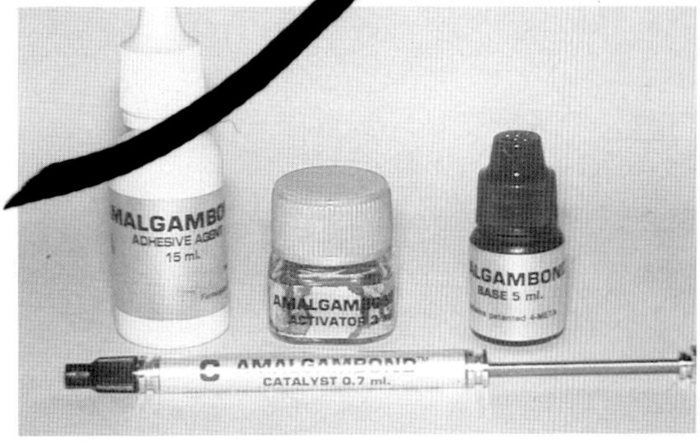

Fig. 3-55 Amalgambond (Parkell), a 4-META-based adhesive resin.

investigators (Van Meerbeek, et al., 1992). By preventing fiber collapse and the resultant shrinkage of the conditioned surface, infiltration of the resin is facilitated. The 4-META/MMA-TBB system is marketed as Amalgambond (Parkell) (Fig. 3-55), which contains conditioner and primer. Cooley, et al. (1992) reported bond strengths of resin to dentin of 21 MPa when using this material. Also available is a luting agent version, which involves mixing the 4-META and TBB liquids with polymethylmethacrylate (PMMA) powder (C&B Metabond, Parkell).

The Clearfil Liner Bond System (Kuraray Co., Ltd.) uses a conditioning solution of 10% citric acid and 20% calcium chloride to condition both enamel and dentin. After rinsing, N-methacryloyl-5-aminosalicylic acid (NMSA) primer is applied. This monomer, a salicylic acid derivative, is designed to promote adhesion to collagen. Adhesive resin (Clearfil Photobond Resin) is then applied. This resin combines Bis-GMA, HEMA and 10-methacryloyloxy decyl dihydrogenphosphate (MDP), an adhesion promoter unique to Kuraray adhesive resins. A fourth step involves placement and polymerization of a microfilled resin liner prior to restorative placement. This liner (Clearfil Protect Liner) has low viscosity and is 42% filled by weight. Barkmeier and Cooley (1992) report bond strengths to dentin of 17.5±6.0 MPa.

The Denthesive System (Kulzer) is designed to bond chemically to both the hydroxyapatite and collagen components of dentin. An EDTA conditioner is used to remove the smear layer. The two-component primer consists of Di-HEMA phosphate (a HEMA derivative) and a functional maleic acid ester (mono-methacryloyloxyethylmaleat or

MMEM). A UDMA bonding resin containing 42% (by weight) silanized microfiller is applied and polymerized as the third and final step. Barkmeier and Cooley (1992) report bond strengths to dentin of 11.6±5.9 MPa.

Syntac (Ivoclar-Vivadent) is supplied with a self-etching primer that contains maleic acid (4%) and TEG-DMA in acetone. Thus, no dentin conditioner is used. After application and drying of the primer, two adhesive resins are applied. The first, referred to in the system as "Adhesive," contains glutaraldehyde (5%) and polyethylene glycol-dimethacrylate in water. Following air drying of the adhesive, Heliobond unfilled resin (Bis-GMA and TEG-DMA) is applied and light-cured. For indirect restorations, the Heliobond step is omitted. Gwinnett, et al. (1992) reported shear bond strengths to dentin of approximately 20 MPa.

Optibond (Kerr) succeeds the XR Bond system described later in this chapter. The components are designed for applicability to many direct and indirect restorative situations. The primer is a single-component light-cured material, containing HEMA, glycerol phosphate dimethacrylate (GPDM) and mono(2-methacryloxy ethyl)phthalate (PAMM) in ethanol and water. If the dentin has not been "etched" with phosphoric acid, a "scrubbing" mode of primer application is used to dissolve the smear layer. Following light curing of the primer, adhesive resin (TEG-DMA, UDMA, and GPDM) is applied. For larger restorations and indirect restorations, a two-component dual cure layer is used instead of the adhesive resin. The mixed dual cure material, containing Bis-GMA, HEMA, fumed silica and fluoride-containing glass, is 48% filled by weight.

The A.R.T. (Advanced Retention Technology) Bond (Coltene/Whaledent) system, like Scotchbond 2 and Syntac, does not utilize a dentin conditioner. The two-component primer is designed to demineralize the smear layer during its application. The mixed primer contains maleic acid, sodium fluoride, HEMA and other methacrylate and maleic acid derivatives. The adhesive resin, primarily Bis-GMA and TEG-DMA, contains maleic acid as well. Directions call for priming and bonding of the dentin prior to etching and bonding of enamel, in a manner similar to that described for Imperva Bond (later in this chapter).

Partial Dissolution of Smear Layer

XR-Bond (Kerr) (Fig. 3-56) is a two-step system that does not include a dentin conditioner. The primer is a 3.75% solution of a phosphonated dimethacrylate ester. It is acidic enough, however, to at least partially dissolve smear debris or essentially remove it in thin areas. A photoiniator is also added to the primer. This solution is not a self-etching primer as it does not contain acidic conditioner, nor does it produce the same surface effects on dentin as these agents. The adhesive resin combines UDMA, TEG-DMA and the phosphonated dimethacrylate ester. Bond strengths to dentin of 15.6± 3.1 MPa have been reported (Barkmeier and Cooley, 1989b). The successor to this system, Optibond, is described earlier in this chapter.

Imperva Bond (Shofu) is designed to produce chelation with and hydrogen bonding to moist dentin. According to the manufacturer, the primer eliminates the need for conditioning of the dentin, as it removes the smear layer, but leaves behind plugs or "caps" of smear debris occluding the tubules. Overconditioning, i.e. demineralization to a depth to which the primer is unable to penetrate, is thus avoided. Directions included with the system, however, state that acid conditioning of the dentin may be performed if desired. Two optional techniques are thus described. In the "3-Step" technique, enamel etching, or etching of both enamel and dentin, is done prior to primer application. In the "4-Step" technique, primer is applied first to protect the dentin during the etching of enamel. The

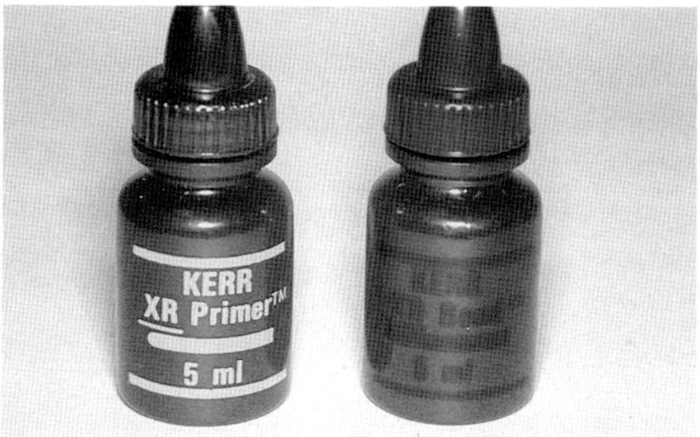

Fig. 3-56 XR-Bond (Kerr) partially dissolves, but does not remove, the smear layer.

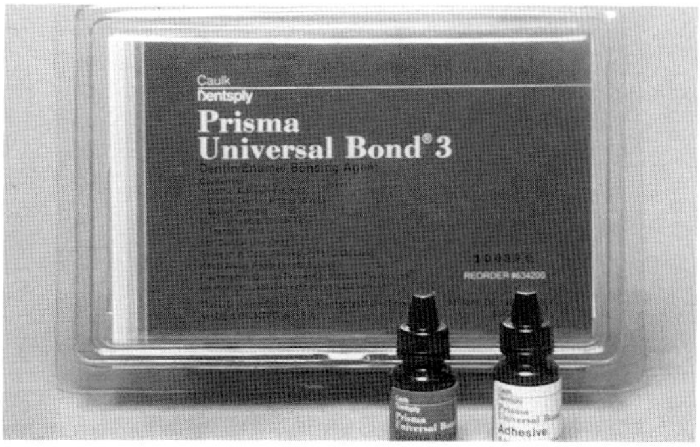

Fig. 3-57 Universal Bond 3 (Prisma) is designed to penetrate the smear layer and bond to the underlying dentin substrate.

single-component primer contains HEMA, silane and acryloxyethyltrimeric acid, in water. It is applied with agitation, air-dried and light-cured. The UDMA adhesive resin also contains the components of the primer. Shear bond strengths (to bovine dentin at 24 hours) of 20 MPa have been reported by the manufacturer.

Preservation or Modification of Smear Layer

All-Bond 2 (Bisco, Inc.), when used with the 20% SA-HEMA (succinic anhydride-hydroxyethyl methacrylate) conditioner, falls into this category. This conditioner, applied and airdried, is weakly acidic and only modifies the smear layer, probably increasing its permeability and reducing its surface tension. The remainder of the technique is identical to that described using the 10% phosphoric acid conditioner. Barkmeier, et al. (1991b) reported bonds to dentin of 14.7±4.3 MPa using this technique.

The Prisma Universal Bond 3 System (Fig. 3-57) does not utilize a conditioner and is the only third-generation system that does not significantly alter the smear layer. The primer is an ethanol solution of 30% HEMA and 6% phosphonated penta-acrylate ester (PENTA). PENTA is described as an adhesion promoter and probably produces slight demineralization of the smear layer, allowing better penetration of the primer into the smear layer. The adhesive resin consists of UDMA, TEG-GMA, PENTA and glutaraldehyde (added to promote bonding to collagen). Barkmeier and Cooley (1992) reported bond strengths to dentin of 18.6±5.3 MPa.

It is significant to note that Van Meerbeek, et al. (1992) reported seeing no hybrid layer for adhesive systems such as these that did not completely remove the smear layer.

REFERENCES

EARLY DEVELOPMENT

Albers, H.F.: Tooth Colored Restoratives (A Text for Selection, Placement and Finishing) (Seventh Edition). (1985). Santa Rosa: Alto Books.

Berglund, A.: Estimation by a 24-hour Study of the Daily Dose of Intra-Oral Mercury Vapor Inhaled After Release from Dental Amalgam. (1990). J. Dent. Res. 69:1646-1651.

Charbeneau, G.T.: Principles and Practice of Operative Dentistry (Third Edition). (1988). Philadelphia: Lea & Febiger.

Craig, R.G.: Restorative Dentals Materials (Ninth Edition). (1993). St. Louis: Mosby-Year Book, Inc.

Fletcher, T.: Fletcher's Patent Porcelain Cement. (1878). Brit. J. Dent. Sci. 21:97-99.

Goldwater, L.J.: Mercury in Dentistry. (1991). Clin. Toxicol. 29: 151-164.

Hoffmann-Axthelm, W.: History of Dentistry. (1981). Chicago: Quintessence.

Joynt, R.B., Wieczkowski, G., Jr., Klockowski, R., and Davis L.: Effects of Composite Restorations on Resistance to Cuspal Fracture in Posterior Teeth. (1987). J. Prosthet. Dent. 57: 431-435.

Landro Olstad, M., Holland, R.I., and Hensten Pettersen, A.: Effect of Placement of Amalgam Restorations on Urinary Mercury Concentration. (1990). J. Dent. Res. 69:1607-1609.

Mackert, J.R.: Dental Amalgam and Mercury. (1991). J. Am. Dent. Assoc. 122:54-61.

Morin, D., DeLong, R., and Douglas, W.H.: Cusp Reinforcement by he Acid-Etch Technique. (1984). J. Dent. Res. 63:1075-1078.

Newman, S.M.L.: Amalgam Alternatives: What Can Compete? (1991): J. Am. Dent. Assoc. 122:67-71.

Paffenbarger, G.C.: Silicate Cement: An Investigation by a Group of Practicing Dentists under the Direction of the A.D.A. Research Fellowship at the National Bureau of Standards. (1940). J. Am. Dent. Assoc. 27:1611-1622.

Ring, M.E.: Dentistry: An Illustrated History. (1985). St. Louis: The C.V. Mosby Co.

Simonsen, R.J., Barovch, E., and Gelb, M.: Cusp Fracture Resistance From Composite Resin in Class II Restorations. (1983). J. Dent. Res. 62 (AADR Abstracts): 297 (Abstract No. 1154).

Skinner, E.W.: Comparison of the Properties and Uses of Silicate Cement and Acrylic Resin in Operative Dentistry. (1959). J. Am. Dent. Assoc. 58:27-36.

Stampalia, L.L., Nichols, J.I., Brudvik, J.S., and Jones, D.W.: Fracture Resistance of Teeth with Resin-Bonded Restorations. (1986). J. Prosth. Dent. 55:694-698.

Sturdevant, C.M., Barton, R.E., Sockwell, C.L., and Strickland, W.D.: The Art and Science of Operative Dentistry (Second Edition). (1985). St. Louis: The C.V. Mosby Co.

Wendt, S.L., Jr.: Microleakage and Cusp Fracture Resistance of Heat-Treated Composite Resin Inlays. (1991). Am. J. Dent. 4:10-14.

COMPOSITE RESINS

Albers, H.F.: Tooth Colored Restoratives (A Text for Selection, Placement and Finishing) (Seventh Edition). (1985). Santa Rosa: Alto Book.

Asmussen, E.: Factors Affecting the Quantity of Remaining Double Bonds in Restorative Resin Polymer. (1982). Scand. J. Dent. Res. 90:490-496.

Asmussen, E.: Restorative Resins: Hardness and Strength vs. Quantity of Remaining Double Bonds. (1982). Scand. J. Dent. Res. 90:484-489.

Baharav, H., Abraham, D., Cardash, H.S., and Helft, M.: Effect of Exposure Time on the Depth of Polymerization of a Visible Light-Cured Composite Resin. (1988). J. Oral. Rehab. 15: 167-172.

Barkmeier, W.W. and Cooley, R.L.: Evaluation of Surface Finish of Microfilled Resins. (1989). J. Esth. Dent. 1:139-143.

Berastegui, E., Canalda, C., Brau, E., and Miquel, C.: Surface Roughness of Finished Composite Resins. (1992). J. Prosth. Dent. 68:742-749.

Berastegui, E., Canalda, C., Braw, E., and Miquel, C.: Surface Roughness of Finished Composite Resins. (1992). J. Prosth. Dent. 68:742-749.

Birdsell, D.C., et al.: Harmful Effects of a Near Ultraviolet Radiation used for polymerization of a Sealant and a Composite Resin. (1977). J. Am. Dent. Assoc. 94:311-314.

Bowen, R.L.: Synthesis of a Silica-Resin Direct Filling Material. (1958). J. Dent. Res. 37:90.

Bowen, R.L.: Development of a Silica-Resin Direct Filling Material. (1959). Washington: National Bureau of Standards, Report 6333.

Bowen, R.L.: Dental Filling Material Comprising Vinyl-Silane Treated Fused Silica and a Ginder consisting of the reaction product of GB-phenol and glycidyl acrylate. (1962). U.S. Patent 3,006,112, November 27.

Bowen, R.L.: Properties of a Silica-Reinforced Direct Polymer for Dental Restorations. (1963). J. Am. Dent. Assoc. 66:71-78.

Charbeneau, G.T.: Principles and Practice of Operative Dentistry (Third Edition). (1988). Philadelphia: Lea & Febiger.

Cook, W.D.: Factors Affecting Depth of Cure of UV Polymerized Composites. (1980). J. Dent. Res. 59:800-808.

Council on Dental Materials, Instruments, and Equipment: Visible Light-Cured Composites and Activating Units. (1985). J. Am. Dent. Assoc. 110:100-103.

Craig, R.G.: Restorative Dentals Materials (Ninth Edition). (1993). St. Louis: Mosby-Year Book, Inc.

Dennison, J.B. and Craig, E.G.: Physical properties and Finished Surface Texture of Composite Restorative Resins. (1972). J. Am. Dent. Assoc. 85:101-108.

Fan, P.L. and Powers, J.M.: In Vitro Wear of Aged Composite Restorative Materials. (1980). J. Dent. Res. 69:2066-2070.

Fan, P.L., Powers, J.M., and Craig, R.G.: In Vitro Wear of Microfilled and Visible Light-Cured Composites. (1979). J. Dent. Res. 58:2116-2119.

Helvatjoglov-Antoniadi, M., Papadogianis, Y., Koliniotov-Kubia, E., and Kubias, S.: Surface Hardness of Light-Cured and Self-Cured Composite Resins. (1991). J. Prosth. Dent. 65:215-220.

Jeffries, S.R., Smith, R.L., Barkmeier, W.W., and Gwinnett, A.J.: Comparison of Surface Smoothness of Restorative Resin Materials. (1989). J. Esth. Dent. 1:169-175.

Kusy, R.P. and Leinfelder, K.F.: Pattern of wear in Posterior Composite Restorations. (1977): J. Dent. Res. 56:544.

Lambrechts, P., Braem, M., and Venherle, G.: Evaluation of Clinical Performance for Posterior Composite Resins and Dentin Adhesives. (1987). Oper. Dent. 12:53-78.

Leung, R.L., Fan, P.L., and Johnston, W.M.: Post-Irradiation Polymerization of Visible Light-Activated Composite Resin. (1983): J. Dent. Res. 62:363-365.

Lewis, G.: In Vivo Occlusal Wear of Posterior Composite Restorations. (1991). Oper. Dent. 16:61-69.

Lutz, F., Imfeld, T., Meier, C., and Firestone, A.R.: Composites Versus Amalgam — Comparative Measurements of In Vivo wear resistance: 1-Year Report. (1979). Quint. Int. 10(3):77-87.

Lutz, F., Phillips, R.W., Roulet, J.F., and Setcos, J.C.: In Vivo and In Vitro wear of Potential Posterior Composites. (1984). J. Dent. Res. 63:914-920.

McCabe, J.F. and Carrick, T.E.: Output from Visible-Light Activation Units and Depth of Cure of Light-Activated Composites. (1989). J. Dent. Res. 68:1534-1539.

Mills, L.F. and Anderson, F.A.: Ultraviolet and Microwave Radiation in Dentistry. (1981). Gen. Dent. 29:481-486.

O'Brien, W.J. and Yee, J.: Microstructure of Posterior Restorations of Composite Resin after Clinical Wear. (1980). Oper. Dent. 5:90-94.

Resin Cements, in Reality (Miller, MB, Ed.-in-Chief). (1992). Vol. 7, No. 2. Houston: Reality Publishing Co.

Roulet, J.F.: Degradation of Dental Polymers. (1987). Basel: S. Karger AG.

Saguchi, R.L., Douglas, W.H., and Peters, M.C.: Curing Light Performance and Polymerization of Composite Restorative Materials. (1992). J. Dent. 20:178-182.

Saguchi, R.L., Peters, M.C., Nelson, S.R., and Douglas, W.H., Poort H.W.: Effects of Polymerization Contraction in Composite Restorations. (1992). J. Dent. 20:178-182.

Seghi, R.R., Gritz, M.D., and Kim, J.: Colorimetric Changes in Composites Resulting From Visible Light-Initiated Polymerization. (1990). Dent. Mater. 6:133-137.

Sturdevant, C.M., Barton, R.E., Sockwell, C.L., and Strickland, W.D.: The Art and Science of Operative Dentistry (Second Edition). (1985). St. Louis: The C.V. Mosby Co.

3M Restorative Z100 Product Profile. (1992). St. Paul (Minn.): Dental Products Division, 3M Health Care.

Wilder, A.D., May, K.N., and Leinfelder, K.F.: Three-Year Clinical Study of UV cured composite resins in Posterior Teeth. (1983). J. Prosth. Dent. 50:26-30.

GLASS IONOMERS

Albers, H.F.: Tooth Colored Restoratives (A Text for Selection, Placement and Finishing) (Seventh Edition). (1985). Santa Rosa: Alto Books.

Causton, B., Sefton, J., and Williams, A.: Bonding Class II Composite to Etched Glass Ionomer Cement. (1986). Br. Dent. J. 163:321-324.

Charbeneau, G.T.: Principles and Practice of Operative Dentistry (Third Edition). (1988). Philadelphia: Lea & Febiger.

Cooley, R.L. and Barkmeier, W.W.: Dentinal Shear Bond Strength, Microleakage, and Contraction Gap of Visible Light Polymerized Liners/Bases. (1991). Quint. Int. 22:467-474.

Coury, T.L., Miranda, F.J., Willer, R.D., and Probst, R.T.: Adhesiveness of Glass Ionomer Cement to Enamel and Dentin: A Laboratory Study. (1982). Oper. Dent. 7:2-6.

Craig, R.G.: Restorative Dentals Materials (Ninth Edition). (1993). St. Louis: Mosby-Year Book, Inc.

DeSchepper, E.J., Berry, E.A., Cailleteau, J.G., and Tate, W.H.: Fluoride Release From Light-Cured Liners. (1990). Am. J. Dent. 3:97-100.

Garcia-Godoy, F.: Glass Ionomer Materials in Class II Composite Restorations: To Etch or Not to Etch? (1988). Quint. Int. 19(3): 241-242.

Hewlett, E.R., Caputo, A.A., and Wrobel, D.C.: Glass Ionomer Bond Strength and Treatment of Dentin with Polyacrylic Acid. (1991). J. Prosth. Dent. 66:767-772.

Hösted-Bindslev, P. and Larsen, M.J.: Release of Fluoride from Light Cured Lining Materials. (1991). Scand. J. Dent. Res. 99: 86-88.

McComb, D., Sirisko, R., and Brown, J.: Comparison of Physical Properties of Commercial Glass Ionomer Luting Cements. (1984). J. Can. Dent. Assn. 9:699-701.

McLean, J.W.: Glass Cermet Cements. (1985). Quint. Int. 16(5): 333-343.

McLean, J.W.: The Use of Glass Ionomers in Bonding Composite Resins to Dentin. (1985). Br. Dent. J. 158:410-414.

McLean, J.W., Wilson, A.D., and Prosser, H.J.: Development and Use of Water-Hardening Glass-Ionomer Luting Cements. (1984). J. Prosth. Dent. 52:175-181.

Mount, G.: The Use of Glass Ionomer Cements in Clinical Practice. (1982). Dental Outlook 8(3):37-65.

Scheper, W. and Barnes, D.: Visible Light-Activated Glass Ionomer Cement: Use of Liners/Bases and Restoratives. (1992). Practical Periodon. Aesthetic Dent. 4:27-30.

Shortall, A.C.: In Vitro Microleakage of Class V Composite Resin Restorations With and Without Light-Cured Glass-Ionomer (Poly Alkenoate) Cement Lining. (1992). Eur. J. Prosthodont. Restor. Dent. 1:7-11.

Sidhu, S.K. and Henderson, L.J.: In Vitro Marginal Leakage of Cervical Composite Restorations Lined With a Light-Cured Glass Ionomer. (1992). Oper. Dent. 17:7-12.

Simmons, J.J.: Post-Cementation Sensitivity Commonly Associated with the "Anhydrous" Forms of Glass Ionomer Luting Cements: A Theory. (1986). Tex. Dent. J. 103:7-8.

Smith, D.C.: Polyacrylic Acid-based Cements: Adhesion to Enamel and Dentin. (1992). Oper. Dent. Supplement. 5:177-183.

Smith, D.C. and Ruse, N.D.: Acidity of Glass Ionomer Cements during Setting and its Relation to Pulp Sensitivity. (1986). J. Am. Dent. Assoc. 112:654-657.

Tam, L.E., McComb, D., and Pulver, F.: Physical Properties of Proprietary Light-Cured Lining Materials. (1991). Oper. Dent. 16:210-217.

Thornton, J.B., Retief, D.H., and Bradley, E.L.: Fluoride Release From and Tensile Bond Strength of Ketac-Fil and Ketac-Silver to Enamel and Dentin. (1986). Dent. Mater. 2:241-245.

Tjan, A.H. and Dunn, J.R.: Microleakage at Gingival Dentin Margins of Class V Composite Restorations Lined With Light-Cured Glass Ionomer Cement. (1990). J. Am. Dent. Assoc. 121: 706-710.

Walls, A.W.G., Adamson, J., McCabe, J.F., and Murray, J.J.: The Properties of a Glass Polyalkenoate (Ionomer) Cement Incorporating Sintered Metallic Particles. Dent. Mater. 3:113-116.

Wilson, A.D. and Kent B.E.: A New Translucent Cement for Dentistry. (1972). Br. Dent. J. 132:133-135.

Wilson, A.D. and McLean, J.W.: Glass Ionomer Cement. (1988). Chicago: Quintessence Publ. Co.

Wong, T.C.C. and Bryant, R.W.: Glass Ionomer Cements: Some Factors in Film Thickness. (1986). Austral. Dent. J. 31:81-85.

RESIN ADHESION TO TOOTH STRUCTURE

Albers, H.F.: Tooth Colored Restoratives (A Text for Selection, Placement and Finishing) (Seventh Edition). (1985). Santa Rosa: Alto Books.

Asmussen, E.: Clinical Relevance of Physical, Chemical and Bonding Properties of Composite Resins. (1985). Oper. Dent. 10: 61-73.

Asmussen, E. and Munksgaard, E.C.: Bonding of Restorative Resins to Dentine: Status of Dentin Adhesives and Impact on Cavity Design and Filling Techniques. (1988). Int. Dent. J. 38:97-104.

Asmussen, E. and Uno, S.: Adhesion of Restorative Resins to Dentin: Chemical and Physiochemical Aspects. (1992). Oper. Dent. Supplement 5:68-74.

Barkmeier, W.W. and Cooley, R.L.: Resin Adhesive Systems: In Vitro Evaluation of Dentin Bond Strength and Marginal Microleakage. (1989a). J. Esth. Dent. 1:67-72.

Barkmeier, W.W. and Cooley, R.L.: Shear Bond Strength, Microleakage, and SEM Study of the XR Bond Adhesive System. (1989b). Am. J. Dent. 2:263-265.

Barkmeier, W.W. and Cooley, R.L.: Laboratory Evaluation of Adhesive Systems. (1992). Oper. Dent. Supplement 5:50-61.

Barkmeier, W.W., Cooley, R.L., and Douville, C.J.: Adhesive Resin Bond Strength to Dentin and Ni-Cr-Be Alloy. (1991b). J. Dent. Res. 70 Special Issue (IADR Abstracts): 526 (Abstract No. 2076).

Barkmeier, W.W., Huang, C.T., Jefferies, S.R., and Hammesfahr, P.D.: Bond Strength, Microleakage, and Scanning Electron Microscopy Examination of the Prisma Universal Bond 2 Adhesive System. (1990). J. Esth. Dent. 2:134-139.

Barkmeier, W.W., Suh, B.I., and Cooley, R.L.: Shear Bond Strength to Dentin and Ni-Cr-Be Alloy with All-Bond Universal Adhesive System. (1991a). J. Esth. Dent. 3:148-153.

Benediktsson, S.: Masters Thesis. (1991). Department of Oral Biology, University of Alabama at Birmingham.

Bertolotti, R.L.: Acid Etching of Dentin. Letters to the Editor. (1990). Quint. Int. 21:77-78.

Bertolotti, R.L.: Total Etch-The Rational Dentin Bonding Protocol. (1991a). J. Esth. Dent. 3:1-6.

Bertolotti, R.L.: Posterior Composite Technique Utilizing Directed Polymerization Shrinkage and a Novel Matrix. (1991b). Prac. Periodont. and Aesthetic Dent. 3:53-58.

Bhaskar, S.N. (Ed.): Dentin (Chap. 4) in: Orban's Oral Histology and Embryology. (1991). St. Louis: Mosby-Year Book, Inc.

Bowen, R.L. and Marjenhoff, W.A.: Development of an Adhesive Bonding System. (1992). Oper. Dent. Supplement 5:75-80.

Bowen, R.L., Cobb, E.N., and Rapson, J.E.: Adhesive Bonding of Various Materials to Hard Tooth Tissues: Improvement in Bond Strength to Dentin. (1982). J. Dent. Res. 61:1070-1076.

Bowen, R.L., Eick, J.D., Henderson, D.A., and Anderson, D.W.: Smear Layer: Removal of Bonding Considerations. (1984). Oper. Dent. Supplement 3:30-34.

Bränström, M.: Dentin and Pulp in Restorative Dentistry. (1982). London: Wolfe Medical Publishers.

Bränström, M. and Nordenvall, K.J.: The Effect of Acid Etching on Enamel, Dentin, and the Inner Surface of Resin Restoration: A Scanning Electron Microscopic Investigation. (1977). J. Dent. Res. 56:917-923.

Bränström, M. and Vojinović, O.: Response of the Dental Pulp to Invasions of Bacteria Around Three Filling Materials. (1977). J. Dent. Child. 43:15-21.

Browne, R.M. and Tobias, R.S.: Microbial Microleakage and Pulpal Inflammation. (1986). Endodon. Dent. Traumatol. 2: 177-183.

Buonocore, M.G.: A Simple Method of Increasing the Adhesion of Acrylic Filling Materials to Enamel Surfaces. (1955). J. Dent. Res. 34:849-853.

Chan, D.C.N. and Jensen, M.E.: Dentin Permeability to Phosphoric Acid: Effect of Treatment with Bonding Resin. (1986). Dent. Mater. 2:251-256.

Charbeneau, G.T.: Principles and Practice of Operative Dentistry (Third Edition). (1988). Philadelphia: Lea & Febiger.

Cooley, R.L., Barkmeier, W.W., and Evans, J.G.: Shear bond Strengths of Resin Adhesive Cements to Dentin and Ni-Cr-Be Alloy. (1992). J. Esth. Dent. 4:117-120.

Cox, C.F., Keall, C.L., Keall, H.J., Ostro, E., and Bergenholtz, T.: Biocompatibility of Surface Sealed Dental Materials Against Exposed Pulps. (1987). J. Prosth. Dent. 57:1-8.

Craig, R.G.: Restorative Dentals Materials (Ninth Edition). (1993). St. Louis: Mosby-Year Book, Inc.

Dental Adhesives in Reality (Miller, MB, Ed.-in-Chief). (1992). Vol. 7, No. 2. Houston: Reality Publishing Co.

Dental Adhesives in Reality Now (Miller, MB, Ed.-in-Chief). (1992). October, No. 38. Houston: Reality Publishing Co.

Dental Adhesives in Reality Now (Miller, MB, Ed.-in-Chief). (1992). November, No. 39. Houston: Reality Publishing Co.

Dental Adhesives in Reality Now (Miller, MB, Ed.-in-Chief). (1993). February, No. 41. Houston: Reality Publishing Co.

Dental Adhesives in Reality Now (Miller, MB, Ed.-in-Chief). (1993). March, No. 42. Houston: Reality Publishing Co.

Eick, J.D., Wilko, R.A., Anderson, C.H., and Sorensen, S.E.: Scanning Electron Microscopy of Cut Tooth Surfaces and Identification of Debris by Use of the Electron Microscope. (1970). J. Dent. Res. 49:1359-1368.

Erickson, R.L.: Mechanism and Clinical Implications of Bond Formation for Two Dentin Bonding Agents. (1989). Am. J. Dent. 2:117-123.

Erickson, R.L.: Surface Interactions of Dentin Adhesive Materials. (1992). Oper. Dent. Supplement 5:81-94.

Eriksen, H.M. and Leidal, T.I.: Monkey Pulpal Response to Composite Resin Restorations in Cavities Treated with various Cleansing Agents. (1979). Scand. J. Dent. Res. 87:309-317.

Fusayama, T., Nakamura, T., Kurosaki, N., and Iwaku, M.: Non-Pressure Adhesion of a New Adhesive Restorative Resin. (1979). J. Dent. Res. 58:1364-1370.

Gwinnett, A.J.: Smear Layer: Morphological Considerations. (1984). Oper. Dent. Supplement 3:3-12.

Gwinnett, A.J.: Structure and Composition of Enamel. (1992). Oper. Dent. Supplement 5:10-17.

Gwinnett A.J., Dickerson W.G., and Yu S.: Dentin Bond Shear Strength and Microleakage for Syntac/Heliomolar: A Comparison Between the Manufacturer's and Total Etch Technique. (1992). J. Esth. Dent. 4:164-168.

Hosoda, H. and Fusayama, T.: A Tooth Substance Saving Restorative Technique. (1984). Int. Dent. J. 34:1-12.

Inokoshi, S., Hosoda, H., Harnirattisai, C., and Shimada, Y.: Interfacial Structure Between Dentin and Seven Dentin Bonding Systems Revealed Using Argon Ion Beam Etching. (1993). Oper. Dent. 18:8-16.

Kanca, J. III: Effect of Dentin Drying on Bond Strength. (1991). J. Dent. Res. 70 Special Issue (IADR Abstracts): 394 (Abstract No. 1029).

Knight, G.T.: Unpublished Data. (1991). University of Texas at San Antonio.

Macko, D.L., Rutberg, M., and Langeland, K.: Pulpal Response to the Application of Phosphoric Acid to Dentin. (1978). Oral Surg. Oral Med. Oral Pathol. 45:930-946.

Nakabayashi, N.: Resin Reinforced Dentin Due to Infitration of Monomers Into the Dentine at the Adhesive Interface. (1982). J. Japanese Soc. Dent. Mater. Devices 1:78-81.

Nakabayashi, N.: Adhesive Bonding with 4-META. (1992). Oper. Dent. Supplement 5:125-130.

Nakabayashi, N., Nakamura, M., and Yasuda, N.: Hybrid Layer as a Dentin Bonding Mechanism. (1991). J. Esth. Dent. 3: 133-138.

Nordenvall, K.-J. and Bränström, M.: In Vivo Resin Impregnation of Dentinal Tubules. (1980). J. Prosth. Dent. 44:630-637.

Pashley, D.H.: Smear Layer: Physiological Considerations. (1984). Oper. Dent. Supplement 3:13-29.

Pashley, D.H.: Interactions of Dental Materials with Dentin; in Setcos, J.C. (editor). Transactions of the Academy of Dental Research, Vol. 3. (1990). Chicago: Academy of Dental Materials. 55-73.

Pashley, D.H., Horner, J.A., and Brewer, P.D.: Interactions of Conditions on the Dentin Surface. (1992). Oper. Dent. Supplement 5:137-150.

Pashley, E.L., Tao, L., Derkson, G., and Pashley, D.H.: Dentin Permeability and Bond Strength After Various Surface Treatments. (1988). J. Dent. Res. 67 Special Issue (IADR Abstracts): 196 (Abstract No. 664)

Roulet, J.F.: Degradation of Dental Polymers. (1987). Basel: S. Karger AG.

Scotchbond Technical Product Profile. (1992). St. Paul (Minn.): Dental Products Division, 3M Health Care.

Shintani, H., Satou, N., and Satou, J.: Clinical Evaluation of Two Posterior Composite Resins Retained with Bonding Agents. (1989). J. Prosth. Dent. 62:627-632.

Sturdevant, C.M., Barton, R.E., Sockwell, C.L., and Strickland, W.D.: The Art and Science of Operative Dentistry (Second Edition). (1985). St. Louis: The C.V. Mosby Co.

Suh, B.I.: All Bond-Fourth Generation Dentin Bonding System. (1991). J. Esth. Dent. 3:129-147.

Tao, L., Pashley, D.H., and Boyd, L.: Effect of Different Types of Smear Layers on Dentin and Enamel Shear Bond Strengths. (1988). Dent. Mater. 4:208-216.

Van Meerbeeck, B., Inokoshi, S., Braem, M., Lambrechts, P., and Vanherle, G.: Morphological Aspects of the Resin-Dentin Interdiffusion Zone with Different Dentin Adhesive Systems. (1992). J. Dent. Res. 71:1530-1540.

Venz, S. and Dickens, B.: Modified Surface Active Monomers for Adhesive Bonding to Dentin. (1990). J. Dent. Res. 69 Special Issue (IADR Abstracts): 116 (Abstract No. 58)

Vojinović, O., Nyborh, H. and Bränström, M.: Acid Treatment of Cavities Under Resin Fillings: Bacterial Growth in Dentinal Tubules and Pulpal Reaction. (1973). J. Dent. Res. 52:1189-1193.

Wang, J.D. and Hume, W.R.: Studies on Diffusive Interactions Between Acids and Alkalis and Dentin. (1988). Int. J. Endodont. 21:17-26.

CHAPTER 4

RESTORATIVE ESTHETIC PROCEDURES: DIRECT COMPOSITE AND GLASS IONOMER

GENERAL CONSIDERATIONS AND ANTERIOR RESTORATIONS

Esthetic adhesive restoratives are the materials of choice for direct restoration of anterior teeth. This chapter contains a discussion of aspects common to all direct esthetic restorative procedures, followed by technique descriptions for specific anterior restorative classifications.

GENERAL CONSIDERATIONS

Advantages and Disadvantages

The advantages and disadvantages of direct adhesive restorative materials are as follows:

Advantages:
- High esthetics
- Conservation of tooth structure (removal of carious/decalcified structure only)
- Adhesion to enamel and dentin (less need for mechanical retention)
- Low microleakage
- Low thermal conductivity

Disadvantages:
- Low resistance to wear and fracture limits used in stress-bearing areas
- Polymerization shrinkage
- Dimensional instability (coefficient of thermal expansion)
- Technique sensitivity

The disadvantages listed here are outweighed by the advantages and can be controlled to some extent, as well. Physical properties continue to improve with the development of new manufacturing techniques, particularly with respect to composition, size distribution and resin loading of filler particles. Incremental layering in large restorations is used to counteract the untoward effects of polymerization shrinkage, including the development of gaps at dentin margins. Current adhesive technology aids in resisting the tendency for microleakage produced by thermally induced dimensional changes. There are, however, no shortcuts for strict adherence to recommended techniques in order to obtain optimal results. Adhesive systems typically contain multiple components and require multiple steps, with each step being critically important to the subsequent ones. Placement and finishing protocols must be carefully followed if maximum longevity and esthetics of composite restorations are to be realized.

Composite resin is the material of choice for most anterior direct restorative situations. Glass ionomer restoratives should be considered as a first choice for root caries due to their fluoride-releasing capabilities, and low levels of microleakage, solubility and dimensional change upon setting. As these lesions occur in non–stress-bearing areas, the lower strength and hardness of glass ionomer as compared to composite is not significant. Newer visible light cured versions of these materials hold significant potential for eliminating many of the challenges associated with the manipulation of chemical-cure glass ionomer restoratives. Longitudinal clinical data will be needed to fully assess their utility and efficacy.

Color and Translucency; Shade Selection

The color perceived in a tooth is the result of combined optical effects of the layers of tooth structure, namely the translucency and thickness of the enamel and the color of the underlying dentin. By developing a restoration in similar fashion, i.e. using layers of composite with differing optical qualities, the restoration can be made to appear very lifelike. The wide selection of colors and opacities available in composite restorative systems facilitates this process. Many systems provide the same colors, or shades, in both opaque (dentin) and translucent (enamel) varieties. Highly translucent shades with little or no pigment are also available for development of incisal translucency. While excellent matching of adjacent tooth structure can often be achieved with a single composite shade in small to medium restorations, layering is useful for achieving optimal results in large restorations.

Shade guides provided with composite resin systems are useful for initial shade selection. These usually consist of plastic tabs formulated to match the shades of the available composites in the kit. Shade guides in some newer systems are fabricated from the actual restorative resin, providing a more accurate representation of the expected shade. Viewing of the shade guides is conducted while holding them adjacent to the teeth to be restored, ideally using indirect sunlight or color-corrected light as the source of illumination. Shade selection must also be completed prior to the application of rubber dam. Desiccation of enamel increases its opacity, resulting in a transient lightening of an isolated tooth's apparent shade. Accurate shade selection under such conditions is not possible.

To verify shade selection, a small amount of the proposed shade is placed on the tooth preoperatively and polymerized. The material is easily removed after viewing as it will not adhere to the unprepared, unetched tooth structure. Trial restorations for larger cases (fractures, direct veneers) can also be quickly placed in this manner to verify shades.

Preparation Design

Cavity designs in restorative dentistry are largely dictated by the properties of the material used to restore the cavity, and esthetic adhesive restorations are no exception to this rule.

Standard outline forms such as those for amalgam and direct gold are not used with adhesive restoratives. Rather, outlines are dictated by the location and extent of carious and decalcified tooth structure. Extension of cavity outlines should be minimal and only to the extent required for access and removal of caries. Undermined enamel should generally not be removed as acid etching and bonding will securely attach it to the restoration. The restorative resin thus replaces the missing dentin and restores the enamel support previously provided by the dentin. Maintenance of undermined enamel also provides for smaller outlines, reducing the amount of restorative exposed to the oral environment. Deterioration related to wear and abrasion is thus limited. Remaining enamel on facial surfaces also improves the esthetics of the final restoration.

Enamel margins of preparations for composite resin are in most cases, finished with bevels. Beveling of enamel margins increases the surface area available for etching at the cavosurface margin, and thus aids in retention and resistance to microleakage. Ends of enamel rods are exposed as result of beveling, which is the optimal orientation for acid etching. Beveling also provides for a gradual transition at the margin between the restorative resin and the tooth structure, making margins more difficult to detect visually. Bevels of 45° and 1 to 2 mm wide are usually employed in visible (facial) areas, with smaller ones (0.5 mm) used in other areas. Larger bevels or chamfers are used for inclusion of decalcified enamel and to increase retention of Class IV restorations. Exceptions to beveling of enamel margins include: cases in which access for beveling would necessitate extension of the preparation outline (e.g. proximal margins in contact with adjacent teeth) and margins of Class I, II, or III preparations in areas of occlusal function.

Dentin margins in composite resin preparations should not be beveled, however. Adhesion of resin to dentin with the same tenacity of that to enamel cannot routinely be produced, and the thin edge of material at a beveled dentin margin would thus be subject to fracture. Margins in dentin are therefore ideally prepared to form a butt joint (90° exit angle), especially if the cavity profile is shallow (e.g. cervical erosions). This modification prepared to a depth of 1 mm allows for adequate bulk of restorative material at the margin. Erosive/abrasive lesions, and caries excavations that approximate butt joint dentin margins, may be left unmodified. For similar reasons of adhesive strength, all margins (enamel and dentin) of preparations for glass ionomer are likewise left unmodified or prepared with 90° exit angles.

Adhesion of composite resin to acid etched enamel provides adequate retention for cases in which the preparation (if any) is largely limited to enamel (incipient caries, direct veneers, Class IV lesions). For carious lesions involving dentin, caries removal will often produce undercuts that provide mechanical retention. Placement of retention grooves at axiogingival and axioproximal line angles has, however, been shown to improve the marginal seal and reduce microleakage at gingival margins (Shahani and Menezes, 1992). It has been suggested that these grooves act as a mechanical brace against shrinkage of resin away from margins (Ben-Amar, et al., 1988). Routine placement of retention grooves adjacent to preparation walls that extend into dentin is thus recommended.

Liners and Bases

The ability of the current generation of adhesive resin to bond and seal conditioned dentin has significantly reduced the need for protective liners and bases. Additionally, contraction forces produced by composite resin polymerization shrinkage can pull conventional glass ionomer liners away from the dentin walls of a cavity preparation (see "sandwich technique" in chapter 3). There are, however, some specific instances in which the placement of a liner is advised.

Calcium hydroxide remains useful for direct pul-capping (application to small pulp exposures) as a stimulus for reparative dentin formation. The amount used should be as minimal as possible, as calcium hydroxide materials dissolve over time, leaving an unsupported area under the restoration.

The notion that dental materials in deep preparations chemically irritate the pulp has been challenged in the scientific literature (Cox, et al., 1992). It is prudent, however, to place liner on thin areas (<1 mm thickness) of dentin near the pulp, as this may prevent mechanical damage to the pulp during restorative material placement. Glass ionomer/resins (light-cured glass ionomers) are the materials of choice for this use, as they exhibit good compressive strength and adhesion to dentin, release fluoride and chemically bond to composite restorative. Glass ionomer liners have also been shown to reduce microleakage at dentin margins of composite restorations when placed at internal line angles adjacent to these margins. Only a minimal amount of liner is used in these applications, leaving as much dentin available as possible to interact with any conditioners adhesive resins used later in the procedure.

Material Placement

Placement of composite resin in increments has several advantages over bulk placement techniques. Thorough polymerization of the resin by visible light is more likely for increments of 2 mm or less in thickness. Increased thickness may result in attenuation of the curing light output, leading to incomplete polymerization of the deeper aspects of an increment.

Incremental placement is also recommended to prevent problems related to polymerization shrinkage. Although greatly reduced by incorporation of large amounts of filler, current composite restoratives remain subject to the polymerization shrinkage common to all acrylate-based resins. As the shrinkage occurs toward the center of an increment of composite, bulk placement produces a tenedency for the composite to pull away from cavosurface margins upon polymerization. Adhesion to etched enamel is usually sufficient to prevent opening of these margins. Shrinkage force has been shown, however, to pull composite away from dentin margins, producing the "contraction gap" phenomenon, and rendering the restoration subject to leakage and secondary caries. Internal dentin walls are also subject to similar gap development. The degree of gap formation is proportional to the size of the composite increment, and becomes negligible in very small increments. By utilizing incremental placement and curing of the composite, with a final small increment used at the dentin margin, shrinkage and gap formation can thus be controlled.

The placement of composite into cavity preparations is facilitated by the use of syringes and other instruments designed for this purpose. Syringe placement aids in the accuracy of placement, minimizes excess and reduces incorporation of air, as compared to freehand placement. Many composite restoratives are supplied preloaded into syringe tips because of these advantages. Hand instruments designed for sculpting and contouring of the composite prior to polymerization can significantly reduce the time required for finishing and polishing. They are also useful for carrying the composite material to the preparation when syringe placement is not used. Such instruments are composed of highly polished stainless steel, or coated with materials designed to prevent the composite from sticking to the instrument surface.

Finishing and Polishing

Attainment and maintenance of a smooth surface on a restoration enhances esthetics while reducing plaque and stain accumulation. Microfill composites have traditionally exhibited the best polishability of all direct adhesive restoratives, due to the extreme fineness of the filler particles used in these materials. Improvements in composite formulations and polishing armamentaria, however, make it possible to produce a finish on the current generation of hybrids that approaches that of microfills. A discussion of instruments and materials used to finish and polish composite restorations follows (it

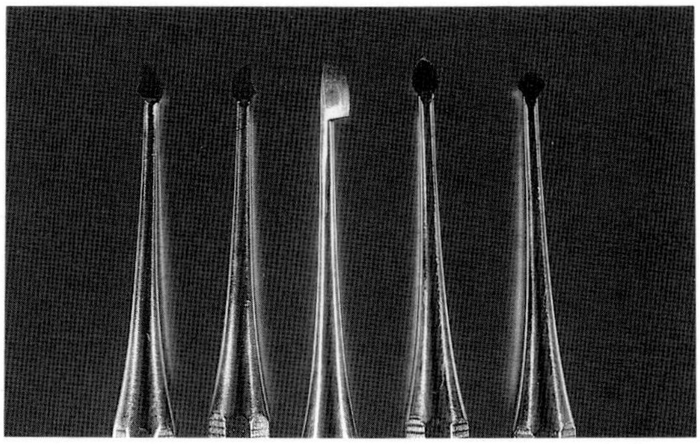

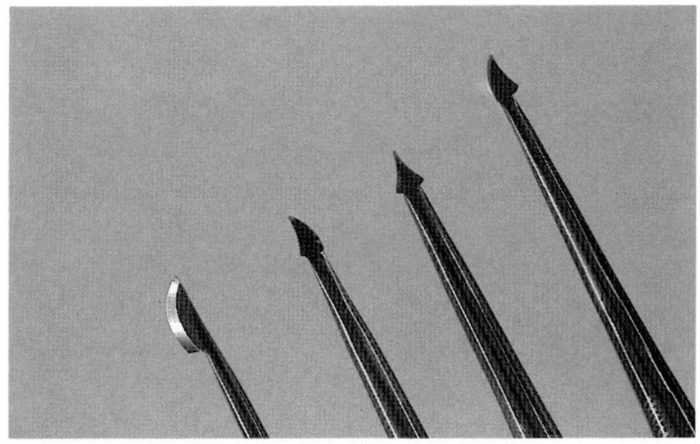

Figs. 4-1a and b Tungsten-carbide carvers for composite resin, useful for excess removal and contouring of embrasures (left: Hu-Friedy; right: Brasseler).

should be noted that items described here are useful on bonded ceramic restorations as well):

Hand instruments. Composite carving instruments are useful for removal of excess and development of contours in areas where finer control than that afforded by rotary instruments is needed. Specifically, areas of difficult access, such as gingival margins, can be instrumented without the potential for damage to cementum and soft tissue encountered with burs and diamonds. While rotary instruments can be used to develop embrasure form, carvers are often necessary for final fine contouring. Instruments of this type are distinguished by their thin, ultra-sharp cutting edges. Disposable scalpel blades (e.g. #12, Bard Parker) are an inexpensive and highly effective option for composite carving. Gold knives, developed for use with direct gold, are useful as well. Tungsten-carbide carvers designed specifically for composite are also available (Fig. 4-1). These generally have cutting edges in various shapes fabricated from tungsten carbide and maintain their sharpness very well.

Burs and diamonds. Rotary instruments designed for use on high speed handpieces are available in an assortment of shapes, sizes and degrees of fineness (see Figs. 6-254a and 6-254b). Used consecutively in increasing order of fineness, they can be applied to all finishing steps from gross excess removal and contouring down to all but the final high polish. Robust shapes are useful in concave areas, i.e. linguals of anteriors and occlusal anatomy of posteriors. Tapered shapes can be applied to general use, with long tapered types especially useful for contouring of large restorations (Class IV, direct veneers). Rounded-end tapered shapes are designed for use at gingival margins as they are less likely to scar cementum than those with pointed tips.

Carbide finishing burs are available in designs of 8, 12, 16 and 30 flutes. The 30-fluted variety have been shown to be particularly effective in intraoral smoothing of ceramic materials following contouring and occlusal adjustment. They also produce a very smooth transition between ceramic, resin cement and tooth structure at the margins of bonded ceramic restorations. Fine finishing diamonds are similarly available in grits ranging from 50 to 8 μm. With the exception of the 30-fluted burs, diamonds are preferable to carbides for finishing ceramics by virtue of their reduced tendency to produce chipping. Copious water spray is recommended when using these burs and diamonds, especially the finer ones, to prevent clogging and premature degradation of the instruments, as well as damage to the composite surface via overheating of the resin.

Some disagreement exists as to which type of instruments, burs or diamonds, are more appropriate for finishing of composite resins. While research studies have been somewhat contradictory, a preference for diamonds over burs is the general trend. Burs are thought to be more damaging to the resin and to producing more "plucking" of filler particles than diamonds. These effects purportedly manifest themselves later as premature staining and loss of surface luster. Many clinicians, however, report the ability to produce a smoother surface with carbide burs. Manufacturers produce both finishing burs and diamonds, often in the same set, allowing individual users to choose their instrument of preference. In practical usage, it appears that either of these instruments when used properly (in sequence, with water spray), and followed by polishing pastes, will produce clinically acceptable results.

Discs. Flexible finishing and polishing discs can be used alone or in combination with burs and diamonds to develop contours and surface smoothness. They are very effective in removing small surface irregularities sometimes left in large restorations by burs and diamonds. On the other hand, they can remove intended surface characterizations such as labial ridges if not used carefully. Discs vary in thickness, with thinner ones adapting to embrasures better than thicker ones. Discs also allow excellent control when "feathering" composite over an etched enamel surface producing a tooth-restorative junction that is visually undetectable.

Finishing strips. Strips remain useful for fine interproximal contouring and finishing of both direct and indirect restorations. Care must be taken to avoid both damage to interdental papillae and inadvertent removal of proximal contacts. Strips with narrow widths and very thin backings are helpful in avoiding these occurrences. Multiple abrasive grits are available, designed to be used in succession, as with finishing burs and diamonds. Coarser grits are also useful for interproximal stain removal and cleaning of enamel prior to acid etching.

Polishing pastes. Microfill composites respond very well to polishing with a thick slurry of tin oxide and water as a final step. Hybrids, however, in addition to the steps described above, require a composite polishing paste to achieve a final high luster similar to that of a microfill. Designed specifically for hybrid composites, these pastes can be used on microfills as well. Several systems contain two pastes, consisting of fine and extra fine grits, to be used in succession.

Pastes are applied with rubber prophylaxis cups, felt wheels or other rotary applicators supplied with some systems. Dental floss can be used to carry polishing paste to proximal surfaces.

CLASS III DIRECT RESIN RESTORATIONS

Restorative Procedure

Material selection: Microfill has traditionally been used for non–stress-bearing restorations replacing facial enamel and hybrid for those involving lingual surfaces and/or proximal contacts. The polishability of currently available hybrids, however, renders them applicable to restoring facial enamel, thereby simplifying material selection and placement. Restoration of root caries with glass ionomer is discussed separately.

Clean teeth with pumice to remove saliva pellicle and surface staining and select shades. Use two shades if the restoration will extend over differently shaded regions of the tooth (e.g. from gingival to incisal). Use an opaque shade (or opaque veneered with translucent) for preparations that extend

Figs. 4-2a and b Preparations for Class III composite.

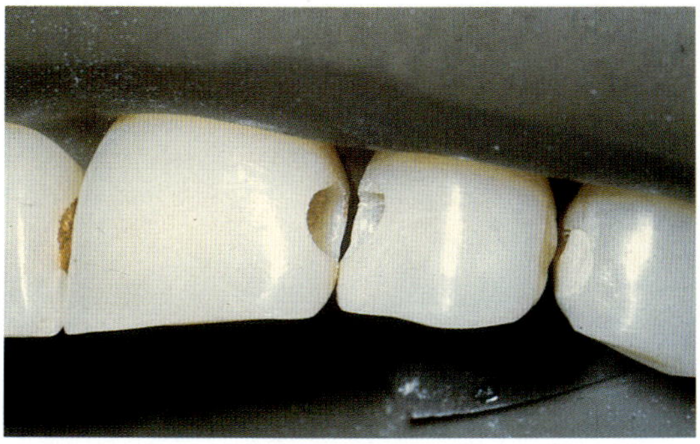

Fig. 4-2a Facial access. Note that undermined enamel is not removed.

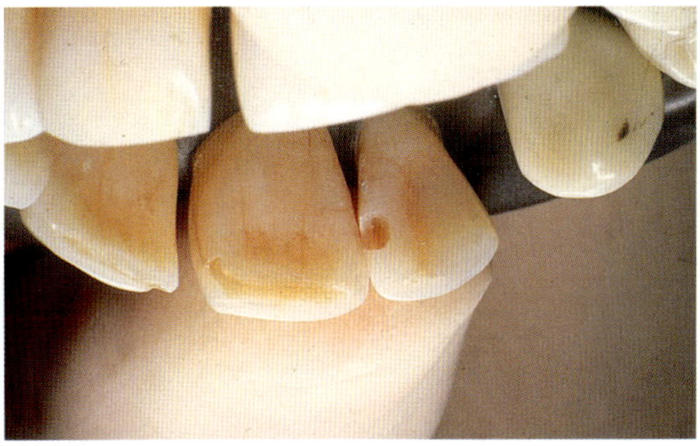

Fig. 4-2b Lingual access, allowing complete preservation of facial enamel (courtesy of Dr. M. Gritz).

through from facial to lingual to block the darkness that results when using translucent alone.

Isolate with rubber dam where possible. For situations where rubber dam impedes access or is otherwise impractical, cheek retractors in conjunction with cotton rolls, gingival retraction cord and warm air dryers provide effective moisture control.

Determine direction of access (facial or lingual). Use facial access if caries breaks through enamel surface and extends into facial embrasure. If facial enamel is intact, use lingual access to preserve facial enamel, thereby enhancing esthetics (Fig. 4-2).

Prepare an outline only large enough to access and remove caries. Incipient lesions (enamel only) need no additional retentive form after removal of discolored and decalcified enamel. For dentinal caries, leave any undermined enamel in place.

Small (0.5-mm-deep) retentive grooves directed incisally and gingivally are used for preparations that extend into dentin, lack undercuts and have minimal enamel at the margins. These will typically occur in the cervical aspect of a tooth.

Apply glass ionomer liner (light cured) to deep dentin areas. Calcium hydroxide is applied directly to small pulp exposures.

Condition enamel and dentin per directions of system being used. Protect adjacent teeth with mylar matrix strips.

Apply primer(s) and adhesive resin, and cure for 20 seconds.

Stabilize the mylar strip with a wedge. A correctly positioned wedge will also aid in controlling extrusion of excess composite beyond the gingival margin.

Use a single increment of composite for small restorations (all margins in enamel, minimal or no dentinal involvement). For lingual access, cure initially from the facial, and vice versa, such that shrinkage of the material will be directed toward tooth structure. Cure from both facial and lingual for 40 seconds.

Restorations extending from facial to lingual are restored incrementally. Place a lingual increment while stabilizing the matrix on the lingual surface with a finger. Condense lingually with an instrument. Cure 40 seconds each from the facial and lingual aspects. Place a facial increment, and wrap the matrix over the facial surface of the tooth. Cure 40 seconds each from the facial and lingual aspects.

For large restorations (deep or with margins extending onto dentin), incrementally restore internal aspects without a matrix, condensing each increment with an instrument. Use a matrix strip for the final increment. Add an additional small increment to the gingival margin, if necessary, after matrix removal.

Remove any gross excess and establish contours with coarse finishing burs, diamonds or discs, using whichever provides best access and control for a given area. Use composite carvers or a scalpel blade to remove excess at the gingival aspect and to refine embrasure form. Contour and smooth proximal surfaces with interproximal finishing strips.

Proceed through successively finer diamonds or discs, followed by composite polishing paste, to produce the final polish. Use dental floss to apply polishing paste to interproximal areas that cannot be accessed with rotary paste carriers.

CLASS V DIRECT RESIN RESTORATIONS

Cervical lesions may be the result of many factors acting independently or in combination, including caries, abrasion, erosion and occlusal disharmony. Flexure of teeth during function, with resultant stress concentration at the cementoenamel junction, has been implicated in the etiology of Class V cervical defects. Examination for and adjustment of occlusal interferences prior to restoration of these areas is therefore prudent. Contributing behavior patterns (oral hygiene technique, diet, parafunctional habits) should also be modified to prevent lesion progression.

Following diagnosis and determination of etiology, decisions to treat cervical lesions must be made. Many such lesions present without symptoms and do not jeopardize the health of adjacent hard and soft tissues. Decisions not to treat in such instances is appropriate. Indications for treatment include:

- Presence of caries
- Intolerable hypersensitivity
- Deep lesions that approximate the pulp and/or structurally weaken the tooth to a significant degree
- Loss of contour affecting hygiene and periodontal health
- Restoration to full contour necessary to facilitate preparation for more extensive restorations (crowns, ceramic veneers)
- Lesions that compromise esthetics in a way that is unacceptable by the patient

Use of microfill composite resins in cervical areas allows for optimal soft tissue response due to the high polishability of these materials. Their lower stiffness, compared to hybrids, is also thought to be advantageous in resisting displacement during tooth flexure. Glass ionomer restoratives should be used when the need for fluoride release is of primary importance (root caries).

Restorative Procedure

Material selection: As stated above, a microfill composite is the resin material of choice for Class V restorations. Restoration of root caries with glass ionomer is discussed separately.

Clean teeth with pumice to remove saliva pellicle and surface staining, and select shades. Use two shades for large restorations that extend over differently shaded regions of tooth (e.g. from gingival to incisal). Shades with slight to moderate translucency (dentin shades) generally blend more readily with cervical tooth structure than do translucent (enamel) shades.

Isolation with rubber dam and retraction of dam and gingiva with a #212 clamp is a very effective means of controlling moisture. In many cases, however, placement of retraction cord combined with cotton rolls and a warm air dryer provide adequate isolation and access, with no trauma to soft tissue (Fig. 4-3). Use plain (nonimpregnated) cord of

Figs. 4-3a to g Class V composite restoration.

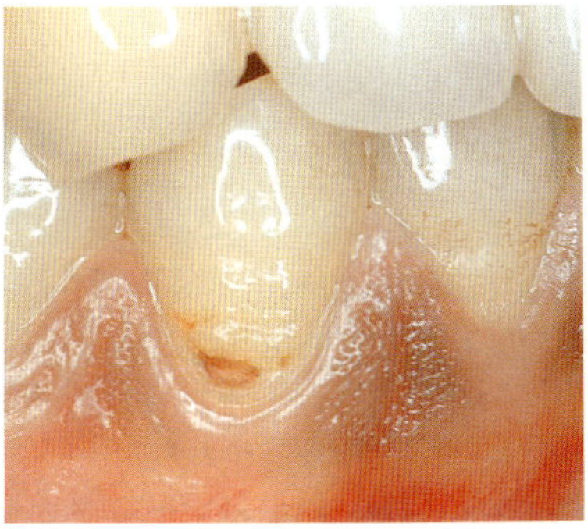

Fig. 4-3a Preoperative erosion with caries.

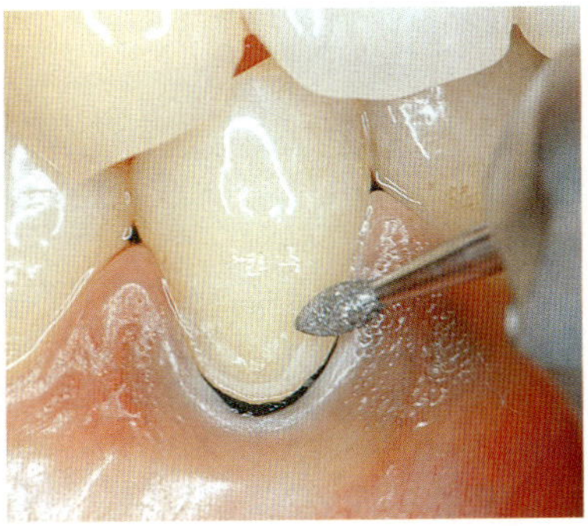

Fig. 4-3b Beveling of enamel margins with diamond. Note placement of retraction cord completely apical to gingival margin.

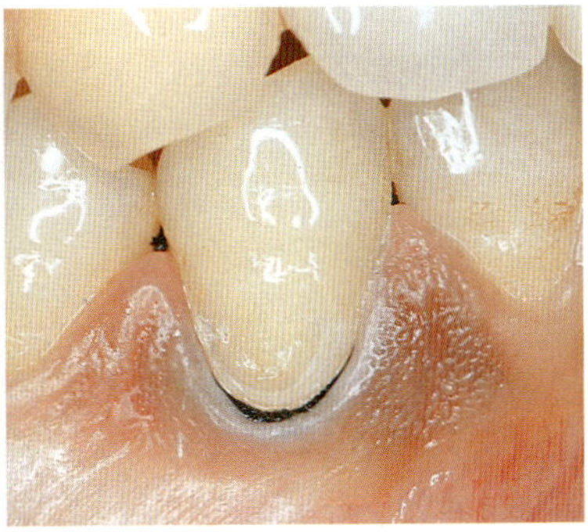

Fig. 4-3c Final preparation.

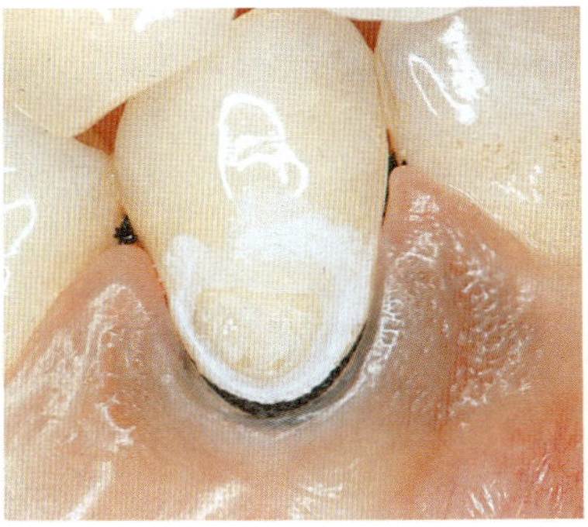

Fig. 4-3d Etched enamel. Note etched areas within preparation, indicating shallow axial depth and minimal dentinal involvement.

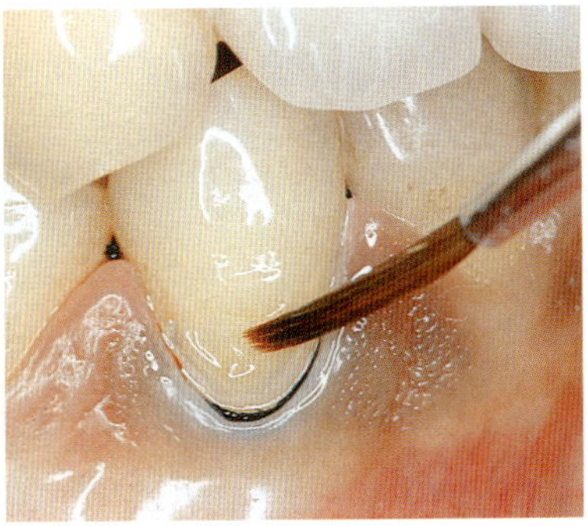

Fig. 4-3e Application of adhesive resin.

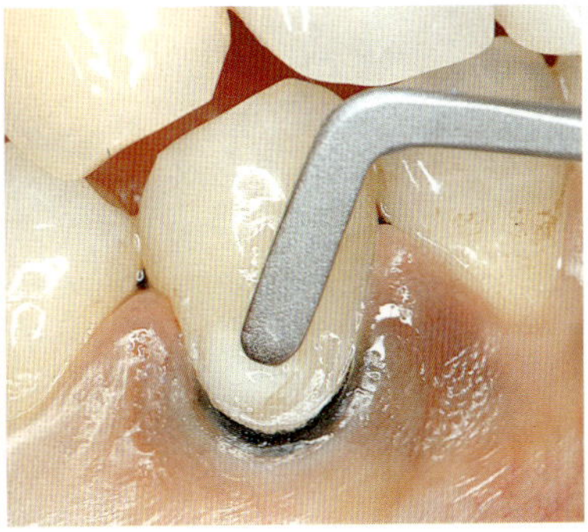

Fig. 4-3f Placement of composite increment. A single increment is used as all preparation margins are in enamel.

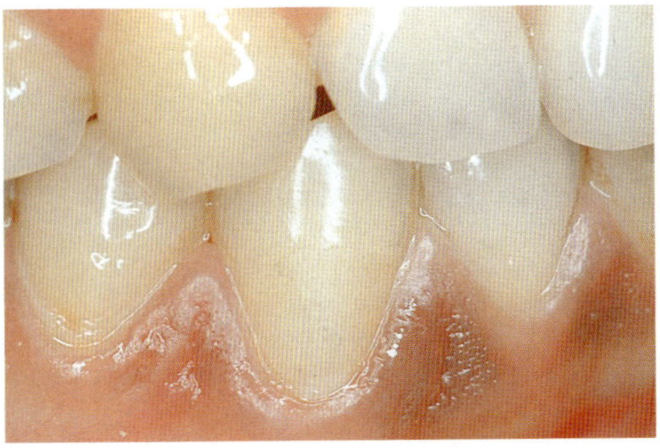

Fig. 4-3g Final restoration.

a size small enough that it remains apical to the gingival margin, allowing it to remain in place throughout the restorative procedure. Margins that are too far subgingival to access with cord can be exposed using electrosurgery, provided that adequate attached gingiva is present. For patients with inadequate attached gingiva, prerestorative periodontal surgery (e.g. apically repositioned flap) may be employed.

Remove any caries present and bevel all enamel margins (Fig. 4-3b). Gingival margins in dentin should approximate a butt joint and should be further prepared, if necessary, to achieve this form. Additionally for such margins, place a small (0.5-mm deep) retentive groove directed gingivally in the adjacent axiogingival line angle.

Noncarious lesions (erosions and abrasions) that are smooth and shiny should be roughened with a diamond or carbide bur prior to bonding. This will remove the highly mineralized surface layer of sclerotic dentin, allowing more predictable conditioning and penetration of primers and resins.

Apply glass ionomer liner (light cured) to deep dentin areas. Calcium hydroxide is applied directly to small pulp exposures.

Condition enamel and dentin per directions of system being used. Protect adjacent teeth with mylar matrix strips, if necessary (Fig. 4-3d).

Apply primer(s) and adhesive resin, and cure for 20 seconds. Protect adjacent teeth, if necessary, with mylar (Fig. 4-3e).

Use a single increment of composite for small restorations, i.e. all margins in enamel, with minimal or no dentinal involvement (Fig. 4-3f). Cure for 40 seconds.

Restorations with gingival margins in dentin are restored incrementally. The coronal portion of the preparation (with enamel margins) is filled to slightly excess contour with an initial increment. For wide or deep preparations, multiple increments may be required for the coronal portion. The initial increment(s) should also cover the entire axial wall, leaving the gingival margin exposed. Cure each increment individually for 40 seconds. Place a small final increment in the gingival aspect to seal the gingival margin, and cure for 40 seconds.

Remove any gross excess and establish contours with coarser finishing burs, diamonds or discs, using whichever provides best access and control for a given area. Care must be taken when using rotary instruments at the gingival margin to prevent damage to cementum and dentin. Remove retraction cord to check for and remove excess composite.

Proceed through successively finer diamonds or discs, followed by composite polishing paste, to produce the final polish.

Treatment of Cervical Hypersensitivity

Many hypersensitive cervical sites are too shallow to retain restorative material without tooth preparation, or present with no other indication for restoration placement. Conservative, noninvasive treatment can be applied to such areas.

According to the most widely accepted theory of pain transmission through dentin, the hydrodynamic theory, tubular fluid movement is affected by temperature changes, desiccation or pressure (mechanical or osmotic). This fluid movement is thought to stimulate nerves closely associated with the odontoblastic processes residing in the tubules. Surface sealing of exposed cervical dentin with resin should prevent fluid movement and produce a reduction or elimination of pain elicited by the above stimuli. This effect is frequently observed clinically when this technique is applied. Periodic sealing in this manner is an option that patients and clinicians may find preferable to more aggressive restorative treatment.

Procedure

Clean areas to be treated with pumice. Rinse, air dry and isolate. Anesthesia may be necessary for patients with extreme response to air and water.

Condition and prime exposed dentin according to manufacturer's protocol for the current generation adhesive system being used. A reduction in the response to air drying is occasionally observed following this step.

Apply a thin layer of adhesive resin and polymerize with light for 20 seconds. Sealed surface should feel smooth and hard when tested with an explorer.

Filled adhesive resins provided with some systems may be substituted for the unfilled adhesive resin as a final step. These materials may exhibit greater longevity via increased resistance to abrasion, although this has not been demonstrated in a controlled study.

GLASS IONOMER RESTORATIONS

Glass ionomer restoratives are not used in a wide range of applications, largely due to the superior properties and utility of the currently available adhesive resin systems. Glass ionomers nonetheless remain useful for the treatment of root caries. Cases involving root caries are typically not limited to a single tooth, but rather tend to occur in individuals with high caries indices. Areas of occurrence are usually difficult to access and maintain. Diminished salivary flow in root caries patients is not uncommon. Additionally, many older patients with impairment of manual dexterity present with poor oral hygiene as a contributing factor to root caries. All of these factors combine to produce a high incidence of secondary caries associated with attempts at restoring root caries. Glass ionomers, then, constitute a useful alternative to adhesive resins for these cases by virtue of their fluoride release and secondary caries inhibition. Advantages in physical properties of composites are not significant as root caries occurs in non–stress-bearing areas. Esthetic considerations regarding root caries also tend to be such that the advantages of composite are irrelevant. It is important, then, to include glass ionomers in a contemporary adhesive restorative armamentarium.

Newer visible light cured glass ionomer restoratives are resin-based, and their handling is thus similar to that of composite resins. The following procedure relates to the use of chemically cured glass ionomers.

Restorative Procedure

Clean tooth with pumice to remove saliva pellicle and surface staining. Scale areas adjacent to lesions, if necessary, to aid in removal of stain and debris in areas inaccessible to prophy cups. Select a shade that closely matches tooth structure if the lesion extends into an esthetically critical area. Otherwise, a slight mismatch between the shades of the glass ionomer and tooth may assist in finishing, as well as in assessment at recall.

Maintenance of a dry field in root caries cases may require combinations of several techniques, including gingival retraction cord, warm air drying, and electrosurgery. Rubber dam is very effective as long as it does not impede access, as is often the case for subgingival Class III lesions. Use plain (nonimpregnated) retraction cord, placed such that it is apical to the gingival extent of the lesion. This allows the cord to remain in place throughout the procedure, aiding in the control of both sulcular fluid flow and extrusion of excess restorative material beyond the margin.

Prepare the tooth by removing caries with a round bur at low speed and spoon excavators. Remove intact tooth structure only if absolutely necessary to gain access, e.g. for posterior interproximal lesions. Cavosurface margins should be approximately 90° butt joints in form. Modify any margins as needed where caries removal has produced bevels. Place mechanical retention, access permitting, if caries removal has not created undercuts.

Apply a small amount of calcium hydroxide directly to pulp exposures. Condition dentin (remove smear layer) by applying 10% polyacrylic solution for 15 seconds. Rinse and dry. Do not, however, desiccate dentin when drying. A slightly moist dentin surface is necessary for optimal glass ionomer adhesion.

Use a matrix where possible — mylar strips with wedges for Class III restorations, preformed cervical matrices for Class V restorations. Matrices prevent dehydration and moisture contamination of the glass ionomer during the critical setting stage.

Mix the glass ionomer per manufacturer's instructions and load into a composite syringe. Encapsulated systems allow delivery of the mixed material directly from the capsule. Inject the material into the cavity, and stabilize the matrix before the material loses its shiny surface appearance. Hold the matrix in place for 4 minutes, allowing the material to reach an initial hard set.

Remove the matrix and immediately coat the restoration with an unfilled light cured adhesive resin. Cure for 20 seconds. This will continue to protect the material from alterations in water balance, and is more effective than varnishes supplied for this purpose. Allow the material to continue to set for the time recommended by the manufacturer (usually 15 minutes).

Contour and polish using fine diamonds with water spray and/or flexible discs lubricated with petroleum jelly or cocoa butter. Scalpel blades, composite carvers and finishing strips are also useful for interproximal contouring. Keep the restoration surface coated with lubricant during finishing to prevent dehydration. Uncured adhesive resin may also be used for this purpose. Apply composite polishing paste as a final polishing step. Use dental floss to apply polishing paste to interproximal areas that cannot be accessed with rotary paste carriers.

Coat the restoration surface again with adhesive resin and light cure for 20 seconds. Translucency will continue to develop in the set material for 24 hours after placement.

CLASS IV DIRECT RESIN RESTORATIONS

Composite resins enable the clinician to conservatively restore anterior teeth in an esthetic and functional manner. Situations described in this section, which in the past required full coverage fixed restorations are now routinely treated with minimal removal of additional tooth structure (Fig. 4-4). Functional forces to be applied to the restoration must nonetheless be carefully considered prior to treatment. Treat the following factors preoperatively should they be present: occlusal disharmonies resulting in excessive lateral forces on the proposed restoration; supereruption preventing adequate space for placement of restorative material; and slight malpositioning of anterior teeth treatable with cosmetic contouring.

Cases involving restoration of large portions of a tooth or treatment of several teeth may best be treated with indirect techniques (e.g. laminate veneers) to achieve optimal esthetics and longevity. Large composite restorations, however, remain viable as a single appointment, lower cost alternative and can be utilized as long term interim restorations pending completion of other procedures, such as orthodontics or perio-

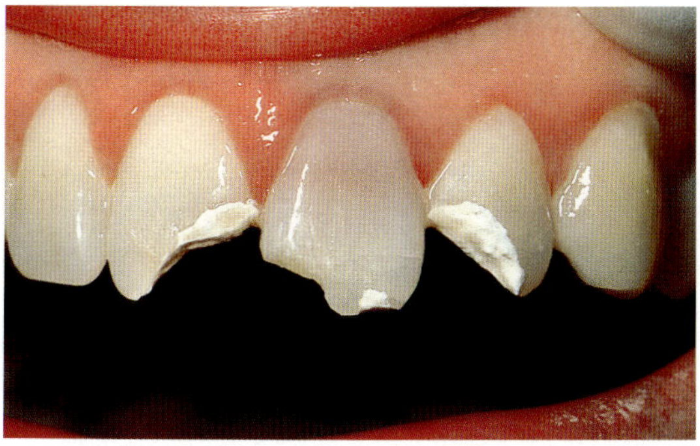

Fig. 4-4a Traumatic fracture of anterior teeth, resulting in loss of vitality of left central incisor.

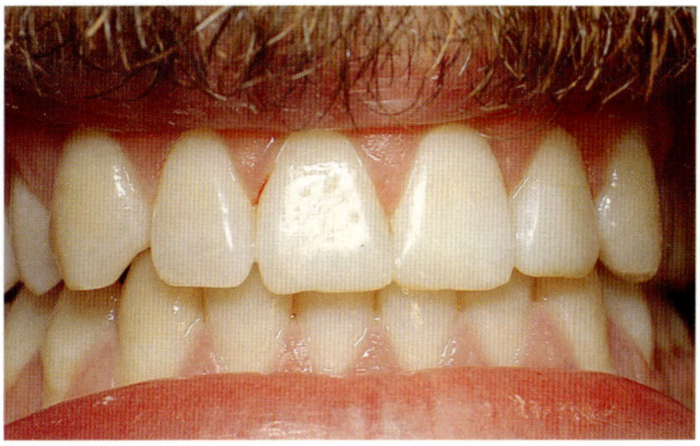

Fig. 4-4b Conservative restoration of fractured teeth with direct composite resin performed in one appointment. Left central incisor was bleached internally prior to restoration.

dontics. Class IV composites also remain the treatment of choice for immediate restoration of traumatic fractures. Full coverage indirect restorations should still be applied to patients with heavy bruxism, or lacking adequate enamel for retention of composite (e.g. severe erosion).

Incisal Fracture

Restorative Procedure

Material selection: Hybrid composite is used for its superior physical properties in restoring stress-bearing (lingual and proximal) areas. Microfill has been recommended for use in labial aspects of the restoration to obtain optimal esthetic results. The polishability of currently available hybrids, however, makes it possible to obtain excellent results using hybrid for the entire restoration. Material selection and placement is thereby simplified.

Clean the teeth with pumice to remove saliva pellicle and surface staining, and select shades. Use two shades if the restoration will extend over differently shaded regions of the tooth (e.g. from gingival to incisal). An opaque (dentin) shade is required to block light transmission through the entire restoration, thereby preventing a dark appearance and inability to match the color of adjacent tooth structure. Select a slightly translucent shade to be applied as a thin (0.5 mm) veneer on the labial surface of the restoration. The goal is to mimic the combined optical effects of enamel and dentin, imparting a quality of depth to the restoration. Use a third, more translucent shade along the incisal edge, if necessary, to match incisal translucency.

Isolate with rubber dam where possible. For situations where rubber dam impedes access or is otherwise impractical, cheek retractors in conjunction with cotton rolls, gingival retraction cord and warm air dryers provide effective moisture control.

Remove any existing restorations or caries adjacent to the fracture site. Preparation is otherwise limited to the margins of the fracture. Prepare a chamfer, using a round-end tapered diamond bur, along all enamel margins, with a depth of approximately one half the enamel thickness (Figs. 4-5 and 4-6a). Place a bevel (0.5 to 1 mm) on the chamfer. The bevel increases surface area for retention and provides for a gradual (and less visible) transition from composite to tooth (Fig. 4-6b). The chamfer depth provides for increased thickness and strength of composite at the tooth-restorative interface. Bevel gingival enamel only slightly to avoid extending the bevel into cementum or dentin. Prepare a 0.5-mm-deep shoulder at gingival

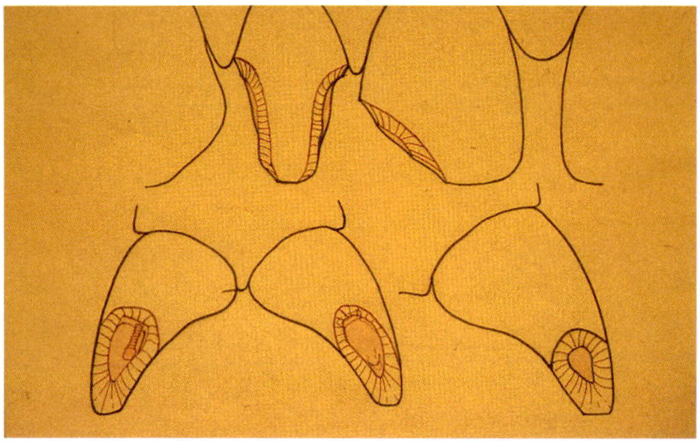

Fig. 4-5 Chamfer preparations for Class IV direct composite restorations (courtesy Dr. M. Gritz).

margins in dentin, and do not bevel. Use a coarse finishing disc to eliminate any enamel staining not removed by pumice or preparation.

If dentin is exposed, apply a small amount of light cured glass ionomer liner only to deep areas approximating the pulp. Use calcium hydroxide for direct application to small pulp exposures. Otherwise leave dentin unlined to improve esthetics and to make it available to the adhesive resin.

Condition enamel and dentin per directions

Figs. 4-6a to q Repair of a Class IV incisal fracture with direct composite resin.

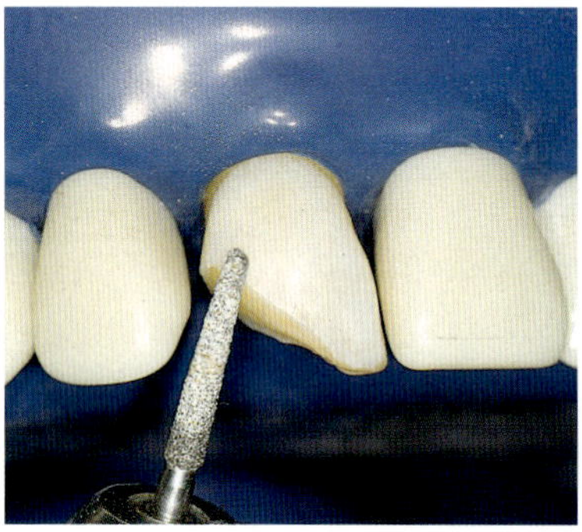

Fig. 4-6a Round-end tapered diamond used to prepare a chamfer in enamel, 2 mm beyond edge of fracture.

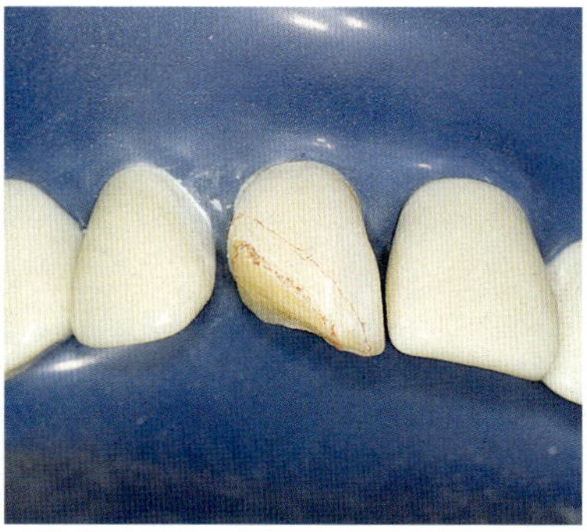

Fig. 4-6b Chamfer margin is beveled to provide gradual transition from restorative to tooth. Prepared area is outlined in red for illustrative purposes.

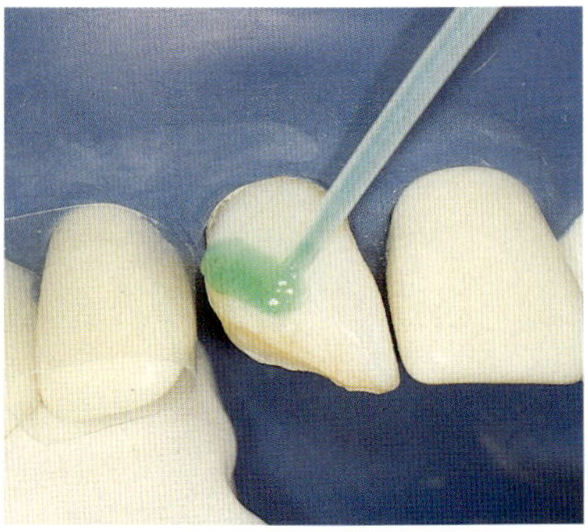

Fig. 4-6c Placement of enamel conditioner. Note protection of adjacent tooth with mylar matrix for both conditioning and application of primers and resins.

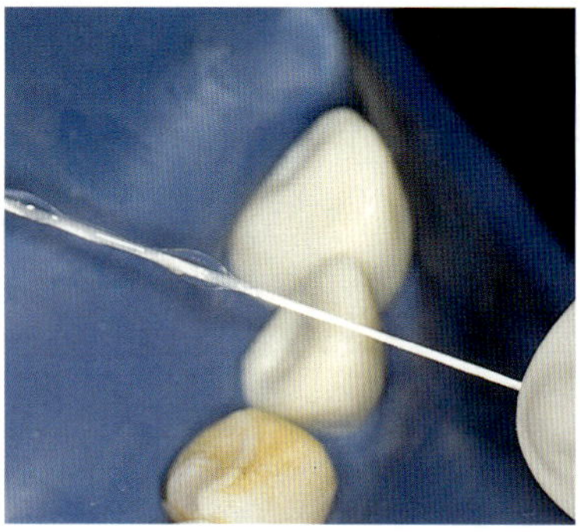

Fig. 4-6d Dental floss coated with water-soluble lubricant. Remove excess before applying to adjacent tooth surface.

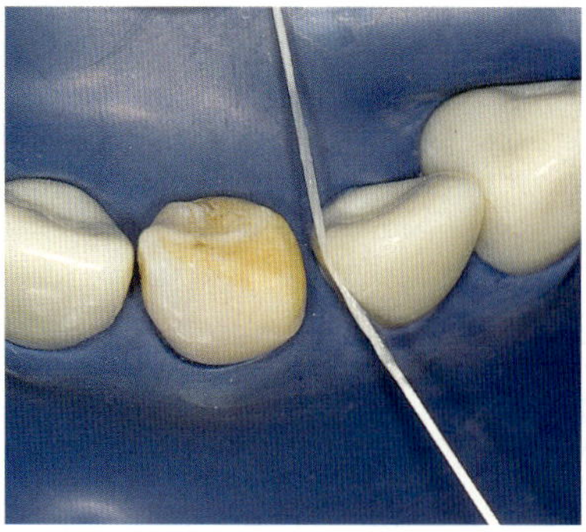

Fig. 4-6e Coating adjacent tooth with lubricant to prevent adhesion of composite, allowing placement of composite without a matrix. Establishment of proximal contact is thus assured.

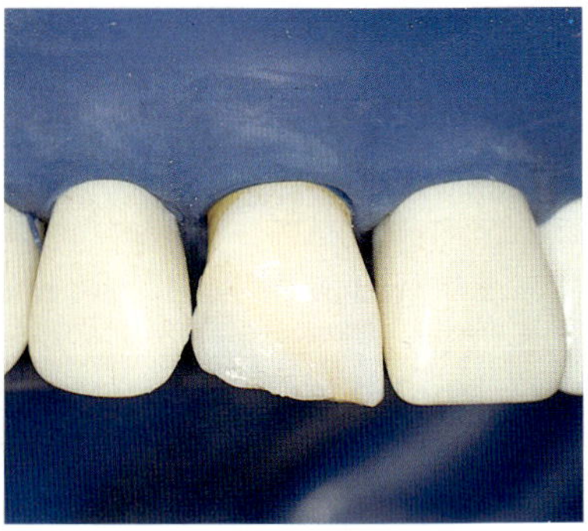

Fig. 4-6f Placement of dentin shade composite, extending to proximal contact area. Labial and incisal aspects are left undercontoured, providing space for enamel shade.

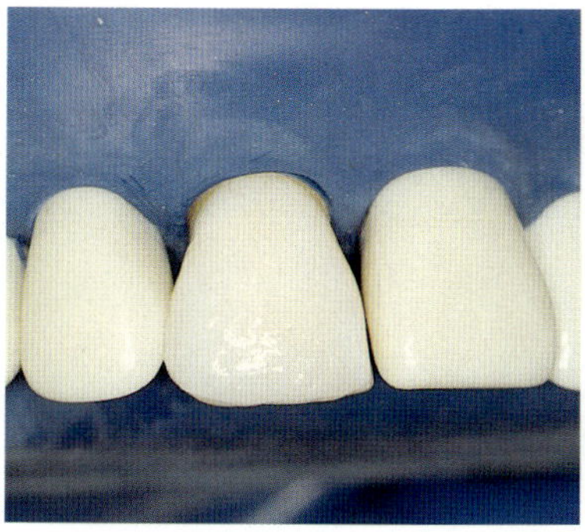

Fig. 4-6g Placement of enamel shade composite, in slight excess of anticipated final contours.

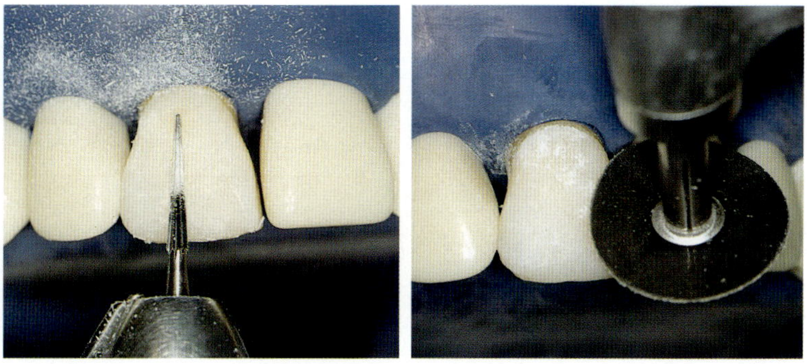

Figs. 4-6h and i Excess removal and contouring using a 12-fluted carbide tapered finishing bur or coarse finishing disc on labial and incisal.

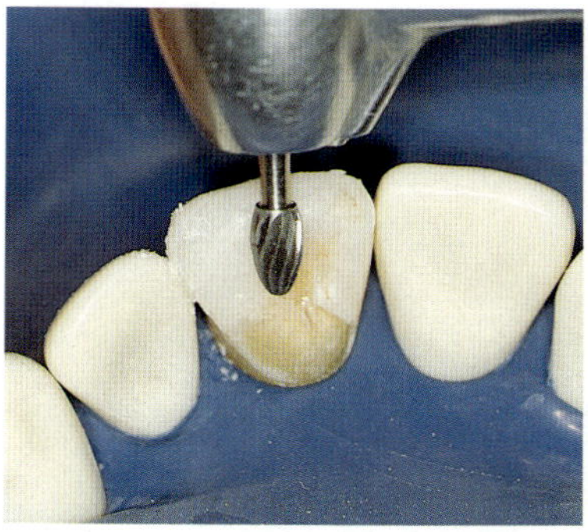

Fig. 4-6j A rounded finishing bur adapts well to the lingual concavity.

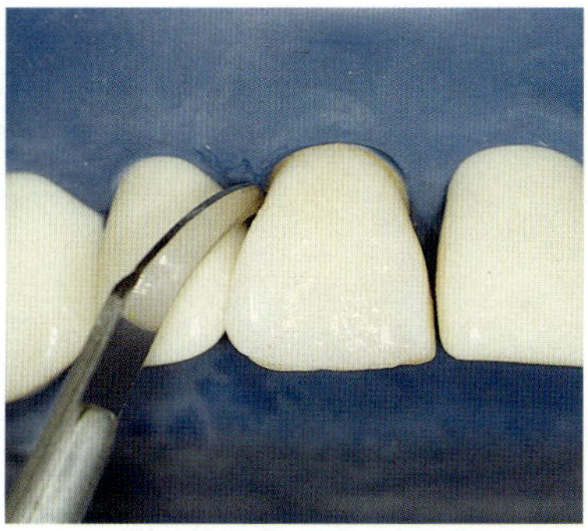

Fig. 4-6k Removal of overhang with a #12 Bard Parker blade.

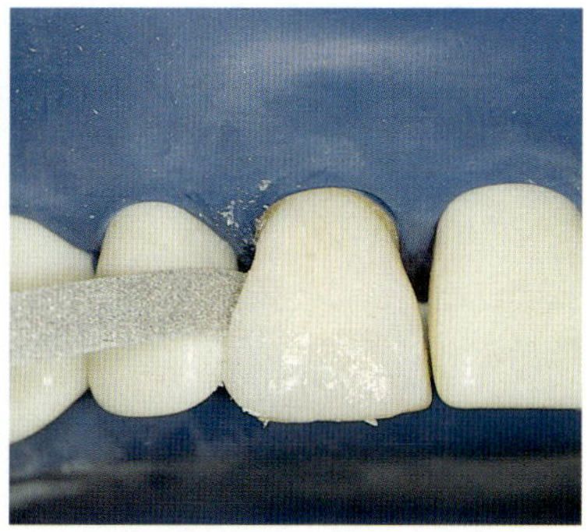

Fig. 4-6l Contouring of proximal surface with a finishing strip, keeping the strip apical to the proximal contact area.

of system being used. Protect adjacent teeth with mylar matrix strips (Fig. 4-6c).

Apply primer(s) and adhesive resin, and cure for 20 seconds. Protect adjacent teeth with mylar.

Incremental buildup with different shades and opacities, as well as establishment of proximal contact, is most conveniently achieved without a matrix strip. This technique also allows for increased control over contour development and reduction of excess material. Permanent bonding to the adjacent tooth is prevented by lack of etching and adhesive resin placement. It is therefore imperative that proximal surfaces adjacent to the restoration site be protected during these steps. To further aid in prevention of bonding, apply a very thin layer of a water-soluble lubricant to the adjacent proximal surface with dental floss immediately prior to composite placement (Figs. 4-6d and e). Caution must be taken to prevent contamination of the preparation if this procedure is employed.

Apply the dentin shade to the lingual aspect of the fracture site, building the restoration into direct contact with the adjacent tooth (Fig. 4-6f). Use multiple increments if necessary, and cure each increment for 20 seconds from the labial and 20 seconds from the lingual. Leave the labial aspect undercontoured by approximately 0.5 mm to allow for placement of the enamel shade(s). Do not restore to full incisal length if incisal translucency is to be developed.

Place the enamel shade layer, leaving a small amount of excess labial and incisal

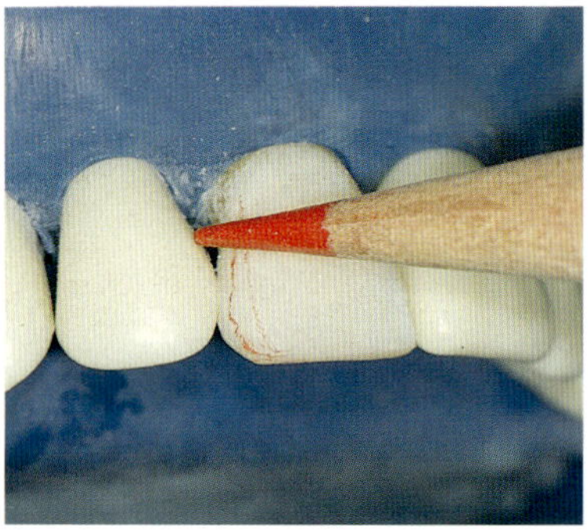

Fig. 4-6m Marking desired location of line angle, to assist in matching contours of contralateral tooth.

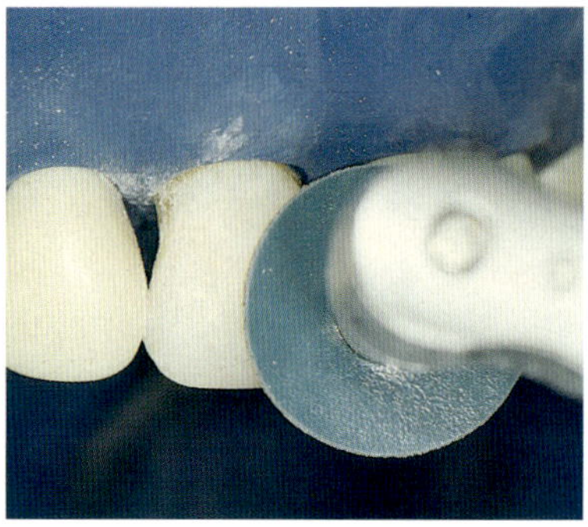

Fig. 4-6n

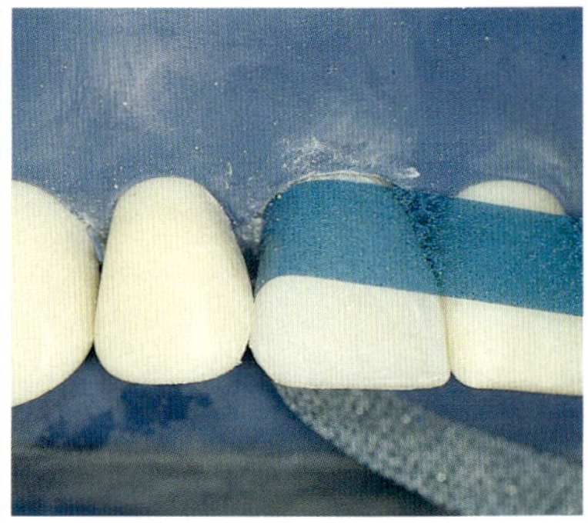

Fig. 4-6o

Figs. 4-6n to p Final polish is achieved with fine diamonds or discs and fine interproximal finishing strips, followed by composite polishing paste.

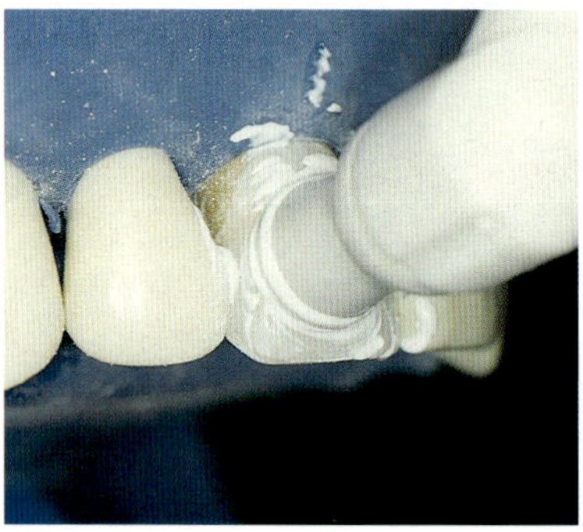

Fig. 4-6p

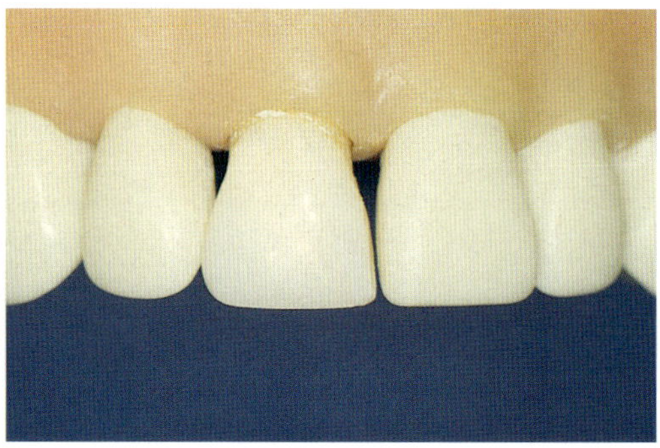

Fig. 4-6q Final restoration.

contour to allow for finishing (Fig. 4-6g). Lubricate the placement instrument with a thin layer of adhesive resin to facilitate contouring and smoothing of the surface. Cure the enamel shade layer for 40 seconds. Apply a separate incisal shade, if necessary, and cure for 40 seconds. Insert a hand instrument into the gingival embrasure, and gently apply a torquing force to break any slight adhesion to the adjacent tooth that may have occurred. Check for separation by passing dental floss through the contact.

A mylar matrix strip may be used as an alternative to the procedure described above. Use of a matrix is convenient for smaller fractures (limited to the incisal angle and not involving the proximal contact) and for those cases that can be restored with a single shade of composite. Place the strip and stabilize with a wedge. A correctly positioned wedge will also aid in controlling extrusion of excess composite beyond the gingival margin. Position the strip against the lingual surface of the tooth with a finger, and inject the dentin shade composite onto the preparation. Use a hand instrument to adapt the composite against the preparation and the matrix, leaving the labial surface undercontoured for placement of the enamel shade. Cure from the labial for 20 seconds, then remove your finger and cure from the lingual for 20 seconds. Add the enamel shade and wrap the matrix around the tooth. Check visually for adequate amount of material to establish contours and for lack of voids. Cure from the labial for 40 seconds. If using only one shade, this procedure may be conducted in a single step, injecting one increment of dentin shade of sufficient volume to restore the entire fracture. Wrap the matrix, ensuring that it remains in contact with the adjacent tooth. Cure for 40 seconds each from the labial and lingual.

Remove gross excess and establish contours with coarse finishing burs or diamonds (Figs. 4-6h to l). Long tapered shapes are useful for labial surfaces, while rounded shapes adapt well to concave lingual areas. Coarse finishing discs may also be used to refine contours and work especially well on labial and incisal surfaces. Remove gingival margin excess with a #12 Bard Parker blade or composite carvers. Use finishing strips for fine contouring and smoothing of proximal areas, taking care to avoid removal of composite from the contact area.

Check for occlusal interferences in the restoration in both centric relation and in excursive movements. Adjust as necessary.

Proceed through successively finer diamonds or discs, followed by composite polishing paste, to produce the final polish (Figs. 4-6n to q). Use dental floss to apply polishing paste to interproximal areas that cannot be accessed with rotary paste carriers.

Diastema Closure

Diastemas are generally closed by adding composite to both teeth adjacent to the space. This is especially true for midline diastemas—central incisors should be exactly the same size for optimal results. Spaces resulting from undersized teeth (peg lateral incisors, retained deciduous teeth) can however be treated by adding only to the affected tooth to increase its apparent size. Measure the length and width of teeth to be restored, as well as the width of the diastema, using a Boley gauge. A length-to-width ratio of 5:4 has been suggested as ideal for anterior teeth. If complete closure of the diastema results in teeth that are as wide or wider than they are long, consider the following options to avoid this unnatural appearance:

- Reduce the diastema without complete closure of the space.
- Increase crown length using soft tissue surgery (gingivoplasty) prior to diastema closure.
- Use laminate veneers to both close the space and increase length, occlusion permitting.
- Remove tooth structure from the opposite side of the tooth to decrease its width, then add composite to close the space and restore proper width. The space created by removal of tooth structure must be closed by adding composite to the tooth adjacent to this space. This technique may necessitate treatment of several teeth in the segment to maintain esthetic length-to-width ratios.
- Treat the patient with orthodontics to eliminate spaces or to distribute a large space evenly throughout the segment. Closure of the resulting small spaces with composite can then be conducted without creating unnatural length-to-width ratios.

Restorative Procedure

Material selection: Hybrid composite is used for its superior physical properties in restoring stress-bearing (lingual and proximal) areas. Microfill has been recommended for use in labial aspects of the restoration to obtain optimal esthetic results. The polishability of currently available hybrids, however, makes it possible to obtain excellent results using hybrid for the entire restoration. Material selection and placement is thereby simplified.

Clean the teeth with pumice to remove saliva pellicle and surface staining, and select shades. Use two shades if the restoration will extend over differently shaded regions of the tooth (e.g. from gingival to incisal). An opaque (dentin) shade is required to block light transmission through the entire restoration, thereby preventing a dark appearance and inability to match the color of adjacent tooth structure. Select a slightly translucent shade to be applied as a thin (0.5 mm) veneer on the labial surface of the restoration. The goal is to mimic the combined optical effects of enamel and dentin, imparting a quality of depth to the restoration. Use a third, more translucent shade along the incisal edge, if necessary, to match incisal translucency.

Isolate with rubber dam where possible. For situations where rubber dam impedes access or is otherwise impractical, cheek retractors in conjunction with cotton rolls, gingival retraction cord and warm air dryers provide effective moisture control.

Slightly roughen proximal enamel using coarse finishing discs and strips. Extend the roughening 1 to 2 mm onto the facial and lingual surfaces, as the composite will be "feathered" onto these areas. Roughen the entire labial surface if the diastema closure is to be combined with direct composite veneers.

Restorative materials are placed and finished one tooth at a time, facilitating contouring and finishing. Etch all enamel areas to be bonded. Rinse and dry. Apply primer(s) and adhesive resin, and cure for 20 seconds. Protect adjacent teeth with mylar matrix strips during these steps.

Incremental buildup with different shades and opacities, as well as establishment of proximal contact, is most conveniently achieved without a matrix strip. This technique also allows for increased control over contour development and reduction of excess material.

Apply the dentin shade to the lingual aspect of the first tooth. The composite must extend to the lingual line angle to develop continuity with existing tooth contours. Pay particular attention to the emergence profile. Increase the width of the tooth by the amount determined with preoperative measurements, and add an additional 0.5 mm to allow for contouring and finishing. Use multiple increments if necessary, and cure each increment for 20 seconds from the labial and 20 seconds from the lingual. Leave the labial aspect undercontoured by approximately 0.5 mm to allow for placement of the enamel shade(s). Do not restore to full incisal length if incisal translucency is to be developed.

Place the enamel shade layer, leaving a small amount of excess labial and incisal contour to allow for finishing. Lubricate the placement instrument with a thin layer of adhesive resin to facilitate contouring and smoothing of the surface. Develop an emergence profile continuous with existing tooth contours, and avoid producing a gingival ledge. Cure for 40 seconds. Apply a separate incisal shade, if necessary, and cure for 40 seconds. Measure the resultant width of the tooth with a Boley gauge to check that adequate material has been added before proceeding.

A matrix may be optionally used to restore the first tooth (Fig. 4-7), especially if only a single shade of composite is being used. Matrix use, however, does not allow as much control over contours as direct placement, particularly with respect to the gingival embrasure. All contouring in this case is done after polymerization, using hand and rotary instruments.

Refine contours and polish with finishing burs or diamonds and discs. Delay finishing of the gingival margin to avoid tissue trauma and bleeding that may interfere with restoration of the adjacent tooth. Use composite polishing paste on all surfaces except the gingival margin. Check the final width with a Boley gauge.

Repeat this procedure, beginning with enamel etching, for the second tooth. Build the restoration into direct contact with the first to assure proper proximal contact development. Permanent bonding to the first tooth is prevented by the high polish on the composite surface, and protection of this surface from exposure to etchants, primers and resin. It is therefore imperative that proximal surface on the first tooth be pro-

Figs. 4-7a to e Optional use of a matrix band to restore the first of two teeth in a diastema closure case.

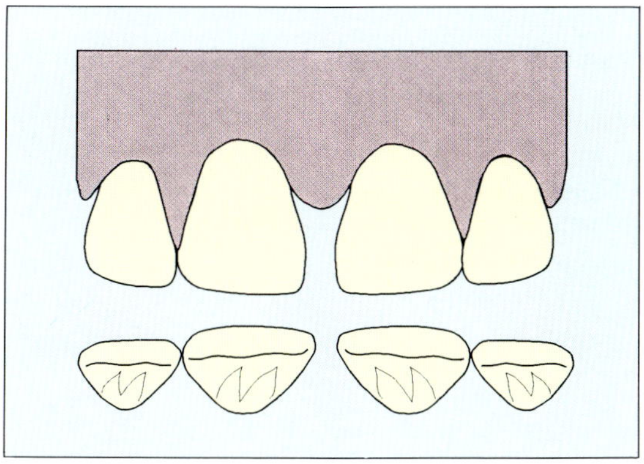

Fig. 4-7a

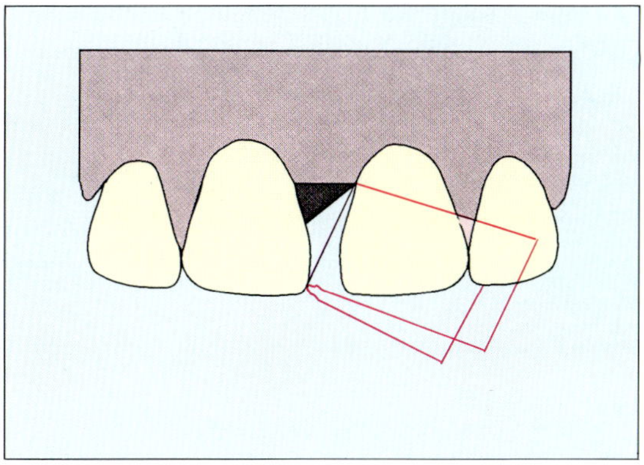

Fig. 4-7b

Fig. 4-7a Preoperative.

Fig. 4-7b Placement of matrix and wedge.

Fig. 4-7c Initial contour following matrix removal.

Fig. 4-7d Final contouring and polishing of the first tooth, performed with hand and rotary instruments. Proximal surface of the restoration is now lubricated to prevent adhesion to the second tooth's restoration.

Fig. 4-7e Final contouring of the second tooth. Composite added to second tooth was built into direct contact with the first, using no matrix.

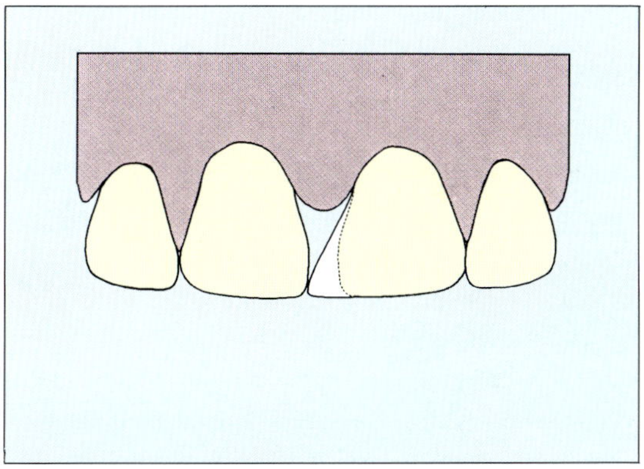

Fig. 4-7c

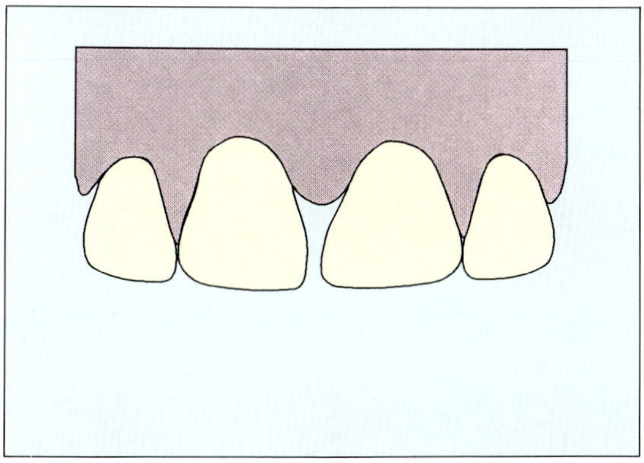

Fig. 4-7d

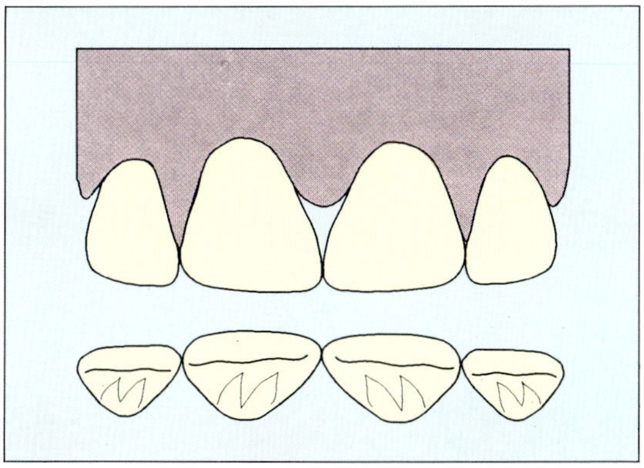

Fig. 4-7e

tected with a mylar strip during these steps. To further aid in prevention of bonding, apply a very thin layer of a water-soluble lubricant to the proximal surface of the first tooth with dental floss immediately prior to restoring the second tooth. Caution must be taken to prevent contamination of the second tooth if this procedure is employed.

Following curing of the final increment on the second tooth, insert a hand instrument into the gingival embrasure and gently apply a torquing force. This will break any slight adhesion to the first tooth that may have occurred. Check for separation by passing dental floss through the contact.

Refine both gingival embrasures and all embrasures of the second tooth using a scalpel blade (#12) or composite carvers. Contour and polish the second tooth. Use finishing strips to refine both gingival margins. Finish again with composite polishing paste, using dental floss to apply paste to interproximal areas that cannot be accessed with rotary paste carriers.

Direct Composite Veneer

Esthetic enhancement of anterior teeth by veneering with a layer of composite resin became an extremely popular procedure shortly after the introduction of visible light cured microfill composites. Laminate veneers now represent the state of the art in this area as they are far more durable, more esthetic, produce better contours and are applicable to a wider range of cases that direct composite. Direct veneers are still useful in some cases, such as: to offer patients a lower-cost alternative to laminate veneers; for patients who refuse to have teeth prepared; for patients who insist on a one-appointment procedure; for adolescent patients, deferring laminate veneers until the dentition matures further; for use as long term interim restorations while completing other treatment (e.g. orthodontics or periodontics).

Both the clinician and patient in these cases must remain aware of the limitations of direct veneers:

1. While effective in changing contour and color, their use in lengthening teeth in function is likely to result in premature failure;
2. They are subject to deterioration processes that will require periodic repair, and ultimate replacement, in order to maintain desired effects.

Restorative Procedure

Cosmetic contouring, if needed, is completed prior to the veneering procedure. Patients' desires regarding change in existing tooth color should be clearly elicited by the clinician at the treatment planning stage.

Material selection: Microfill composite resin is the material of choice due to its excellent polishability. Smooth surface attainment is needed to give the illusion of natural enamel and to reduce irritation of marginal gingiva. Additionally, as the material will be limited to non–stress-bearing areas, the superior physical properties of hybrid composite are not critical to the success of these restorations. For cases combining direct veneering with diastema closure (Fig. 4-8) or restoration of a fracture, use a hybrid composite for lingual, proximal and incisal edge areas.

Clean the teeth with pumice to remove saliva pellicle and surface staining, and select shades. Use different shades for the gingival two thirds and incisal one third to produce a more natural and vital appearance. Opaque shades are required to lighten teeth.

Use selected shades to place a trial veneer on one of the teeth. Spread the composite in a thin (0.5 mm) layer over the labial surface. Lightly lubricate the placement instrument with adhesive resin to assist in developing a smooth labial surface. Cure for 40 seconds, and allow the patient to view and approve the proposed shades. The veneer can be easily lifted off of the unetched tooth with a hand instrument.

Isolation with rubber dam may impede access to labial areas adjacent to the gingival crest. Use cheek retractors, cotton rolls, gingival retraction cord and warm air dryers to control moisture.

Placing direct veneers without tooth preparation renders the procedure reversible, and assures that maximum enamel will be present if more definitive treatment (e.g. laminate veneers) is elected in the future. Limiting veneer thickness to 0.5 mm and contouring all gingival aspects to a feather edge precludes the need to prepare teeth by

Figs. 4-8a and b Modification of peg lateral contours using direct composite resin.

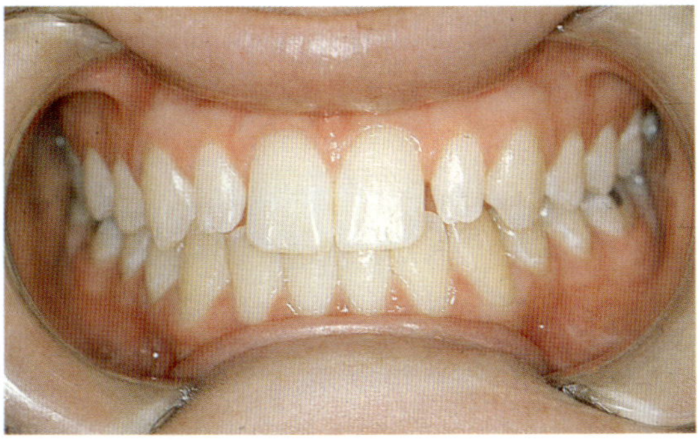

Fig. 4-8a Preoperative.

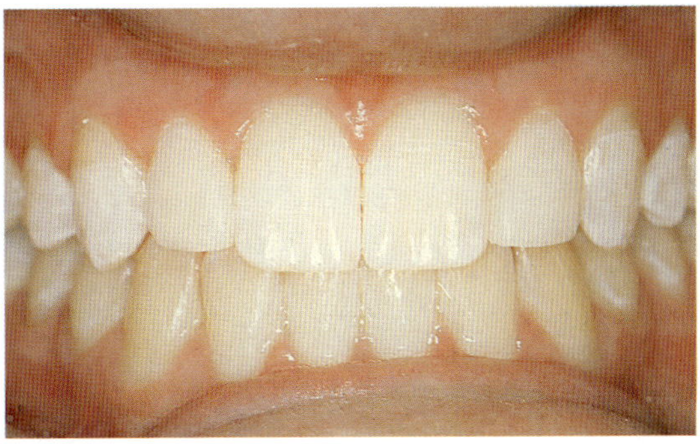

Fig. 4-8b Final restorations (courtesy of Dr. M. Gritz).

removing intact enamel. Slightly roughen labial enamel with a coarse finishing disc to enhance adhesion of composite.

Darkened teeth may require preparation to create space for adequate thickness of composite to produce the desired lighter shade. Preparation should be considered to prevent overcontour, especially at the gingival margin, if the veneer must be more than 0.5 mm in thickness. The need for preparation can be determined with the trial veneer placed on unetched enamel. Preparation form is similar to that for a laminate veneer: uniform reduction of labial enamel, up to a maximum of 0.5 mm in depth, extending from mesial to distal line angles and from gingival crest to inciso labial line angles; chamfer finish line at gingival margin; extend preparation over the incisal and onto lingual if tooth is to be lengthened, terminating in a chamfer placed 2 mm apical to the linguo-incisal line angle.

Separate each tooth to be veneered from adjacent teeth with mylar matrix strips. Etch all enamel areas to be bonded. Rinse and dry. Apply primer(s) and adhesive resin, and cure for 20 seconds. Matrix strips are now removed to allow greater control over forming proximal contours with composite.

Apply the gingival shade evenly and smoothly. Create an irregular junction between gingival and incisal shades by scalloping the gingival material in this area. The junction will thus be more gradual and more difficult to perceive. Slightly overcontour to allow for finishing. Cure for 40 seconds.

Apply and contour the incisal shade, also with slight overcontour. Cure for 40 seconds.

If veneering adjacent teeth, take care to prevent bonding the veneers together. Prior to curing increments that extend to line angles, use a fine explorer or carver to separate any contact with freshly placed composite on an adjacent tooth. A scalpel or carver may also be used to separate any small amount of inadvertent adhesion between veneers after curing.

Refine contours with finishing burs or diamonds and discs. Long tapered shapes and discs are useful for labial surfaces, while rounded shapes adapt well to concave lingual areas. Use a #12 scalpel or composite carver to eliminate gingival excess interproximally and to modify emergence profile. Use retraction cord or a hand instrument to slightly displace labial gingiva for finishing. Develop a smooth feather-edge transition from composite to tooth in this area.

Proceed through successively finer diamonds and discs to smooth and polish. Apply composite polishing paste as a final step.

Direct composite veneering combined with diastema closure is illustrated in Fig. 4-9.

Figs. 4-9a to i Diastema closure and labial veneering with direct composite resin.

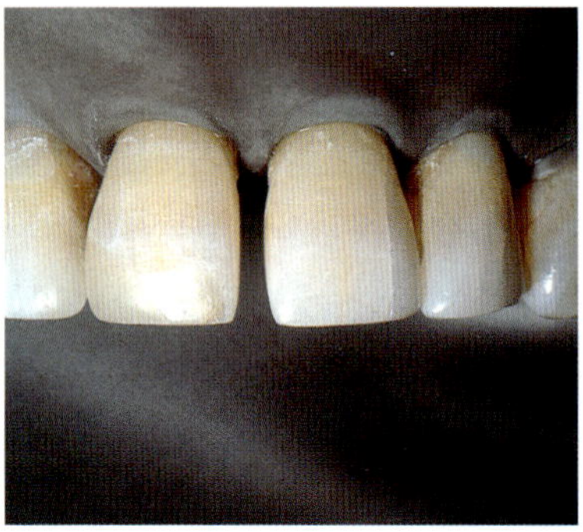

Fig. 4-9a Preoperative. No tooth preparation is used in this case.

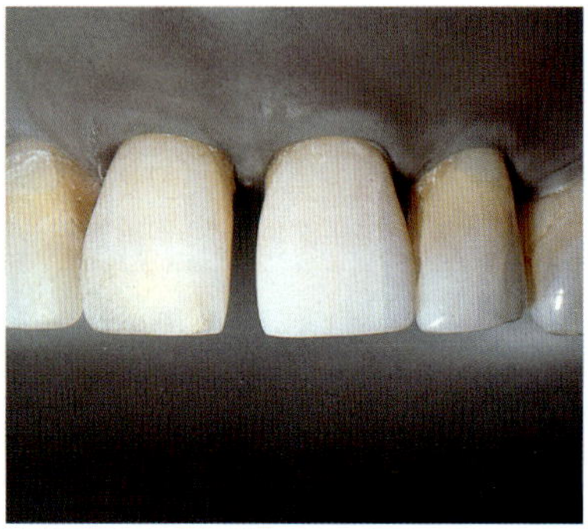

Fig. 4-9b Etched enamel.

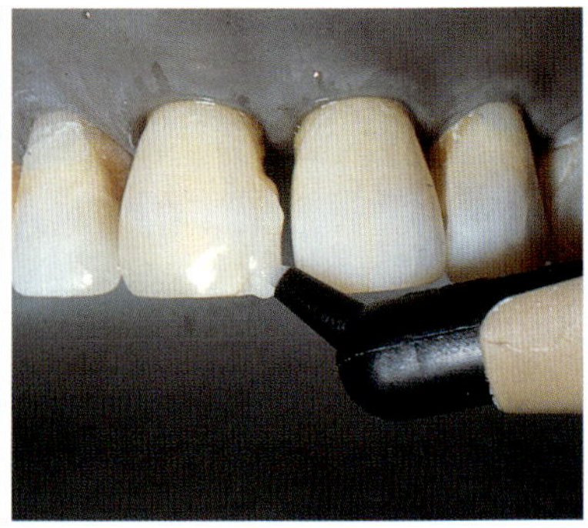

Fig. 4-9c Placement of dentin shade hybrid composite on first tooth in diastema closure sequence.

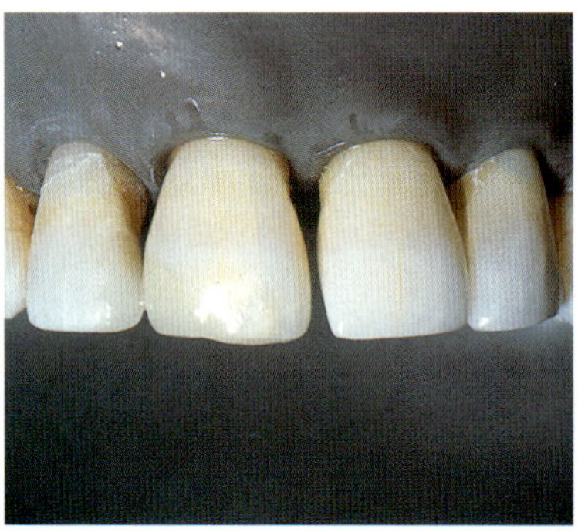

Fig. 4-9d Proximal composite on first tooth is finished and polished before proceeding.

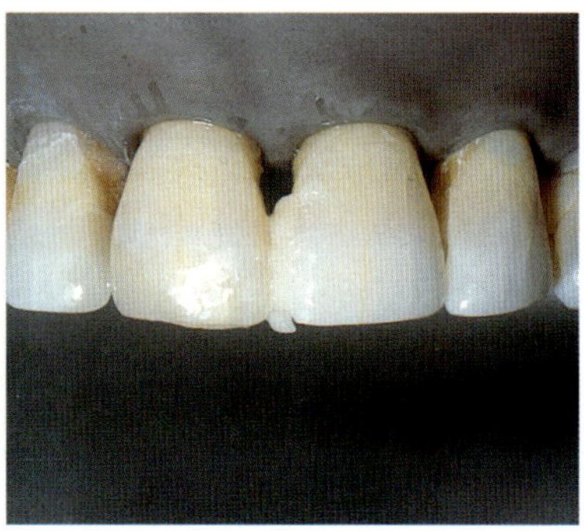

Fig. 4-9e Application of hybrid to second tooth, building into direct contact with polished restoration on first tooth. The high polish should prevent permanent adhesion between the teeth.

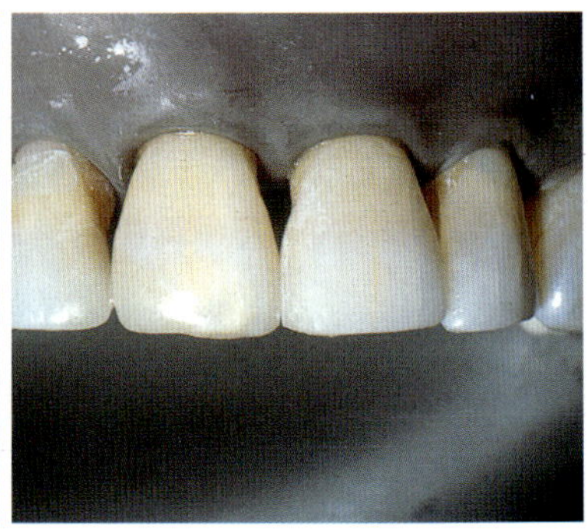

Fig. 4-9f Final finishing of proximal addition to second tooth is deferred until veneering is completed.

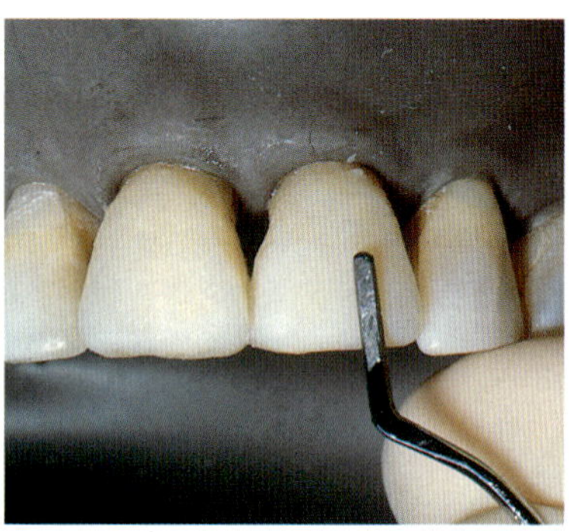

Fig. 4-9g Placement of microfill composite resin for veneering.

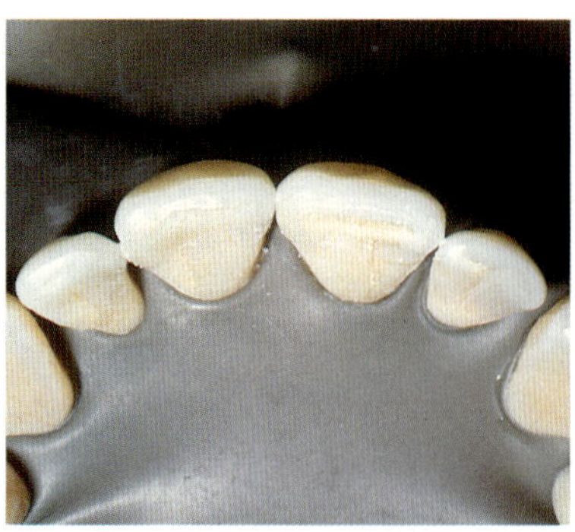

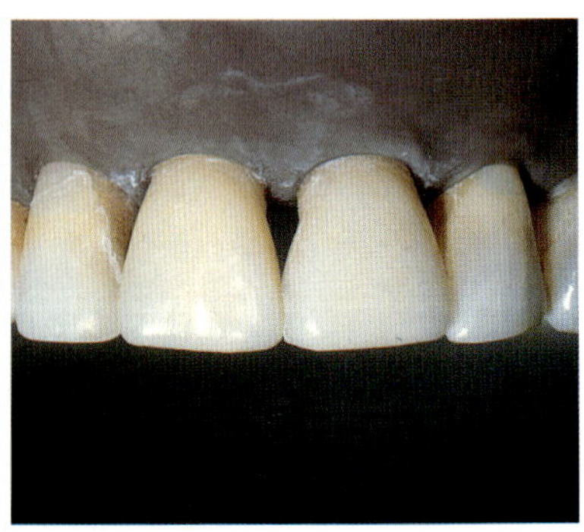

Figs. 4-9h and i Final restorations.

POSTERIOR RESTORATIONS

An esthetic restorative material suitable for routine use in posterior segments continues to be actively sought by the dental materials industry. Wear resistance of composite resins, while markedly improved over that of earlier formulations, continues to raise questions as to their suitability for replacing medium and large amalgams, especially in molar teeth.

Initial treatment of small-to-medium Class I and II lesions, however, can be carried out using composite resin very conservatively and predictably. The adhesive qualities of composite allow for preparation designs involving minimal removal of tooth structure (see chapter 4), unlike more invasive conventional designs for nonadhesive materials. More residual tooth structure imparts greater resistance form to the restored tooth. Small outline forms limit the area of composite exposed to functional stresses, minimizing wear resistance as a factor in the restoration's longevity. Control of microleakage associated with composite resin restorations continues to improve as adhesive resin systems evolve and become more effective.

CLASS I DIRECT RESTORATIONS

Pit and Fissure Sealants

Sealants represent the most conservative application of adhesive resins for Class I locations (Fig. 4-10). The efficacy of sealants as a preventive measure in juveniles has been demonstrated repeatedly in clinical studies. While routine sealing of unrestored adult posterior teeth is not widely recommended, sealants should be considered in some situations. Changes in health, diet and oral hygiene can alter caries susceptibility and lead to new caries in teeth that had remained unrestored for many years. An adult patient with a clinical presentation such as this would be well served by sealing of pits and fissures that have yet to develop caries.

Restorative Procedure

Material choice: Visible light cured sealants are available in translucent and opaque

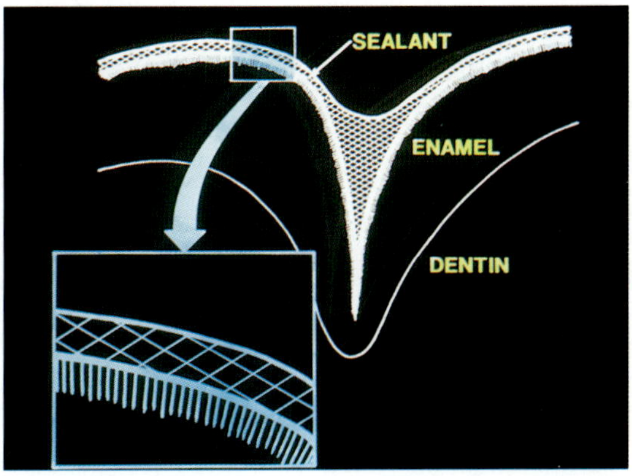

Fig. 4-10 Narrow pits and fissures are sealed with low viscosity adhesive resin. Acid etch (inset) provides excellent retention and resistance to microleakage.

Figs. 4-11a to c Application of sealants to occlusal pits and fissures of molar teeth.

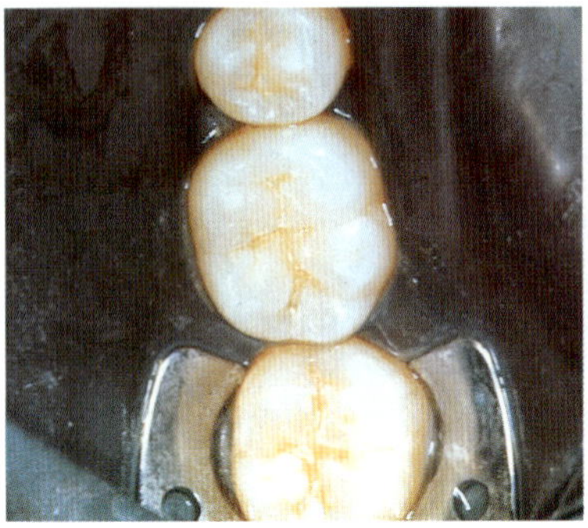

Fig. 4-11a Conservative widening of fissures performed with a 1/4 round carbide bur.

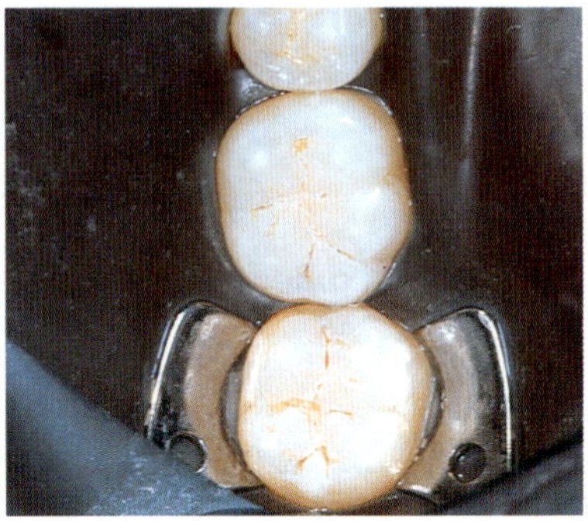

Fig. 4-11b Etched enamel.

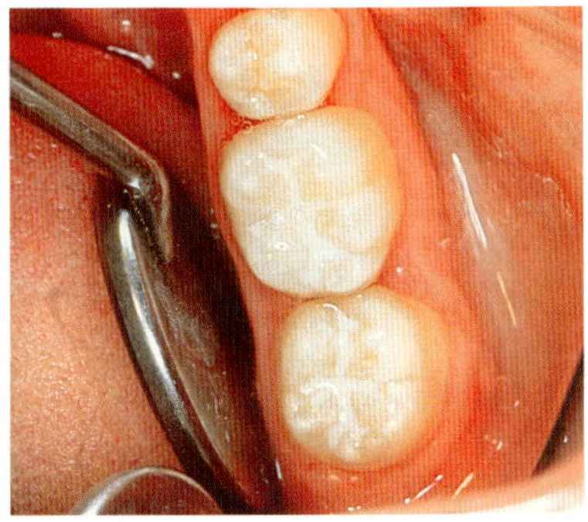

Fig. 4-11c Final sealant placement. Material is largely limited to fissures, minimizing need for occlusal adjustment (courtesy of Dr. M. Greitz).

varieties. Translucent sealants are virtually invisible to the casual observer. Opaque sealants, however, are easier to visually evaluate at recall with very little trade-off in esthetics.

Rubber dam isolation is the most effective means of moisture control, especially for mandibular teeth. Adequate moisture control can also be achieved with cotton rolls, warm air dryers and high volume evacuation. In any event, it is imperative that enamel remains absolutely uncontaminated during all steps from etching to occlusal adjustment of the sealant.

Clean the teeth with pumice on a tapered prophylaxis brush to remove saliva pellicle and staining in grooves. Air abrasive prophylaxis units are also extremely effective for this purpose. Rinse and dry. Re-examine grooves visually and with a sharp explorer to verify that no caries is present. Use a 1/4 round bur on a high speed handpiece to remove any remaining stain and debris, and to slightly open very narrow grooves to allow penetration of etchant and sealant (Fig. 4-11a).

Etch enamel for 15 to 30 seconds, rinse and dry thoroughly (Fig. 4-11b). Liquid etchants of watery viscosity are supplied with some etchant kits, and are effective in penetrating intricate occlusal anatomy. Gel etchants may be used if a liquid version is not available, but should be gently directed into grooves with an explorer.

Apply sealant with the applicator included in the kit or with a small brush. Use an explorer to work the sealant into grooves and to eliminate any air bubbles. Sealant should fill all grooves but should not form a large pool over the entire occlusal surface, as this will necessitate extensive occlusal adjustment (Fig. 4-11c). Remove excess sealant by absorption with a cotton roll. Cure for 40 seconds.

Check occlusion with articulating paper, and remove any premature contacts in the sealant with a rounded composite finishing diamond.

Preventive Resin Restoration

This technique adds the use of composite resin to the sealant procedure to restore small carious lesions in pits and fissures.

Restorative Procedure

Material selection: In addition to a sealant, use a hybrid composite resin for placement in the cavity preparation. Shade is not critical.

Proceed as described for sealants with

Figs. 4-12a to f Preventive resin restoration.

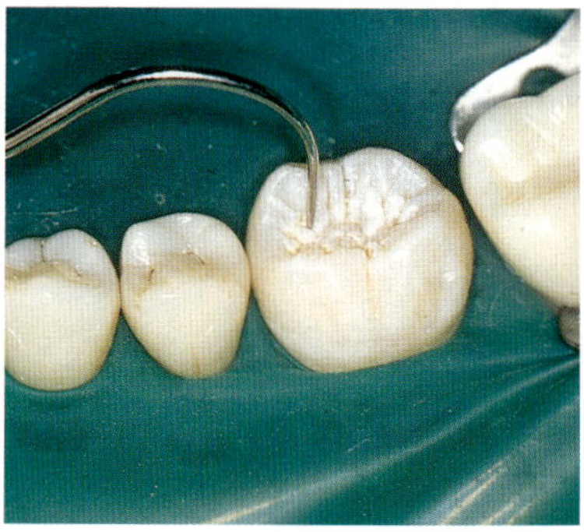

Fig. 4-12a Location of isolated caries with explorer.

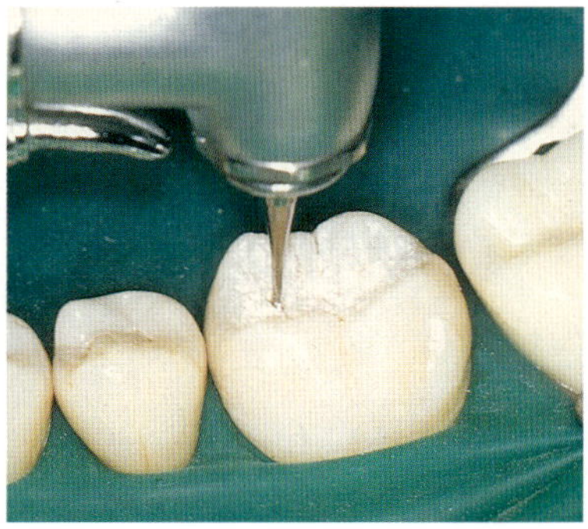

Fig. 4-12b Conservative removal of tooth structure with a small (1/2 to 1/4) round bur.

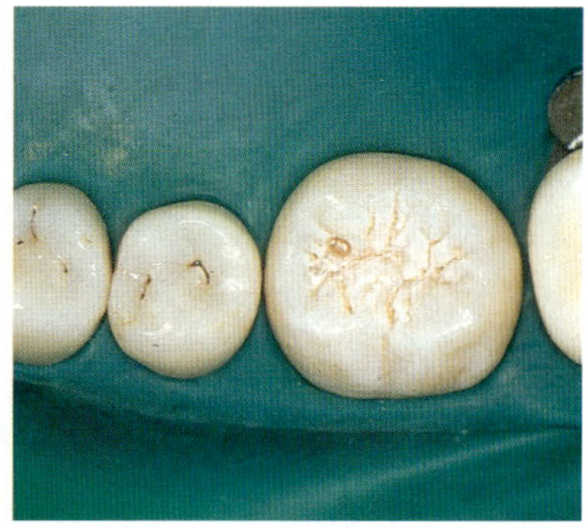

Fig. 4-12c Final preparation.

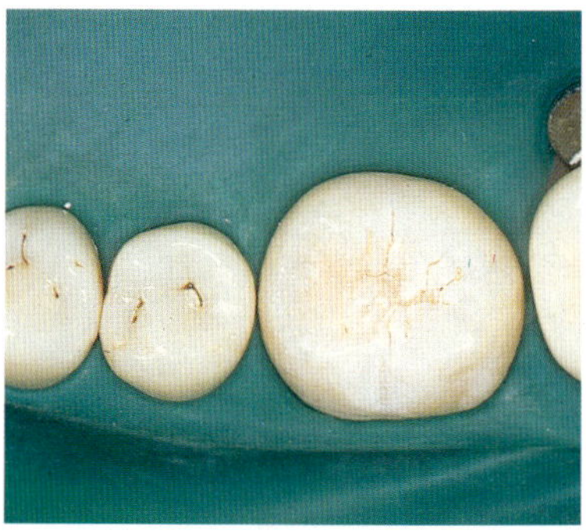

Fig. 4-12d Composite placement. Surface is left unfinished.

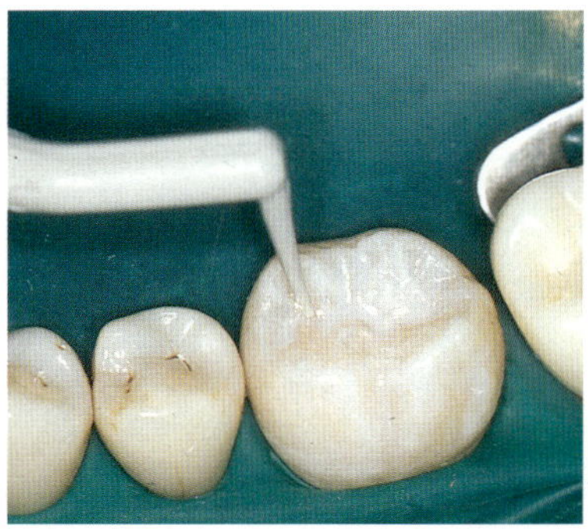

Fig. 4-12e Sealant placement over composite and into pits and fissures.

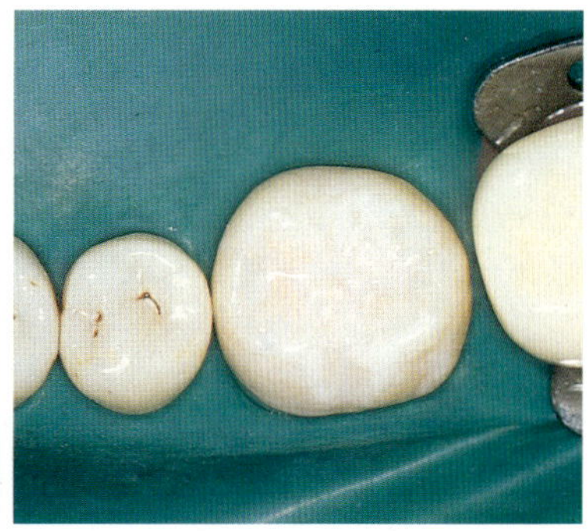

Fig. 4-12f Final restoration (courtesy of Dr. M. Gritz).

isolation, cleaning and groove preparation. Locate carious areas by tactile means with a sharp explorer (Fig. 4-12a). Use small round burs to remove only decalcified enamel and dentin, leaving all noncarious tooth structure intact (Figs. 4-12b and c). Check the preparation with an explorer to verify caries removal.

Etch enamel, condition dentin and apply primer and adhesive resin to the cavity preparation per directions for the system being used. Cure for 20 seconds.

Fill the cavity with hybrid composite, using a small ball burnisher to condense the material and eliminate any excess from the margins. Cure for 40 seconds. Finishing of the surface is unnecessary (Fig. 4-12d).

Apply sealant to occlusal grooves as described previously, covering the composite surface as well (Figs. 4-12e and f). Cure for 40 seconds.

Check occlusion with articulating paper, and remove any premature contacts in the sealant with a rounded composite finishing diamond.

Class I Composite

Restorative Procedure

Material selection: Use a dentin shade hybrid composite with high filler content.

Select composite shade. Exact matching of adjacent tooth structure is not critical. Use of a shade slightly lighter than that of the tooth facilitates removal of excess prior to contouring and finishing.

Rubber dam isolation is the most effective means of moisture control, especially for mandibular teeth. Adequate moisture control may also be achieved with cotton rolls, warm air dryers and high volume evacuation. In any event, it is imperative that the occlusal surface remain absolutely uncontaminated during all steps from enamel etching through curing of the final composite increment.

Clean the teeth with pumice on a tapered prophylaxis brush to remove saliva pellicle and staining in grooves. Air abrasive prophylaxis units are also extremely effective for this purpose.

Outline form, extensions and depth are established only to the extent necessary for removal of caries and existing restorations. Do not "extend for prevention" into non-carious pits and fissures. Small undercuts resulting in unsupported enamel may be left in place. Do not bevel enamel margins, as the thin area of composite covering the bevel may fracture under function.

Apply glass ionomer liner (light cured) to deep dentin areas. Calcium hydroxide is applied directly to small pulp exposures.

Etch enamel, condition dentin and apply primer and adhesive resin per directions for the system being used. Cure for 20 seconds.

Inject a first increment of composite and condense against the pulpal wall, as well as the buccal wall. The increment should extend to and cover the buccal margin. Place the curing light tip against the buccal surface of the tooth, and cure from the buccal direction for 40 seconds. Shrinkage is thus directed buccally. Cure for an additional 40 seconds from the occlusal.

Place and condense a second increment along the lingual wall, covering the lingual margin and filling the remainder of the preparation. Cure from the lingual, then from the occlusal for 40 seconds each. The directed shrinkage of the buccal and lingual increments is designed to prevent cuspal flexure produced by polymerization shrinkage toward the center of the tooth.

Use finishing burs or diamonds to remove excess and develop contours. Rounded and tapered ovoid shapes are best for developing and refining occlusal contours and anatomy.

Remove rubber dam or other isolation materials and check occlusion with articulating paper. Remove any premature contacts or interferences with the finishing bur or diamond. Proceed with finishing using progressively finer finishing diamonds.

Dry the occlusal surface, isolate with cotton rolls and apply enamel etchant to the restoration and adjacent enamel for 15 to 30 seconds. Rinse and dry. Brush on a thin layer of a surface-sealing resin (e.g. Fortify, Bisco) and cure for 20 seconds. Postfinishing sealing in this manner is thought to reduce early wear by sealing surface microcracks produced during finishing.

Apply composite polishing paste as a final polishing step.

CLASS II DIRECT RESTORATIONS

Tunnel Preparation

This technique represents another radical departure from traditional cavity designs that reflect the adhesive capabilities of current esthetic restoratives. It involves "tunneling" under marginal or oblique ridges to remove small caries, leaving the undermined ridge in place. Proximal contact in natural tooth structure is also maintained, facilitating restoration of the cavity. Adhesion of the restorative to the undermined area provides reinforcement, making it unnecessary to remove these areas.

Use of the tunnel preparation is not recommended for routine treatment of proximal caries, as access to and visualization of caries is often difficult. It does however serve as a useful alternative to proximal box preparation in many cases, especially when removal of an existing occlusal restoration provides adequate access.

Restorative Procedure

Material selection: Use a dentin shade hybrid composite with high filler content.

Select composite shade. Exact matching of adjacent tooth structure is not critical. Use of a shade slightly lighter than that of the tooth facilitates removal of excess prior to contouring and finishing.

Rubber dam isolation is the most effective means of moisture control, especially for mandibular teeth. Adequate moisture control with other means may be difficult to achieve with respect to proximal surfaces. Use cotton rolls, warm air dryers and high volume evacuation if rubber dam cannot be placed. In any event, it is imperative that the occlusal surface remain absolutely uncontaminated during all steps from enamel etching through curing of the final composite increment.

Clean the teeth with pumice on a tapered prophylaxis brush to remove saliva pellicle and staining in grooves. Air abrasive prophylaxis units are also extremely effective for this purpose. Insert a metal matrix band interproximally to protect the adjacent tooth during preparation.

Occlusal outline form, extensions and depth are initially established only to the extent necessary for removal of caries and existing restorations. Do not "extend for prevention" into noncarious pits and fissures. In the absence of occlusal restorations or caries, use a #330 carbide bur to enter the occlusal at an oblique angle, aimed toward the proximal lesion.

Extend the occlusal outline, if necessary, to visualize proximal caries. Remove caries with a round bur at low speed. If caries removal cannot be ascertained, or if the marginal ridge is thinned to the point of transparency, preparation of a more conventional proximal box will be necessary.

Remove the metal matrix band, and bevel any accessible buccal and lingual proximal margins with a narrow tapered diamond. Do not bevel other margins, including occlusal.

Place a mylar matrix strip and transparent wedge, as these will allow curing from the buccal and lingual directions.

Placement of enamel etchant on dentin cannot be avoided when etching interproximal enamel from the internal aspect of the preparation. Etching should thus be limited to 15 seconds, or an adhesive system should be used that employs a single agent for conditioning of enamel and dentin. Apply primer and adhesive resin per directions for the system being used. Cure for 20 seconds.

Place and condense an increment of composite to fill the proximal portion of the preparation. Cure from the buccal and lingual each for 20 seconds to direct shrinkage toward proximal margins. Cure from the occlusal for 20 seconds.

Place and condense a single occlusal increment if the outline extensions are minimal. Cure from the occlusal for 40 seconds. For larger occlusal outlines, place separate vertical wall increments buccally and lingually as described in the restoration procedure for a Class I composite restoration.

Remove wedge and matrix, and remove proximal excess with a #12 scalpel blade or composite carver.

Use finishing burs or diamonds to remove excess and develop contours. Rounded and tapered ovoid shapes are best for developing and refining occlusal contours and anatomy.

Remove rubber dam or other isolation materials and check occlusion with articulating paper. Remove any premature contacts or interferences with the finishing bur or diamond. Check for overhangs with dental floss. Proceed with finishing using progressively finer finishing diamonds.

Dry the occlusal surface, isolate with cotton rolls and apply enamel etchant to the restoration and adjacent enamel for 15 to 30 seconds. Rinse and dry. Brush on a thin layer of a surface-sealing resin (e.g. Fortify, Bisco) and cure for 20 seconds. Postfinishing sealing in this manner is thought to reduce early wear by sealing surface microcracks produced during finishing.

Polish any accessible proximal margins with fine finishing discs. Apply composite polishing paste to all surfaces as a final polishing step.

Class II Composite

Restorative Procedure

Material selection: Use a dentin shade hybrid composite with high filler content. The directed polymerization shrinkage technique also calls for the use of a dual cured or chemically cured composite for placement along the gingival margin. The chemical polymerization reaction is thought to begin along the surface adjacent to the gingival wall, as the temperature should be slightly higher at this interface than at the surface of the increment exposed to air. Polymerization shrinkage should then occur in a gingival direction toward the initial reaction site, thus minimizing the marginal gap produced by shrinkage in the opposite direction. This technique may be of particular value when the gingival margin of the preparation has little or no enamel.

Select composite shade. Exact matching of adjacent tooth structure is not critical. Use of a shade slightly lighter than that of the tooth facilitates removal of excess prior to contouring and finishing.

Rubber dam isolation is the most effective means of moisture control, especially for mandibular teeth. Adequate moisture control with other means may be difficult to achieve with respect to proximal surfaces. Use cotton rolls, warm air dryers and high volume evacuation if rubber dam cannot be placed. In any event, it is imperative that the occlusal surface remain absolutely uncontaminated during all steps from enamel etching through curing of the final composite increment.

Insert a wedge snugly into the gingival embrasure of the proximal surface to be restored. This prewedging aids in developing the tooth separation necessary to establish a proximal contact with the composite. Use two wedges if both proximal surfaces are to be restored.

Clean the teeth with pumice on a tapered prophylaxis brush to remove saliva pellicle and staining in grooves. Air abrasive prophylaxis units are also extremely effective for this purpose. Insert a metal matrix band interproximally to protect the adjacent tooth during preparation.

Outline form, extensions (occlusal and proximal) and depth are established only to the extent necessary for removal of caries and existing restorations (Figs. 4-13a and b). Otherwise, do not extend proximal margins to break contact. Do not "extend for prevention" into noncarious pits and fissures. Small undercuts resulting in unsupported enamel may be left in place. Do not bevel enamel margins. The thin area of composite covering the bevel may fracture under function, and a tightly adapted matrix may prevent coverage of proximal bevels.

Apply glass ionomer liner (light cured) to deep dentin areas. Calcium hydroxide is applied directly to small pulp exposures.

Place matrix. Several types of matrices are available. A Tofflemire retainer may be used in combination with a clear mylar strip (Figs. 4-13c and d) . The Cure-Thru system (ESPE-Premier) (Fig. 4-14a) provides individual clear matrices as well as plastic wedges. The wedges are designed to both transmit light and reflect light onto the gingival aspect of the restoration. The Sectional Matrix

Figs. 4-13a to d Class II composite restoration.

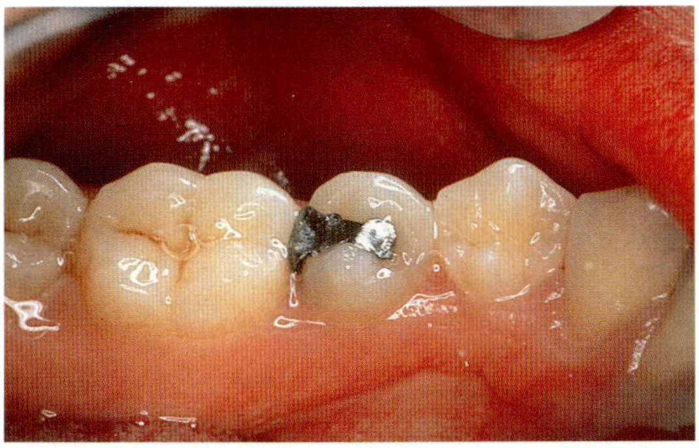

Fig. 4-13a Preoperative, existing amalgam to be replaced with direct composite resin.

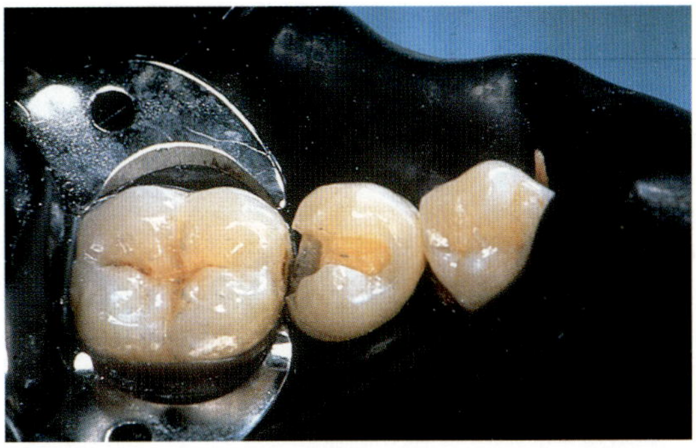

Fig. 4-13b Final preparation.

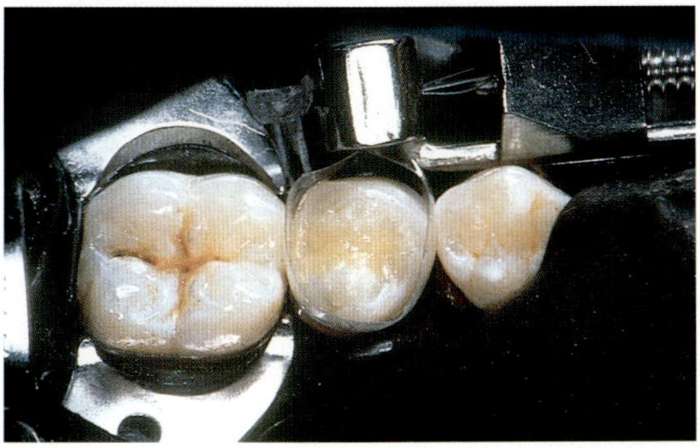

Fig. 4-13c Tofflemire matrix retainer used with clear mylar strip.

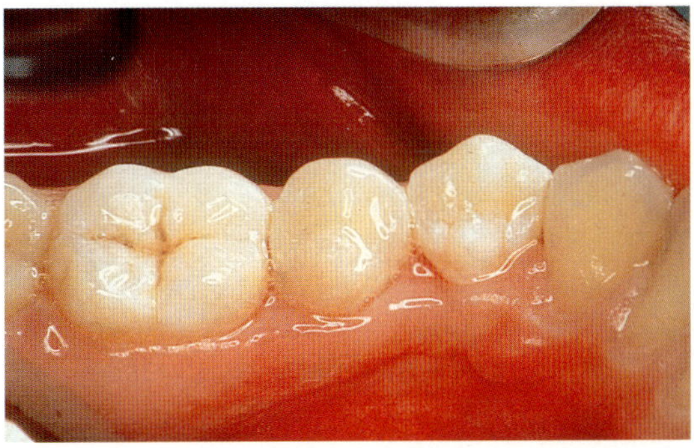

Fig. 4-13d Final restoration (courtesy of Dr. M. Gritz).

Figs. 4-14a to c Additional matrices for Class II composite.

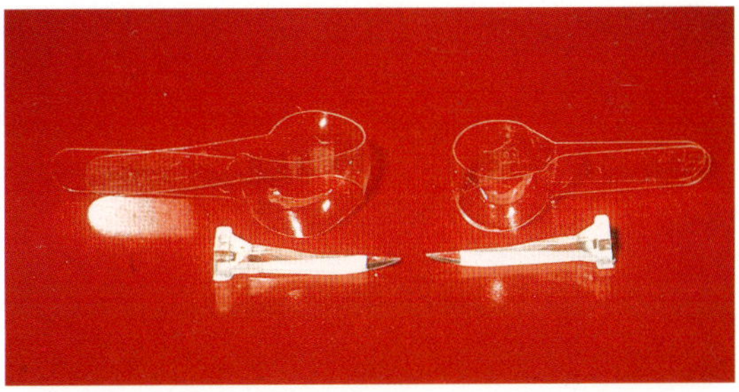

Fig. 4-14a Cure-Thru system, with clear matrices and reflective wedges (ESPE-Premier).

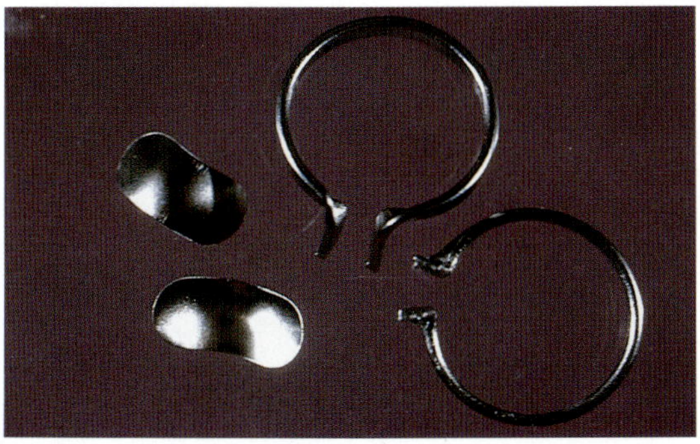

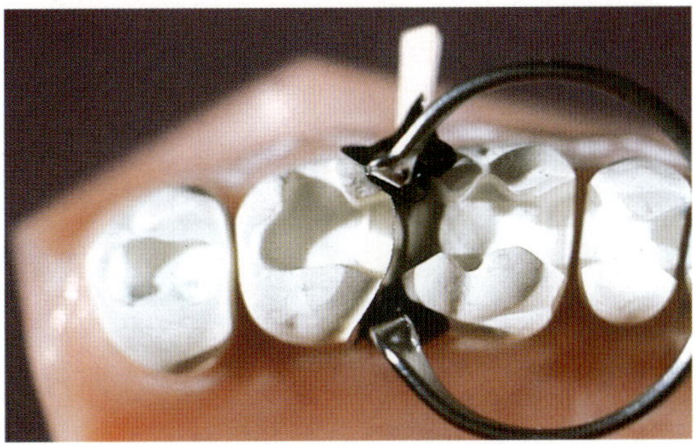

Figs. 4-14b and c Sectional Matrices (Palodent).

(Palodent) (Figs. 4-14b and c) is simple to use, and the biconcave shape of the matrix is designed to prevent flattening of proximal contours that may occur with an over-tightened Tofflemire. A wooden wedge is used for tooth separation, and the Bitine Ring is placed using rubber dam forceps to stabilize the small matrix. All light curing must be done from the occlusal direction with this system.

Etch enamel, condition dentin and apply primer and adhesive resin per directions for the system being used. Cure for 20 seconds. Protect adjacent teeth during these steps with a matrix strip.

Inject and condense an increment of composite covering the gingival wall, 1 mm in thickness. If a dual cure or chemical cure material is being used as described in the directed polymerization shrinkage technique (see the discussion on material selection at the beginning of this procedure), allow the reaction to commence before proceeding. Test the increment with an explorer, and irradiate dual cure material for 40 seconds only after initial chemical set renders the increment hard.

Inject a first occlusal increment of composite and condense against the pulpal wall, gingival increment and buccal wall. The increment should extend to and cover the buccal margin. Place the curing light tip against the buccal surface of the tooth, and cure from the buccal direction for 40 seconds. Shrinkage is thus directed buccally. Cure for an additional 40 seconds from the occlusal.

Place and condense a second increment along the lingual wall, covering the lingual margin and filling the remainder of the preparation. Cure from the lingual, then from the occlusal for 40 seconds each. The directed shrinkage of the buccal and lingual increments is designed to prevent cuspal flexure produced by polymerization shrinkage toward tho contor of tho tooth.

Remove matrix and check the proximal contact with dental floss. If contact is inadequate, it will be necessary to add composite. Remove composite from the proximal area, preparing a small box within the newly placed composite. Protect the adjacent tooth with a matrix strip. Apply enamel etchant to the prepared area for 15 seconds, rinse and dry. Place a thin layer of adhesive resin and cure for 20 seconds. Remove matrix, insert a wedge tightly and inject and condense composite, building into direct contact with the adjacent tooth. Permanent bonding to the adjacent tooth will be prevented as it has not been etched or treated with resin. Contour the added material, removing excess from embrasures with a carver or explorer. Cure from the occlusal for 40 seconds. Insert a beavertail burnisher into the gingival embrasure, and gently torque the teeth to break adhesion. Use floss to recheck the contact and to check for overhangs.

Eliminate proximal excess and refine embrasures as necessary with a #12 scalpel or composite carvers. Use finishing burs or diamonds to remove excess and develop contours occlusally. Rounded and tapered ovoid shapes are best for developing and refining occlusal contours and anatomy.

Remove rubber dam or other isolation materials and check occlusion with articulating paper. Remove any premature contacts or interferences with the finishing bur or diamond. Proceed with finishing using progressively finer finishing diamonds.

Dry the occlusal surface, isolate with cotton rolls and apply enamel etchant to the restoration and adjacent enamel for 15 to 30 seconds. Rinse and dry. Brush on a thin layer of a surface-sealing resin (e.g. Fortify, Bisco, Fig. 4-15) and cure for 20 seconds. Post-finishing sealing in this manner is thought to reduce early wear via sealing surface micro-cracks produced during finishing.

Polish any accessible proximal margins with fino finiching dicoo. Apply oompocito

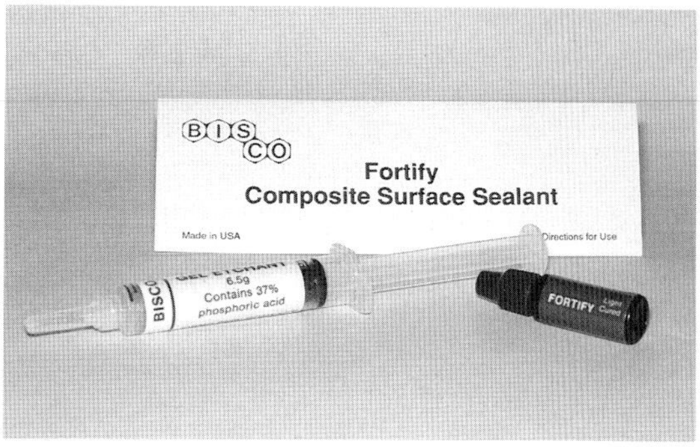

Fig. 4-15 Fortify (Bisco), a low viscosity unfilled resin used to seal the occlusal surfaces of newly placed direct posterior composite restorations.

polishing paste to all surfaces as a final polishing step.

REFERENCES

GENERAL CONSIDERATIONS AND ANTERIOR RESTORATIONS

Albers, H.F.: Tooth Colored Restoratives (A Text for Selection, Placement and Finishing) (Seventh Edition). (1985). Santa Rosa: Alto Books.

Ben-Amar, A., Liberman, R., Nordenberg, D., and Metzger, Z.: The Effect of Retention Grooves on Gingival Marginal Leakage in Class II Posterior Composite Resin Restorations. (1988). J. Oral Rehab. 15:325-331.

Boghosian, A.A.: Restoration of Class V Abrasions with a New Light-Cured Glass Ionomer Restorative. (1992). Practical Periodont. Aesthetic Dent. 4:43-48.

Charbeneau, G.T.: Principles and Practice of Operative Dentistry (Third Edition). (1988). Philadelphia: Lea & Febiger.

Cox, C.F., White, K.C., Ramus, D.L., Farmer, J.B., and Snuggs, H.M.: Reparative Dentin: Factors Affecting its Deposition. (1992). Quint. Int. 23:257-270.

Hansen, E.K.: Three Year Study of Cervical Erosions Restored with Resin and Dentin Bonding Agent. (1989). Act. Odont. Scand. 47:301-306.

Hergoff, A.M., Ziemiecki, T.L., and Dennison, J.B.: An Evaluation of Different Composite Resin Systems Finished with Various Abrasives. (1989). J. Am. Dent. Assoc. 119:729-732.

Kaim, J.M.: Current Composite Resin Techniques. (1988). N.Y. State Dent. J. 54:56-59.

Kaplan, I., Mincer, H.H., Harris, E.F., and Cloyd, J.S.: Microleakage of Composite Resin and Glass Ionomer Cement Restorations in Retentive and Non-retentive Cervical Cavity Preparations. (1992). J. Prosth. Dent. 68:616-623.

Kemp-scholte, C.M. and Davidson, C.L.: Marginal Sealing of Curing Contractions Gaps in Class I Composite Resin Restorations. (1988). J. Dent. Res. 67:841-845.

Krejci, I., Lutz, F.: Marginal Adaptation of Class V Restorations Using Different Restorative Techniques. (1991). J. Dent. 19: 24-32.

Larson, T.D.: Techniques for Achieving Realistic Color Distribution in Large Composite Resin Restorations. (1986). J. Am. Dent. Assoc. 112:669-672.

Leclaire, C.C., Blank, L.W., Hargrave, J.W., and Pelleu, G.B., Jr.: Use of a Two-Stage Composite Resin Fill to Reduce Microleakage Below the Cementoenamel Junction. (1988). Oper. Dent. 13:20-23.

Lee, W.C. and Eakle, W.S.: Possible Role of Tensile Stress in the Etiology of Cervical Erosive Lesions of Teeth. (1984). J. Prosth. Dent. 52:374-380.

Lutz, F., Setcos, J., and Phillips, R.: New Finishing Instruments for Composite Resins. (1983). J. Am. Dent. Assoc. 107:575-580.

Miller, M.B., Ed.-in-Chief. Section 2: The Techniques, in Reality. (1992). Vol. 7, No. 2. Houston: Reality Publishing Co.

Saguchi, R.L., Douglas, W.H., Peters, M.C.: Curing Light Performance and Polymerization of Composite Restorative Materials. (1992). J. Dent. 20:178-182.

Saguchi, R.L., Peters, M.C., Nelson, S.R., Douglas, W.H., and Poort H.W.: Effects of Polymerization Contraction in Composite Restorations. (1992). J. Dent. 20:178-182.

Shahani, D.R. and Menezes, J.M.: The Effect of Retention Grooves on Posterior Composite Resin Restorations: An In Vitro Microleakage Study. (1992). Oper. Dent. 17: 156-164.

Shortall, A.C.: In Vitro Microleakage of Class V Composite Resin Restorations With and Without Light-Cured Glass-Ionomer (Poly Alkenoate) Cement Lining. (1992). Eur. J. Prosthodont. Restor. Dent. 1:7-11.

Sidhu, S.K. and Henderson, L.J.: In Vitro Marginal Leakage of Cervical Composite Restorations Lined With a Light-Cured Glass Ionomer. (1992). Oper. Dent. 17:7-12.

Smales, R.J.: Effect of Rubber Dam Isolation on Restoration Degradation. (1992). Am. J. Dent. 5:277-279.

Stoddard, J.W. and Johnson, G.H.: An Evaluation of Polishing Agents for Composite Resins. (1991). J. Prosth. Dent. 65: 491-495.

Tjan, A.H. and Dunn, J.R.: Microleakage at Gingival Dentin Margins of Class V Composite Restorations Lined With Light-Cured Glass Ionomer Cement. (1990). J. Am. Dent. Assoc. 121: 706-710.

vanDijkin, J.W. and Horstedt, P.: Effect of the Use of Rubber Dam versus Cotton Rolls on Marginal Adaptation of Composite Resin Fillings to Etched Enamel. (1987). Acta. Odontol. Scand. 45:303-308.

Vanherle, G., Lambrechts, P., and Braem, M.: An Evaluation of Different Adhesive Restorations in Cervical Lesions. (1991). J. Prosth. Dent. 65:341-347.

Whitehead, S.A. and Wilson, N.H.: The Native and Effects of Composite Finishing Pastes. (1989). J. Dent. 17:234-40.

Zalkind, M. and Heling, L.: Composite Resin Layering: An Esthetic Technique for Restoring Fractured Anterior Teeth. (1992). J. Prosth. Dent. 68:204-205.

POSTERIOR RESTORATIONS

Albers, H.F.: Tooth Colored Restoratives (A Text for Selection, Placement and Finishing) (Seventh Edition). (1985). Santa Rosa: Alto Books.

Bertolotti, R.L.: Posterior Composite Technique Utilizing Directed Polymerization Shrinkage and a Novel Matrix. (1991). Practical Periodont. Aesthetic Dent. 3:53-58.

Buonocore, M.G.: Caries Prevention in Pits and Fissures Sealed with an Adhesive Resin Polymerized by Ultraviolet Light: A Two-Year Study of a Single Adhesive Application. (1971). J. Am. Dent. Assoc. 82:1090-1093.

Charbeneau, G.T.: Principles and Practice of Operative Dentistry (Third Edition). (1988). Philadelphia: Lea & Febiger.

Dickinson, G.L., Leinfelder, K.F., Mazer, R.B., and Russell, C.M.: Effect of Surface Penetrating Sealant on Wear Rate of Posterior Composite Resins. (1990). J. Am. Dent. Assoc. 121:251-255.

Handleman, S.L.: Effect of Sealant Placement on Occlusal Caries Progression. (1982). Clin. Prev. Dent. 4:11-16.

Hill, F.J. and Halaseh, F.J.: A Laboratory Investigation of Tunnel Restorations in Premolar Teeth. (1988). Br. Dent. J. 165: 364-367.

Hunt, P.R.: A Modified Class II Cavity Preparation for Glass Ionomer Restorative Materials. (1984). Quint. Int. 15(10): 1011-1018.

Kaim, J.M.: Current Composite Resin Techniques. (1988). N.Y. State Dent. J. 54:56-59.

Kays, B.T., Sneed, W.D., and Nuckles, D.B.: Microhardness of Class II Composite Resin Restorations with Different Matrices and Light Positions. (1991). J. Prosth. Dent. 65:487-490.

Lewis, G.: In Vivo Occlusal Wear of Posterior Composite Restorations. (1991). Oper. Dent. 16:61-69.

Lutz, E., Krejci, I., and Oldenburg, T.R.: Elimination of Polymerization Stresses at the Margins of Posterior Composite Resin Restorations: A New Restorative Technique. (1986). Quint. Int. 17:777-784.

Lutz, F., Krejci, I., Liischer, B., and Oldenburg, T.R.: Improved Proximal Marginal Adaptation of Class II Composite Resin Restorations by Use of Light Reflecting Wedges. (1986). Quint. Int. 17:659-664.

Lutz, F., Phillips, R.W., Roulet, J.F., and Setcos, J.C.: In Vivo and In Vitro Wear of Potential Posterior Composites. (1984). J. Dent. Res. 63:914-920.

Miller, M.B., Ed.-in-Chief: Section 2: The Techniques in Reality. (1992). Vol. 7, No. 2. Houston: Reality Publishing Co.

Ratanapridakul, K., Leinfelder, K.F., and Thomas, J. : Effect of Finishing on the In Vivo Wear Rate of a Posterior Composite Resin. (1989). J. Am. Dent. Assoc. 118:333-335.

Saguchi, R.L., Peters, M.C., Nelson, S.R., Douglas, W.H., and Poort H.W.: Effects of Polymerization Contraction in Composite Restorations. (1992). J. Dent. 20:178-182.

Simonsen, R.J.: Preventive Resin Restoration: Five Year Results. (1982). J. Am. Dent. Assoc. 102:323-327.

Simonsen, R.J.: Preventive Resin Restorations. Innovative Use of Sealants in Restorative Dentistry. (1982). Clin. Prev. Dent. 4:27-29.

Smales, R.J.: Effect of Rubber Dam Isolation on Restoration Degradation. (1992). Am. J. Dent. 5:277-279.

vanDijkin, J.W. and Horstedt, P.: Effect of the Use of Rubber Dam versus Cotton Rolls on Marginal Adaptation of Composite Resin Fillings to Etched Enamel. (1987). Acta. Odontol. Scand. 45:303-308.

Warren, J.A., Jr. and Clark, N.P.: Posterior Composite Resin: Current Trends in Restorative Techniques. Part 1: Pre-preparation considerations, Preparation, Dentin Treatment, etching/ Bonding. (1987). Gen. Dent. 35:368-372.

Warren, J.A., Jr. and Clark, N.P.: Posterior Composite Resin: Current Trends and Restorative Techniques. Part 2: Insertion, Finishing, and Polishing. (1987). Gen. Dent. 35:497-499.

CHAPTER 5

INDIRECT AND DIRECT COMPOSITE RESTORATIONS

INDIRECT COMPOSITE RESTORATIONS

The use of composite resin as an indirect restorative material has its roots in efforts to improve the physical properties and clinical performance of composite restorations. By fabrication and polymerization of the restoration indirectly (i.e. in the laboratory), heat, light and pressure can be utilized to achieve a higher degree of polymerization than is possible in direct applications. More thorough polymerization is thought to impart increased wear resistance over direct restorations, but clinical research has yet to substantiate this claim. Additionally, polymerization shrinkage occurs prior to placement, potentially reducing gap formation at dentin margins and walls, as well as flexure forces on cusps.

Techniques utilizing bonded ceramic have supplanted those involving indirect composite, particularly with respect to anterior veneers. The following considerations, however, have resulted in the continued use of indirect composite inlays as an alternative to bonded ceramic in posterior teeth:

- Reduced abrasion of opposing teeth for composite vs. ceramic (especially porcelain).
- Ease of fabrication — in-office fabrication is more feasible for composite systems.
- Lower hardness and brittleness renders composite easier to adjust, finish and polish than ceramic.
- Intraoral repair of composites can be performed with virtually the same material used for the original restoration.

With respect to posterior inlays, then, indirect composite represents a restorative material alternative to ceramic. The restorative procedures for indirect composite inlays are not outlined here, as they are essentially the same as those for ceramic inlays (see CERAMIC INLAY-ONLAY chapter).

The remainder of this chapter describes a technique that combines the advantages of extraoral polymerization of the restoration with the one-appointment convenience of direct placement: the direct/indirect composite inlay.

THE DIRECT COMPOSITE INLAY

INTRODUCTION

The increased demand for amalgam alternatives has been a major motivation for manufacturers to develop substitutes that will provide a restoration with a good long term prognosis and are relatively easy to place. In addition, patients are demanding tooth colored materials that create a more natural and esthetic result. Manufacturers initially answered these demands by developing composite resin restorative materials that supposedly could be easily manipulated, were esthetic and would provide many years of service. Unfortunately, the manufacturers failed on all three accounts. The materials were very difficult to use due to "stickiness" and poor handling, limited in shades, difficult to polish and proved to be clinically unacceptable due to their poor wear resistance and high polymerization shrinkage.

The manufacturers, however, continued to market these substitutes and they were used by many clinicians with poor results. These early problems frightened many clinicians away from using composite resin materials in posterior teeth and has led to its guarded acceptance as a restorative material by many leading clinicians and researchers. Poor wear resistance, marginal leakage and staining, high polymerization shrinkage, poor interproximal contacts and high early failure rates became synonymous with posterior composites (Fig. 5-1).

Fortunately, research and development continued by dental manufacturers and as a result many outstanding composite resins have been developed for use in both anterior and posterior teeth. Handling characteristics have been significantly improved and wear resistance values of new composite resins are approaching the wear rates of traditional amalgam alloys. Unfortunately, factors such as high polymerization shrinkage and poor wear resistance are still a concern today and leading clinicians and researchers continue to develop new materials and techniques that will improve restorative results (see chapter 3).

The advantages of using a composite resin restoration over gold or amalgam in posterior teeth include improved esthetic results and conservation of tooth structure because retention is achieved through bonding, not mechanical means. It has also been shown that the fracture resistance of resin restored teeth exceeds that of those restored with alloy or gold inlays. Reduced fracture potential may lead to a decreased incidence of larger restorations in the future (Figs. 5-2 and 5-3).

Clinically, direct filled posterior composite resin restorations are very technique sensitive, which may lead to problems and premature failure. Frequent causes of failure include postinsertion sensitivity, excessive occlusal wear, lack of adequate interproximal contacts and leaking or staining margins. It has become evident that these materials do not often meet the demands required for long term posterior application. Studies have shown that one of the major problems with these large composite resin restorations is polymerization shrinkage. The composite resins shrink toward the light source, breaking the bond between the composite resin and the tooth surfaces, leaving marginal gaps. This gap results in a restoration that is not in direct contact with the tooth and thus microleakage is prevalent, especially at the gingival margin, which may have minimal enamel for bonding (Fig. 5-4). Contraction shrinkage has also been suggested as a cause of unfavorable intercuspal deformation, resulting in postoperative sensitivity.

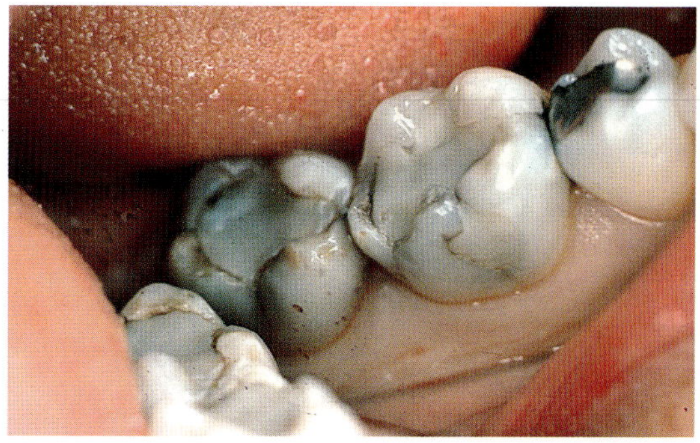

Fig. 5-1 Direct light cured only posterior composites placed only 2 years previously. Note staining and ditching of margins and wear of occlusal surface.

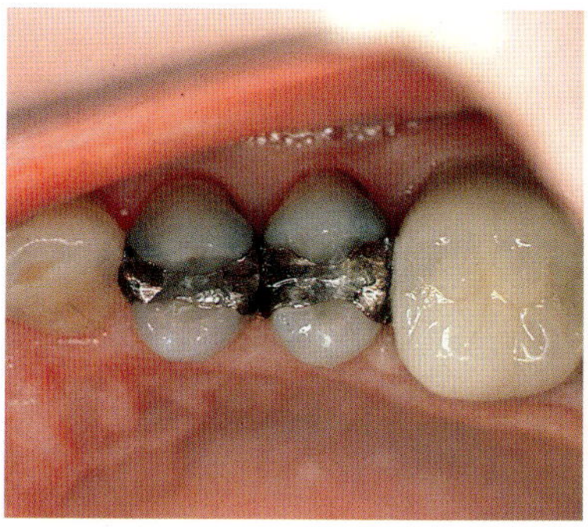

Fig. 5-2a Preoperative view.

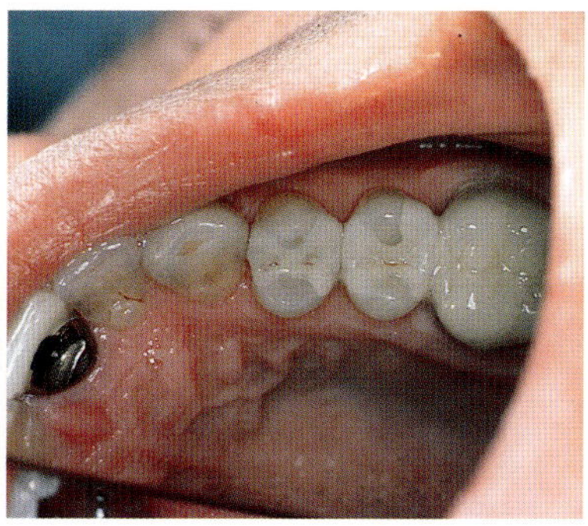

Fig. 5-2b Three surface direct resin inlays were used to replace defective alloys.

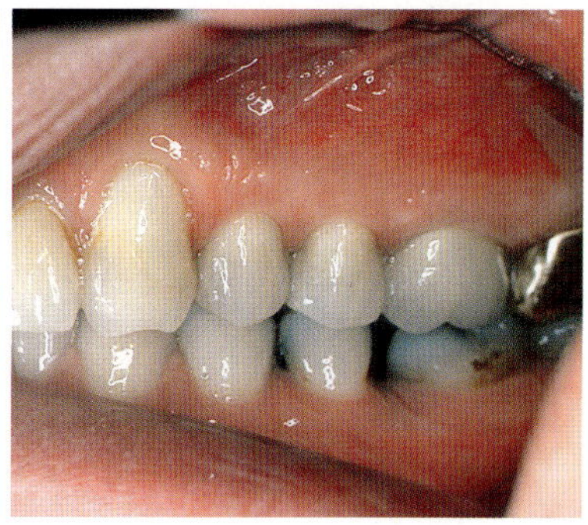

Fig. 5-2c Opacity difference is noticeable from the occlusal view, but blend very esthetically when seen from the facial aspect.

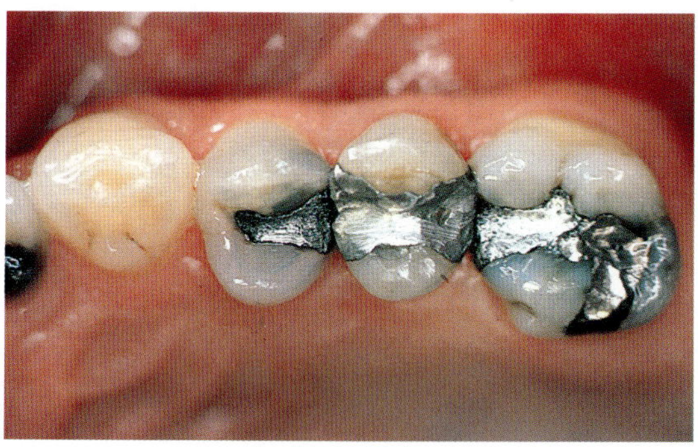

Fig. 5-3a Preoperative view.

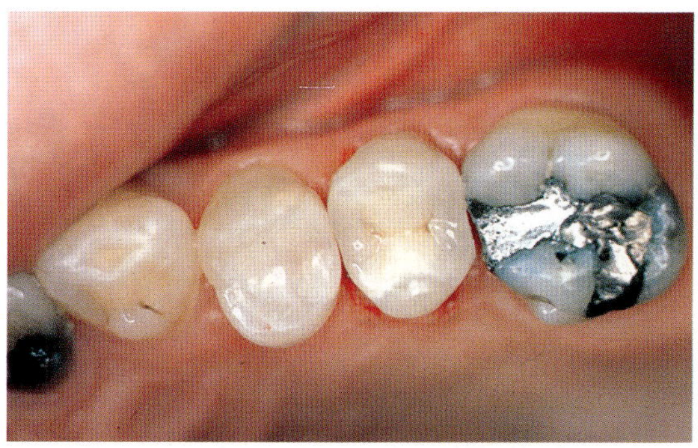

Fig. 5-3b

Fig. 5-3b The ability to bond the inlay into place allows for less aggressive restorative treatment, as seen by these direct resin inlays on maxillary premolars. Notice the minimal amount of lingual cusp present on tooth 4. This restoration was placed 4 years ago.

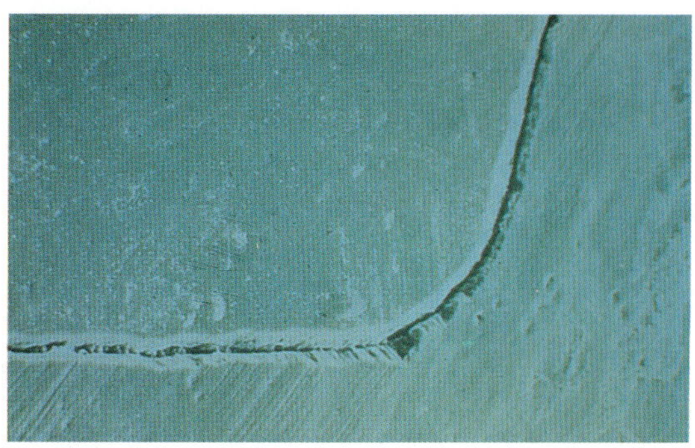

Fig. 5-4

Fig. 5-4 Scanning electron micrograph of a traditional light cured composite resin bonded to tooth structure. Notice gap caused by polymerization shrinkage of resin. This gap is responsible for leakage, sensitivity and premature failure of these types of restorations.

Finally, it has been shown that resins polymerized with traditional hand-held visible light sources exhibit incomplete polymerization, which may account for lower surface hardness and decreased abrasion resistance.

It has been postulated by many, and proven in several studies, that if most of the polymerization shrinkage could take place outside the mouth, many of the negative aspects of posterior composite resin restorations could be overcome. Other researchers have shown that by subjecting the composite resin to heat and more intense light, the surface hardness is greatly enhanced, thus increasing wear resistance. It is with this in mind that the technique for the direct composite resin inlay has evolved.

This technique utilizes the prepared tooth as the "working die" eliminating the need for impressions and models. The composite resin is placed, polymerized, removed form the prepared tooth and then treated extraorally with heat and additional light. This "enhanced" composite inlay is then bonded back into the tooth utilizing a composite resin cement. Additional advantages of this technique include the elimination of laboratory costs associated with indirect composite and porcelain inlays/onlays and the ability to start and finish the restoration in a single visit.

MATERIAL REQUIREMENTS

The "ideal" direct inlay composite resin should have the following properties: high condensability, high filler load, large assortment of shades, different degrees of opacity, radiopacity and convenient packaging to allow for easy placement into the cavity preparation. Many hybrid composites have been developed that meet these criteria. The presence of glass filler particles allows for the etching of the internal surfaces of these restorations with hydrofluoric acid that increases the bond strength between the resin and the tooth.

INDICATIONS

A direct resin inlay can be utilized wherever an existing one, two or three surface amalgam or gold inlay would be treatment planned. Their ability to reinforce or strengthen teeth may indicate their use in larger restorations not normally considered appropriate for amalgam or gold inlays. They are especially appropriate for use in maxillary and mandibular premolars where an esthetic restoration is necessary (Fig. 5-5). It has also proven to be an excellent restoration for the distolingual surface of maxillary canines where resistance to wear and esthetics are equally important (Fig. 5-6). Unlike an unbonded restoration, direct composite resin inlays can be used in situations where a large isthmus is present, as long as the cusps have adequate dentinal support. The decision as to when cuspal coverage is needed becomes a personal one based on the clinician's judgment and experience. Many clinicians, including the author, have provided very successful direct resin inlays where minimal functional cusp tooth structure remains, without the need to cover the cusp. These circumstances would definitely warrant cuspal coverage if an unbonded restorative material were used (Fig. 5-7).

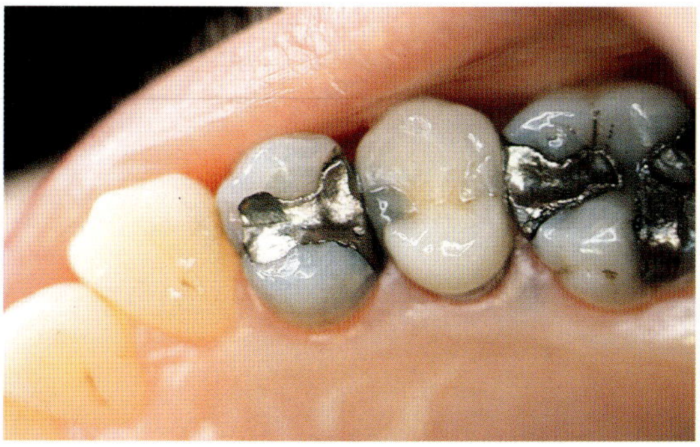

Fig. 5-5a Preoperative view.

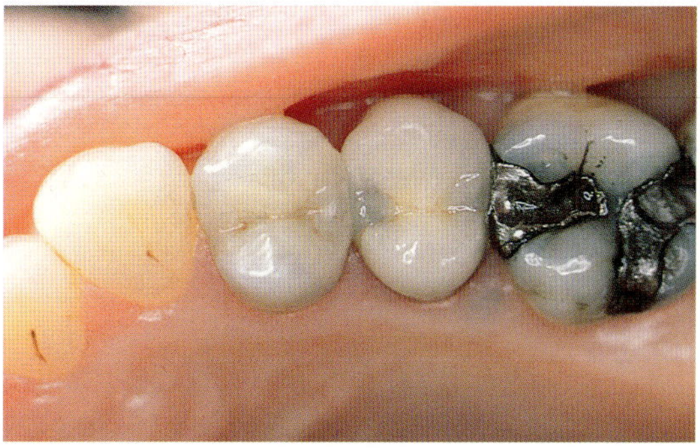

Fig. 5-5b Large defective alloy replaced with conservative direct resin inlay in tooth 12. Notice custom staining on mesial of porcelain crown to mimic preexisting alloys in adjacent teeth.

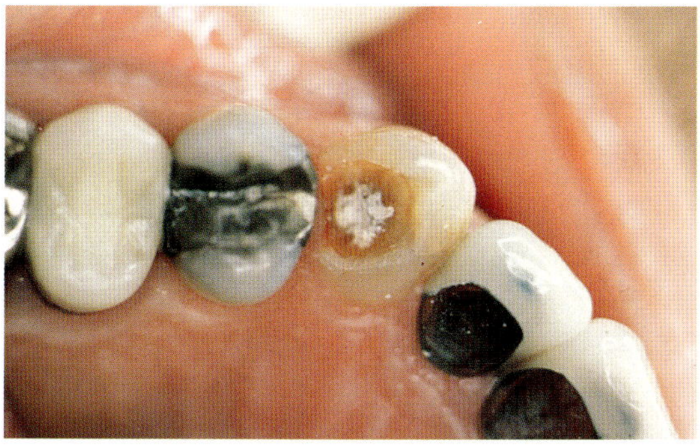

Fig. 5-6a Preoperative view.

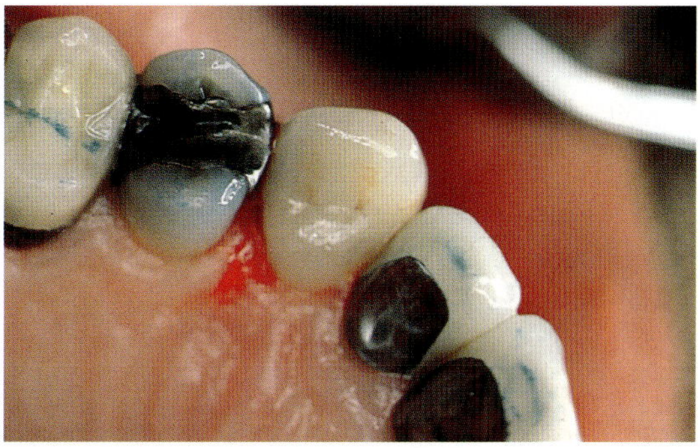

Fig. 5-6b Direct resin inlay used to replace defective distolingual composite in maxillary canine. Esthetics are excellent and wear of opposing dentition is less than with porcelain.

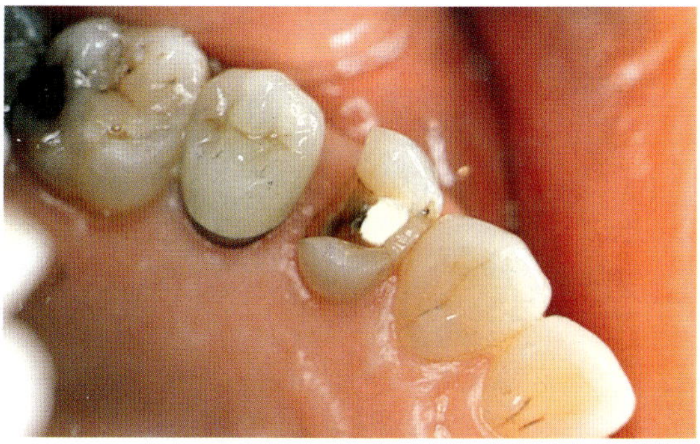

Fig. 5-7a Preoperative view.

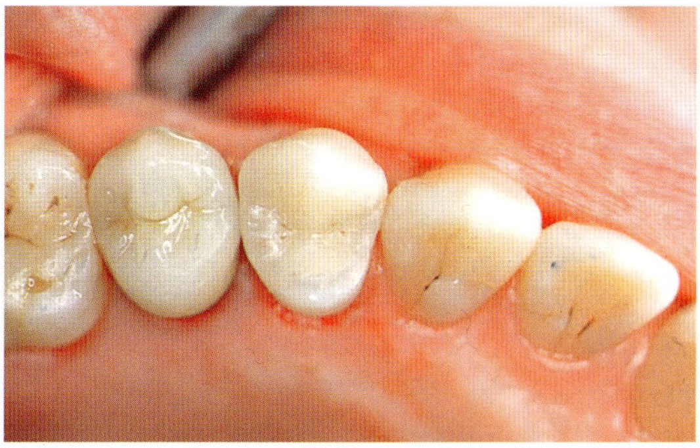

Fig. 5-7b Large distocclusal direct composite resin inlay used to restore premolar.

CLINICAL PROCEDURES

Prepreparation

Prior to tooth preparation, determine which shade of resin will produce the best esthetic results. Fabricating custom shade tabs using the resin itself provides a more predictable color match since many of the shade tabs included with the resin kits are not a very accurate representation of the actual composite color. The custom shade tabs can be stored in water for several days to mimic hydration occuring in the oral cavity. Since these restorations will blend into the surrounding dentition, shade choice is not as critical as with full coverage porcelain crowns. A lighter shade is usually preferred as it tends to mimic adjacent tooth enamel more readily. The use of a very translucent enamel shade for the final layer will produce more realistic results.

Since these restorations are being "bonded" into place using a composite resin cement, proper moisture barrier controls are mandatory. It is recommended to utilize a rubber dam whenever possible. This should be placed prior to the preparation but following shade selection to minimize shade alterations caused by desiccation.

Tooth Preparation

The preparation for a direct resin inlay is similar to that for a gold inlay, except there are no beveled margins (see chapter 6 for detailed preparation designs). Unlike a gold inlay preparation, bevels placed at the gingival floor or occlusal surface may cause unwanted thin areas in the composite resin restoration and should be avoided. Remove the previous restoration or caries. The walls of the preparation should diverge occlusally 15° to 20° to allow for an adequate line of draw to facilitate easy removal of the resin inlay after light curing intraorally. All undercuts do not have to be eliminated after removing existing amalgam restorations at this time since they can be blocked out using a glass ionomer base material prior to composite resin placement.

Depth of the preparation should be approximately 1.5 mm to allow space for the composite resin inlay and cement. All internal line angles should be slightly rounded. The walls of the proximal box should diverge occlusally and the isthmus of the preparation should be at least 1.5 mm wide to avoid fracture of the inlay during removal (Fig. 5-8).

Blocking Out Undercuts

Since most direct amalgam restorations utilize slight undercuts in the preparation to provide retention, a more conservative inlay preparation can be made by blocking out these undercut using a flouride-releasing base material, rather than excessive flaring. The new light cured glass ionomer liners and bases have substantially increased their ease of placement. The use of glass ionomer as a liner/base has several advantages. Glass ionomers have been shown to release flouride, provide thermal diffusion, have a coefficient of thermal expansion similar to dentin, and bond reasonably well to both dentin and composite resin. Use according to its manufacturer's recommendations and place the material only where undercuts exist. Avoid placement of the glass ionomer on the enamel margins. In very deep areas of the preparation where near mechanical exposures of the pulp exists, a thin layer of a glass ionomer liner should be utilized as well. After the glass ionomer liner has set, the preparation is redefined and enamel margins are cleaned of any overextended glass ionomer.

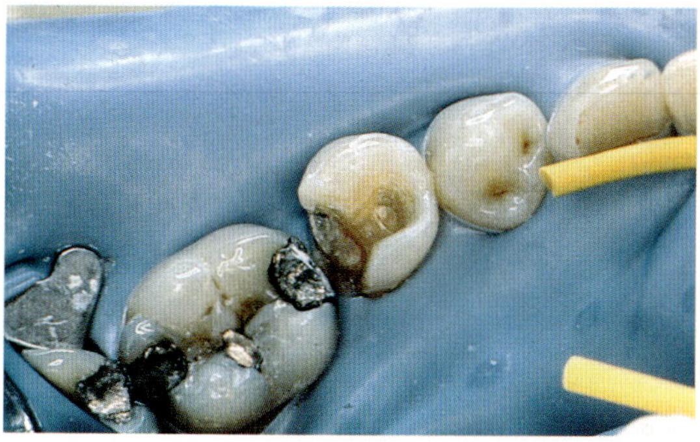

Fig. 5-8 Resin inlay preparation after defective alloy was removed.

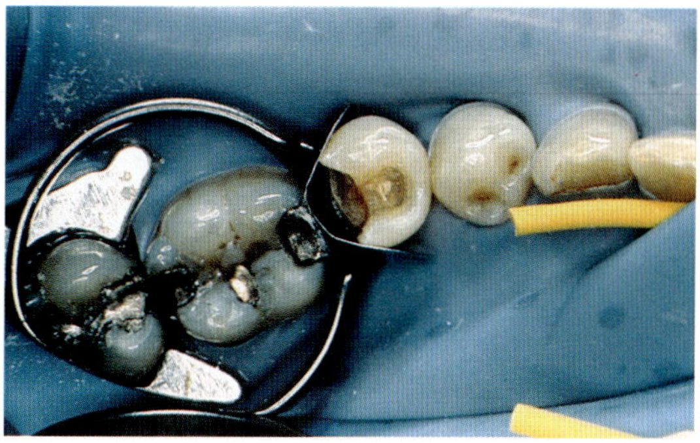

Fig. 5-9 Sectional Matrix and Bitine Ring in place.

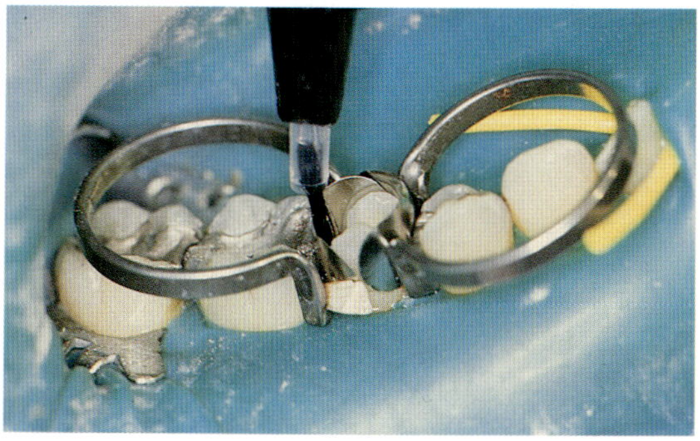

Fig. 5-10 If an MOD preparation is to be done, two Bitine Rings and Sectional Matrices will be needed.

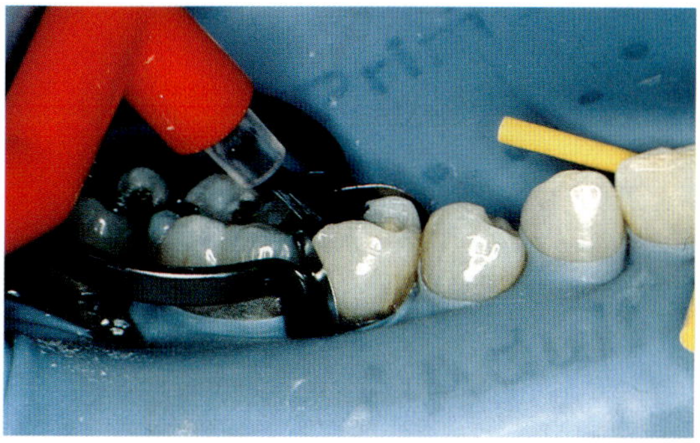

Fig. 5-11 A separating medium is painted into the preparation to avoid bonding of the composite resin to the tooth structure at this stage.

Matrix Band Placement

Because most composite resin materials do not condense as easily as amalgam, properly shaped and adequate proximal contacts have always been a problem. The use of Sectional Matrices (Palodent, Portola Valley, CA) and Bitine Rings (Palodent) have provided a very predictable method to overcome previous proximal contact problems. The matrix is a contoured, kidney-shaped metal band approximately 0.0015 inches thick. One band is needed for each proximal surface, so two bands will be required for an MOD preparation (Figs. 5-9 and 5-10). The band is positioned in the proximal space, followed by wooden wedge placement. A Bitine Ring, which is similar in appearance to a rubber dam clamp, is placed over the adjacent tooth, engaging the line angles of the prepared tooth, holding the matrix firmly in place. This ring creates pressure between the two teeth resulting in an excellent proximal contact and a secure, well contoured matrix. This matrix system often results in a superior proximal contact compared to other systems.

If a standard retainer band and matrix system is to be used, it may be advisable to prewedge the tooth prior to preparation. An anatomically contoured wooden wedge placed interproximally between the tooth to be prepared and the adjacent tooth causes a slow separation of the teeth which creates a very slight space that will compensate for the thickness of the matrix band. After the inlay is completed, the teeth will move into their original position causing a tighter contact than if prewedging were not done. Place the wedge after rubber dam placement and prior to preparation. The wedge can be used as a guide to determine the extent of gingival preparation and may also eliminate damage to the proximal surface of the adjacent tooth during preparation.

Separating Medium

The preparation is now lubricated with a thin layer of a lubricant, such as Separator (Coltene/Whaledent, New York) or Insulating Gel (Kulzer, Irvine, CA) (Fig. 5-11). The lubricant is used to eliminate bonding of the resin to the glass ionomer base and to facilitate removal of the inlay. After placement, the preparation should be blown with compressed air to create a very thin film of lubricant and to eliminate pooling of excess lubricant in the proximal boxes where it could be incorporated into the composite resin during placement.

Composite Placement

Place the composite resin into the proximal box, filling about 2 to 3 mm of the box, overlapping onto the pulpal floor (Fig. 5-12). The composite resin should be condensed into the proximal boxes and adapted to the walls of the preparation using composite hand instruments. The recommended composite resin is one of the hybrids due to strength and polishability. A microfill resin can be used, except handling properties are usually not as good as the hybrids. The microfills tend to be stickier and more difficult to condense. A compule tip allows for easy composite resin placement and initial condensation. This first increment should be light cured from the occlusal for at least 40 seconds. Since the restoration will be bonded back into the tooth using a composite resin cement, the amount of polymerization shrinkage at the gingival margin is not a concern at this time. Since this first increment is replacing dentin, a dentin shade should be used first.

Lightly coat this first increment with a very thin coat of an unfilled resin to aid in the adaption of the overlying occlusal increment. Fill the remainder of the preparation with composite resin that matches the enamel and contour as much as possible using composite condensers and contouring instruments (Figs. 5-13 and 5-14). Overfill slightly at the occlusal-lingual and occlusal-buccal line angles to provide an area where a margin trimmer or spoon excavator can engage the resin to help in removing the inlay from the preparation. Light cure the occlusal portion for 60 seconds.

When optimal natural esthetics is mandatory, composite resin tints can be used between the two increments to produce occlusal staining or color modification. After curing the first increment, place a small amount of yellow or brown modifier on the pulpal floor using the tip of an explorer, cure for 20 seconds and then place the second increment. The entire restoration should now be light cured for at least 60 seconds to eliminate deformation, due to underpolymerization, during removal.

Inlay Removal

Remove the matrix assembly and wedge. Insert a spoon excavator or margin trimmer under the marginal ridges or any area where excess composite may be present and gently lift out the restoration (Fig. 5-15). Do not use forced removal because a cusp could fracture if there are any undercuts present. If it cannot easily be removed, section the restoration, check the preparation carefully for any possible undercuts, modify and repeat the above procedures.

After removal of the composite resin inlay,

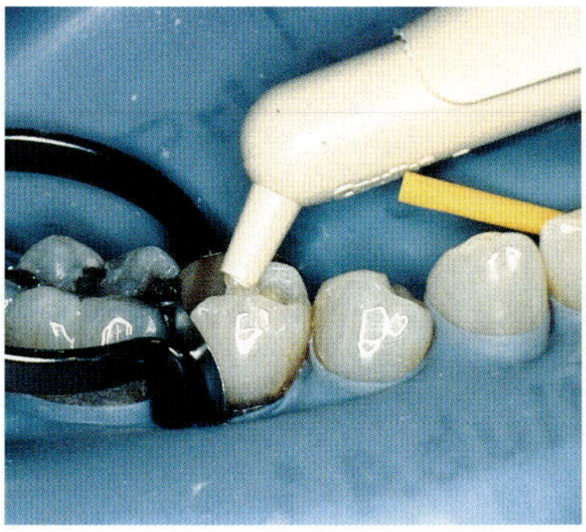

Fig. 5-12 The first increment of composite is injected into the proximal box and then light cured.

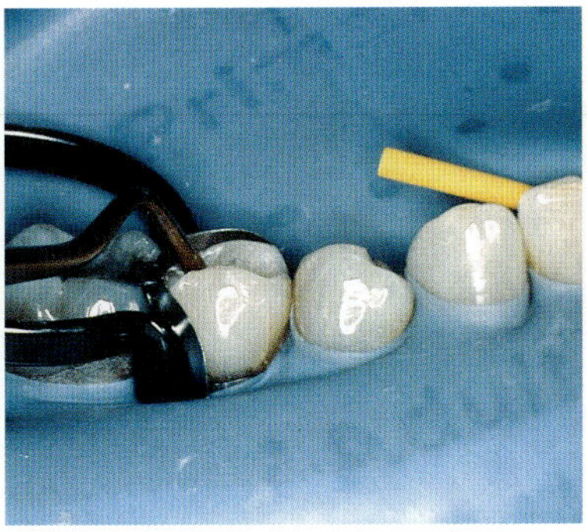

Fig. 5-13 A composite condenser or carving instrument can be used to create occlusal anatomy after the second increment is placed.

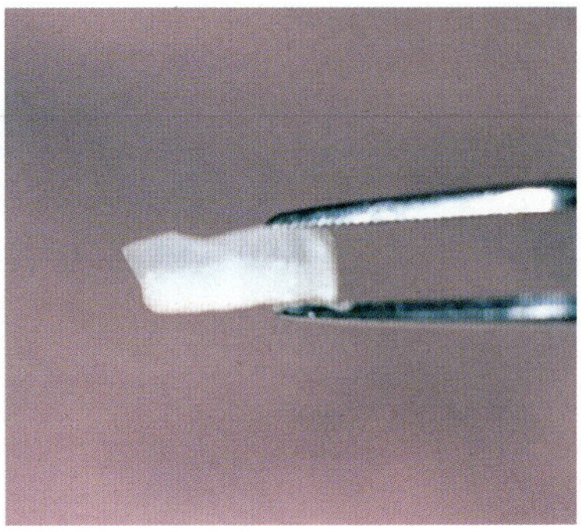

Fig. 5-14 A direct composite resin inlay after removal from the tooth. Notice the difference between the "dentin-like" opacity of the first increment and the more translucent "enamel-like" top layer.

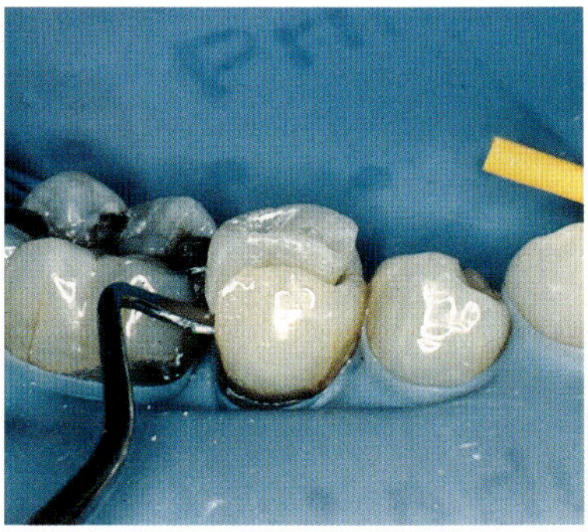

Fig. 5-15 Remove the inlay with a spoon excavator or margin trimmer after curing.

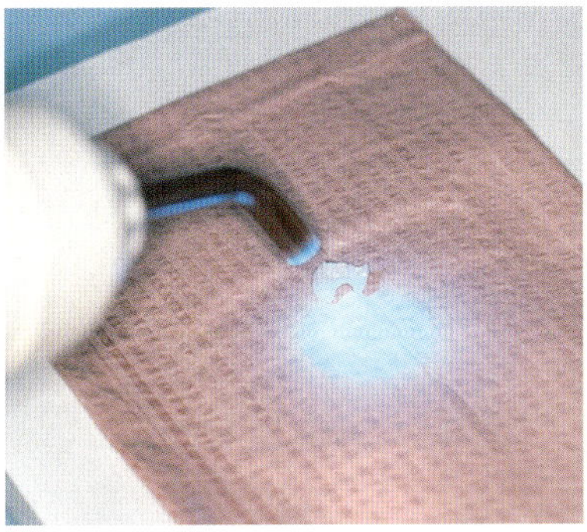

Fig. 5-16 Light cure the resin inlay for 1 minute from both the internal and external aspects before placing in a curing oven.

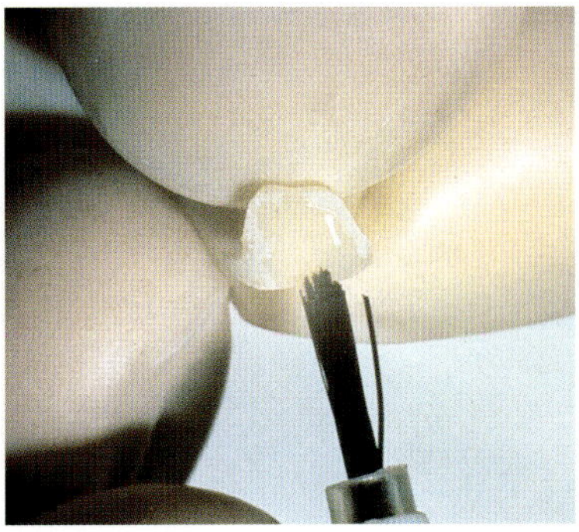

Fig. 5-17a

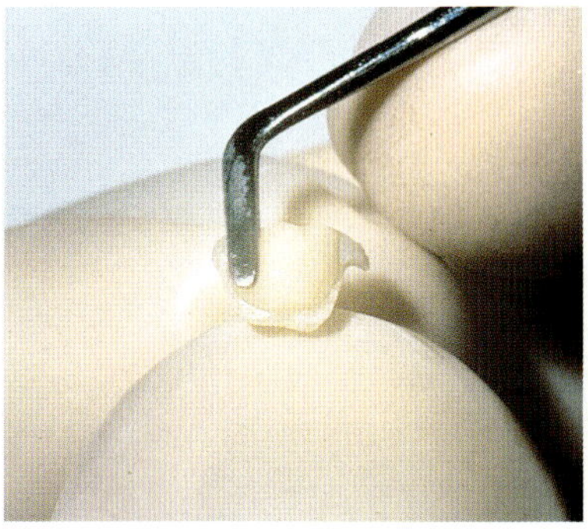

Fig. 5-17b

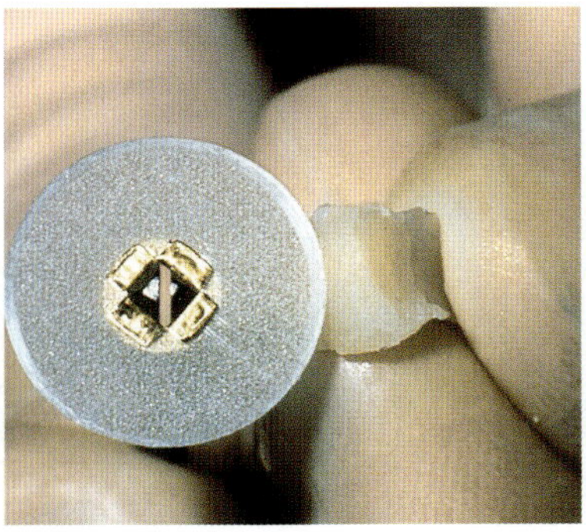

Fig. 5-17c

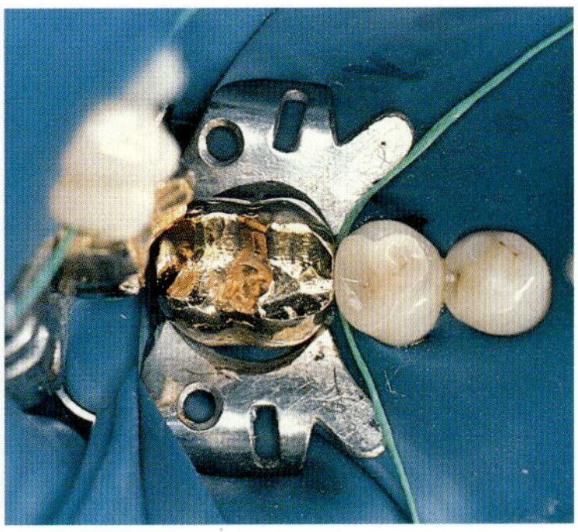

Fig. 5-17d

Figs. 5-17a to d If the interproximal contact is light, roughen the proximal surface of the inlay with air abrasion or a diamond bur, apply a low viscosity resin, followed by additional composite resin, and then light cure. Contour and polish this new contact with discs and polishing points. After polishing, retry the inlay back into the mouth to verify adequate interproximal contact.

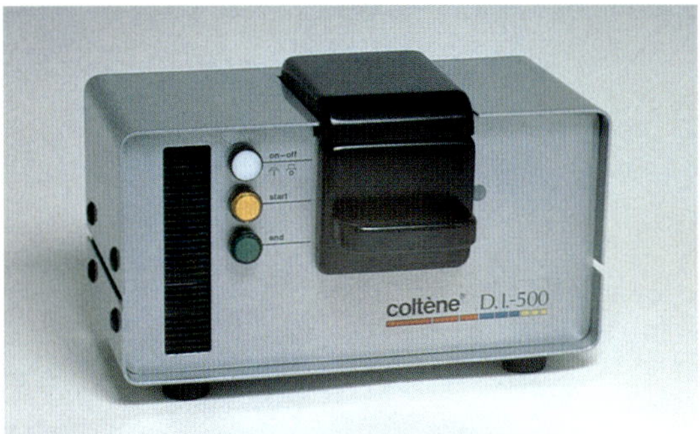

Fig. 5-18a The resin inlay is now polymerized additionally using an extraoral curing oven.

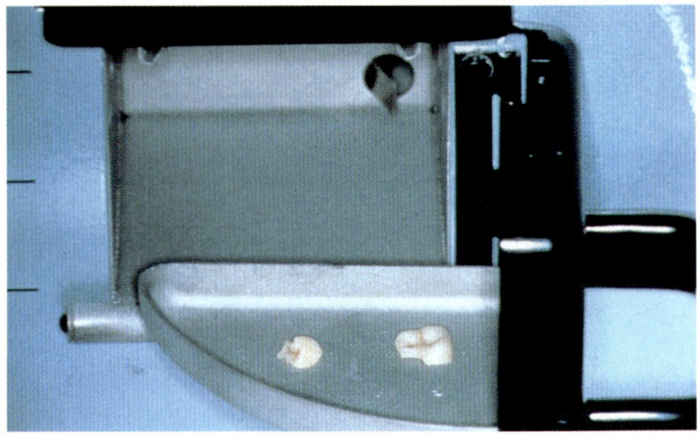

Fig. 5-18b View of internal aspects of oven.

cure the restoration on the bench top for 60 seconds from both the internal and external directions (Fig. 5-16).

Restoration Contouring

Place the inlay back into the preparation and contour the interproximal surface using carbide finishing burs and composite finishing discs. Check for adequate interproximal contacts with dental floss and for marginal discrepancies. If the interproximal contacts are undercontoured, remove the restoration, roughen the contact area with a diamond bur or air abrasion with aluminous oxide, rinse, dry, place an unfilled resin, add more composite and light cure for 40 seconds. Recontour with discs to establish the desired contours and embrasure form (Figs. 5-17a to c). Place back into the preparation and recheck the interproximal contacts (Fig. 5-17d). If a marginal discrepancy is present, modify the area using this same technique. Place a small amount of resin into the preparation at the site of the marginal discrepancy. Completely seat the restoration, making sure all margins are seated. Contour the new composite resin with a thin instrument such as an interproximal carver or gold knife and cure for 40 seconds. Remove the inlay and polish with discs and polishing cups.

Extraoral Polymerization

Place the completed inlay into an extraoral curing oven that generates heat in the range of 125°C to 150°C (Fig. 5-18). This heat range corresponds to the glass transition temperatures and creates changes in the filler-matrix interactions that enhances the physical properties of the composite resin. Although some authors have suggested the use of a toaster oven designed for cooking purposes, consistency of heat and the time it takes to reach the desired temperatures may be a drawback. There are extraoral heating units available designed specifically for this purpose.

Inlay Cementation

After the inlay has been polymerized in the oven, it is tried into the preparation to verify fit. Sharp internal line angles may need to be reduced slightly to facilitate easy seating. The internal aspects of the restoration are now carefully etched with a 9% to 10% hydrofluoric acid for 30 seconds and then rinsed thoroughly. This will result in a surface pattern similar to etched porcelain and will increase the bond strength between the composite resin inlay and the composite resin cements (Fig. 5-19). It is advisable not to use a darkly tinted hydrofluoric acid as it has been shown

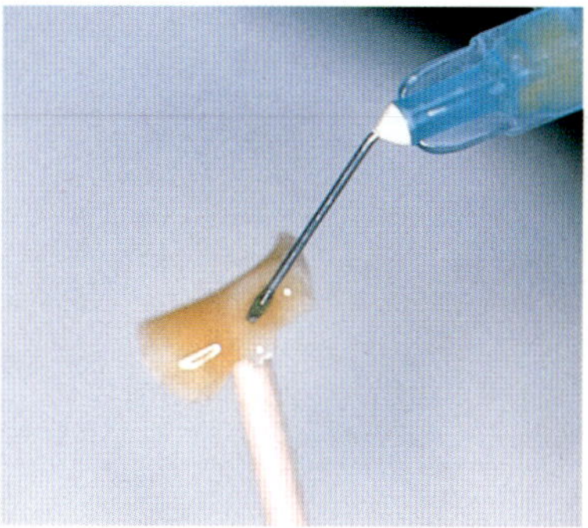

Fig. 5-19a After removal from the curing oven, the internal aspect of the inlay is etched with hydrofluoric acid.

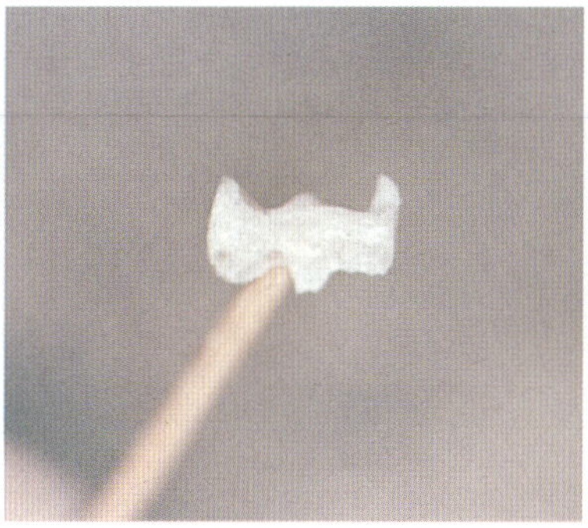

Fig. 5-19b Notice the frosted appearance of the resin after etching.

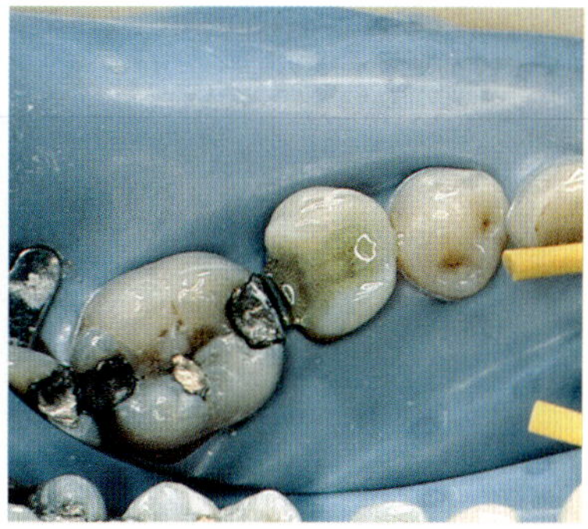

Fig. 5-20a The preparation is etched with phosphoric acid.

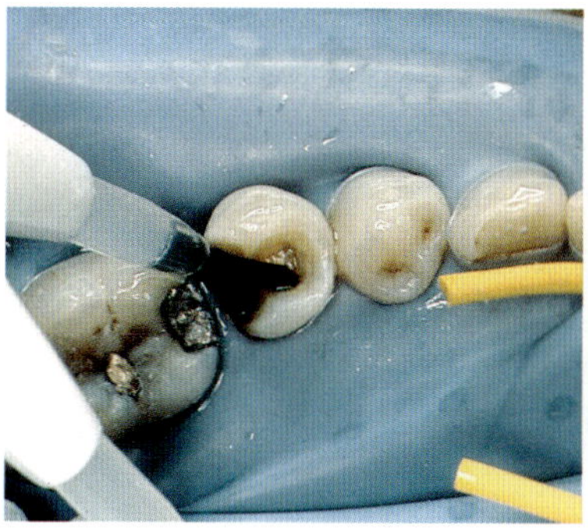

Fig. 5-20b A multipurpose bonding agent and low viscosity bonding resin are lightly applied to all internal surfaces of the preparation and etched surfaces of the inlay.

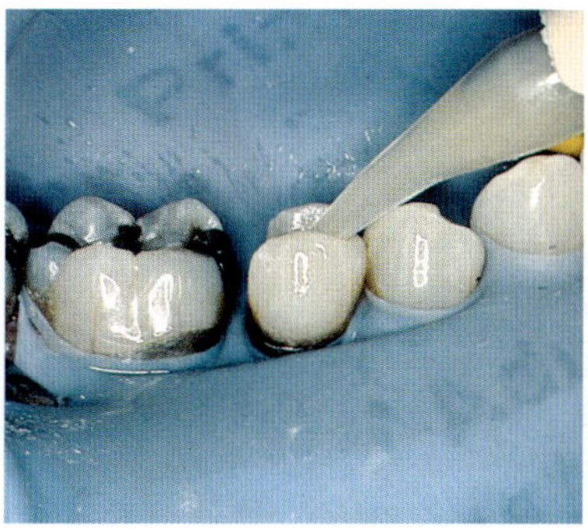

Fig. 5-20c A dual cured luting resin is mixed and then injected into the preparation.

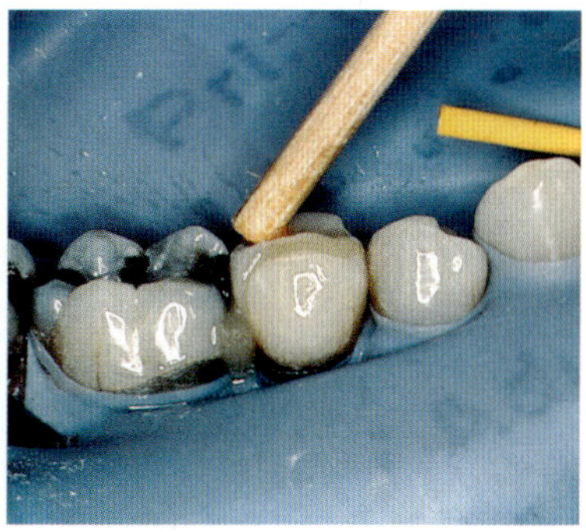

Fig. 5-20d The inlay is seated gently. A wooden stick is "sticky-waxed" to the occlusal surface for easier handling and removed once the inlay is seated.

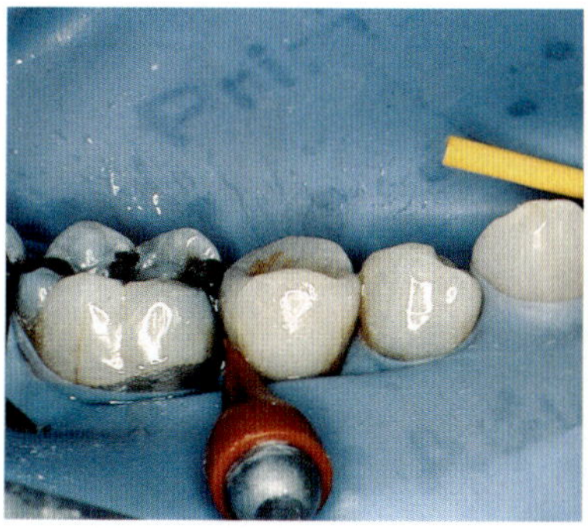

Fig. 5-20e A rubber tipped instrument is excellent to remove excess cement before light curing.

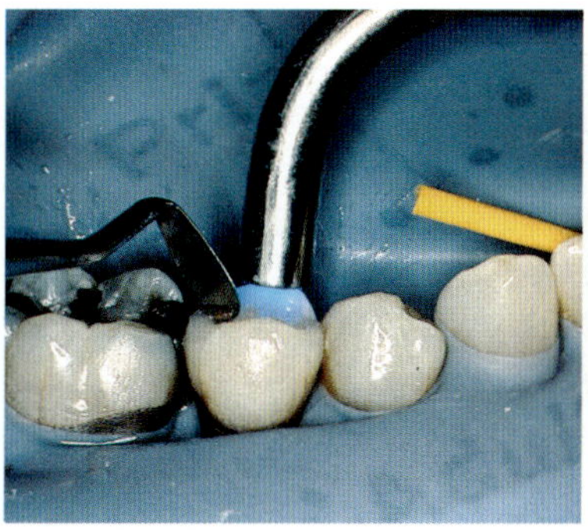

Fig. 5-20f Using a 3-mm light tip, the inlay is "tacked" into place for 20 seconds.

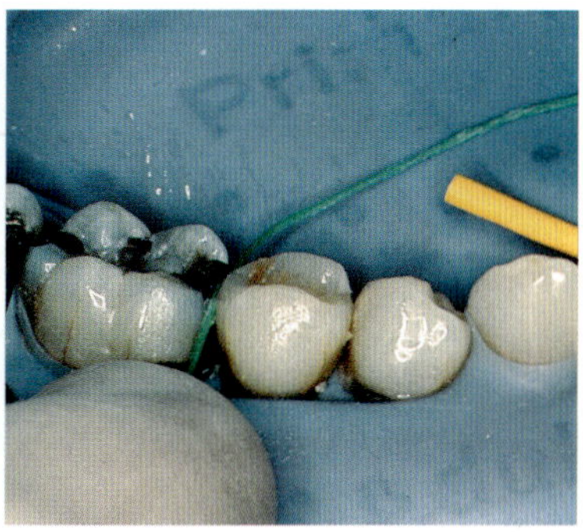

Fig. 5-20g Flossing the proximal contact removes excess resin interproximally.

to stain some hybrid composites. A silane coupling agent is applied to the etched surface of the inlay. The silane acts as a bond enhancer between the etched glass in the inlay and the composite resin cement. If a microfill resin was used instead of a hybrid, there is no need to etch with the hydrofluoric acid since they do not contain any glass particles. A resin primer, such as Special-Bond II (Vivadent, Amherst, NY), is recommended because the microfill resin is so densely cured with the extraoral polymerization. The resin primer opens double bonds in the composite resin inlay to allow for improved bonding between the composite resin cements and the inlay.

The tooth is now prepared for bonding. The internal surfaces of the preparation should be scrubbed with a chorhexidine soap/pumice mixture. This mixture can be used on a cotton pellet and easily manipulated within the preparation. Wash thoroughly for 30 seconds. The entire preparation, both enamel and dentin, is etched with phosphoric acid for 15 seconds, rinsed and dried (Fig. 5-20a). Clear matrix strips should be placed interproximally to keep excess etchant off adjacent teeth.

A newer generation "multi purpose" dentinal bonding agent should be used immediately according to manufacturer's instructions on all dentin and enamel surfaces. A system that includes a dual cure or chemical cure unfilled resin must be used since the unfilled resin layer is not light polymerized prior to placement of the inlay. The bonding agents and low viscosity resins should be applied to all surfaces to be bonded, including the glass ionomer liner, as well as the internal aspect of the resin inlay (Fig. 5-20b). These materials will act as wetting agents and ensure intimate contact between the inlay and the preparation. Mix a dual cure composite resin cement and place it into the preparation using a composite syringe (Fig. 5-20c). Gently seat the restoration and remove most of the excess resin with a small brush or rubber tip instrument while firmly holding the inlay in place using a blunt instrument (Figs. 5-20d and e). "Tack" the restoration in place by curing from the occlusal for 20 seconds using a small diameter (2- to 3-mm) curing light tip, keeping it away from the interproximal areas (Fig. 5-20f). Gently floss through the interproximal cement (Fig. 5-20g). The restoration should be held firmly in place during flossing. The rest of the excess unset composite cement is removed with a fine brush. Cure all restored surfaces of the tooth for 1 minute on each surface to ensure a complete cure. Also cure the gingival margins if accessible.

Finishing and Polishing

After the composite resin cement has fully polymerized, remove gingival excess using a #12 scalpel blade, gold knife or cleoid instruments (Fig. 5-21a). Tungsten carbide tipped composite finishing hand instruments are especially useful for removing excess cured cement. Contour the restoration using composite finishing discs, diamonds or carbides (Fig. 5-21b). The gingival margin should be finished using aluminum oxide finishing strips.

Remove the rubber dam and check occlusal contacts. Adjust the occlusion as necessary using finishing diamonds and polish with rubber points and cups.

Sealing the Restoration

Isolate the tooth again, using cotton rolls or svedopter, and re-etch the entire occlusal surface of the restoration for 30 seconds with phosphoric acid. Rinse thoroughly, dry and apply a thin layer of Fortify (Bisco, Itasca, IL.) to the occlusal surface of the inlay. Cure with a curing light for 20 seconds. Fortify is a surface-penetrating sealant which readily flows across the surface of the resin inlay and penetrates into the microstructural defects

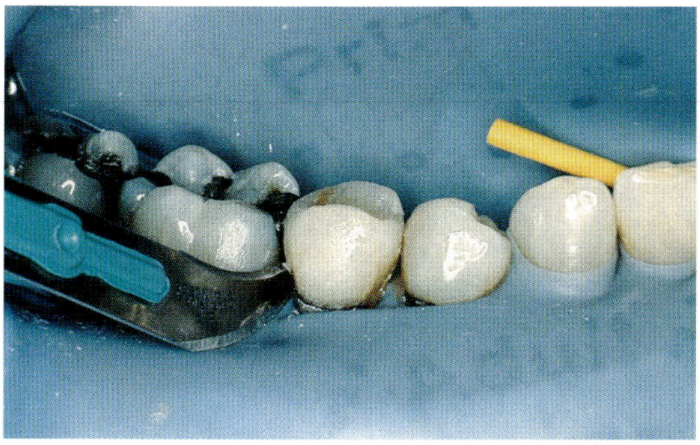

Fig. 5-21a

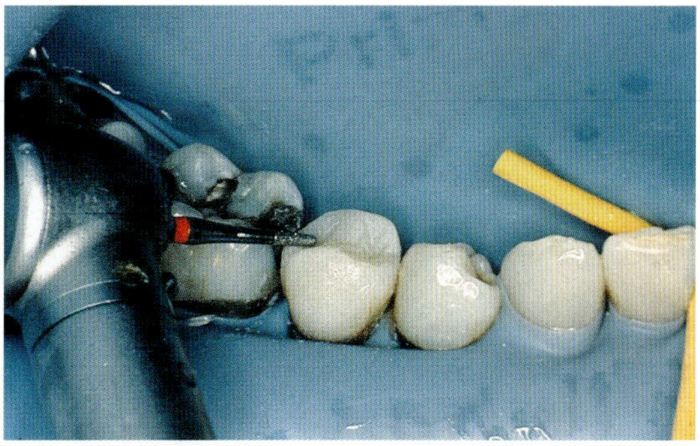

Fig. 5-21b

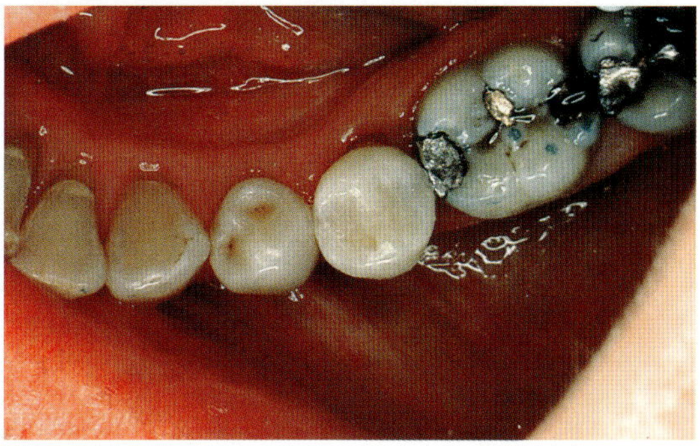

Fig. 5-21c

Fig. 5-21a After curing the inlay for 1 minute from all sides, the excess cement can be removed using a #12 scalpel blade or tungsten carbide instruments.

Fig. 5-21b Defining anatomy and final contouring is achieved with diamond finishing and fluted carbide burs.

Fig. 5-21c The final direct resin inlay after polishing with rubber points and composite polishing paste.

caused during finishing of the resin. The finishing process of composite resin causes microcracks that extend across and below the surface and decrease the wear resistance of the resin. When properly applied, Fortify can reduce the wear rate by as much as 50%. At the margins, a thin band of composite resin cement will always show increased wear compared to the inlay. Sealing this band may decrease wear and ditching of the margin.

Obtain the final high polish using a composite polishing paste on a rubber cup or point. Floss through the contact with the polishing paste moving it back and forth along the gingival margin to polish this area (Fig. 5-21c).

THE FLEXIBLE MODEL TECHNIQUE

The flexible model technique is an alternative to using the natural tooth as the die for inlay fabrication. The technique starts by making a polyvinylsiloxane impression of the preparation (Fig. 5-22a). After the impression is made, a silicone releasing agent is sprayed onto this impression (Fig. 5-22b). A heavy bodied polyvinylsiloxane is now placed into the impression to make the flexible working model. Although many techniques can be used, the author prefers injecting a heavy bodied (high viscosity) material into the preparation impression, followed immediately with a putty material (Fig. 5-22c). The putty is mixed by the dental assistant while the dentist injects the heavy bodied material into the impression and is used to force the less viscous heavy body material into the details of the impression. This is allowed to set for

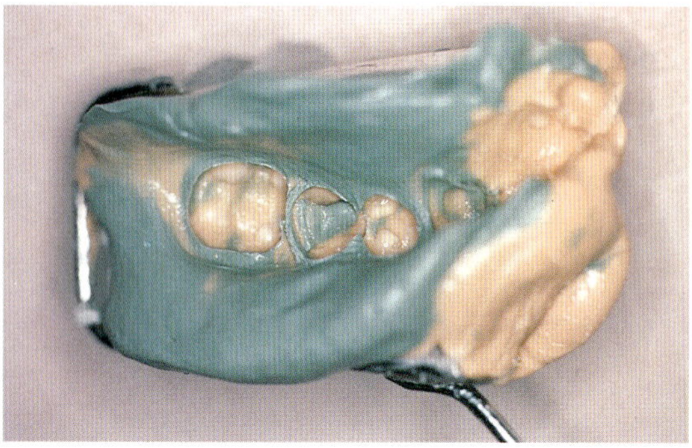

Fig. 5-22a An impression is taken of the prepared tooth with a polyvinylsiloxane material.

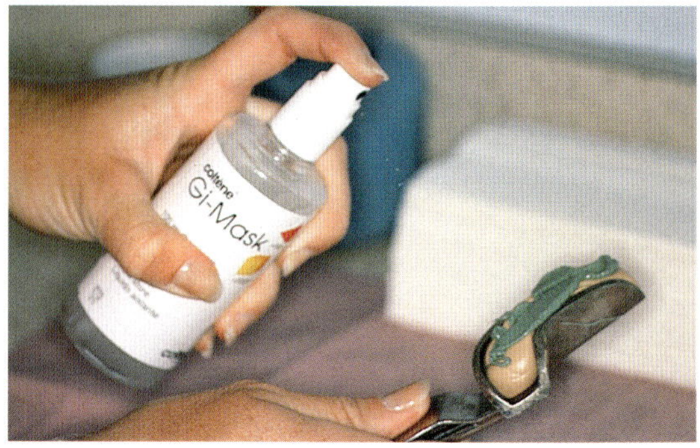

Fig. 5-22b The initial impression is then sprayed with a silicone releasing agent.

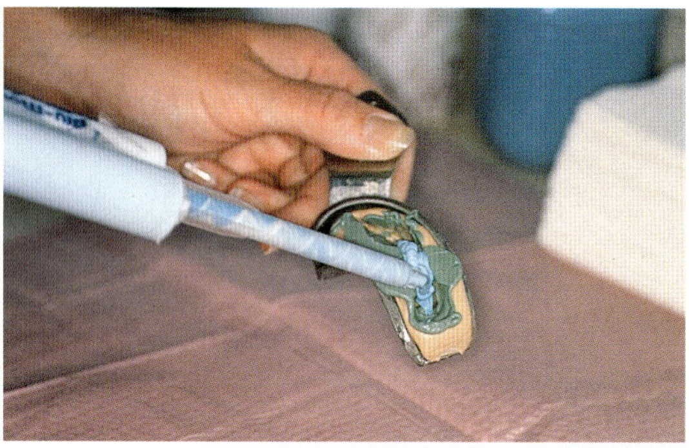

Fig. 5-22c A heavy bodied vinyl impression is injected into the original impression.

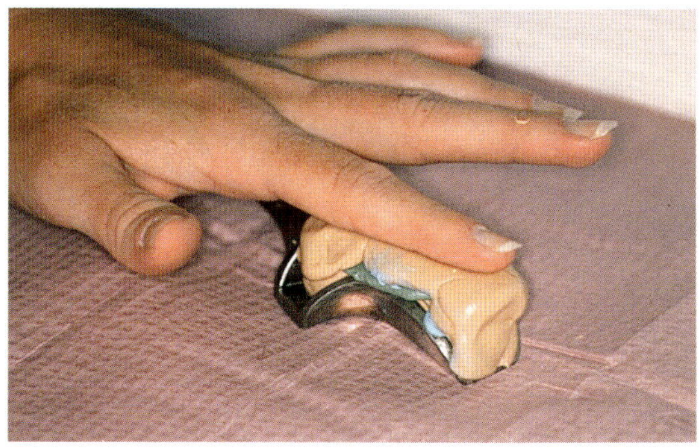

Fig. 5-22d A putty is applied forcing the impression material into the original impression.

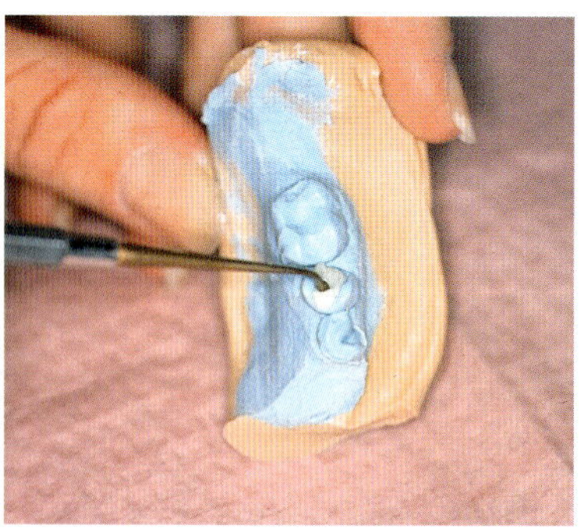

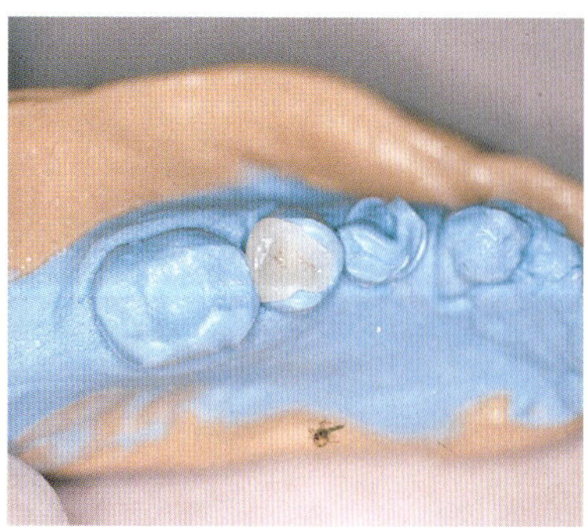

Figs. 5-22e and f The composite resin inlay is then fabricated on the flexible model using composite instruments.

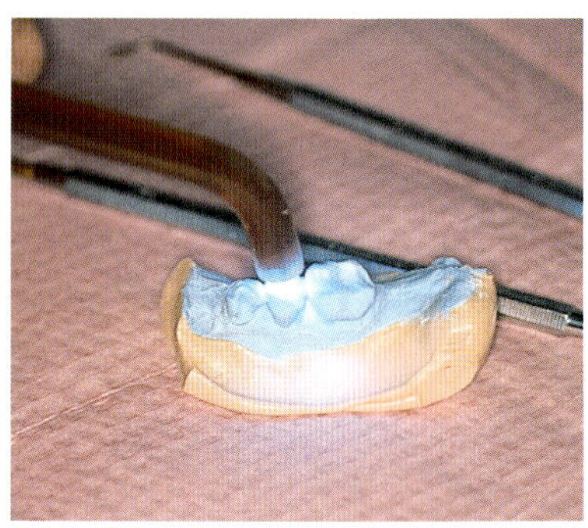

Fig. 5-22g The inlay is light cured for 1 minute from all surfaces.

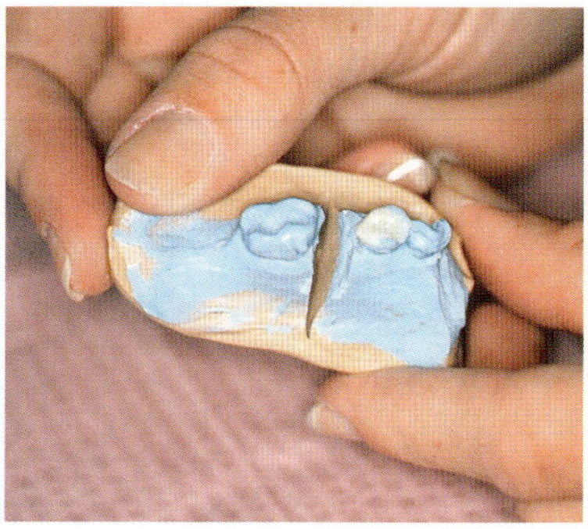

Fig. 5-22h The model can be sectioned to allow proximal access for contouring. After light curing, the inlay is removed from the flexible model and placed in the extraoral curing oven.

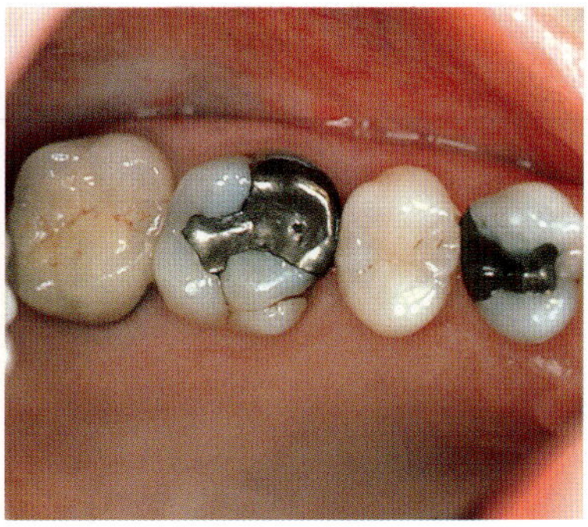

Fig. 5-23a Preoperative view.

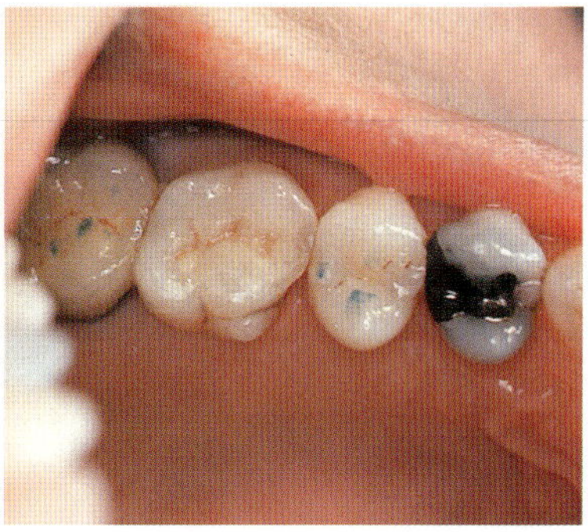

Fig. 5-23b A composite resin inlay made on a flexible model was used to replace a defective MOB alloy on the first molar. Extraoral manipulation of the composite is easier than direct manipulation in the tooth when the restoration involve cusps.

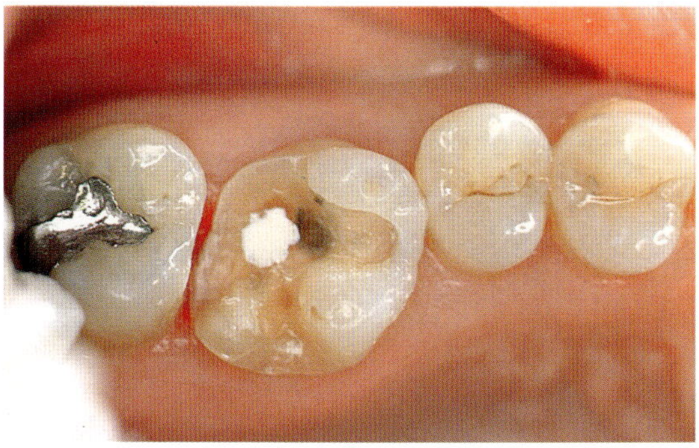

Fig. 5-24a Preoperative view.

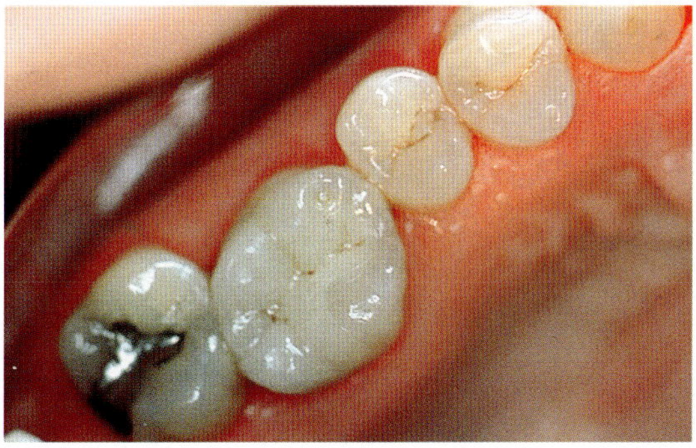

Fig. 5-24b A large composite resin inlay was made using the flexible model technique.

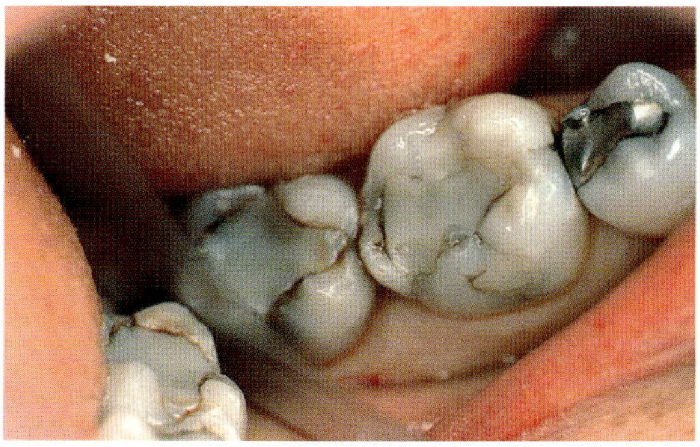

Fig. 5-25a Preoperative view.

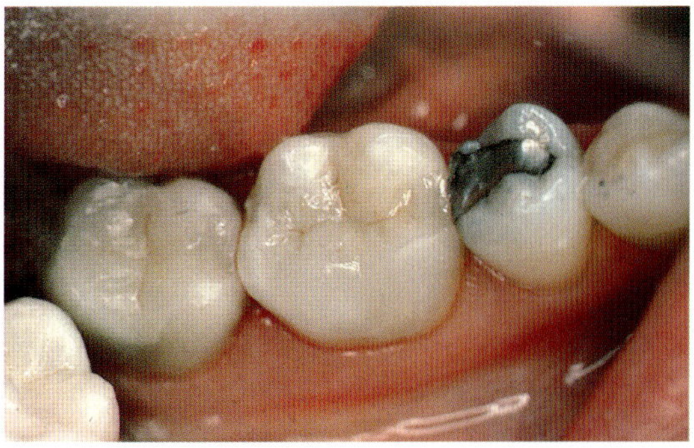

Fig. 5-25b Multiple restorations, such as these two defective composite resins, are frequently more easily done using a flexible model technique.

the manufacturer's recommended time and the impressions are separated. The use of the silicone releasing agent facilitates separation. If this agent were not used, the two silicone impression materials would bond together. The resin inlay is now fabricated as with the direct technique (Figs. 5-22e to g). Many clinicians find the flexible model technique easier because it provides greater control extraorally. To aid in proximal contouring, the model can be partially sectioned (Fig. 5-22h). Curing times, cementation and finishing procedures are all identical to those used with the direct composite inlay technique described previously.

The disadvantages of this technique are the cost of impression materials, the time needed for impression material to set and possible deformation of the original impression when making the flexible die. Advantages include the ability to achieve improved contours, improved esthetic results and minimal finishing times. This extraoral technique also allows the dentist to delegate the fabrication of the inlay to a competent auxiliary.

Although the author has utilized this technique many times, he prefers the ease and accuracy of the direct resin inlay utilizing the natural tooth as the working die. When a larger restoration is required or if the preparation involves cuspal coverage, the flexible model technique facilitates contour of the restoration (Figs. 5-23 to 5-25).

DISCUSSION

Direct composite inlays offer the dentist an opportunity to provide patients with an excellent esthetic restorative option without many of the drawbacks associated with other posterior esthetic restorations. The lack of laboratory costs and the need for a second appointment are a benefit for the dentist, and for the patient in terms of chairtime, time away from work or family and comfort. The demand for esthetic restorative materials in posterior teeth is increasing. The use of the direct resin inlay has many advantages over directly placed light cured posterior composites. These advantages include improved physical properties, excellent marginal adaptation and elimination of problems associated with intraoral polymerization shrinkage. The use of the direct composite resin inlay also eliminates some of the limitations of porcelain inlays such as cost, number of appointments, laboratory variation and wear of opposing dentition.

REFERENCES

Bakke, J.C., Duke E.S., and Norling B.K., et al.: Fracture Strength Of Class II Preparations With Posterior Composites. (1985). J. Dent. Res. Vol. 64, p. 350, (abstr. 1578).

Bertolotti, R.: Total Etch: The Rational Dentin Bonding Protocol. (1991). J. Esth. Dent. Vol. 3, p. 1.

Bertolotti, R.: Personal Communication.

Boksman, L., Jordan, R.E. Suzuki, M., and Charles, D.H.: A Visible Light-Cured Posterior Composite Resin: Result of a 3-Year Clinical Evaluation. (1986). J.A.D.A. Vol. 112, p. 627.

Bowen, R.L.: Use Of Epoxy Resin In Restorative Materials. J. Dent. Res. Vol. 35, p. 360.

Bowen, R.L., Cobb, E.N., and Rapson, J.E.: Adhesive Bonding Various Materials To Hard Tooth Tissues. Improvement In Bond Strength To Dentin. (1982). J. Dent. Res. Vol. 61, p. 1070

Buonocore, M.G.: A Simple Method Increasing the Adhesion of Acrylic Filling Materials to Enamel Surfaces. (1955). J. Dent. Res. Vol. 34, p. 849.

Christensen, G.J.: A Look At State-Of-The-Art Tooth-Colored Inlays and Onlays. (1992). J.A.D.A. Vol. 123, p. 66.

Cook, W. and Johnson, M.: The Influence Of Post-Curing On The Fracture Properties Of Photo-Cured Dimethacrylate Based Dental Composite Resin. (1987). J. Biomed. Mater. Res. Vol. 21, p. 979.

Darbyshire P.A., Messer L.B., and Douglas W.H.: Microleakage in Class II Composite Resin Bonded to Dentin Using Thermal and Load Cycling. (1988). J. Dent. Res. Vol. 67, p. 585.

Daniel, C.N.: The Extraoral System Technique for Fabrication Indirect Composite Inlay. (1992). Esth. Dent. Update Vol. 3, (1).

Eakle, W.S. and Nakamoto, D.: Microleakage In Mod Composites with Three Dentin Bonding Agents. (1988). J. Dent. Res. (Abstract No. 1584) (special issue) Vol. 67, p. 311.

Ehrnford, L. and Derand, T.: Cervical Gap Formation In Class II Composite Resin Restorations. (1984). Swed. Dent. J. Vol. 8, p. 15.

Erickson, R.L. and Glasspoole, E.A.: Comparison of Microleakage and Bond Strength for Dentin Adhesive Materials. (1986). J. Dent. Res. (Abstract) Vol. 65, p. 848.

Erickson, D. and Derand, T.: Reduction of Cervical Gap in Class II Composite Resin Restorations. (1991). J. Prosth. Dent. Vol. 65, p. 33.

Fayyad, M.A. and Shortall A.C.C: Microleakage of Dentin-Bonded Posterior Composite Restorations. (1987). I. Dent. Vol. 15, p. 67.

Feigenbaum, N.L.: The Perfect Material: The Restorative Maturation of Resin Inlays and Onlays. (1992). Dent. Today Vol. 11, (5) p. 42.

Feilzer, A.J., DeGee, A.J., and Davison, C.L.: Curing Contraction of Composites and Glass Ionmer Cements. (1988). J. Prosth. Dent. Vol. 59, p. 297.

Ferracane, J.L.: Using Posterior Composites Appropriately. (1992). J.A.D.A. Vol. 123, p. 53.

Forsten, L., Kuusisto, E., and Ruokolainen, R., et al.: Marginal Leakage in Vitro of Composite Fillings in Posterior Human Teeth. (1982). Proc. Finn. Dent. Soc. Vol. 78, p. 155.

Gelb, M.N., Barouch, E., and Simonsen, R.J.: Resistance to Cusp Fracture in Class II Prepared and Restored Premolars. (1986). J. Prosth. Dent. Vol. 55, p. 184.

Gross, J.D., Retief, D.H., and Bradley, E.L.: Microleakage of Posterior Composite Restorations. (1985). Dent. Mater. Vol. 1, p. 7.

Hornbrook, D.S. and Pai, N.D.: Direct Composite Resin Inlay Techniques and Materials. (1990). Esth. Dent. Update, Vol. 1, (1), p. 7.

Jackson, R.D. and Ferguson, R.W.: An Esthetic, Bonded Inlay/Onlay Technique for Posterior Teeth. (1990). Quint. Int. Vol. 21, (1), p. 7.

Jensen, M.D., Redford, D.A., and Williams, B.T., et al.: Posterior Etched Porcelain Restorations: An In Vivo Study. (1987). Compend. Contin. Educ. Dent. Vol. 8, p. 615.

Jones, G.B.: Posterior Composite Restorations: A Review of the Literature. (1989). Tex. Dent. J. Vol. 106, p. 13.

Jordan, R.E. and Suzuki, M.: Direct Hybrid Composite Inlay Technique. (1988). J. Esth. Dent. Oct, p. 57.

Jordan, R.E. and Suzuki, M.: Posterior Composite Restorations: Where and How They Work Best. (1991). J.A.D.A. Vol. 122, p. 31.

Joynt, R.B., Wieczkowski, G., Klockowski, R., and Donis, E.L.: Fracture Resistance of Teeth Restored with Amalgam Versus Composite Resin. (1985). J. Dent. Res. (Abstract No. 1579) Vol. 64, p. 350.

Kanca, J.: Dental Adhesion And The All-Bond System. (1991). J. Esth. Dent. Vol. 3, p. 129.

Kanca, J.: The Single Visit Heat Processed Composite Resin Inlay. (1988). J. Esth. Dent. Oct., p. 31.

Kandil, A.H., et al: Effect of Temperature and Aging on the Mechanical Properties of Dental Polymeric Composite Materials. (1989). Biomat. Vol. 10 (8), p. 540.

Kusy, R.P. and Leinfelder, K.F.: Pattern of Wear in Posterior Composite Restorations. (1987). J. Dent. Res. Vol. 56, p. 544.

Lacy, A.M., Zhang, K., and Koh, A., et al: Marginal Leakage Around Class II Resin and Dicor Inlays. (1988). J. Dent. Res. (Abstract No. 669) Vol. 67, p. 196.

Lamabrechts, P., Braem, M., and Vanherle, G.: Evaluation of Clinical Performance for Posterior Composite Resins and Dentin Adhesives. (1987). Oper. Dent. Vol. 12, p. 53.

Landy, R.A. and Simonsen, R.J.: Cusp Fracture Strength in Class II Composite Resin Restorations. (1984). J. Dent. Res. (Abstract No. 40) Vol. 63, p. 175.

Leinfelder, K.F.: Evaluation of Criteria Used for Assessing the Clinical Performance of Composite Resin in Posterior Teeth. (1987). Quint. Int. Vol. 18, p. 531.

Leinfelder, K.F., Sluder, T.B., and Sockwell, C.L., et al.: Clinical Evaluation of Composite Resins as Anterior and Posterior Restorative Materials. (1975). J. Prosth. Dent. Vol. 33, p. 406.

Leinfelder, K.F.: Using Composite Resin as a Posterior Restorative Material. (1991). J.A.D.A. Vol. 122, p. 65.

Lutz, F., Krejci, I., and Oldenburg, T.R.: Elimination of Polymerization Stresses at the Margins of Posterior Composite Resin Restorations: A New Restorative Technique. (1986). Quint. Int. Vol. 17, p. 777.

Nakabayashi, N., Nakamura, M., and Yasuda, N.: Hybird Layer as a Dentin-Bonding Mechanism. (1991). J. Esth. Dent. Vol. 3, p. 133.

Peutzfeldt, A. and Asmussen, E.: Retention of Composite Inlays in Enamel Dentin Cavities. (1991). Dent. Mater. Vol. 7, p. 11.

Rada, R.E.: In-Office Fabrication of Indirect Composite-Resin Restorations. (1992). Pract. Perio. Aesth. Dent. Vol. 4, (3), p. 25.

Reality. (1992). Section 2. Reality Pub. Co., Houston, TX.

Rees, J.S. and Jacobson, P.H.: The Polymerization Shrinkage of Composite Resins. (1987). J. Dent. Res. (Abstract No. 119) Vol. 66, p. 848.

Robinson, P.B., Moore B.K., and Swartz, M.L.: Comparison of Microleakage in the Direct and Indirect Composite Resin Restorations in vitro. (1987). Oper. Dent. Vol. 12, p. 113.

Ruge, G.: Clinical Criteria. (1980). Int. Dent. J. 30, p. 347.

Scherer, W., Caliskan, F., Kaim, J., Moss, S., and Vijayaraghavan, T.: Comparison of Microleakage Between Direct Placement Composites and Direct Composite Inlays. (1990). Gen. Dent. May-June, p. 209.

Sheth, J.J., Fuller, J.L., and Jensen, M.E.: Cuspal Deformation and Fracture Resistance of Teeth With Dentin Adhesives and Composites. (1988). J. Prosth. Dent. Vol. 60, p. 560.

Sheth, P.J., et al.: Comparative Evaluation of Three Resin Inlay Techniques: Microleakage Studies. (1989). Quint. Int. Vol. 20 (11), p. 831.

Shintani, H. Satou N., and Satou J.: Clinical Evaluation of Two Posterior Composite Resins Retained With Bonding Agents. (1989). J. Prosth. Dent. Vol. 62, p. 627.

Shortall, A. and Asmussen, E.: Influence of Dentin-Bonding Agents and a Glass-Ionomer Base on the Cervical Marginal Seal of Class II Composite Restorations. (1988). Scand. I. Dent. Res. Vol. 96, p. 590.

Simonsen, R.J., Barouch, E., and Gelb, M.: Cusp Fracture Resistance From Composite Resin in Class II Restorations. (1983). J. Dent. Res. (Abstract No. 761). Vol. 62, p. 254

Smith, L.A., O'Brien, J.A., and Retief, D.H., et al: Microleakage of Two Dentinal Bonding Restorative Systems. (1988). IADR J. Dent. Res. (Abstract No. 1568). Vol. 67, p. 309.

Sneed, W.D. and Looper, S.W.: Shear Bond Strength of a Composite Resin to an Etched Glass Ionomer. (1985). Dent. Mater. J. Vol. 1, p. 127.

Stoffels, L.S.: Posterior Composite Resins: An Update. August (1991). Esth. Dent. Update, Vol. 2, p. 67.

Suzuki, M., Jordan, R.E., and Boksman, L.: Posterior Composite Restoration-Clinical Considerations. In Posterior Composite Resin Dental Restorative Materials. (1985). Vanherle, G. & Smith, D.C., (eds.) P. Szule Publishing Co., Utrecht., The Netherlands, p. 455.

Swartz, M.L., Phillips, R.W., and Clark, H. E.: Long Term Fluoride Release From Glass Ionomer Cements. (1984). J. Dent. Res. Vol. 63, p. 158.

Tay, W.M. and Braden, M.: Thermal Diffusivity of Glass Ionomer Cements. (1987). J. Dent. Res. Vol. 66, p. 1040.

Torstenson, B. and Brannstrom, M.: Contraction Gap Under Composite Resin Restorations-Effect of Hygroscopic Expansion and Thermal Stress. (1988). Oper. Dent. Vol. 13., p. 24.

Torstenson, B. and Brannstrom, M: Composite Resin Contraction Gaps Measured With a Fluorescent Resin Technique. (1988). Dent. Mater. Vol. 4, p. 238.

Walls, A.W.G., McCabe, J.F., and Murray, J.J.: The Polymerization Contraction of Visible-Light Activated Composite Resins. (1988). J. Dent. Vol. 16, p. 177.

Wendt, S.L. and Leinfelder, K.F.: Clinical Evaluation of a Heat-Treated Composite Resin Inlay: 3-Year Results. (1992). Am. J. Dent. Vol. 5 (5), p. 258.

Wendt, S.L. and Leinfelder, K.F.: Clinical Evaluation of a Heat-Treated Composite Resin Inlay. (1990). J.A.D.A. Vol. 120, p. 171.

Wendt, S.L.: The Effect of Heat Used as Secondary Cure Upon the Physical Properties of Three Composite Resins II. Wear, Hardness and Color Stability. (1987). Quint. Int. Vol. 18 (5), p. 351.

Wilson, N.H.F., Wilson, M.A., and Smith, G.A.: A Clinical Trial of New Visible Light-Cured Composite Restorative-Initial Findings and One Year Results. (1985). Quint. Int. Vol. 16, p. 281.

Wilson, M.A. and Norman, R.D.: An Investigation Into the Incidence of Voids in Indirect Composite Inlays Formed Using Different Packing Techniques. (1991). J. Dent. Vol. 19, p. 296.

CHAPTER 6

ESTHETIC CERAMIC RESTORATIVE MATERIALS AND TECHNIQUES

DENTAL CERAMIC MATERIALS

HISTORICAL BACKGROUND

In the search for more stable and esthetic restorative dental materials, ceramics were first mentioned for use by Pierre Fauchard (1678-1761), a French dentist. He described the application of jewelers' enamel to artificial teeth of thin gold plate. Another French dentist named Chemant, pursuing the idea of an apothecary named Alexes, developed "incorruptible teeth of mineral paste" in the 1790s. These "mineral paste" dentures led to the development of "Ferro Metallic Teeth" by an Italian dentist named Fonzi who practiced in Paris. These were the first successfully manufactured individual teeth and small blocks of teeth in porcelain.

With the industrial revolution, the manufacture of porcelain denture teeth increased and by the middle to late 19th century, with the advent of the vulcanite process, dentures with porcelain teeth became more affordable for the average individual. The use of porcelain for crowns was delayed until more efficient tooth preparation instrumentation was developed. Improved dental cements (oxyphosphate of zinc), the introduction of gutta percha for root canal fillings and smaller sized porcelain ovens all preceded the use of porcelain for crown and bridge work.

The first porcelain jacket crown is attributed to Dr. C.H. Land, who patented his platinum matrix technique in 1887. The use of high, medium and low fusing porcelains was debated. Many ceramic inlay and crown techniques were used and abused. By the early 1900s porcelain use for dental restorations was declining due to this abuse. By the 1920s, successful results, demonstrated by clinicians and researchers, led to a renewed popularity. In the 1950s, with the development of acrylic resins in dentistry, the use of porcelain again declined and along with it the skilled porcelain technicians. The development and successful use of porcelain fused to metal in the 1960s restored the use of porcelain in fixed prosthodontics. Porcelain fused to metal restoration will continue to be the most popular restoration for fixed prosthodontics. Superior strength and good esthetics provide a predictable and long-lasting solution to most esthetic fixed prosthodontic problems. During the 1970s and 1980s, porcelain fused to metal restorations became the primary restoration of choice for many clinicians. Porcelain fused to metal techniques are well covered in other texts and will not be detailed in this book.

In the 1980s and early 1990s, patient demands for improved esthetic results have led to the development of many ceramic systems. This chapter will provide a basic introduction to and classification of these systems.

COMPOSITION

Dental ceramics have their origin in a traditional triaxial porcelain (white ware) with three components consisting of clay or kaolinite (AL_2O_3, SiO_2, $2H_2O$), feldspar (K_2O, AL_2O_3, $6SiO_2$) and quartz (SiO_2). The demand for higher translucency led to the virtual elimination of clay and an increase in the feldspar to about 80%. Currently dental ceramics are essentially feldspathic glasses with oxides added (B_2O_3, K_2O, Na_2O, and CaO) to lower the firing temperature and modify thermal expansion, which is needed for bonding to metal. In addition, other metallic oxides such as Fe_2O_3 and TiO_3 are contained in the ceramic and impart color and opacity. In the production of dental ceramic powders, the raw materials and additives are heated together at high temperatures and quenched in water. This breaks up the ceramic mass or frit, which is subsequently milled into a powder. This powder can be mixed with a liquid and modeled into the shape of a tooth. Multiple ceramic frit combinations yield powders of various color and translucency which, when layered, create the many esthetic features making up a tooth. These modeled ceramic teeth are brought to the appropriate temperature where the edges start to melt and fuse together (Fig. 6-1). This process is known as sintering and results in partial fusion of the particles and a minimum change in the shape of the mass. Heating the ceramic under vacuum yields minimal porosity and maximum optical translucency. Ultimately, a composition material is formed in which crystallized and noncrystallized inorganic oxides are fused together in a glass

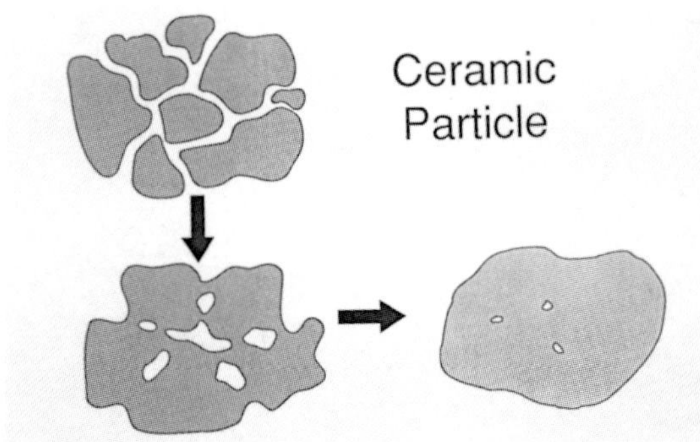

Fig. 6-1 Sequential illustration showing how ceramic particles, when heated, fuse (sinter) together, but small voids remain.

matrix to form a heterogenous solid mass. This is similar to a composite resin material that contains glassy particles held together by a resin matrix instead of glass.

The composition of the many ceramic materials used in dentistry is a complex of many variable components that modify strength and esthetic properties. The perfect ceramic material has not been discovered, but the creative and artistic ability of dental technicians allows for the close duplication of most teeth.

FAILURES

Dental ceramic materials are essentially borosilicate and/or feldspathic glasses that may contain dispersed crystalline metallic oxide components. These crystals are stronger than corresponding noncrystalline structures because the atoms are in a state of maximum packing density. Most ceramic dental restorations are the result of the fusion of small frit particles and not made from a glass melt as in the production of most industrial glass objects. Imperfections in the fused dental ceramic caused by incomplete fusion result in reduced strength. The

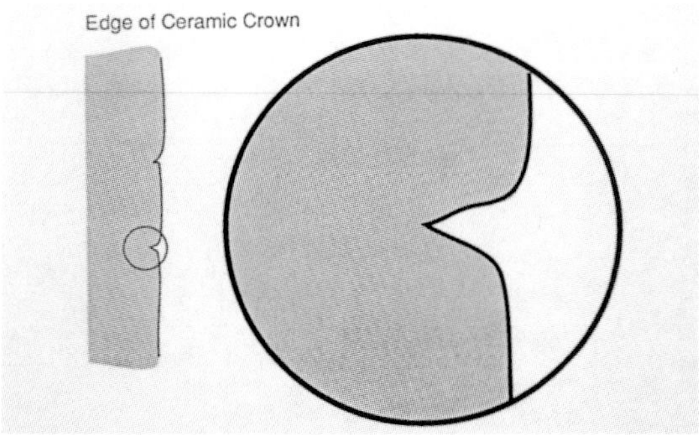

Fig. 6-2a Griffith flaw in the surface of a ceramic material.

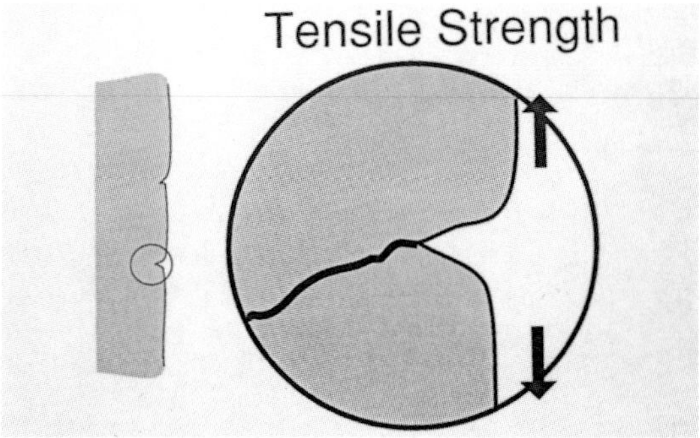

Fig. 6-2b Stress yields crack growth from Griffith flaw.

presence of these surface cracks and flaws was established by Griffith in 1920 and these are often referred to as "Griffith flaws." When the ceramic is stressed, these flaws provide the start of a crack (Fig. 6-2). Ceramic materials have a "critical strain" of about 0.1%. Increasing the strength of dental ceramics often involves an increase in the modulus of elasticity, which results in the need for a greater stress to reach the critical 0.1% strain. Reduction of surface flaws will also result in improved strength characteristics.

Another factor that may effect the long term prognosis of a dental ceramic is called "static fatigue." This time dependent process of static fatigue is due to the influence of water in moist ambient conditions upon the ceramic. A stress dependent chemical reaction between the water and surface flaws causes the flaw to grow to a critical dimension, which then allows for spontaneous crack propagation. The chemical environment may have an even greater effect on the long term strength of a ceramic restoration than surface flaws. It has been shown that ceramic samples in vacuum dry air require about 33% more stress to fracture than moist samples.

Clinically, ceramic failures are often reported as resulting from a minimal stress or trauma. The combination of flaw propagation and static fatigue allow the restoration to reach the point that a minimal stress can cause a noticeable ceramic fracture. In reality, the failure process has occurred over an extended period of time. Protecting a ceramic material from moisture contamination would also increase the potential long term strength.

STRENGTHENING

Dental ceramic materials are capable of producing highly esthetic restorations that closely resemble the natural dentition. These materials are harder than enamel but in general are comparatively weak in tension compared to gold alloys. Surface flaws play a major role in the longitudinal performance of a ceramic restoration. Stronger, more flawed ceramic restorations may perform poorly compared to weaker but less flawed restorations. Ceramic restorations fail when strain is about 0.1%. Minimizing strain by increasing the elastic modulus of a ceramic material or eliminating surface flaws will provide improved strength. Several methods have been used over the last three decades to strengthen dental ceramics. Some of these are:

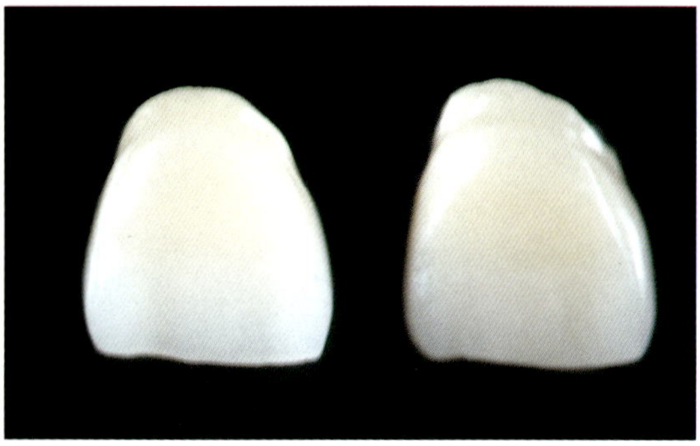

Fig. 6-3 Note brighter ceramometal crown on the left compared to the more natural-looking opalescent ceramometal crown on the right.

1. Enameling of metals
2. Dispersion strengthening
3. Crystallization of glasses
4. Chemical toughening by ion exchange
5. Bonding to metallic foils
6. Bonding to natural tooth structure

Enameling of Metals

Weinstein described the first successful metal ceramic restoration in 1962. Since that time the use of high expansion glasses bonded to metal has become the primary choice for predictable and esthetic fixed restorations. The introduction of higher levels of K_2O into the ceramic frit resulted in the elevated production of leucitic crystals, which increased the ceramic's thermal expansion and made it compatible with the higher thermal expansion of certain metals. These ceramic materials will bond to the exterior oxide layer of metallic alloys and provide an extremely strong restoration.

Metal ceramic restorations have become the primary restoration of choice over the last three decades due to their strength, adequate esthetic qualities and predictable clinical results. Increased esthetic demands and limited esthetic results, for selective situations, have lead to a continuing development of all ceramic systems and improved methods of strengthening. Newer ceramics have been developed that scatter light better and have significantly improved the esthetic results achievable with metal substructures. These opalescent type ceramic materials combined with more conservative metal designs minimize the brightness typically seen in the gingival one third or other thin areas of the ceramometal crown (Fig. 6-3).

Dispersion Strengthening

If ceramic crystals of high strength and elasticity are dispersed in the glassy phase of dental ceramics, the resultant glass-crystal composite will also have an increased strength and elasticity. These harder masses interfere with crack propagation, thus a greater stress is necessary for fracture. This increase strength is relative to the concentration of the crystalline phase (Fig 6-4). McLean and Hughes in 1965 developed a high strength core porcelain used to significantly increase the strength of all ceramic crowns. This core porcelain contained 50% fused alumina crystals by weight. The finer the crystal size, the greater their strength. Improved materials have been developed in relationship to the original aluminous porcelain by optimizing the crystal-glass size relationship in order to improve the sintering characteristics, strength and also optical properties of a typically opaque core.

Dispersion strengthened, alumina reinforced feldspathic ceramic materials have poor esthetic properties and are used as a core to strengthen an all ceramic crown

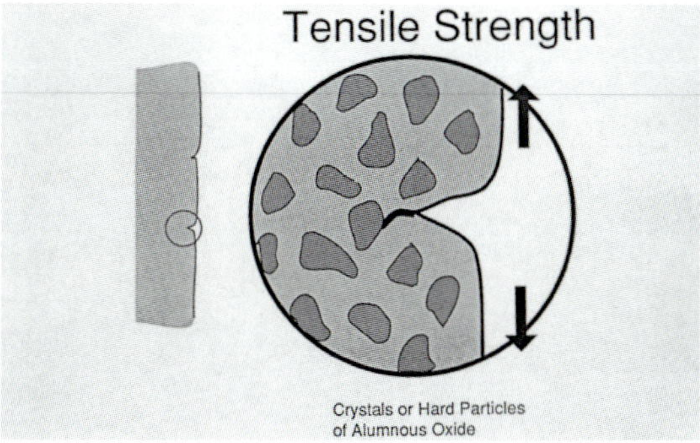

Fig. 6-4 Dispersion strengthening. Harder masses interfere with crack propagation.

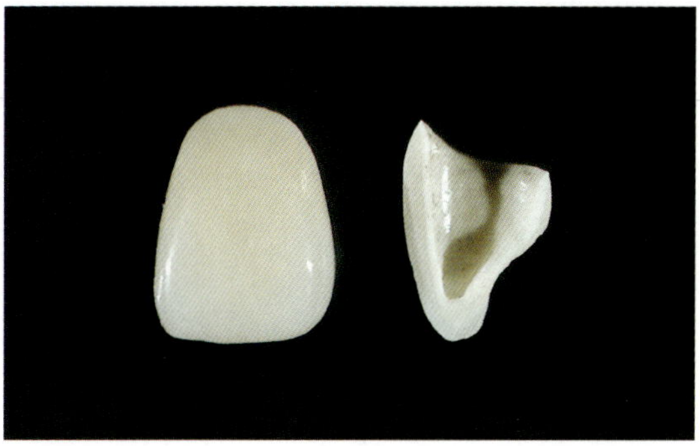

Fig. 6-5 Frontal view and cross section of aluminous oxide core strengthened crown. Note opaque core.

much like a metal coping strengthens a ceramometal crown (Fig. 6-5). The original aluminous porcelain material, VITADUR-N Core (Vita Zahnfabrik, Bad Säckingen, Germany), has since been improved with the development of Hi-Ceram (Vita Zahnfabrik) and more currently the development of In-Ceram (Vita Zahnfabrik). In-Ceram, developed by Saadoun (1989) in France, is one of the more significant developments in dental ceramics. Saadoun refined a technique known as slip-casting, which has been used for over 200 years in forming clay bodies. Slip-casting generally involves small aluminous oxide particles ranging in size from 1 to 5 μm, which results in a very high strength alumina core material.

A pure alumina coping is made by slowly heating it on a special refractory die to 1100°C for 2 hours and holding. This very accurate but poorly fused alumina core can be shaped and finally infused with shade matched low viscosity glass. Capillary action draws this glass into the porous alumina resulting in an extremely strong and dense alumina/glass composite structure. This core material contains at least 70% alumina and is currently the strongest dental ceramic available, developing flexural strengths in excess of 400 MPa. They may also have slightly improved optical properties than the previous aluminous core materials. Unfortunately this strength still does not compare to cast metal alloys.

O'Brien in the mid 1980s described the use of magnesia crystals to reinforce a glass resulting in a high coefficient of thermal expansion similar to that of ceramics used to enamel metals. This high thermal expansion core porcelain has a modulus of rupture similar to that of the conventional alumina reinforced porcelain (131 MPa). The strength of this magnesia core can be significantly improved by treating the surface with a suitable glaze. This surface glass glaze is thought to penetrate surface flaws and possibly put the surface layer in compression. The effect of use of this glaze in the internal aspect of the restoration on core fit is unclear. This magnesia core material is to be introduced by Leach and Dillon for use with their high expansion dental ceramic materials. The advantage of this core material over others may be its compatibility with the more commonly used and available high expansion ceramometal dental ceramic materials.

Crystallization of Glasses

The principles of glass ceramics and the controlled crystallization of glass is another method by which dental ceramics are strengthened. By definition, glass is a ceramic material. Glass is unique among

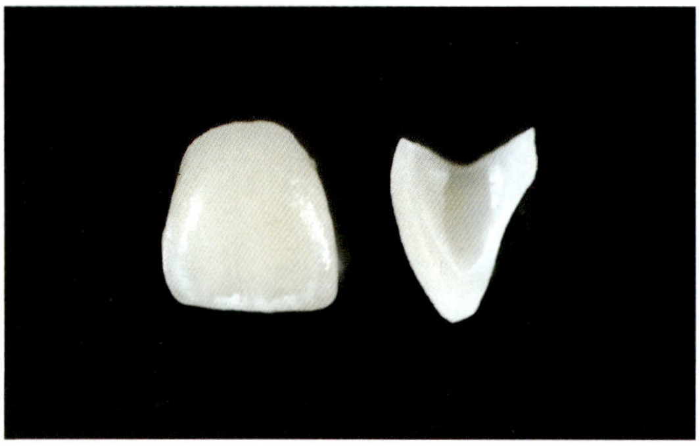

Fig. 6-6 Frontal view and cross section of Dicor core strengthened crown. Note translucent core.

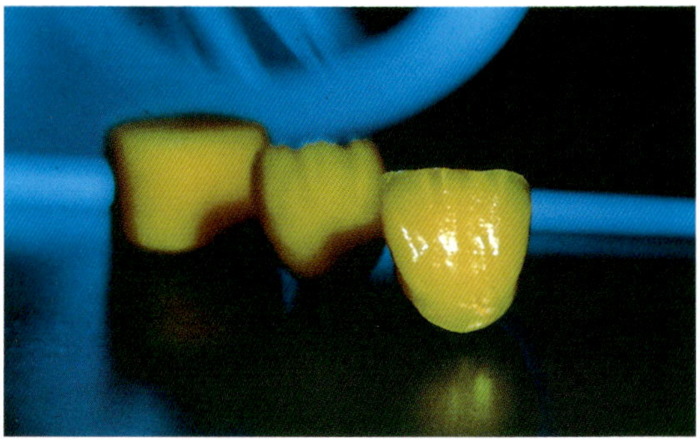

Fig. 6-7 IPS Empress ceramic pellet background (courtesy of Williams-Ivoclar).

ceramics in that it has no crystallinity. It has been called a supercooled liquid and is formed by melting or softening. Softening in the case of glass is not a physical change like it is with metals that change from an amorphous liquid to a crystalline solid. Glass is amorphous in both the solid and liquid states. Softening in glass is only a change in viscosity. In hardening it becomes so viscous that it has many physical attributes of a solid with the exception of crystallinity. The viscosity is so great that the molecules cannot realign themselves into crystals in a reasonable length of time. Based upon the work of Grossman and Adair, Dicor (Densply International Inc, York, PA), a crystallized glass used for dental restorations has been developed. Using the lost wax process, dental restorations made of thin silica-based glass can be accurately cast. Magnesium fluoride acts as a nucleating agent for crystal formation. These amorphous cast glass restorations nucleate at temperatures between 650°C and 1075°C, in a process called "ceramming," forming a network of overlapping tetrasilicic fluormica crystals ($K_2Mg_5Si_2O_{20}F_4$) within the glass matrix. These tetracyclic crystals add strength and resistance to fracture propagation. The strength of Dicor is approximately that of the original aluminous porcelain. Unlike the very opaque aluminous porcelain, it is very translucent (Fig. 6-6).

Another glass ceramic restoration formed using the lost wax process is IPS Empress® (Ivoclar, Amherst, NY). This unique leucite reinforced glass ceramic is supplied in cylindrical pellets that are made by sintering the ground particles of the precerammed glass with additives, altering esthetic properties. They are available in a variety of opacities and dentin shades (Fig. 6-7).

Chemical Toughening by Ion Exchange

Failure of ceramic restorations often occurs when surface flaws are placed in tension and crack growth occurs. If a ceramic surface can be put in a compressed state, this compression stress must first be overcome before such a tensile condition exists. Thus a greater force would be necessary to fracture such a ceramic restoration than an untreated restoration (Fig. 6-8). A process known as "ion exchange" has been proven to significantly strengthen dental ceramics. This process involves the chemical displacement of smaller surface sodium ions in a ceramic by larger potassium ions (Fig. 6-9). The resultant ceramic surface is put in compression due to crowding of the silicate network, resulting in a 23% to 140% increase in strength.

Traditionally ceramic crowns were placed in platinum crucibles containing molten

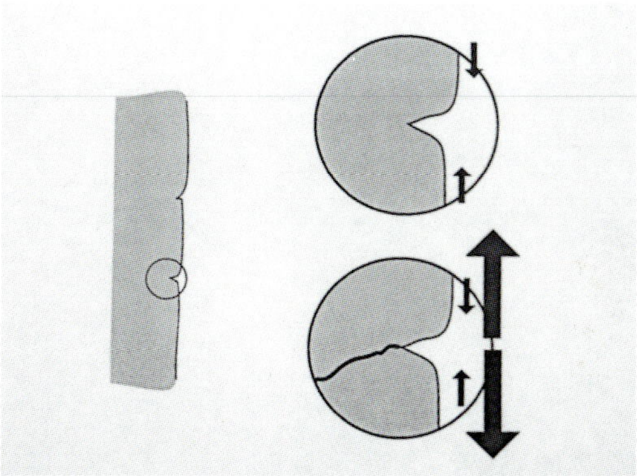

Fig. 6-8 Placing the surface of a ceramic material in compression requires a greater tensile force for crack propagation.

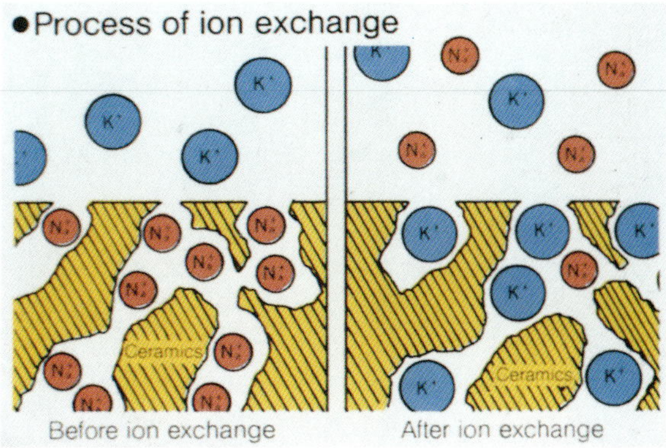

Fig. 6-9 Ion exchange of larger potassium atoms for smaller sodium atoms on the ceramic surface (courtesy of G.C. International, Chicago, IL, Tuf-Coat).

potassium nitrate for 24 to 48 hours. These extended treatment times may have discouraged its utilization. Currently new commercially available products have been developed to significantly reduce the treatment time to approximately 1 hour. Such surface treatment does not appear to alter translucency and may also improve the ceramic's chemical durability, fracture toughness, hardness, abrasion resistance and reduce plaque adhesion. Time and temperature variables need continued investigation to optimize treatment techniques for each individual ceramic material.

Ion exchange may prove to be especially beneficial for use on bonded ceramic restorations that are fabricated with lower strength and nonreinforced ceramic materials.

Bonding to Metallic Foils

Bonding ceramic materials to cast metallic substrates provides for maximum strength and minimizes the potential for internal flaw and crack propagation. Attempts to strengthen crowns using thinner metallic substrates have been made. An initial approach was developed in the mid 1970s by McLean and Sced, who used tin plated platinum foil copings as the crown substrate (Fig. 6-10). Technique variables and questionable strength advantages led to a decline in popularity. Preformed platinum alloy copings were described by McLean and Sced (1987) to provide an economic alternative to copings fabricated using the lost wax process.

Another technique, described by Schössow in 1984, used a laminated foil. The outer layer of pure gold melts and solders an umbrella-like coping together. The inner three layers consist of a gold, platinum and palladium layer, a pure palladium layer and an inner gold, platinum and palladium layer. These Renaissance® copings are easy to fabricate but their strength and resistance to thermal distortion has been questioned (Fig. 6-11).

Gold foil copings (Sunrise Crowns) have also been described by Tanaka. Esthetic results appear to be excellent.

The use of the various foil reinforcement techniques provide an easily fabricated alternative to cast copings. Their ability to strengthen ceramic restorations varies but the esthetic result appears to be improved over that of cast metal reinforced crowns.

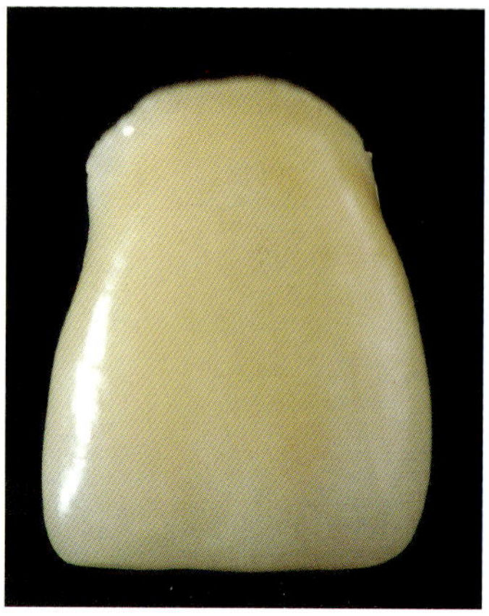

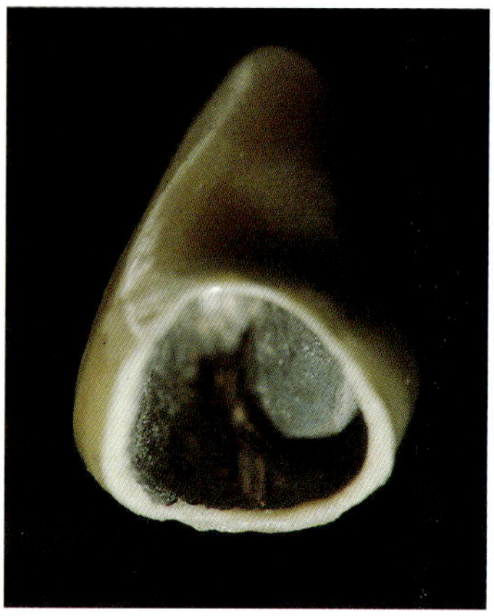

Figs. 6-10a and b Crown with a tin plated platinum foil substrate.

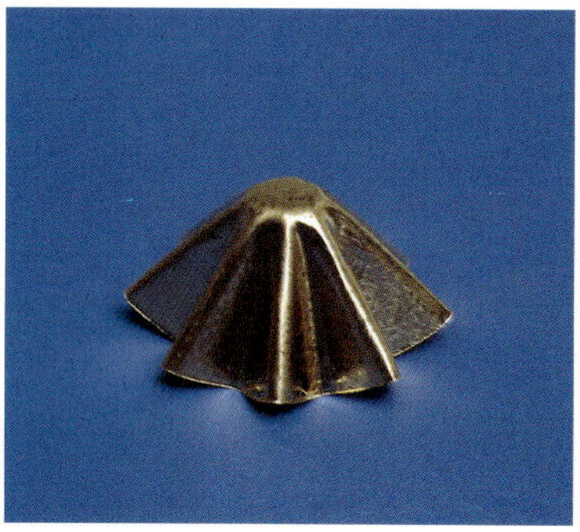

Fig. 6-11a Renaissance® foil coping before adaptation to a die.

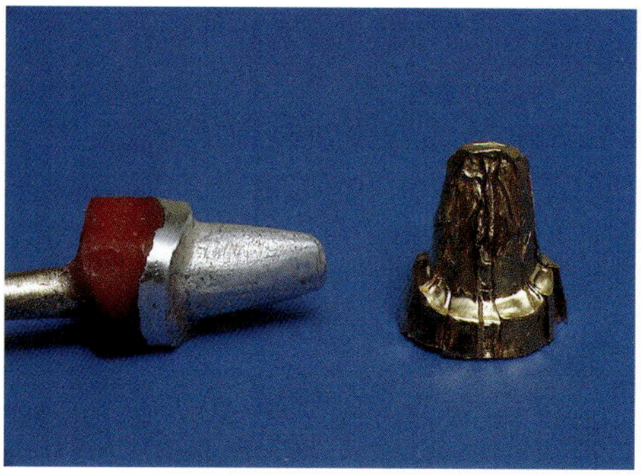

Fig. 6-11b Renaissance coping after adaptation.

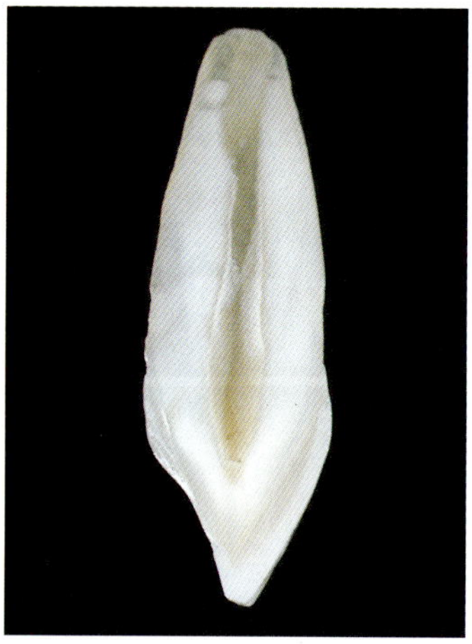

Fig. 6-12 Cross section of ceramic veneer bonded to a tooth.

Bonding to Enamel and Dentin

One of the most significant advances in contemporary esthetic restorative dentistry has been the ability to bond ceramic materials to enamel and dentin. The bond strengths of ceramic to enamel are well documented. The bond strengths of ceramics to dentin are constantly increasing and may soon rival that of bonding to enamel.

By bonding to enamel, the relatively weak ceramic restorations are significantly strengthened. The necessity to remove intact tooth structure during preparation is minimized. The high success rate of bonded porcelain veneers has established bonded ceramic restorations as a conservative and highly esthetic alternative to traditional fixed prosthodontics (Fig. 6-12).

To put it in perspective, most dental ceramic materials are stronger than enamel would be if it were removed from dentin. Enamel gets much of its strength through its attachment to dentin. Thus, if ceramic restorations can be adequately bonded to tooth structure, the potential result should be a restoration with at least the strength of the original tooth. While this view may be somewhat optimistic, the time is rapidly approaching when only the defective portion of a tooth will have to be removed and replaced with a bonded restoration. The conservative nature of such restorations will minimize tooth destruction and iatrogenic periodontal disease and maximize longevity of the dentition. This form of ceramic strengthening will play an even greater role as bonding techniques and materials improve. Universal acceptance of these bonded ceramic restorations will require clinical research to substantiate their longevity.

CLASSIFICATION

The chemical composition and structure of dental ceramic materials are complex and difficult to understand. A simple classification system that can be used to categorize materials for the purpose of defining utilization is more helpful to the practicing dentist. The following is a categorization outline based primarily on strengthening techniques. These categories will be referred to in the clinical sections and should prove useful in the selection of appropriate ceramic materials for various situations and applications.

Conventional Ceramic

Conventional ceramic materials are any low strength ceramics that provide an esthetic veneer. These materials are traditionally bonded to metal or strengthened ceramic cores. They provide the esthetic portion of a restoration but generally lack sufficient strength without one of the strengthening techniques in order to resist functional occlusal stresses and a resultant high failure rate.

Examples:

Most porcelain jacket and ceramometal veneering ceramics, feldspathic porcelains.

Core Strengthening Ceramic

These ceramic materials have high strength compared to conventional ceramics but generally are quite opaque and do not have adequate esthetic properties by themselves. They are used as internal substructures for ceramic restorations and are veneered with conventional ceramic materials for maximum esthetics. Core strengthening ceramics can significantly increase the strength of a ceramic restoration. They require adequate bulk and preparations must provide adequate thickness for layering the two ceramic materials in order to achieve adequate strength and esthetics.

Examples:

Aluminous porcelain, Hi-Ceram®, In-Ceram®, Cerestore®, Alceram®.

Strengthened Ceramic

Strengthened ceramic materials have been developed to provide a combination of strength and esthetic properties in one material. These materials are stronger than conventional ceramic materials and achieve this improved strength in a variety of ways. In general they are feldspathic ceramics that contain aluminous oxide, leucite crystals or

ceramic fiber whisks. These materials are used to fabricate the entire dental restoration and possess sufficient properties to satisfy most esthetic demands.
Examples:
Cerinate®, Optec®, Mirage II®.

Glass Ceramic

Glass ceramics can be centrifuged or pressed into an investment void form using a lost wax process because they are a super-cooled liquid. These materials possess the approximate strength of the strengthened ceramics and some of the core strengthening ceramics. Because they are fabricated using a lost wax process, the entire void in the mold is filled with only one material and esthetic modifications must be achieved by layering with surface colorants or veneering with conventional ceramics. Thus, glass ceramic materials may also be used for core strengthening.

Machinable Ceramic

Pre-made conventional ceramic and glass ceramic blocks have also been used successfully with CAD-CAM and copy-milling systems. These new ceramic applications have improved strength and wear properties due to controlled manufacturing techniques.
Examples:
Dicor MGC®, Vita Mark II®, Vita Celay Blanks®.

MATERIALS, ANALYSIS AND SELECTION

Introduction

The abundance of ceramic systems and materials available today, along with the continuous development of new ones, makes the selection process for the optimal material confusing at best. No single ceramic system will universally satisfy all requirements. By understanding the make up of the various ceramic systems, their physical properties and esthetic parameters, the dentist can make appropriate material selections for various situations. The purpose of this section is to analyze how ceramic materials meet various dental demands and to provide guidelines for selection. In addition, techniques for successful all ceramic crown fabrication and clinical application will be presented.

The appropriate material for a ceramic crown should be dictated by the dentist and not exclusively by laboratory availability. The dentist must analyze the patient's esthetic, functional and physiologic demands and select the optimal material. A basic understanding of the esthetic and physical properties of the various ceramic categories is essential in order to select an optimal material for each patient requirement. During the diagnostic phase, patient demands and needs must be prioritized and considered in finalizing the selection of the most appropriate ceramic material.

Esthetic Analysis

Treatment Goals

When a tooth is to be crowned, diagnosis of how much of the tooth is visible during normal communication is essential. Demonstrating to the patient how much of a tooth is visible when they talk and smile, using a video camera or minimally a hand mirror, is essential for proper patient understanding and decision making. When a tooth is highly visible, maximum esthetics is often required (Fig. 6-13). In selected instances other priorities such as periodontal health or conservation of tooth structure may take precedence. Less visible teeth should be clearly demonstrated to the patient and beneficial but less esthetic modifications may be planned (Fig. 6-14). For instance, when gingival crown margins are not visible, supragingival margin

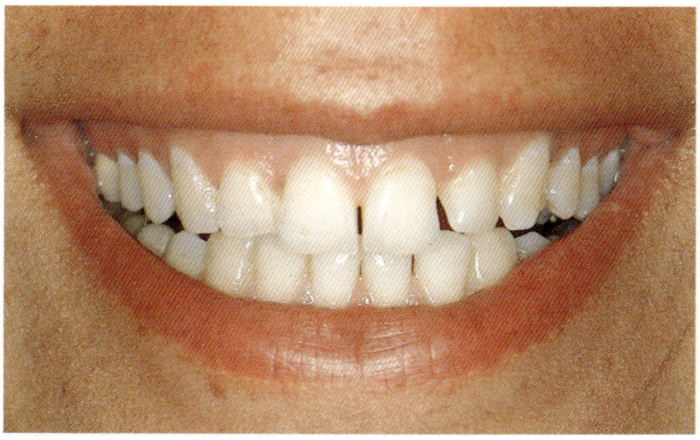

Fig. 6-13 Smile with maximum exposure of maxillary teeth.

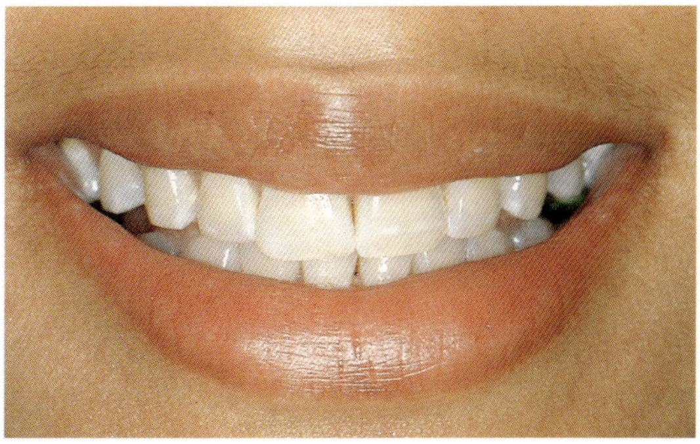

Fig. 6-14 Smile with minimal gingival areas showing.

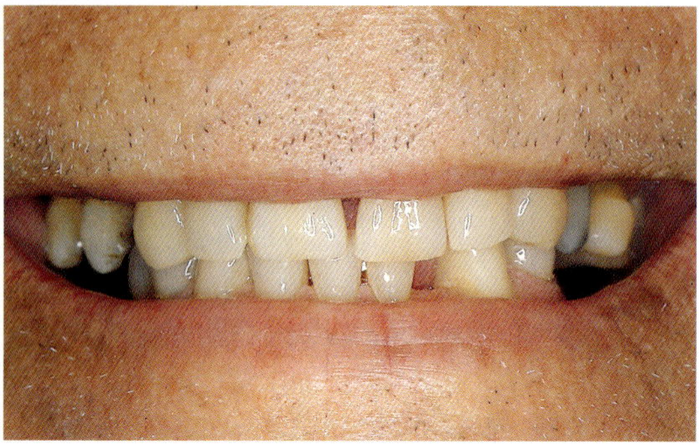

Fig. 6-15a Smile covering gingival of tooth 8.

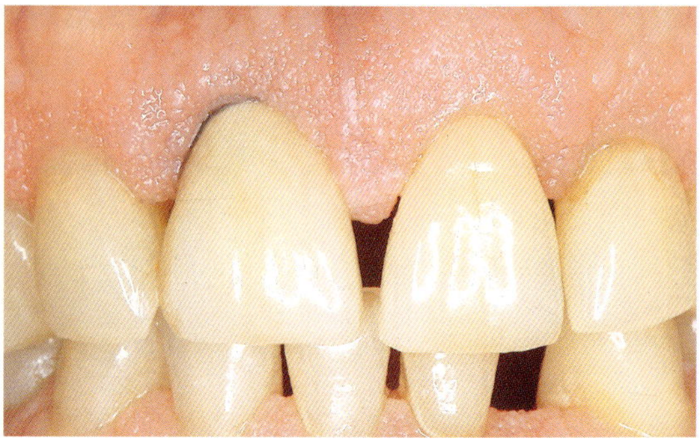

Fig. 6-15b Close up showing supragingival margin placement on tooth 8 crown.

placement may be treatment planned with the patient's consent (Fig. 6-15). A thorough diagnosis of esthetic demands based upon an educated patient's input will establish pretreatment esthetic goals. The materials and technique that best meet these goals can then be treatment planned.

Limitations

During the treatment planning phase, limitations to achieving esthetic goals must be made clear to the patient.

1. Single vs. multiple restorations: When restoring a single tooth, the difficulty in achieving an acceptable esthetic match is generally greater than with multiple units. This should be made clear to the patient. Single unit esthetic restorations should be treatment planned at a slightly higher fee to compensate for the additional chair time and laboratory costs that are often necessary.
2. Homogenous vs. heterogeneous tooth color: Restorations that must match teeth with unique and variable color distributions will require additional procedures to obtain an optimal shade match (Figs. 6-16 and 6-17). Custom shade guides, patient trips to the laboratory, photographs and other visual aids as well as custom tinting in the office may also be necessary. Again, patient understanding of the problems is critical and fee adjustment may be necessary.
3. Thin vs. thick teeth: Teeth that have adequate bulk may be restored with a variety of materials. When 1.25 to 1.50 mm

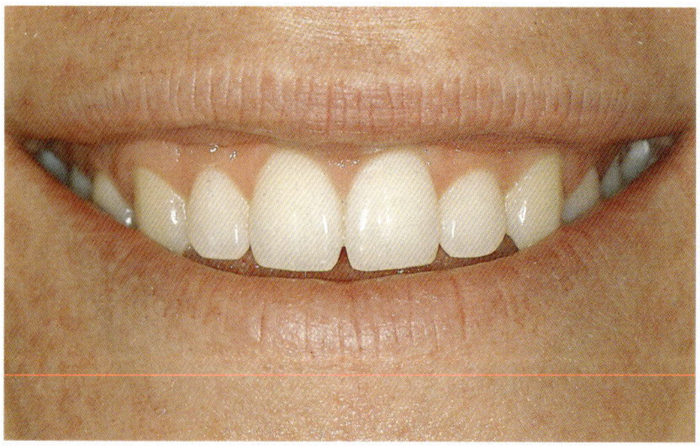

Fig. 6-16 Homogenous teeth with little color are easier to match.

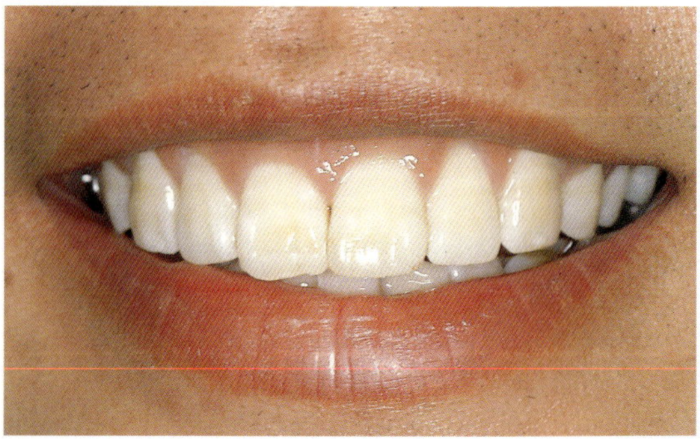

Fig. 6-17 Heterogenous teeth with distinctly colored areas are more difficult to match.

EXAGGERATED SMILE (MANDIBULAR)
% Not Showing

	Central %	Lateral %	Cuspid %
Gingival 1/3	52.7	51.3	64.7
Middle 1/3	9.4	9.9	12.7
Incisal 1/3	1.9	2.1	2.1

Fig. 6-18a

EXAGGERATED SMILE (MAXILLARY)
% Not Showing

	Central %	Lateral %	Cuspid %
Gingival 1/3	25.9	16.0	24.2
Middle 1/3	1.9	2.1	3.3
Incisal 1/3	0.7	0.5	0.5

Fig. 6-18b

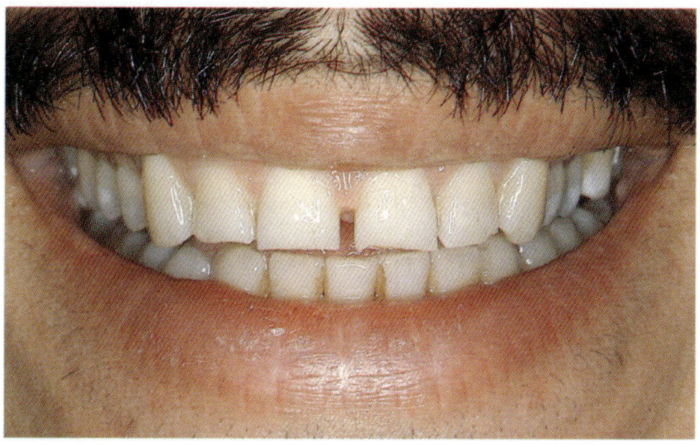

Fig. 6-19 Worn teeth with minimal to no incisal characteristics.

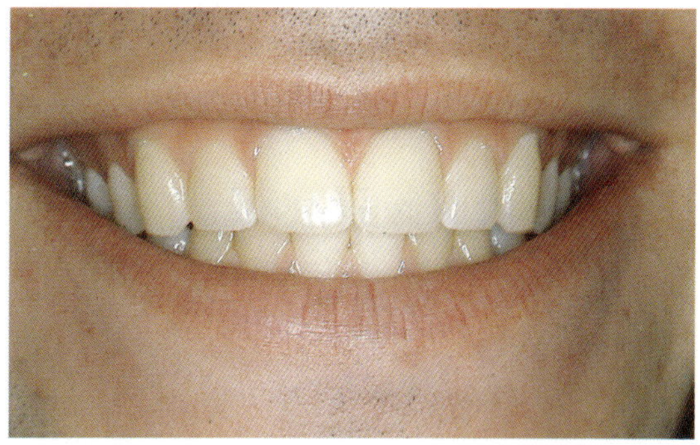

Fig. 6-20 Teeth with indistinct transition between incisal and gingival portions (similar to shade guides).

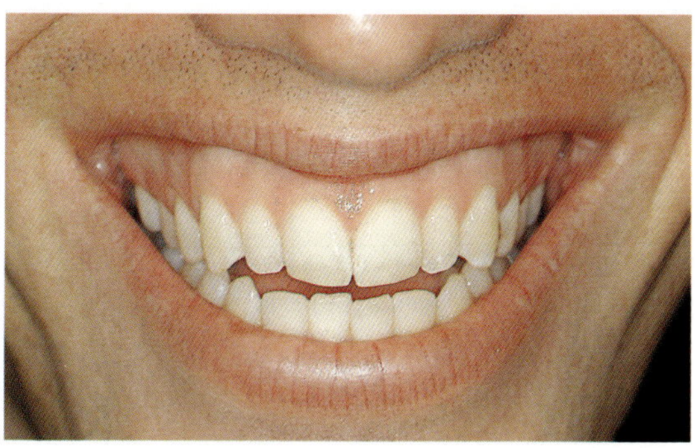

Fig. 6-21 Teeth with a distinct, well defined transition adjacent to incisal area.

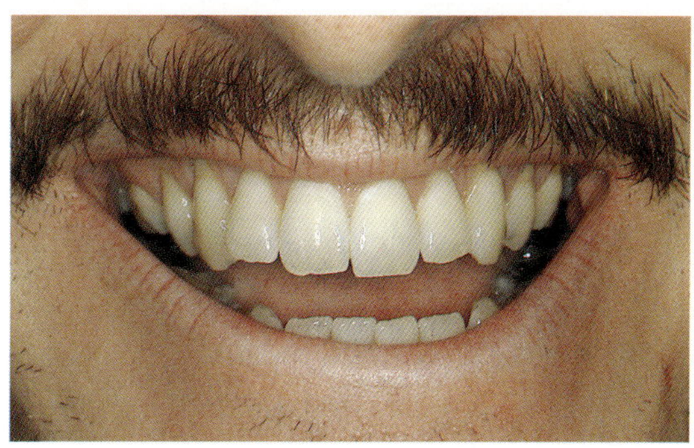

Fig. 6-22 Teeth with distinct incisal characteristics and colors.

of uniform tooth reduction can be accomplished, good esthetic results are possible with many esthetic ceramic systems. When teeth are small, thin or have large pulp chambers, the amount of tooth reduction may be limited. Ceramic systems requiring thickness for strength or core strengthening may be contraindicated or esthetic results may be compromised. Utilizing bonded ceramic techniques has greatly alleviated this problem by providing strength to a conservative ceramic restoration without compromising esthetic results.

4. Incisal characteristics: According to a study by Crispin et al., while the gingval

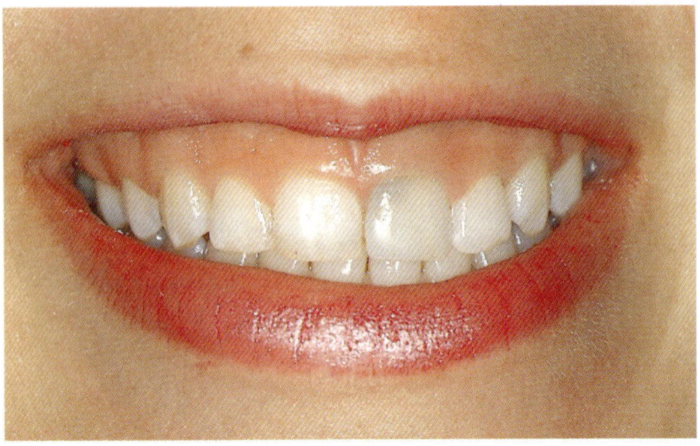

Fig. 6-23a Preoperative view of teeth 8 and 9; note short clinical crowns.

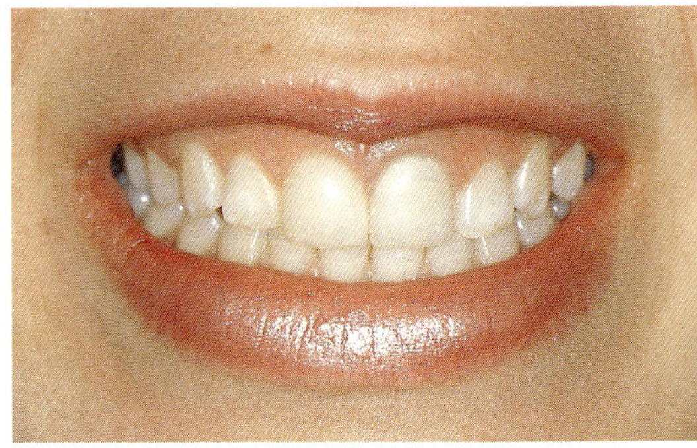

Fig. 6-23b Postoperative view of teeth 8 and 9; crown elongation and ceramic veneers placed.

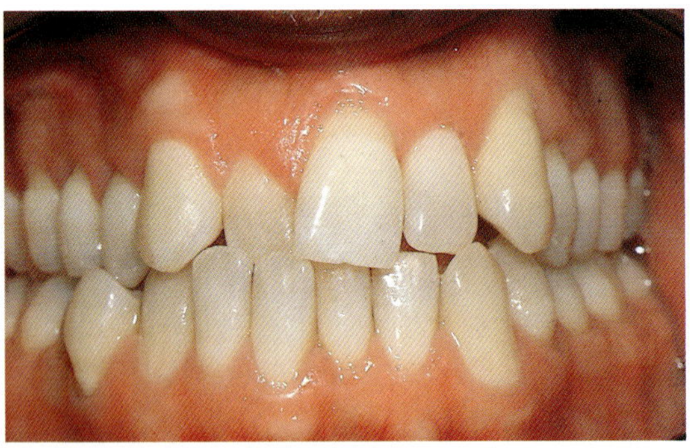

Fig. 6-24

Fig. 6-24 Preoperative view; tooth 8 is missing.

Fig. 6-25a Postorthodontic view; note tissue asymmetries.

Fig. 6-25b Postoperative view after periodontal surgery to improve tissue symmetry, and placement of ceramic veneers on teeth 8 and 9.

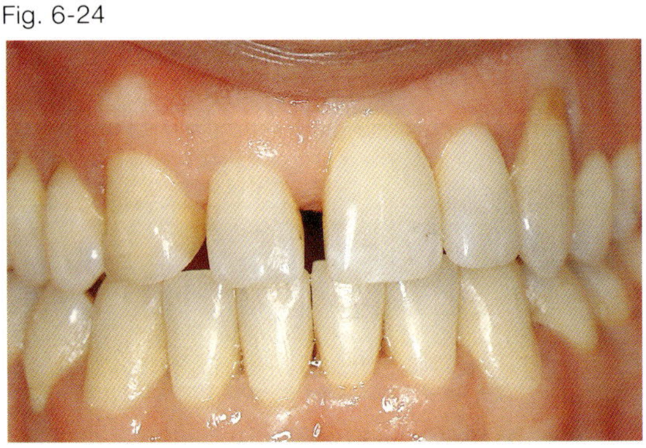

Fig. 6-25a

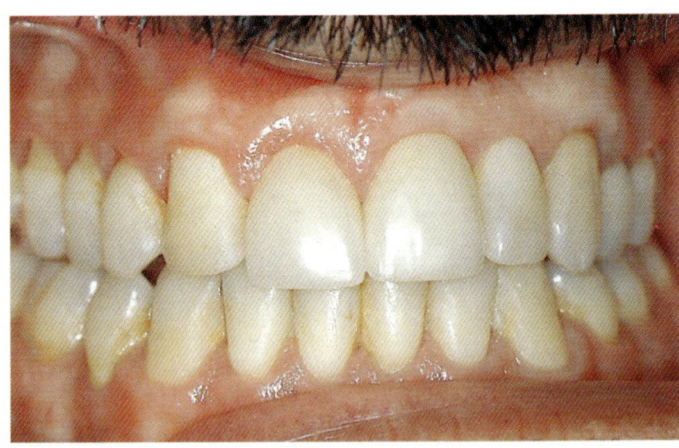

Fig. 6-25b

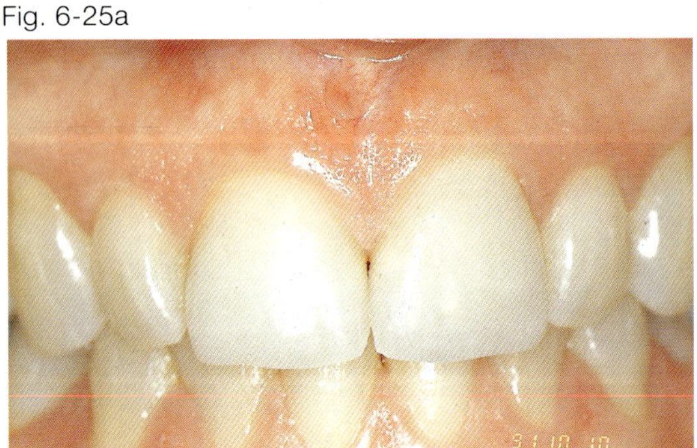

Fig. 6-26a Excellent tissue health adjacent to bonded ceramic veneers on teeth 8 and 9.

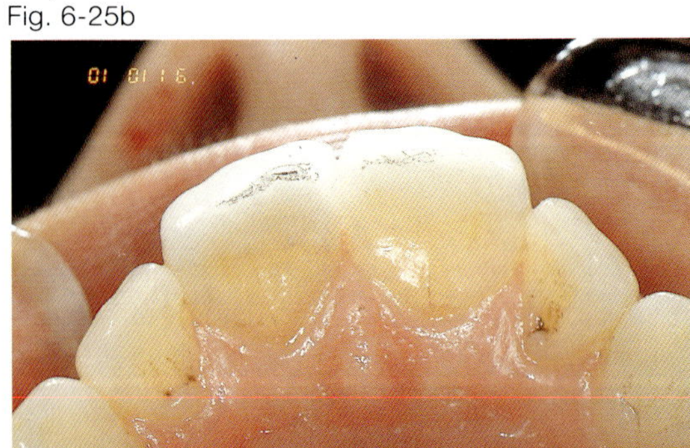

Fig. 6-26b Lingual view showing conservative margin extension of bonded ceramic veneers.

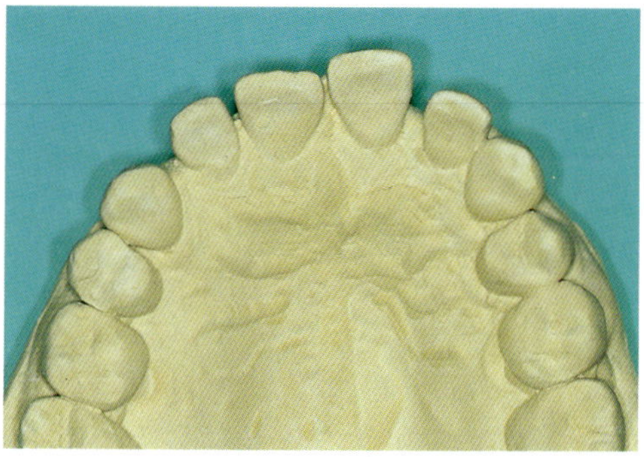

Fig. 6-27a Preoperative study model of malaligned teeth.

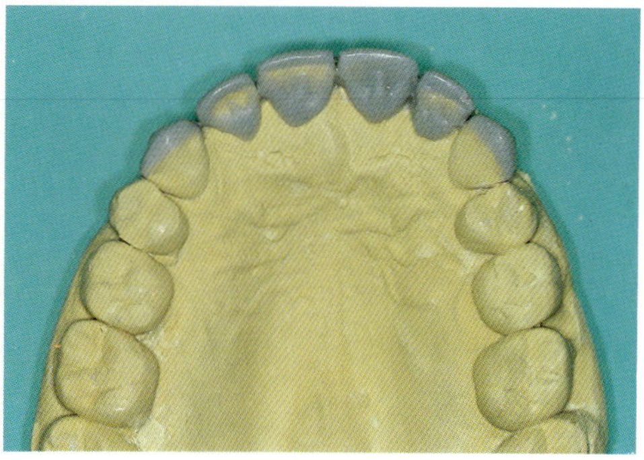

Fig. 6-27b Diagnostic waxup to align teeth.

third of a tooth is often not visible, almost everyone shows the incisal one third of their anterior and often the posterior teeth (Fig. 6-18). A comprehensive analysis and description of incisal characteristics to be matched is essential for optimal esthetic results. In older patients, incisal enamel is often worn or nonexistent (Fig. 6-19). Prescriptions should request that only dentin porcelain should be used in such instances. In situations where incisal enamel exists but no special characteristics are evident, the transition or junction between the incisal enamel and that supported by dentin must be defined. When this junction is indistinct, these teeth look like shade buttons and are relatively easy to match (Fig. 6-20). In contrast, when distinct incisal to dentin transitions exist (Fig. 6-21) or unique incisal characteristics are obvious (Fig. 6-22), precise matching will require greater communication and laboratory skills as well as chair time. Patients should be fully informed of these limitations.

5. Surrounding periodontal structures: Periodontal contour and health will often modify or restrict esthetic results and must not be overlooked during the diagnostic phase. Insufficient crown length may require clinical crown elongation, and this can often be accomplished by a simple tissue plasty (Figs. 6-23a and b). Asymmetrical periodontal contours may necessitate modification when visible (Fig. 6-24). Many innovative periodontal plastic surgical procedures are possible and significantly contribute to an optimal esthetic restorative result (Figs. 6-25a and b). Contemporary esthetic ceramic techniques are potentially much kinder to periodontal tissues. All ceramic restorations, in conjunction with bonding techniques, require less tooth reduction and if finished properly, result in excellent postoperative tissue health (Figs. 6-26a and b). Lack of patient acceptance of appropriate periodontal modifications will limit esthetic results and must be clearly explained to the patient before starting restorative therapy.
6. Positional relationships: Malaligned teeth often present an esthetic compromise that may or may not be correctable restoratively (Fig. 6-27a). Careful preoperative analysis of diagnostic casts and waxups will assure optimal results (Fig. 6-27b). In selected situations, orthodontic treatment should be recommended or esthetic limitations will be inevitable. Often patients, especially older patients, are reluctant to accept prerestorative orthodontic therapy. A thorough analysis of treatment limitations can often persuade patients to at least get an orthodontic consultation.

Failure to have the necessary orthodontic therapy may result in unusual restorative approaches that modify materials selection and compromise the prognosis. The patient must be thoroughly informed and the records carefully documented.

Functional Analysis

In addition to a thorough esthetic analysis and consultation, functional factors must also be diagnosed and discussed prior to finalizing a treatment plan. Increased functional demands may modify the treatment approach or material selection. Patients with obvious signs of excessive wear, for their age, present a potential problem (Fig. 6-28). Functional loading potential increases from the incisor region to posterior teeth in the arch. Materials with adequate strength for incisors and even canines may be inadequate for bicuspids and molars.

Occlusal abnormalities may also modify function. Edge to edge occlusion, crossbites and malpositioned teeth may all increase the functional demands on a restoration and must be recognized.

In addition, environmental or personal factors must be explored. Individuals who use their teeth in their work, such as carpenters or glass blowers, may have increased functional demands. Patients active in contact sports or activities with the potential for dental trauma must be consulted. Treatments can be developed for maximum esthetics but patients may prefer an option of maximum strength over optimal esthetics if they understand the situation and are given a choice. Patients with the potential for excessive post-operative functional demands should receive some type of protective device. An occlusal splint and/or custom made vinyl mouthguard should be included in the treatment plan of any vulnerable ceramic restoration that may be subjected to potentially destructive post-operative forces.

Physiologic Factors

Patients differ in their response to dental restorations. Functional factors may require enhanced strength while signs of wear may also dictate selection of a potentially less abrasive ceramic material. Ceramic materials may vary greatly in their abrasion potential based upon the type of material and the surface treatment of the ceramic restoration. Generally smoother ceramic surfaces have a lower wear potential. In addition, the castable glass ceramic, Dicor, has been shown to have a lower wear potential than most other ceramic materials. Glazing or tinting the

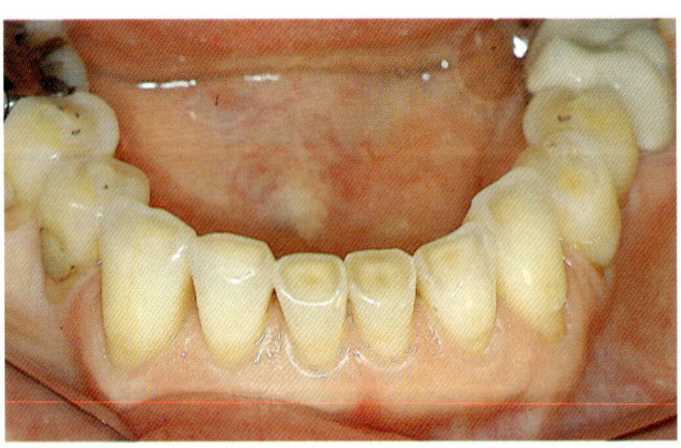

Fig. 6-28 Excessive wear for age.

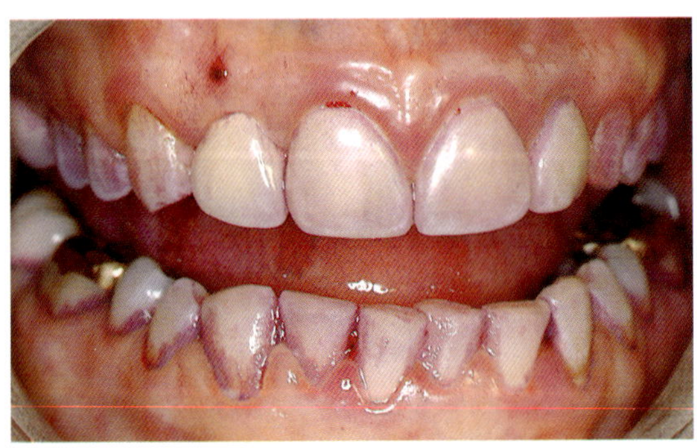

Fig. 6-29 Teeth 7 to 10 have Dicor crowns; note that they have less plaque accumulation than adjacent natural teeth.

occlusal surface results in a layer of conventional ceramic material that increases the wear potential compared to a polished Dicor surface.

Periodontal response to dental materials also varies significantly from patient to patient. An analysis of the periodontal response around preexisting restorations can indicate a potential problem. When an adverse periodontal response to dental restorations is evident, a ceramic material with a minimal potential for plaque accumulation should be selected. The castable ceramic Dicor, if properly glazed, has been shown to accumulate less plaque than enamel (Fig. 6-29). In addition, factors such as supragingival margin placement, contours maintaining normal emergence profiles and meticulous surface finishing, polishing and glazing techniques must be used. Marginal accuracy is also important.

Physiologic factors may play an important role in the success and longevity of a ceramic restoration. Esthetic goals may sometimes be modified in order to ensure maximum health. Patients must understand and agree to any modification that may change the final esthetic result.

Selection of the Optimal Ceramic Material

The final selection of a ceramic material is too often based upon accepting what our favorite laboratory uses. With the many ceramic alternatives available today, several laboratories might have to be utilized in order to provide optimal results using a variety of ceramic materials. This section will recommend the types of ceramic materials that might be appropriate for various situations. In most instances, several choices exist and results are significantly modified by the skill and knowledge of the dentist-laboratory technician team. It is recommended that each dentist establish a laboratory support network that uses a variety of materials that can be utilized as needed. The selections may vary from dentist to dentist but appropriate material selection will optimize the restorative results.

1. Esthetic priority: Optimal esthetic results should always be a high priority. Esthetic dentistry is truly the "artistic application of science." The level at which it can be accomplished will be dictated by the expertise of the laboratory technician and perfected by the aptitude and skill of the dentist. A coordinated team effort is essential for consistent esthetic results.

   Most of the ceramic systems can provide excellent esthetic results for certain situations. A few technician-dentist teams may be capable of using only one ceramic system and still provide excellent results for most situations. For the majority of dentists, it will be necessary to use different ceramic systems to maximize esthetic and functional results in the most predictable way.

   For ceramic crowns, maximum esthetic results may be achieved using almost any "conventional ceramic system" that has a full compliment of porcelains that can be layered to mimic natural tooth characteristics. Full ceramic crowns made with conventional ceramic systems alone are relatively weak when cemented with luting cements such as zinc phosphate, polycarboxylate and glass ionomer cements. Strength can be significantly improved by using composite resin cements and modern porcelain bonding techniques. Because most conventional ceramics are relatively translucent, composite resin cements may also be used to make generalized color changes. This cementation technique is recommended for maximum strength and esthetics. Conventional ceramic crowns should be used selectively. Ideally, they may be used for single

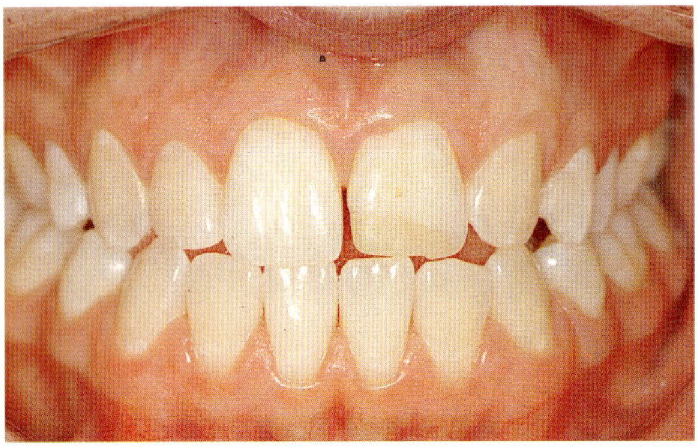

Fig. 6-30a Preoperative view.

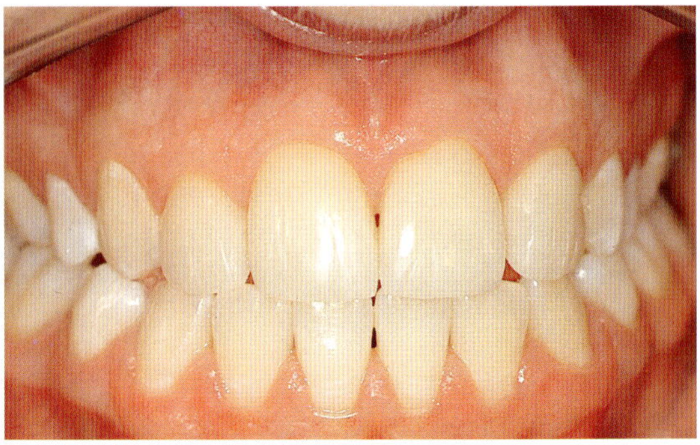

Fig. 6-30b Ceramic crown on tooth 9, porcelain veneers on teeth 7, 8, 10.

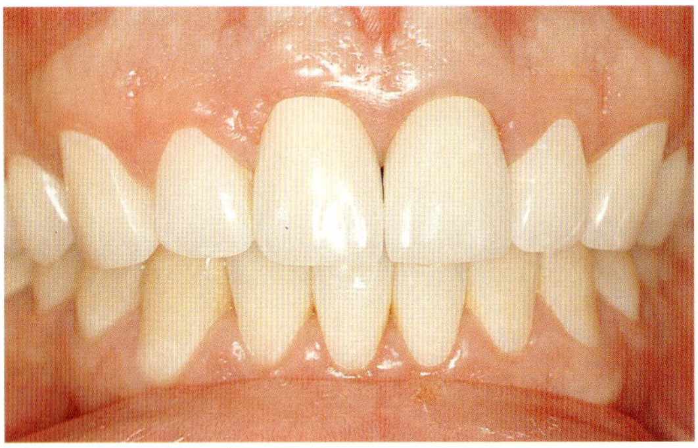

Fig. 6-31 Bleached natural teeth with aluminous porcelain crowns on teeth 8 and 9.

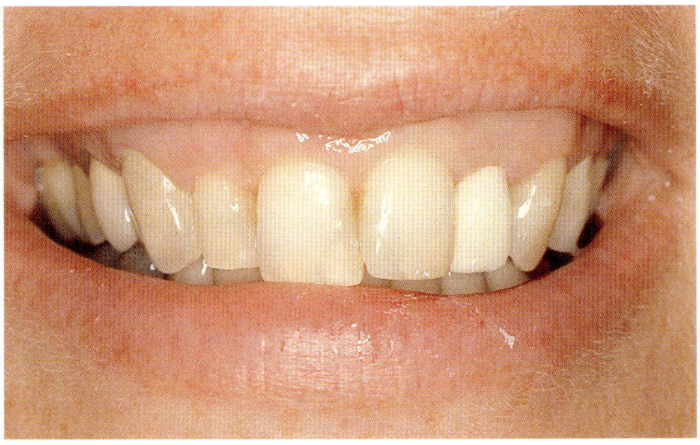

Fig. 6-32 Dicor crown on tooth 6; note translucency similar to that of tooth 11.

anterior esthetic crowns or when a crown is used in conjunction with porcelain veneers (Fig. 6-30). Use of the same ceramic system is advisable when fabricating adjacent crown and porcelain veneer restorations. Conventional ceramic systems are also used extensively for porcelain veneers, inlays and onlays.

In addition to poor strength, the other major problem with the use of conventional ceramic crowns is difficulty in modifying the final esthetic results. When generalized shade modifications using tinted cements are inadequate for a satisfactory shade match or when localized characterizations like cracks or opacities must be added, extrinsic staining techniques must be used. Extrinsic staining of conventional ceramic crowns is complicated. First, because of the translucency of this type of crown, a cement or try-in paste must be placed under the crown before final staining. This can be messy and, the try-in paste must be kept off external surfaces being stained. Once the stained ceramic crown has been through the appropriate thermal cycle, the cement residue in the restoration must be removed prior to cementation using air abrasives or steam cleaning. Re-etching internal surfaces is recommended to avoid a possible reduction in bond strength.

A second problem is that of staining temperature. Normally, ceramic stains are applied to the surface of a ceramic crown and it is placed in the oven and run through a normal glazing cycle. If conventional ceramic restorations are heated to normal glazing temperature, the fine margins will be rounded and the potential

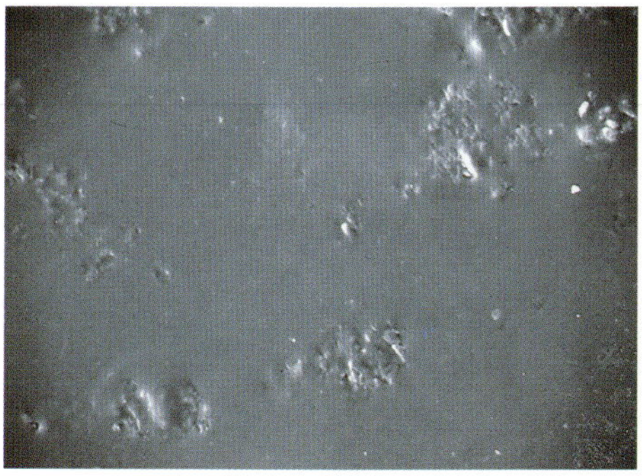

Fig. 6-33

Fig. 6-34

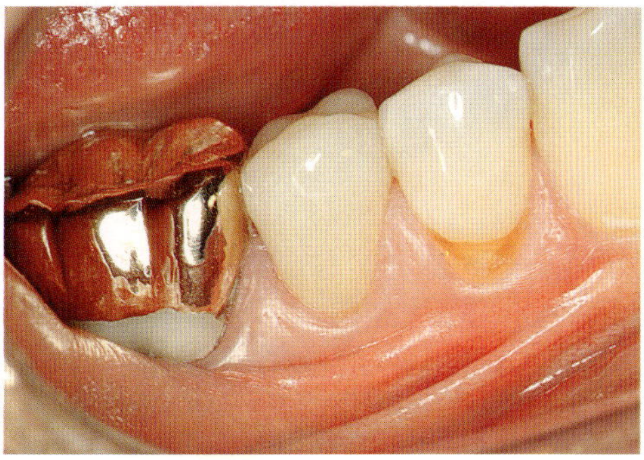

Fig. 6-35

Fig. 6-33 Glazed conventional ceramic 1500×.

Fig. 6-34 Glazed Dicor 1500×.

Fig. 6-35 Supragingival facial margin on tooth 29 with all ceramic crown.

for distortion is high. To avoid this, ceramic staining must be done at lower temperatures. Low fusing (lower temperature) ceramic stains must be utilized for this process. Higher temperature high fusing stains mixed with lower temperance clear glazes have also been reported as a successful alternative. The development of more esthetic shoulder porcelains has minimized this problem for crowns of adequate margin depth. For shallow veneer depth restorations the problem remains.

In contrast, when high temperature "core strengthened ceramics" are used under a conventional ceramic, this second problem is eliminated. The core material sinters at a higher temperature and supports the margins with less chance of distortion. When are core strengthened ceramics advisable? In addition to esthetic results, the primary reason for utilization of core strengthened ceramics should be a desire for higher potential strength. Selection can be divided into two basic esthetic categories. The first category is the need for lighter more opaque teeth. The whiter less translucent shades are easier to match when using lighter more opaque cores made of aluminous porcelain (Fig. 6-31). Any of the aluminous porcelain core materials that have been discussed will have greater opacity than conventional ceramics and "whiter" or "brighter" crowns are more easily fabricated. In contrast, when a more translucent, lower value restoration is desired, a more translucent material such as Dicor may be a more appropriate core material. Ceramic crowns made with Dicor copings and veneered with an appropriate conventional ceramic provide highly esthetic restorations with high translucency and lower value (Fig. 6-32).

Greater ceramic strength can also be achieved with the utilization of one of the

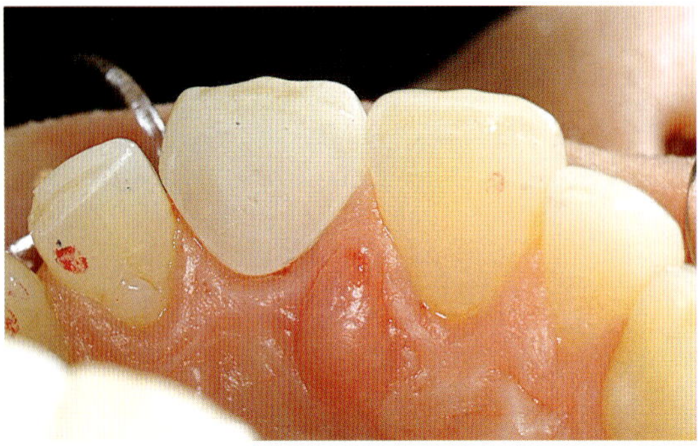

Fig. 6-36 Dicor core strengthened crown with unglazed Dicor exposed on the lingual for minimum wear of opposing natural teeth.

"strengthened ceramic systems." The advantage here is that the entire restoration is fabricated out of a stronger ceramic material. Several of these systems have been developed and the esthetic components of each system have been expanded. The ability of the individual laboratories to work with these systems in achieving esthetic results varies and must be evaluated. Also the translucency range of each system is variable. As with conventional ceramics, extrinsic staining must be done at lower temperatures than that used for natural glazing.

2. Periodontal priority: When poor periodontal results have been achieved with conventional ceramics, another alternative may be advisable. The stained surface of the cast ceramic, Dicor, has been shown to be extremely smooth (Figs. 6-33 and 6-34). Clinical studies have shown that these smooth surfaces of Dicor will accumulate plaque less than natural tooth enamel. Dicor crowns may be the restoration of choice in such instances when minimal plaque adherence is a high priority.

One of the advantages of all ceramic crowns in general is the option to keep margins supragingival or minimally subgingival due to their excellent esthetic properties (Fig. 6-35). When finalizing the margins in preparation for a ceramic crown, deep subgingival margins should be avoided to maximize the potential for a favorable periodontal response.

3. Functional factors: Ceramic materials occluding with natural teeth or other nonceramic restorations have been shown to have a higher abrasion potential than metallic or composite materials. In clinical situations where the potential for wear exists and must be minimized, selection of the least abrasive ceramic may be desirable. Unglazed Dicor has been shown in vitro to be less abrasive to enamel than conventional and strengthened ceramics. Initial studies have shown that the glass ceramic IPS Empress also has a low wear potential. The use of these glass ceramic materials in functional areas such as the linguals of maxillary anteriors and posterior occlusal areas may provide a more functionally compatible ceramic alternative in areas where esthetic considerations are less demanding. (Fig. 6-36). Those materials provide an esthetic alternative to metal and a functional alternative to traditional sintered ceramic restorations.

A second functional factor that must be considered is strength. Almost any of the core strengthened, strengthened and glass ceramic materials have sufficient strength for conventionally luted anterior crowns. With the use of bonding techniques, even conventional, lower strength, ceramic crowns are highly successful. For posterior teeth, the occlusal stresses are significantly higher and the incidence of failure for posterior all ceramic crowns has been much higher. The use of bonding techniques has improved the success of posterior all ceramic crowns but not to the level of porcelain fused to metal. With the introduction of In-Ceram, a ceramic core material has been introduced that is significantly stronger than all others. For posterior crowns where an all ceramic restoration is desirable, In-Ceram may be a more predictable alternative. As with other core strengthened restorations, adequate preparation depth must be achieved to provide space for both the In-Ceram core and the esthetic conventional ceramic veneering materials. Long term clinical data are needed to substantiate that the all ceramic systems are viable alternatives to porcelain fused to metal when sufficient tooth loss warrants a full esthetic crown for posterior teeth.

CLINICAL PROCEDURES

Introduction

This section will describe clinical techniques to be used for all ceramic crowns or what is commonly called "the porcelain jacket crown." Ceramic veneer restorations that cover a majority of the tooth will be covered in the section on ceramic veneers and referred to as "full veneers." The term "full veneer" refers to full ceramic crowns that are fabricated to the approximate depth of a porcelain veneer. The all ceramic techniques discussed in this section will describe all ceramic crowns of more traditional thickness. When using any of the core strengthening ceramic systems, adequate preparation depth is mandatory to provide room for core and esthetic veneering materials. When replacing existing ceramo-metal crowns, preparation depth may be preestablished. When preparing relatively sound teeth or those with only small restorations and a significant amount of existing intact enamel, more conservative restorations such as ceramic veneers or full veneers should be considered.

Preparation Techniques

One of the primary goals of any preparation technique is to ensure uniform and consistent tooth reduction that will allow sufficient room for the restorative materials to be used. All ceramic crowns that have uneven thick and thin areas may have compromised esthetics and strength. When luting cements are used, inadequate crown thickness is one of the main causes of crown failure in function (Fig. 6-37).

The preparation dimensions for anterior and posterior all ceramic crowns are shown in Figs. 6-38 and 6-39. Note that these dimensions are similar to those of ceramo-metal crowns. When using luting cements, significant ceramic bulk must be provided to resist functional stresses. Newer bonding procedures appear to reduce the necessity for such deep preparations but additional longitudinal clinical research is needed for this to be substantiated. A shoulder finish line is placed around the entire circumference of the preparation to provide sufficient bulk of porcelain for marginal strength and esthetics.

The preparation technique used is called the "silhouette technique." Half of the tooth is prepared leaving an unprepared half as a point of reference. Once completed, the prepared half becomes the point of reference for the unprepared half.

Starting with an unprepared central incisor (Fig. 6-40), a groove is placed in the mid-facial surface of the tooth from the free gingival margin to the incisal edge (Fig. 6-41) using a long chamfer diamond (Fig. 6-42). A

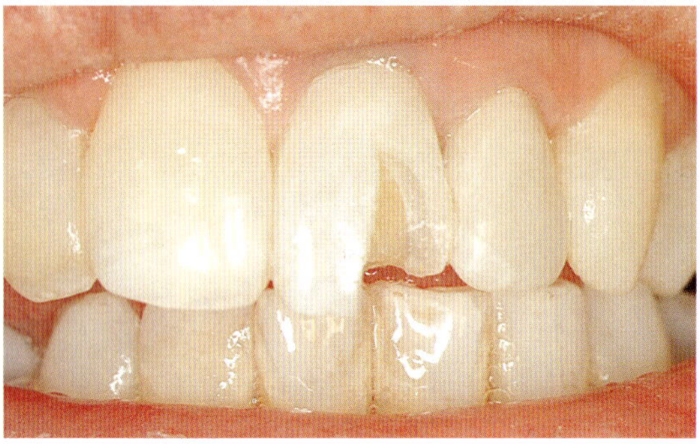

Fig. 6-37a Facial view of fractured Dicor core strengthened crown.

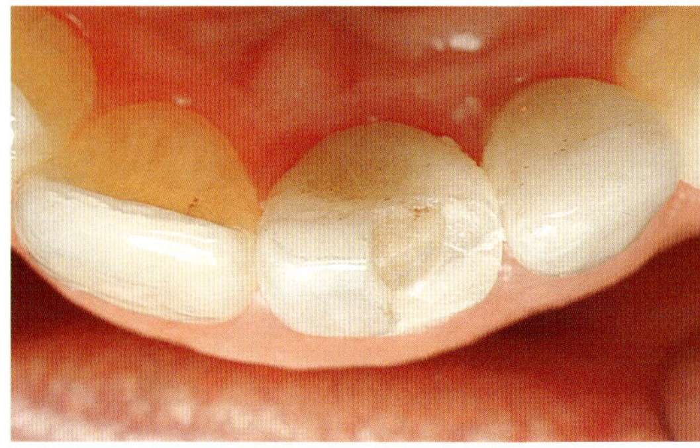

Fig. 6-37b Incisal view; note thin lingual area in fracture.

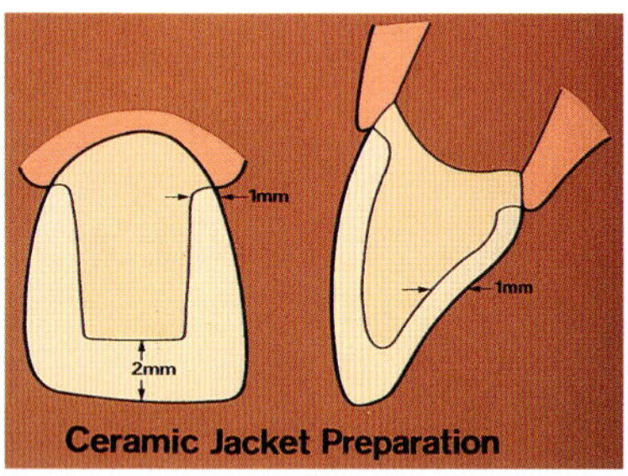

Fig. 6-38 Anterior ceramic crown recommended preparation depths.

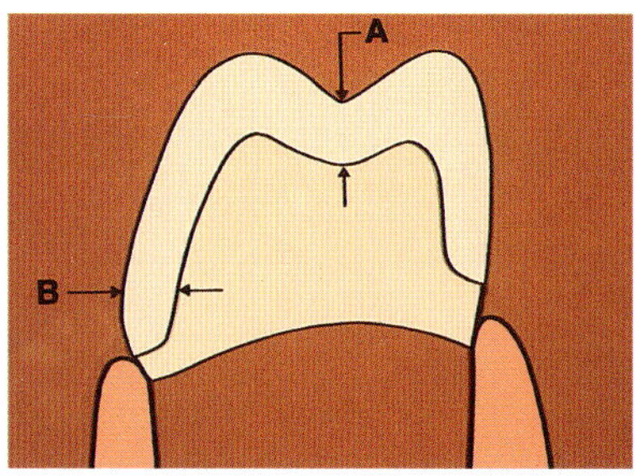

Fig. 6-39 Posterior ceramic crown recommended preparation depths.

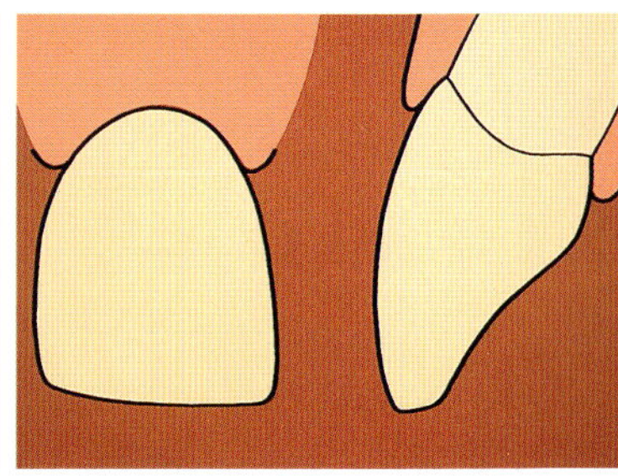

Fig. 6-40 Unprepared maxillary central.

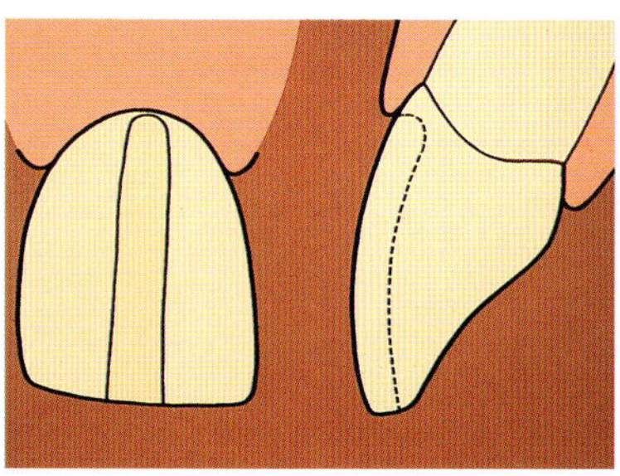

Fig. 6-41 Midfacial depth groove.

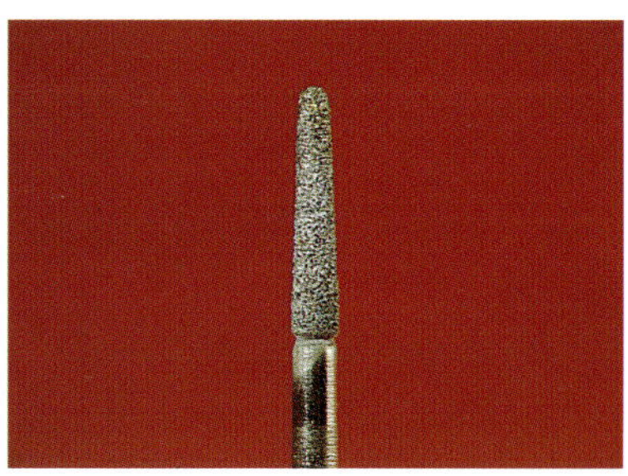

Fig. 6-42 Chamfer diamond used.

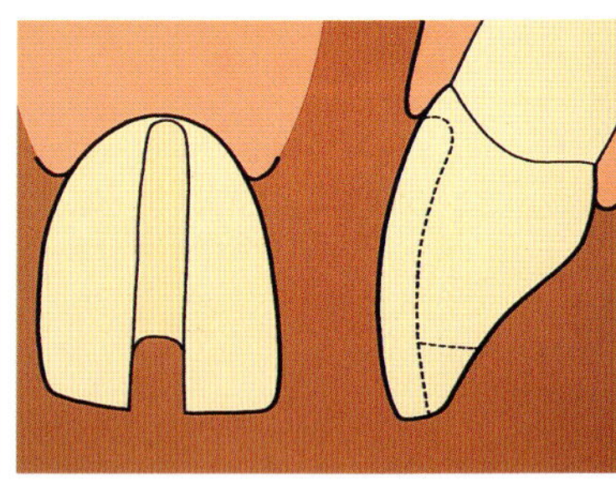

Fig. 6-43 Incisal depth groove.

groove can now be placed through the incisal edge (Fig. 6-43). The depth of this groove should be related to the desired length of the final crown. About 1.5 to 2.0 mm of space for incisal ceramic is necessary. The depth of these grooves should be approximately 0.25 mm less than the final desired depth. Thus when finishing the preparation, final depth is achieved without overreduction. The depth cutting diamonds described in the CERAMIC VENEER section are very useful here as well. Next, half of the incisal edge is reduced to the depth of the incisal groove (Fig. 6-44). Now one half of the facial is reduced to the preestablished depth (Fig. 6-45). At this point the prepared half is easily compared to the unprepared half (Fig. 6-46). Preparation symmetry and depth are easily verified by comparing the "silhouette" of the prepared and unprepared halves. The incisal surface of the

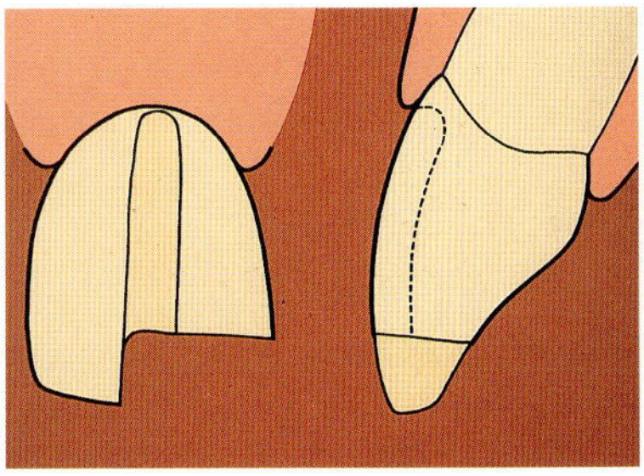

Fig. 6-44 Reduce first half of incisal edge.

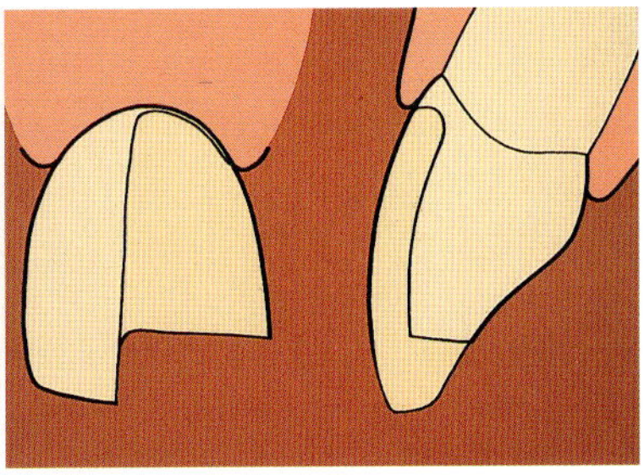

Fig. 6-45 Reduce first half of facial surface.

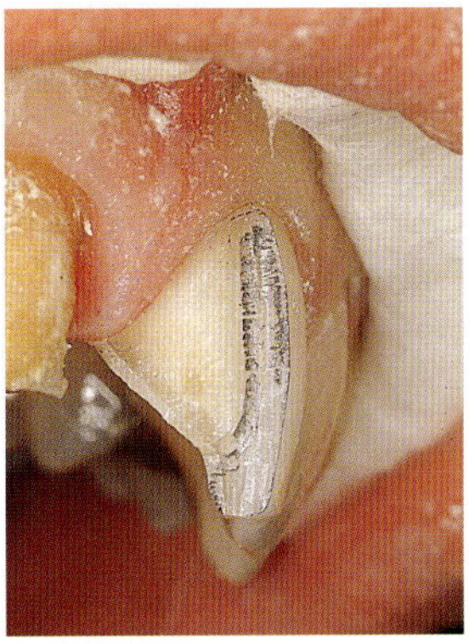

Fig. 6-46 Clinical view comparing prepared and unprepared sides.

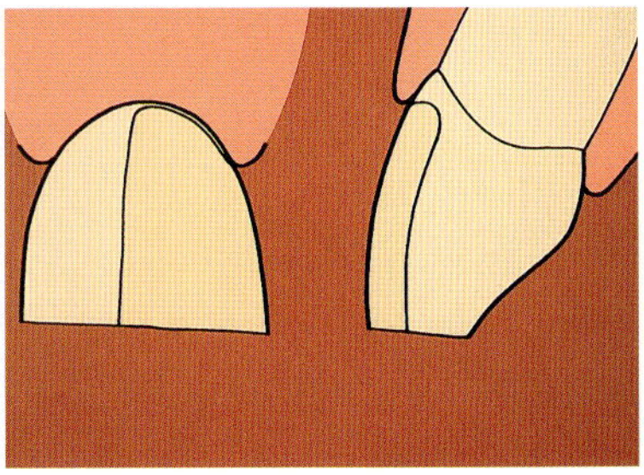

Fig. 6-47 Reduce remaining incisal edge.

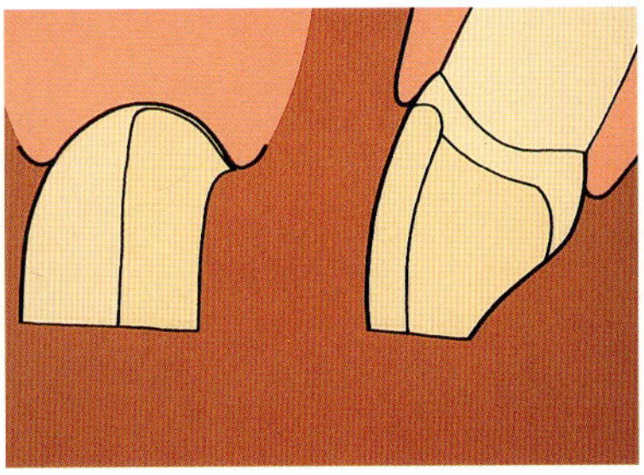

Fig. 6-48 Prepare interproximal.

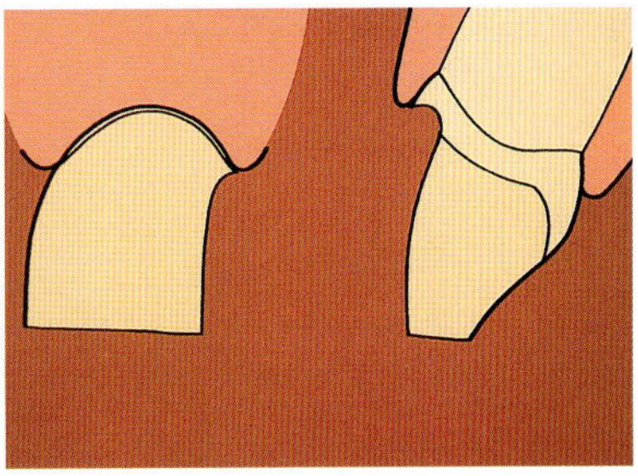

Fig. 6-49 Reduce the remaining facial surface to a depth of the first half.

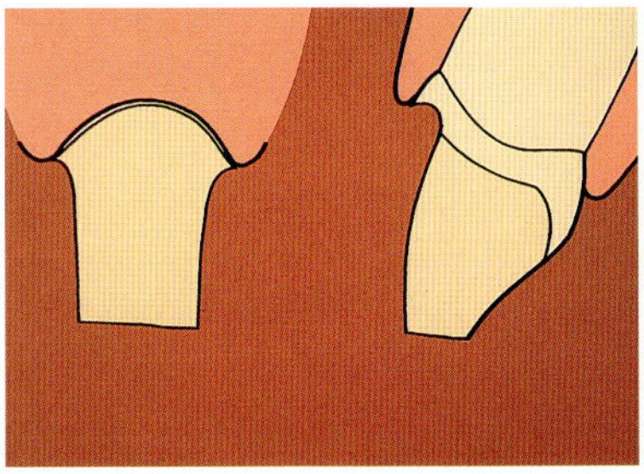

Fig. 6-50 Prepare second proximal surface.

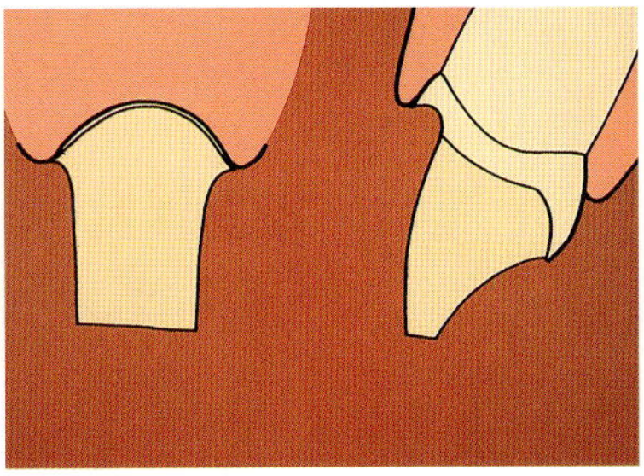

Fig. 6-51 Reduce lingual surface to provide a minimum of 1 mm of occlusal clearance.

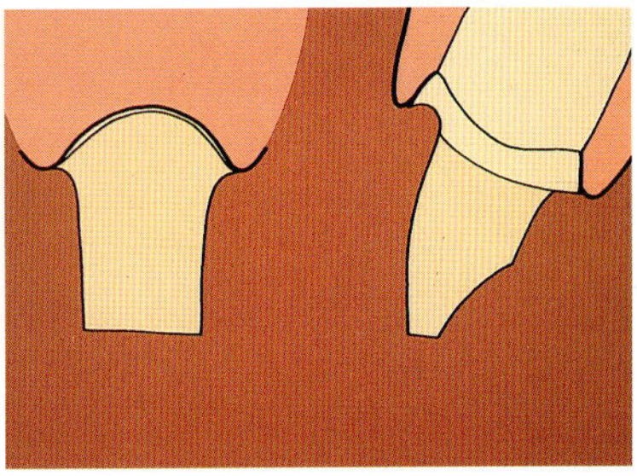

Fig. 6-52 Prepare lingual shoulder continuous with proximals.

unprepared half may be prepared at this point (Fig. 6-47) or the proximal contact on the prepared side completed (Fig. 6-48). Interproximal reduction should be deep enough to provide at least a 1-mm shoulder width and about 6° of axial wall convergence incisally. Now the facial and interproximal surfaces of the unprepared half are prepared to a depth and contour symmetrical with the prepared half (Figs. 6-49 and 6-50). The lingual wall and lingual cavosurface areas are now prepared (Figs. 6-51 and 6-52). The lingual surface must be prepared to allow for a minimum of 1 mm of ceramic thickness in functional areas. The lingual shoulder should be placed supragingivally if possible and should be a uniform 1 mm in depth.

Once the initial preparation is complete, desired depth dimensions can be finalized. The facial shoulder, because of its greater

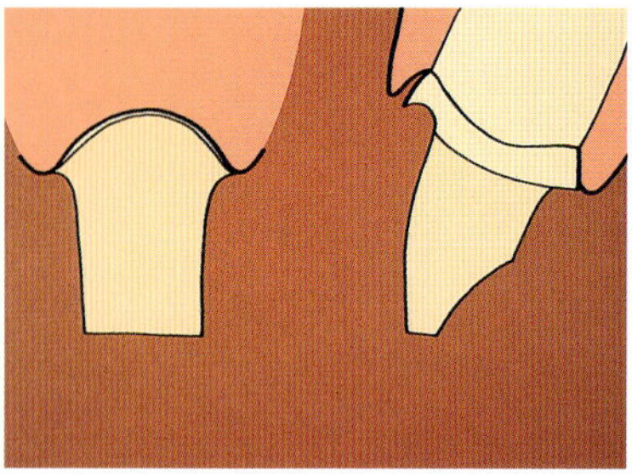

Fig. 6-53 Retract facial gingival tissues to minimize trauma when preparing subgingival margin.

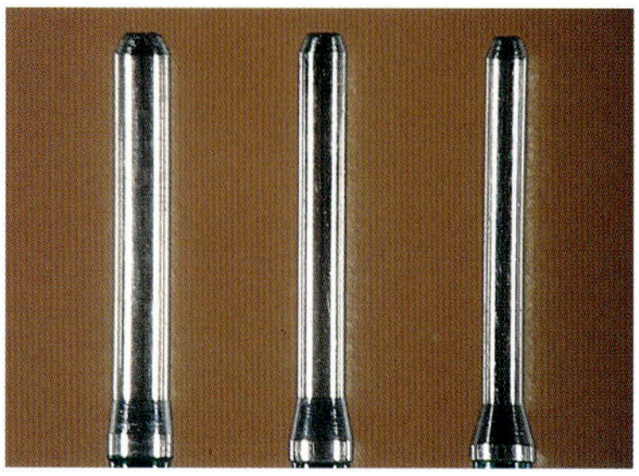

Fig. 6-54 End cutting diamonds.

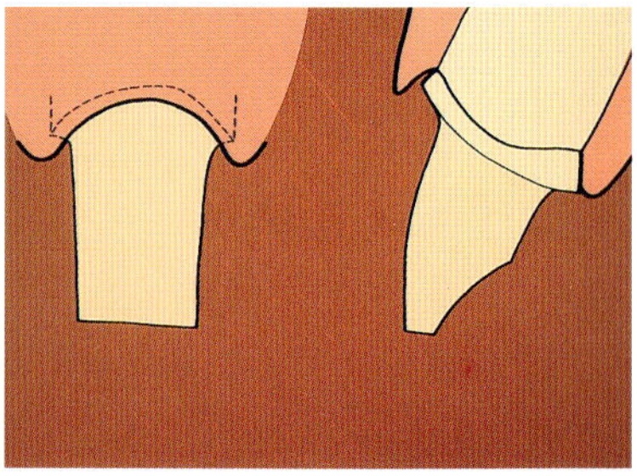

Fig. 6-55 Prepare facial shoulder finish line slightly subgingivally.

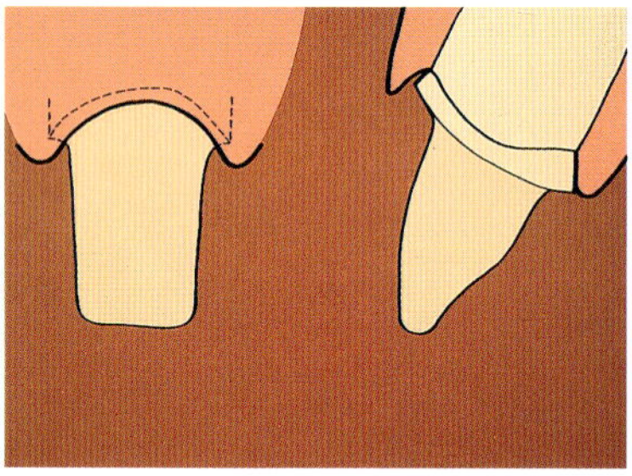

Fig. 6-56 Round all line angles.

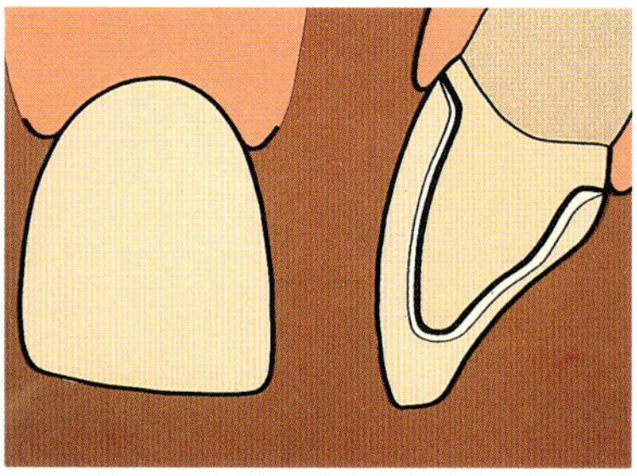

Fig. 6-57 Cross section of aluminous porcelain crown on finished preparation.

depth, will be slightly concave. The rough facial cavosurface margin should extend to the free gingival margin externally with the shoulder slightly deeper internally. This depth should be at the desired subgingival position. At this point the soft tissues should be retracted using mechanical, chemical or electrosurgical means as preferred by the operator and dictated by the tissue type (Fig. 6-53). Using an end cutting diamond (Fig. 6-54) the facial cavosurface margin can be prepared to the desired subgingival position and a flat shoulder established. The end cutting diamond can be used circumferentially to ensure the smooth sharp cavosurface margins necessary for all ceramic crowns (Fig. 6-55). Irregular margins are to be avoided because they complicate fabrication and may make the ceramic margins more vulnerable to fracture if they are not of uniform thickness and bulk. Finally, all internal sharp line angles are rounded to minimize die abrasion and potential stress concentrations (Fig. 6-56). At this point, soft tissues must be evaluated for stability prior to making the final impression. Free gingival tissues that are inflamed due to pre-existing restorations or are extremely thin and vulnerable may not be good candidates for a final impression at this appointment. A well designed and accurately fitting provisional restoration should be placed and tissues allowed to heal. In 1 to 4 weeks, the health and stability of the tissues are re-evaluated and any final marginal modifications made. The final impression can now be made with greater assurance of tissue stability and less chance of undesirable esthetic changes. The crown is now finalized (Fig. 6-57).

Laboratory Communications

Many texts, chapters and papers have been written on laboratory communications. Clearly this is an area that has many approaches, techniques and devices that vary with the materials used, technician's needs and the esthetic demands of the case. No single approach has been shown to be ideal for communicating information and no device has yet been developed that exactly measures the complicated blends of tooth color and translucencies. The purpose of this section will be to outline a few simple techniques that will assist in the communication process between the dentist and ceramist. Through improved communications, a clearer picture of the desired restoration is transmitted to the ceramist, increasing the potential for esthetic success.

For some multiple unit situations, crowns must only match crowns and an esthetic match is not difficult. A more difficult challenge is to match a single anterior restoration to the adjacent teeth. An all ceramic crown is often selected to make this matching process easier. The appropriate ceramic material, based upon natural tooth translucency, shade and functional demands must be selected as described earlier. The subtleties of shade, incisal translucency and specific characterizations must be transmitted to the ceramist. Rarely does a shade guide exactly match the shade of a tooth. So simply putting a shade button number on a prescription is usually inadequate.

Shade guides or ceramic tabs (Fig. 6-58) are simply a means of communicating the perceived appearance of various portions of the tooth. A prescription should include a tooth drawing and a specific ceramic tab identified that closely matches each area of the tooth being matched (Fig. 6-59). This will provide the ceramist with the basic color information for crown fabrication. The more difficult problem is describing how shades overlap and blend. There are an infinite number of possibilities for how the various esthetic components of teeth combine and this is further modified by age, environment and function. Visualization is the key to communicating effectively. Color slides, color prints, computer imaged prints and Polaroid prints are a few methods that provide the ceramist with an image of the actual tooth being matched (Fig. 6-60). This image, combined with the accurate shade tab data provided for each specific area of the tooth, will lead to accurate esthetic results by an experienced ceramist. An additional technique that is helpful for accurate shade matching is shade tab modification. Shade tabs may be modified using systems designed to characterize provisional restorations and can provide a very accurate custom shade guide for use by the ceramist (Fig.

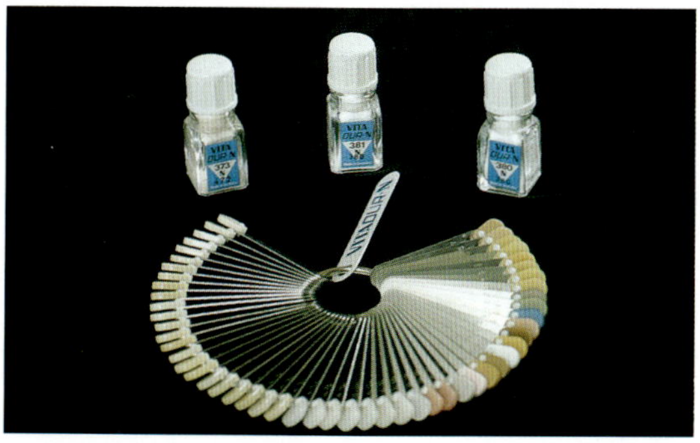

Fig. 6-58a Individual ceramic shade tabs.

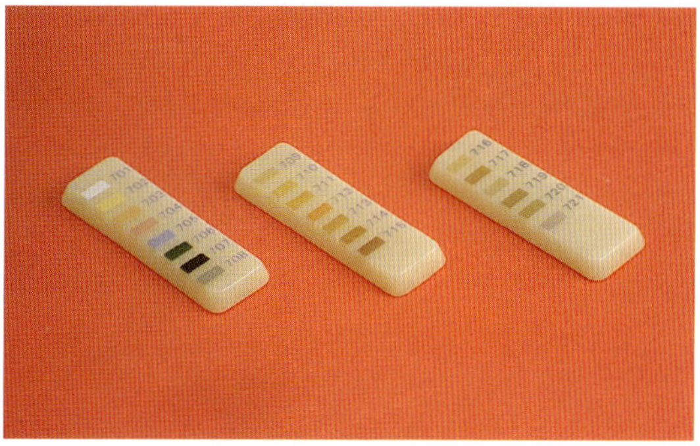

Fig. 6-58b Ceramic stain guides.

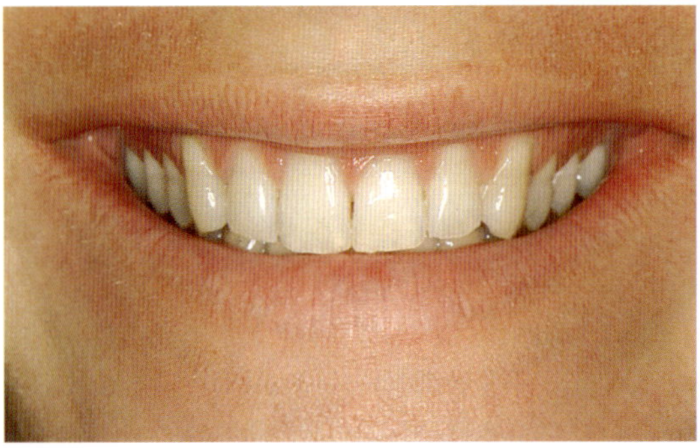

Fig. 6-59a

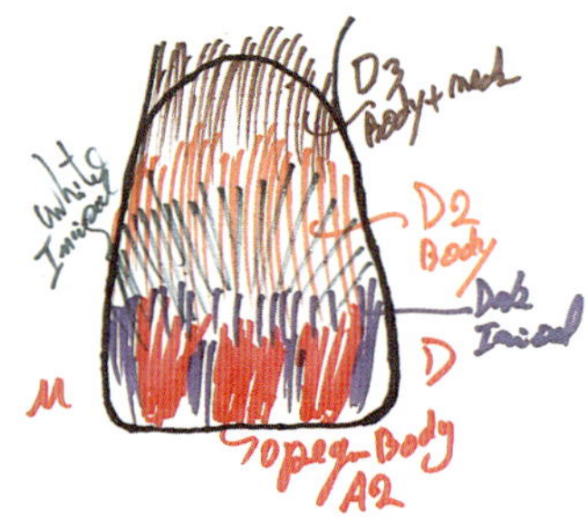

Fig. 6-59b

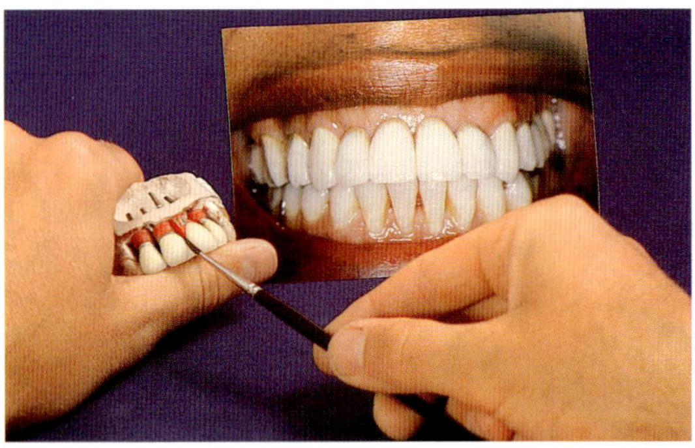

Fig. 6-60

Fig. 6-59a Anterior smile.

Fig. 6-59b Tooth diagram of Fig. 6-59a using colored pens for different areas and specific shades (courtesy of Uri Yarovesky, da Vinci Studios).

Fig. 6-60 Photographic aid to ceramist.

Fig. 6-61a Natural tooth and unaltered shade tab.

Fig. 6-61b Natural tooth and modified shade tab.

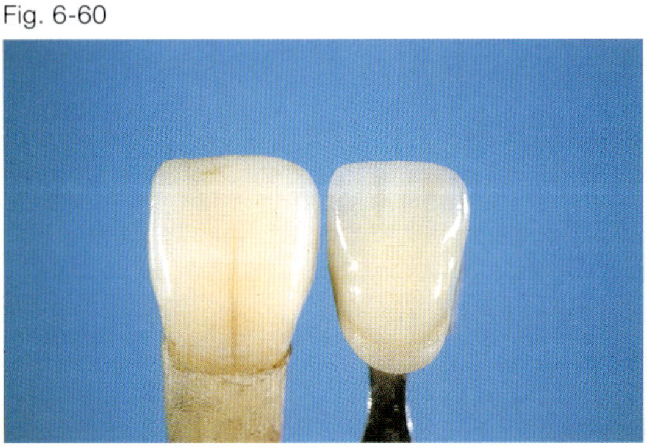

Fig. 6-61a

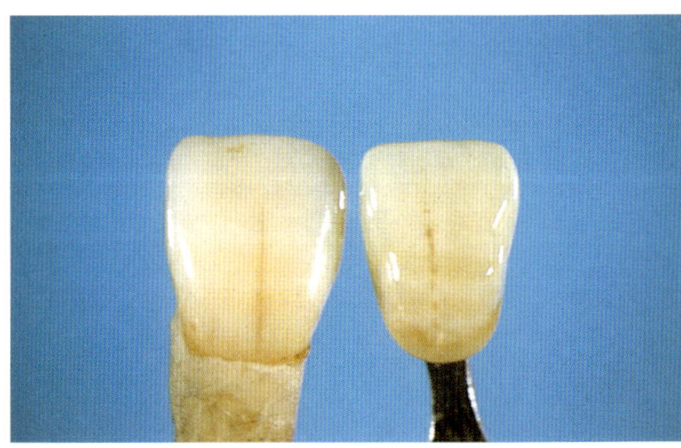

Fig. 6-61b

6-61). Ceramic stains may also be mixed with clear unfilled light cure resins and used as shade guide modifiers.

Sending the patient to the laboratory can be helpful but visual memory is short lived. Ceramists can choose their own shades and make notes when directly visualizing the patient and an ideal communication system is established. Accurate photographic visualization techniques are most effective and should be routinely provided for esthetically demanding cases.

Finally, matching a single crown to adjacent teeth is very difficult and the exact translucency, color and blending of the various ceramic components is often not achieved on the first attempt. The ability to make subtle shade modifications using resin color modifiers for translucent crowns is helpful. The ability to make specific shade modifications and place specific characterizations requires the use of ceramic stains during the delivery appointment. Appropriate use of chairside ceramic staining technique is a must for all practices that wish to achieve optimal esthetic results. All of these techniques require additional time, skills and materials. Providing esthetic crowns that must match natural teeth should demand an adequate fee to compensate for these additional requirements.

Finalizing the Esthetic Results

By properly communicating esthetic requirements to a skilled ceramist, and selecting the most appropriate ceramic material, the dentist will make the task of finalizing the esthetic match of an all ceramic crown to a natural tooth minimal and achievable using simple chairside procedures. Subtle generalized shade modifications may be made using shaded luting cement or using more versatile resin cements and composite resin color modifiers (tints). In addition, extrinsic ceramic stains may be used to make both generalized shade modifications and more specific localized characterizations chairside. The handling of different ceramic crown systems will be summarized.

1. Aluminous oxide core strengthened ceramic crowns are handled much like porcelain fused to metal crowns. If fabricated properly, the higher temperature aluminous core or shoulder porcelains are used to fabricate the margins and support the outer conventional ceramic veneer. Because these cores are relatively opaque, the shade of the cement will have little esthetic effect (Figs. 6-62a and b). Chairside shade modification is accomplished using conventional ceramic stains. The core material will prevent distortion during normal glazing temperatures so higher temperature extrinsic stains may be used to finalize the esthetic results (Fig. 6-62c).

The ability to do chairside shade modification with extrinsic ceramic stains is a necessity for the practice desiring maxi-

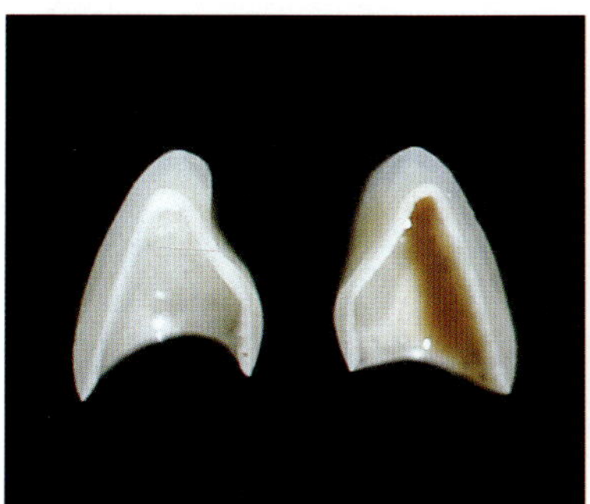

Fig. 6-62a

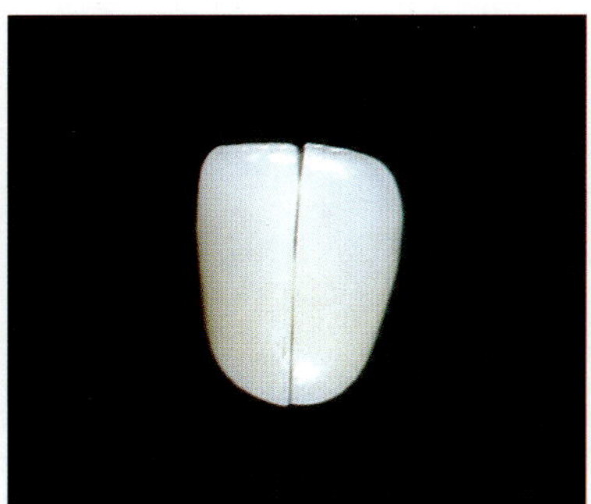

Fig. 6-62b

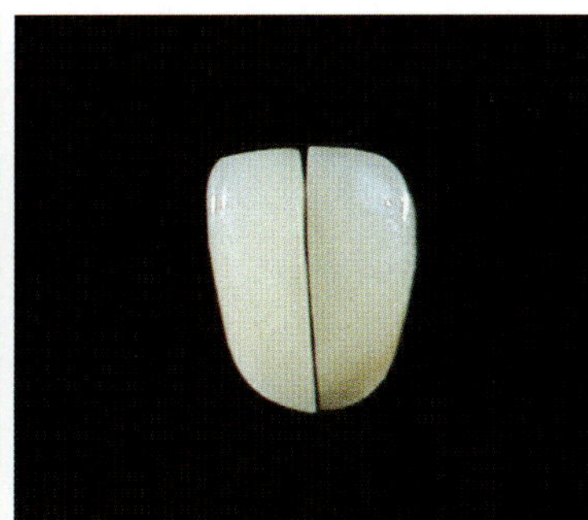

Fig. 6-62c

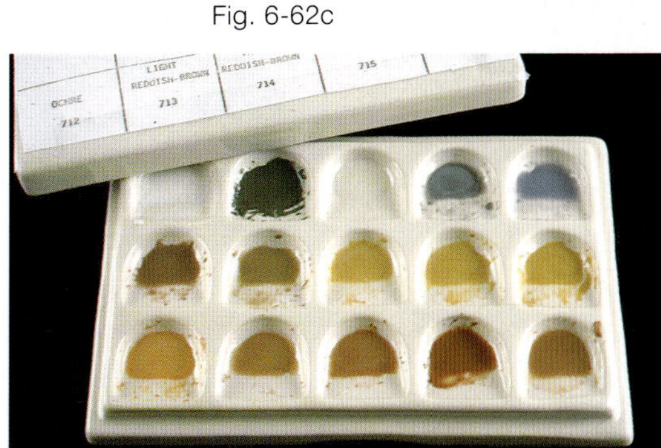

Fig. 6-63

Fig. 6-62a Cross section of aluminous oxide crown; right side has facial composite resin tint.

Fig. 6-62b Crown assembled; note tint's minimal effect on color.

Fig. 6-62c Extrinsic ceramic stain used to modify color.

Fig. 6-63 Ceramic staining palate and basic colors used.

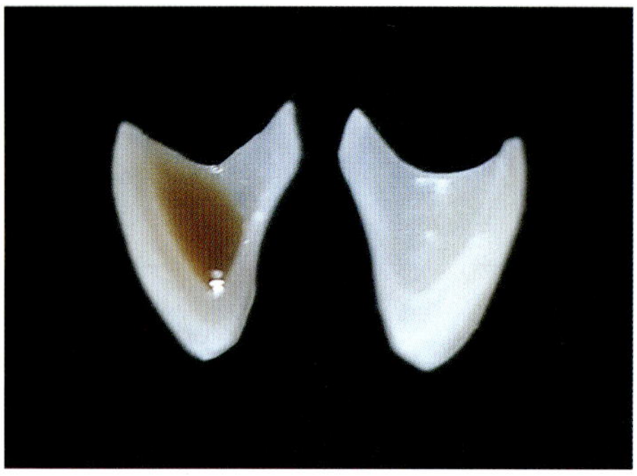

Fig. 6-64a Cross section of glass ceramic core strengthened crown; left side has facial composite resin tint.

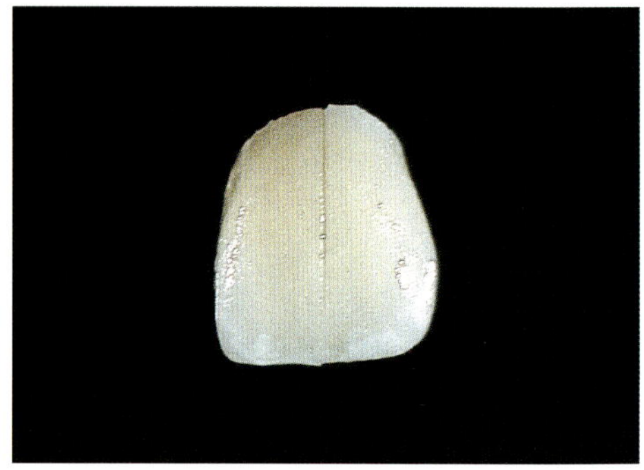

Fig. 6-64b Crown assembled; note obvious color change of left side with a translucent core material.

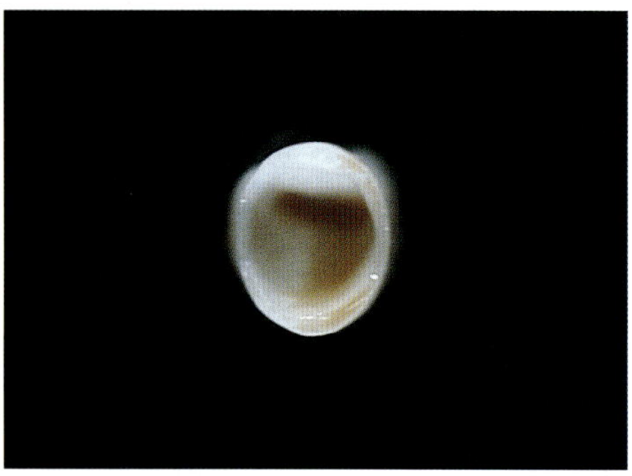

Fig. 6-65a Conventional ceramic crown with tint on right half.

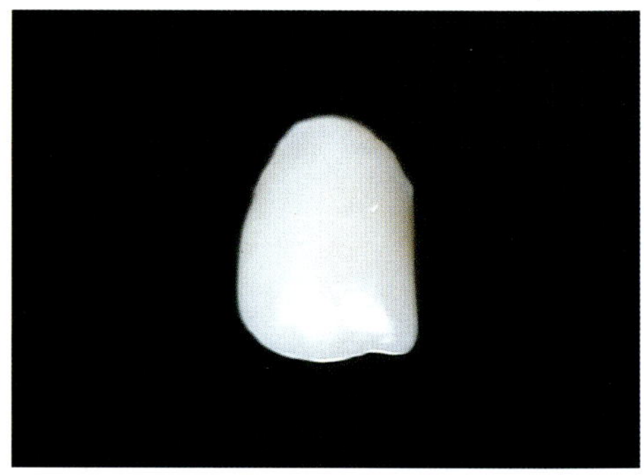

Fig. 6-65b Facial view of conventional ceramic crown; note color penetrating through right half.

mum esthetic results without the need to return crowns routinely to the laboratory. A ceramic staining kit and glazing oven are mandatory armamentaria for any esthetic dental practice (Fig. 6-63).

2. Glass ceramic or glass ceramic core strengthened crowns allow for two methods of shade alteration. Because the glass ceramic has a high melting range, conventional ceramic stains may be used externally. The glass ceramic will not significantly distort using normal glazing temperatures. In addition, the high translucency of the glass ceramic will transmit color from both the natural tooth and the cement itself when optically connected to the tooth. Cements may be used to make subtle generalized shade and opacity modifications (Fig. 6-64).
3. Conventional ceramic crowns made of conventional ceramic materials are more translucent than aluminous porcelain crowns but variable opacities may be built in similar to ceramic veneers. Because these are the weakest of the all ceramic crowns, composite resin cements and dentinal bonding techniques should be used to maximize strength. Composite resin color modifiers (tints) can be used to create subtle generalized shade modifications but the effect will diminish with increased opacity and thickness of the conventional ceramic crown (Fig. 6-65).

The use of extrinsic staining techniques is often necessary to achieve the best esthetic results. If higher temperature

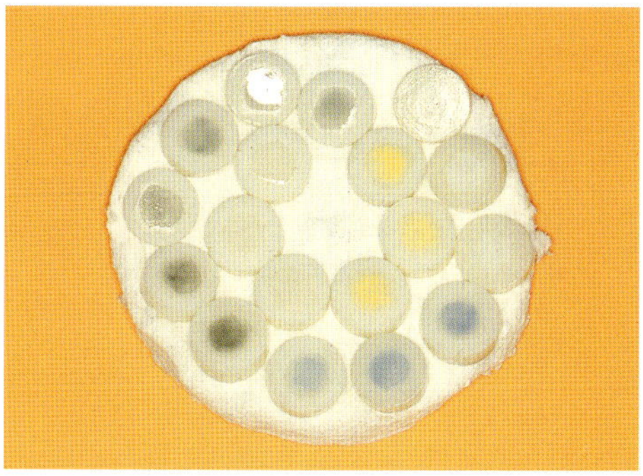

Fig. 6-66a Ceramic stains on ceramic tabs before glazing thermal cycle.

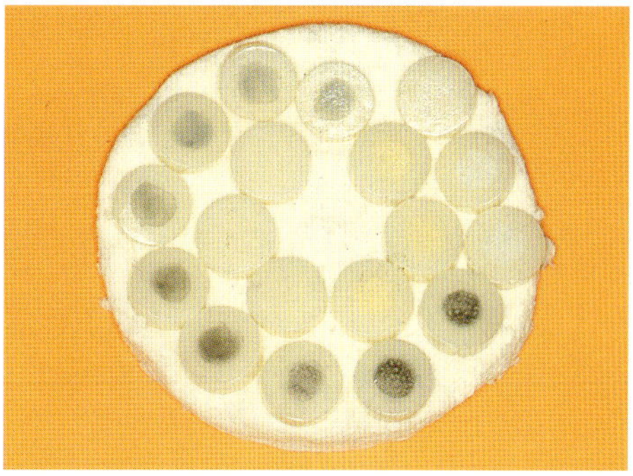

Fig. 6-66b After glazing thermal cycle. Note color change on some stains.

stains are used, they fuse to the crown at a temperature similar to the glazing temperature of the ceramic used to make the crown, resulting in distortion and rounded margins. Consequently, lower (fusing) temperature stains must be used. Alternative methods used to prevent distortion include investing the crown in a custom ceramic sager tray material or use of higher fusing stains mixed with low fusing clear ceramic glazes. When both internal and external color modifiers are used, the process can get complicated. Composite resin cements or try-in cement and composite resin color modifiers are used initially and the crown is seated intraorally. Once a maximum color modification is achieved, low fusing ceramic stains can be used to finalize the esthetic match. The crown is lifted out of the mouth with an explorer and placed on a sager pillow without touching the stain. Removing the try-in cement at this point is difficult so the crown is run through the appropriate thermal cycle in the porcelain oven and the stain fused to the crown. The high temperatures will burn out the organic component of the composite resin cement leaving only the inorganic filler particles that can be air abraded away. It has been shown by Crispen and Hewlett that some ceramic stains change color when fired so the above cycle might have to be repeated to obtain an optimal color match (Fig. 6-66).

4. Strengthened ceramic crowns made entirely from one of the various strengthened ceramic materials are modified esthetically much like conventional ceramic crowns using composite resin color modifiers internally and lower fusing stains externally.

The ability to achieve excellent esthetic results with these techniques is well within the abilities of any dentist with minimal equipment and training.

CEMENTATION PROCEDURES

Prior to the clinical appointment, inspect the finished restoration for an even internal etch, fit and contour (Figs. 6-67a and b).

1. The provisional crown is removed and the tooth cleaned with pumice or an appropriate cavity cleaner (Figs. 6-67c and d).
2. The crown is tried in, interproximal contacts are adjusted with a fine rotary stone and margins are checked for accuracy and complete seating (Figs. 6-67e to i).
3. The crown is esthetically contoured, the occlusion adjusted and the surface texture

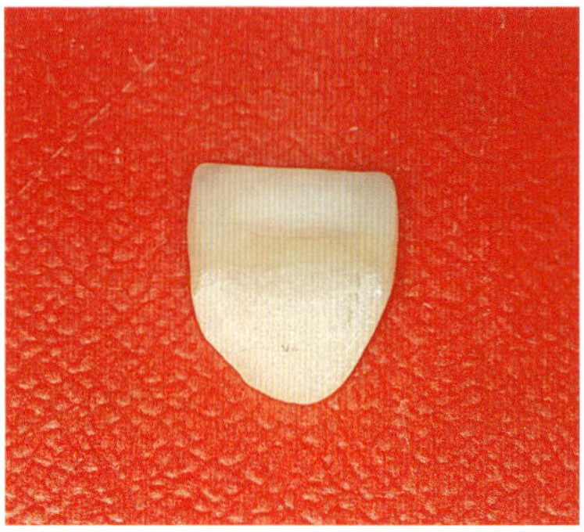

Fig. 6-67a Inspect internal etch of conventional ceramic crown.

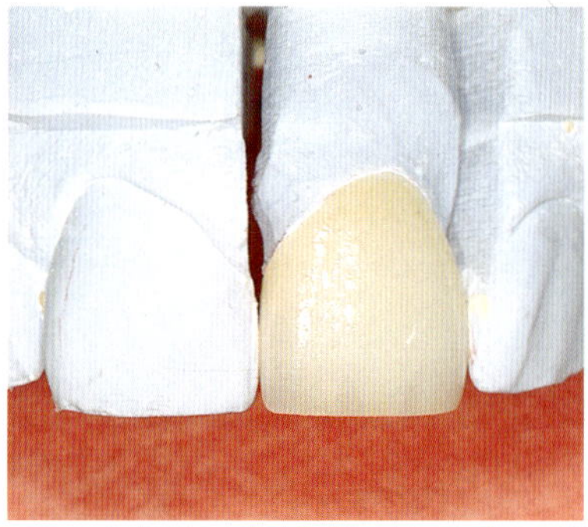

Fig. 6-67b Check crown on die for fit and contour.

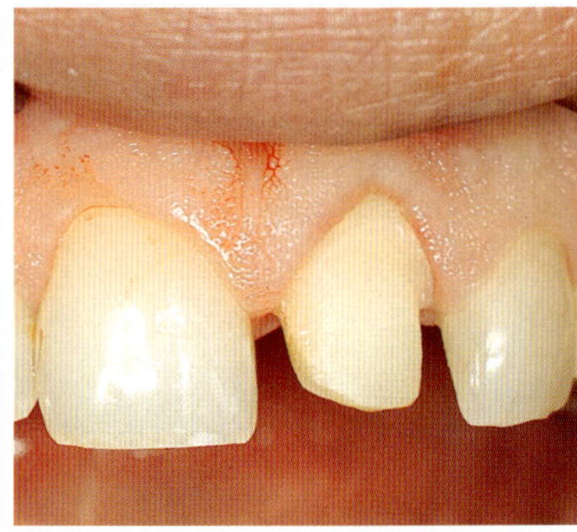

Fig. 6-67c Facial view of cleaned preparation.

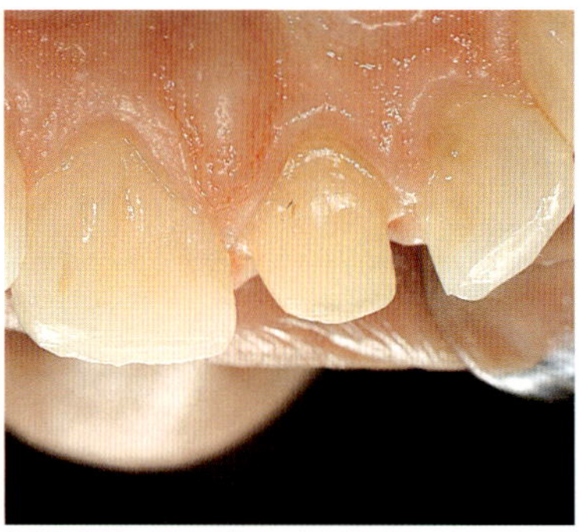

Fig. 6-67d Incisal view of cleaned preparation.

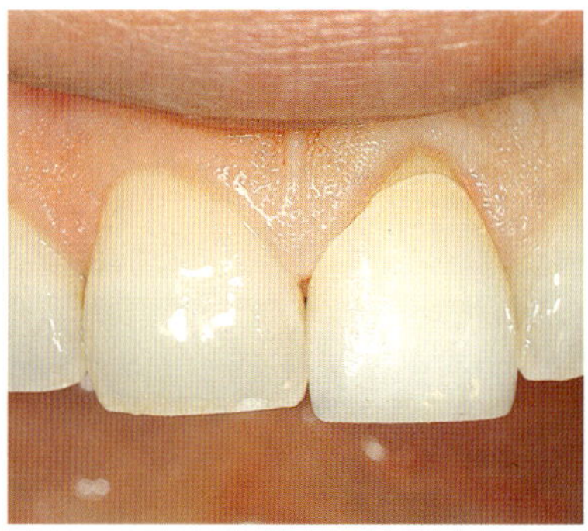

Fig. 6-67e Gently seat crown; if not fitting, check proximal contacts.

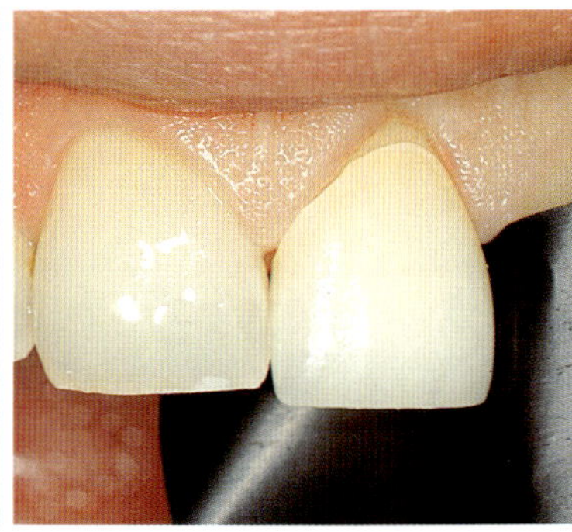

Fig. 6-67f Marking proximal contact with thin mylar carboned ribbon.

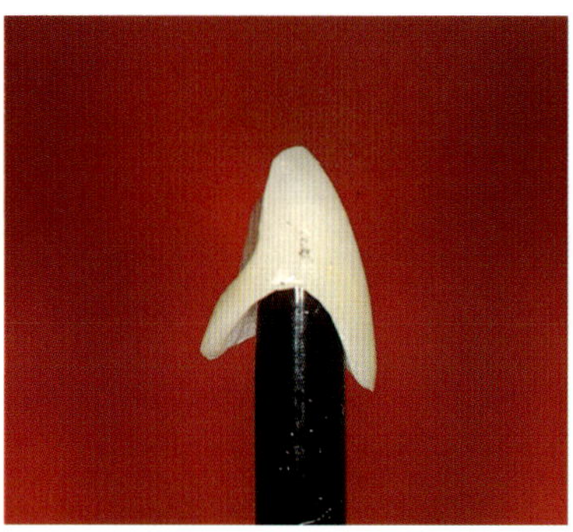

Fig. 6-67g Black mark showing high spot.

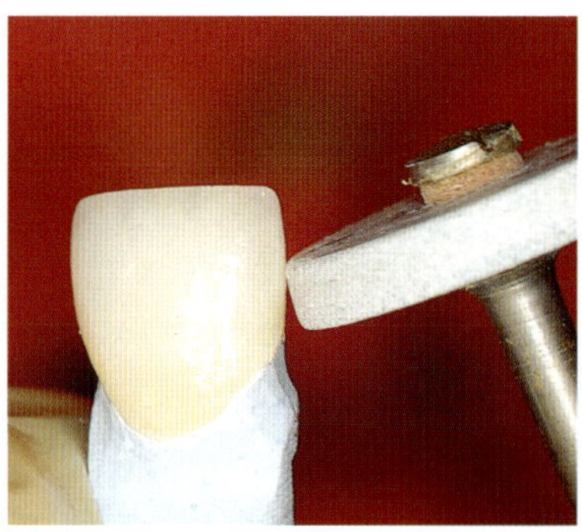

Fig. 6-67h Use fine ceramic adjusting stone to reduce proximal.

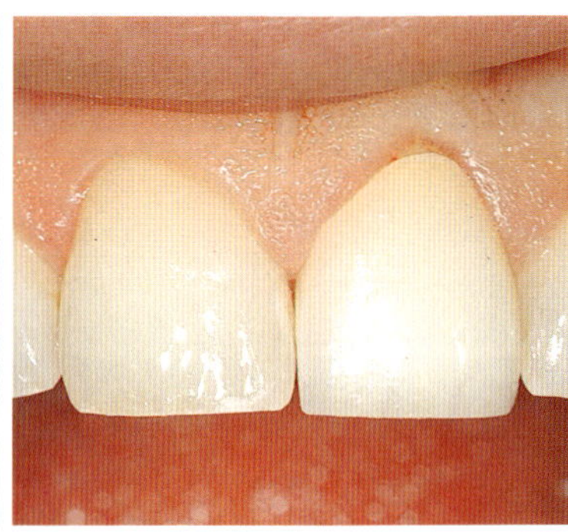

Fig. 6-67i Completely seated crown.

adjusted if necessary using appropriate rotary instruments. The crown is now polished using sequentially finer diamonds or stones followed by porcelain polishing rubber wheels (Figs. 6-67j to m). The final texture and resultant light reflection are critical for maximum esthetic results and may be achieved by a combination of natural glazing in a porcelain oven and/or polishing with extrafine abrasives and a buffing wheel.

4. If color modifications are necessary, the appropriate procedures are used, as outlined on pages 181 to 183, for the crown

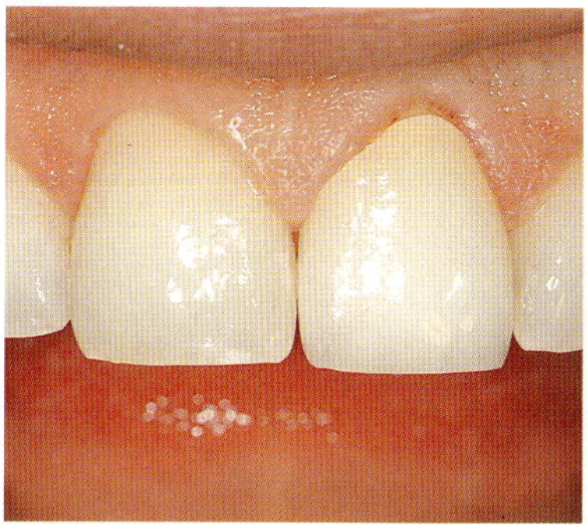

Fig. 6-67j Adjust to final contour.

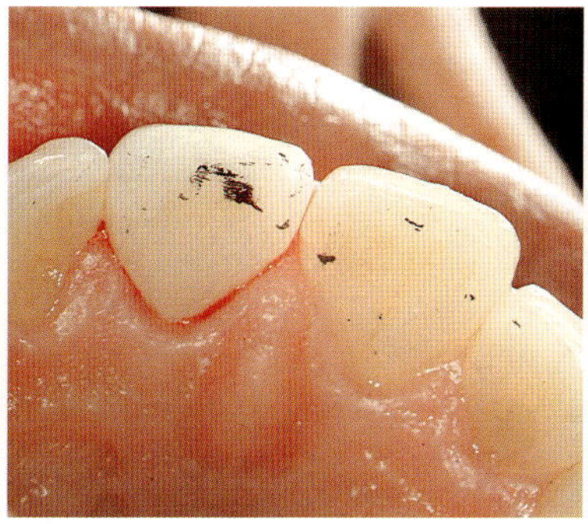

Fig. 6-67k Adjust occlusal contacts.

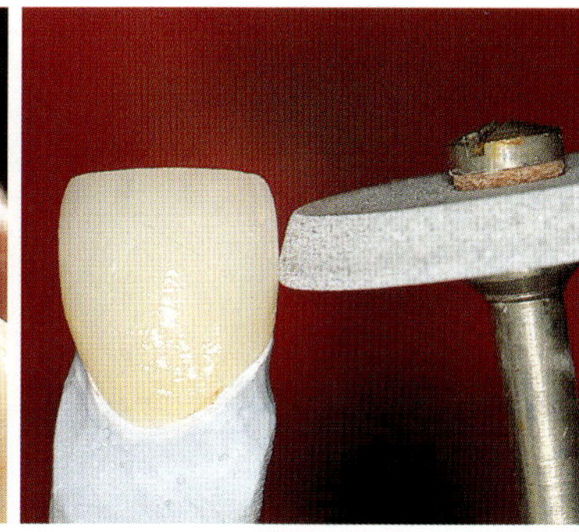

Fig. 6-67l Fine porcelain polishing wheel.

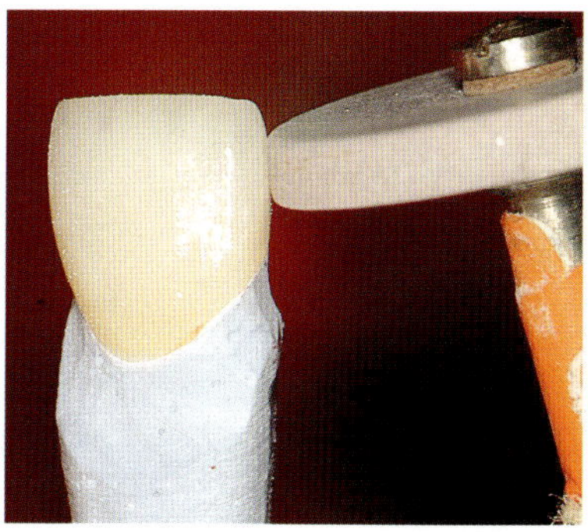

Fig. 6-67m Final porcelain polishing wheel.

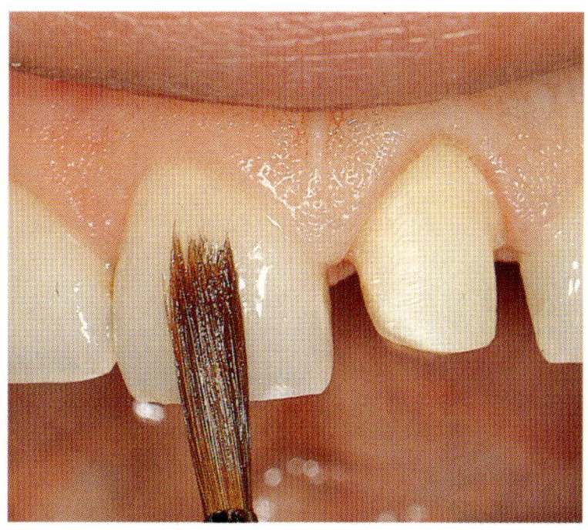

Fig. 6-67n Coat adjacent tooth with clear staining liquid to prevent desiccation and color change.

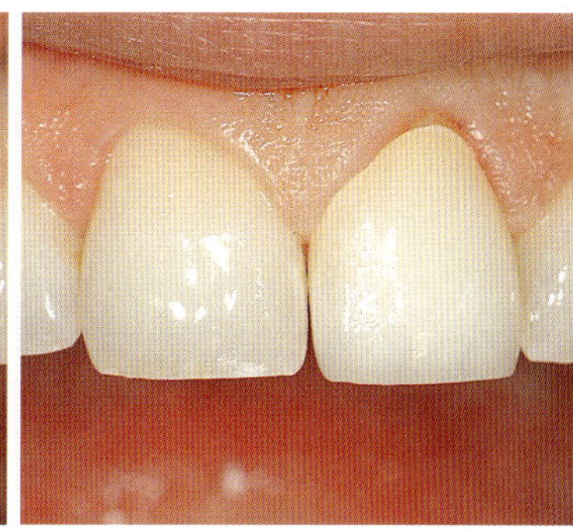

Fig. 6-67o Crown seated with air between crown and tooth; note opaque appearance.

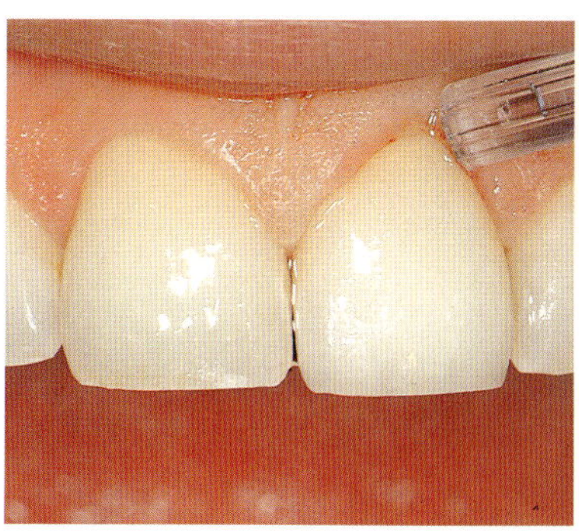

Fig. 6-67p Flow water under crown.

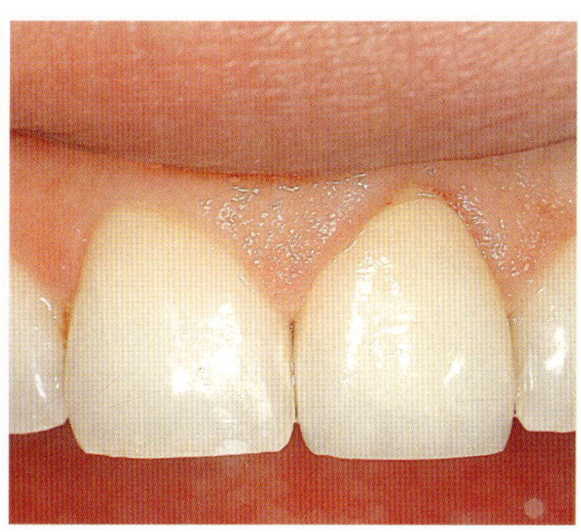

Fig. 6-67q Note color change when air space is removed and crown is "optically connected."

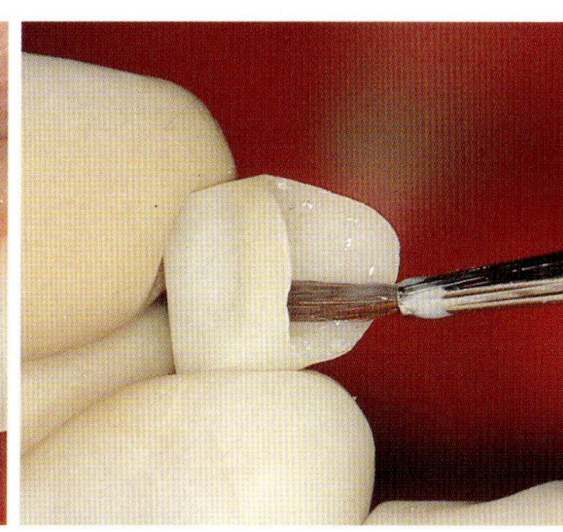

Fig. 6-67r Tints are placed and trial cement is used to finalize precementation esthetic analysis.

type used. Be sure to coat the adjacent tooth with clear stain liquid to prevent dehydration and color change (Fig. 6-67n). The crown must be optically connected to the prepared tooth with water or water-soluble gel to evaluate color (Figs. 6-67o to q). The color is finalized, the correct cement is selected, and the cementation process continues (Figs. 6-67r and s).

5. The internal surface of the crown should be lightly air abraded and ultrasonically or steam cleaned prior to cementing with luting cements. When using composite resin cements, the internal surface of the

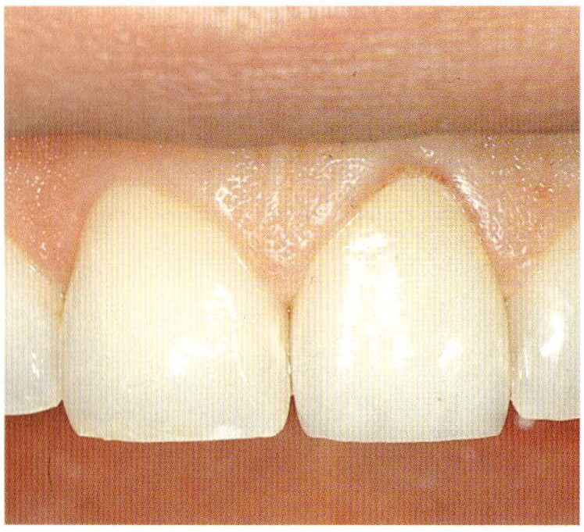

Fig. 6-67s Final esthetic results achieved during try-in.

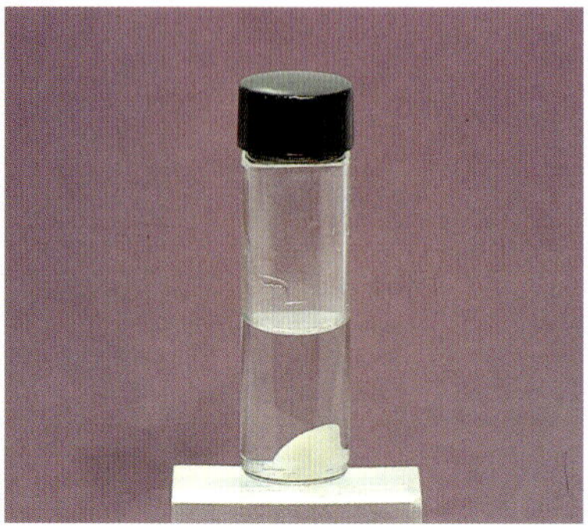

Fig. 6-67t Place crown in acetone-filled bottle and float in ultrasonic cleaner.

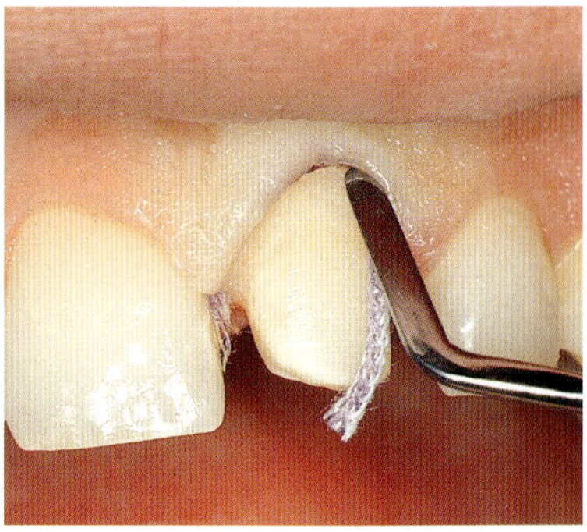

Fig. 6-67u Retract tissues with cord if necessary.

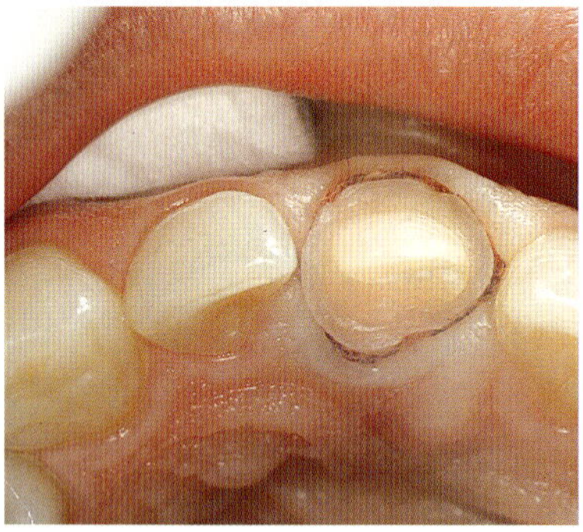

Fig. 6-67v Incisal view of retracted tissues.

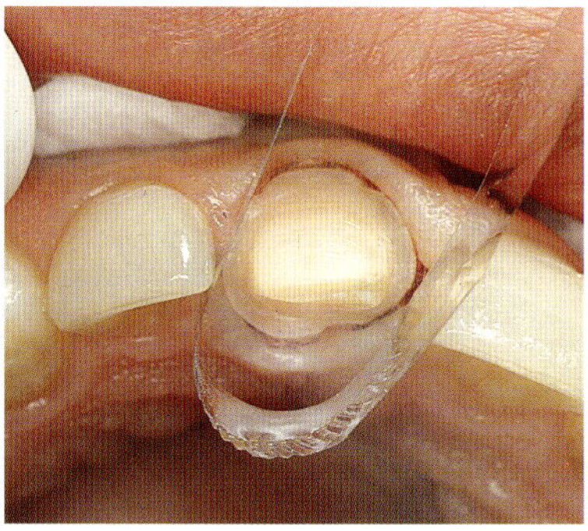

Fig. 6-67w Thin mylar strip stuck to copal varnish coated on adjacent contacts.

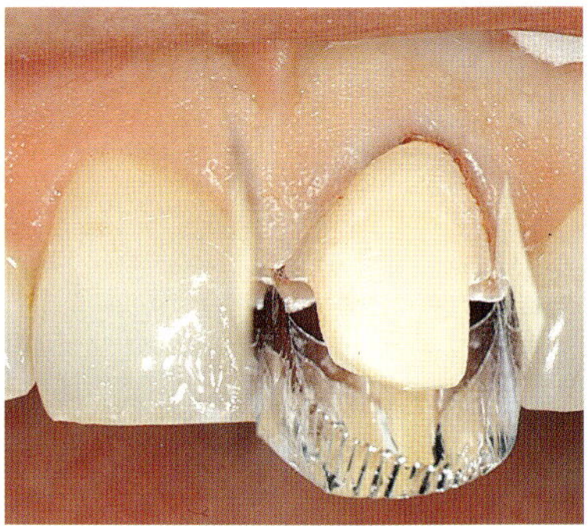

Fig. 6-67x Facial view.

crown must be treated differently depending upon the ceramic used. Aluminous porcelain core materials do not etch so they are only air abraded to roughen. The conventional and strengthened ceramic materials are etched with hydrofluoric acid. Dicor is etched with ammonium bifluoride. Etching procedures should precede the try-in appointment.

The try-in resins must be thoroughly cleaned out with acetone in an ultrasonic cleaner prior to cementation. Placing the restoration in a small screw top bottle of acetone and floating it in the ultrasonic cleaner works efficiently (Fig. 6-67t). Phosphoric acid is also an effective cleaner. Once the crown is cleaned, the inner bonding surface is coated with silane. It is recommended that Dicor be coated with silane 24 hours prior to placement. Other ceramics may be treated differently and manufacturer's recommendations should be followed.

6. When composite resin cements are used, the procedures are more demanding and time consuming. Isolation is critical and a dry field must be maintained throughout the procedures. Tissue retraction with cord is recommended (Figs. 6-67u and v). Paint a thin layer of copal varnish on adjacent teeth. A thin mylar matrix will stick to the copal coated teeth and prevent their etching, which would lead to a more difficult cement cleanup (Figs. 6-67w and x). Enamel margins are etched for 15 to 20 seconds with phosphoric acid (Fig. 6-67y). Dentin surface are conditioned (etched) as recommended in the

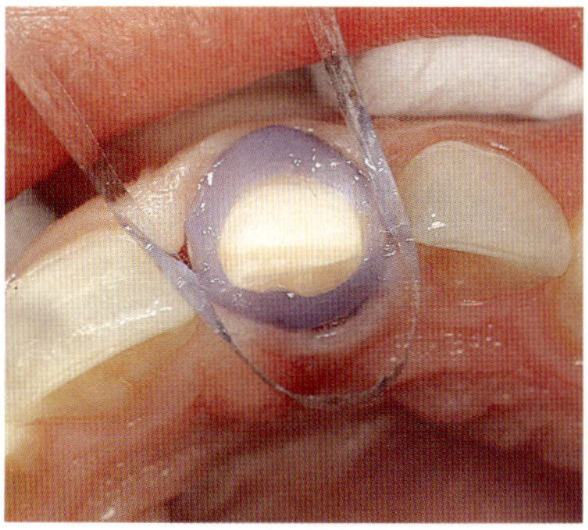

Fig. 6-67y Etch enamel margins with 37% phosphoric acid.

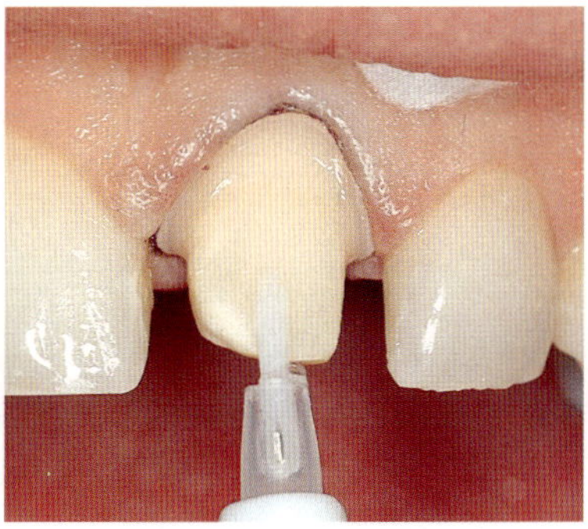

Fig. 6-67z Apply multi-purpose bonding agent to the preparation and the crown.

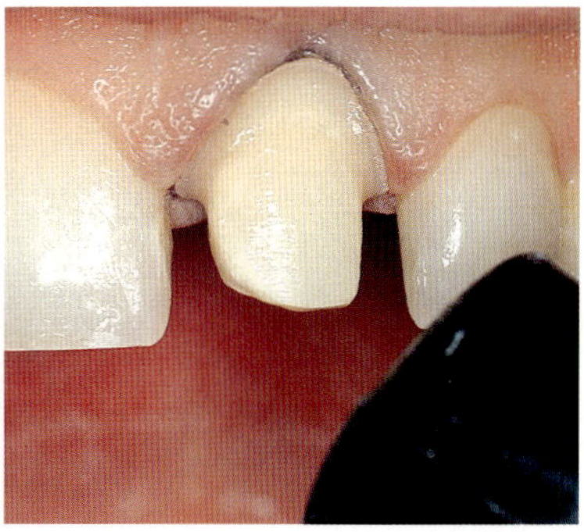

Fig. 6-67aa Use warm air gun to dry.

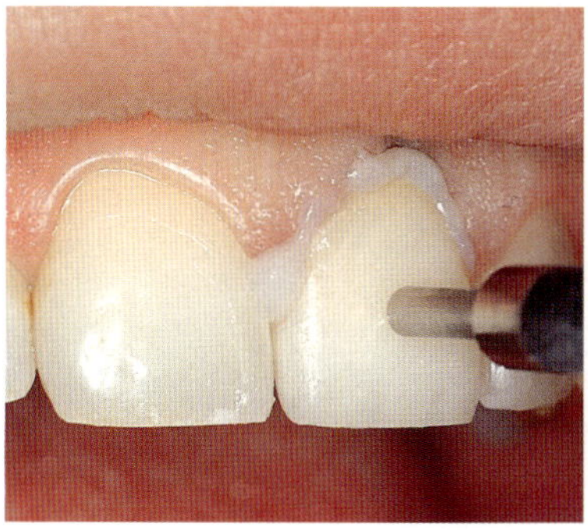

Fig. 6-67bb Tack in place with small curing tip.

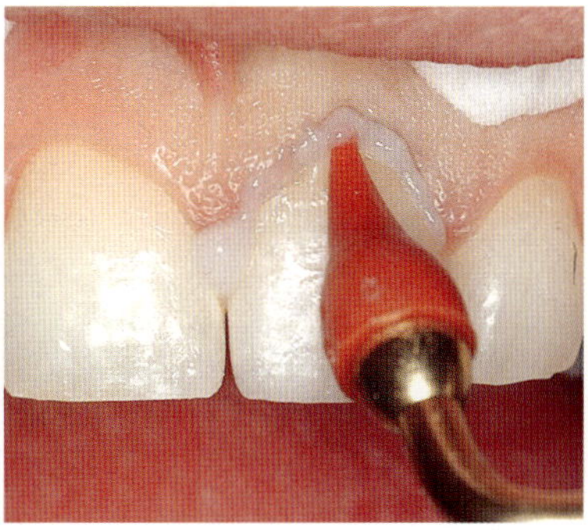

Fig. 6-67cc Remove gross excess and leave slight excess.

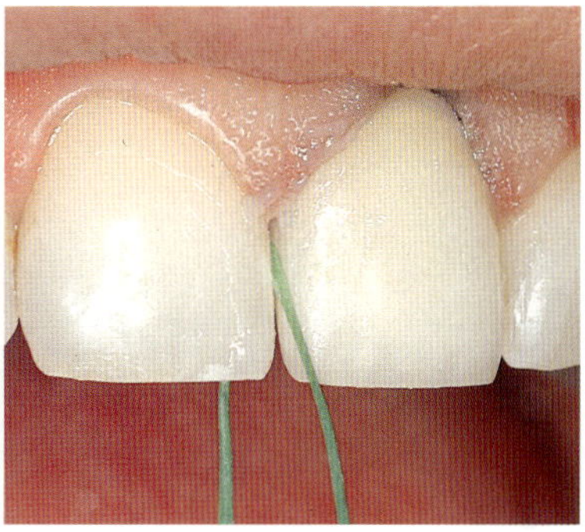

Fig. 6-67dd Floss away proximal cement excess.

dental bonding system. The desired multipurpose dentinal bonding system is applied to both the tooth and crown and dried with a warm air dryer (Figs. 6-67z and aa). The internal surfaces of the crown are prepared with the predetermined composite resin cement and color modifiers and seated. More opaque crowns require dual curing or chemical curing cements to ensure complete polymerization. The resin cement should be polymerized in the midfacial portion of the crown with a 2- or 3-mm curing light tip for 10 to 20 seconds (Fig. 6-67bb). The excess cement is removed with a fine brush or a rubber stimulator tip and the proximal contacts are flossed in a gingival direction to remove additional cement excess. (Figs. 6-67cc and dd). Note that a slight amount of excess should remain around the margins to compensate for polymerization shrinkage. Completely cure with a large curing tip (8 to 13 mm) from both the buccal and lingual for 1 to 2 minutes each (Fig. 6-67ee).

7. All ceramic margins may not routinely be as accurate as metal margins. If excess cement is chipped out with a hand instrument, a marginal void may be created. Use of a 30-fluted carbide bur to amputate or cut off the excess cement flush with the margin will prevent these voids (Fig. 6-67ff). This bur is minimally abrasive and will remove excess cement safely without damaging the tooth or crown. Interproximal excess can be removed with a #12 scalpel (Fig. 6-67gg).
8. If ceramic margins require contouring

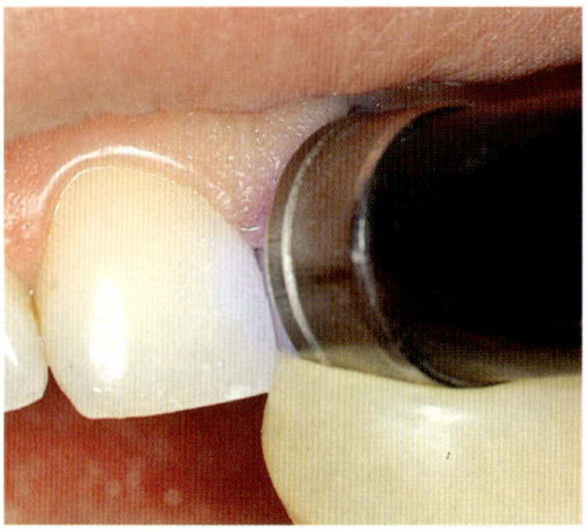

Fig. 6-67ee Cure crown completely.

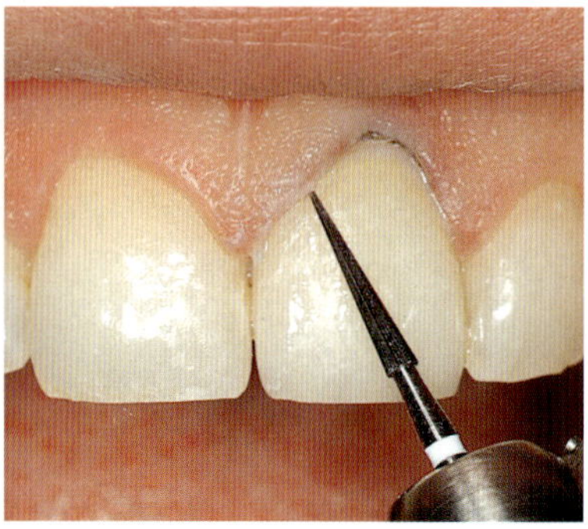

Fig. 6-67ff Remove excess with 30-fluted finishing bur.

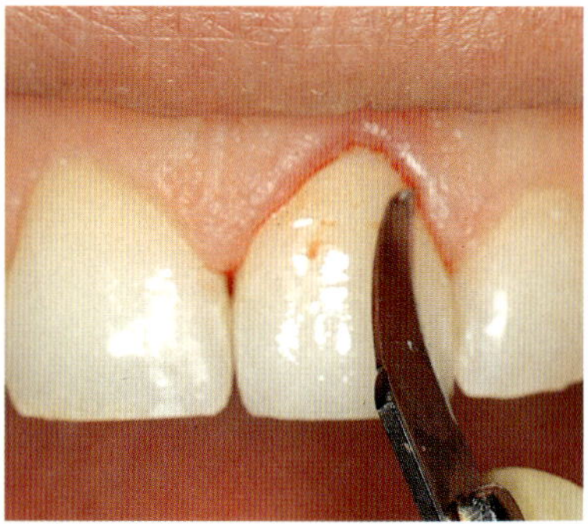

Fig. 6-67gg Use scalpel with a #12 blade to remove interproximal excess.

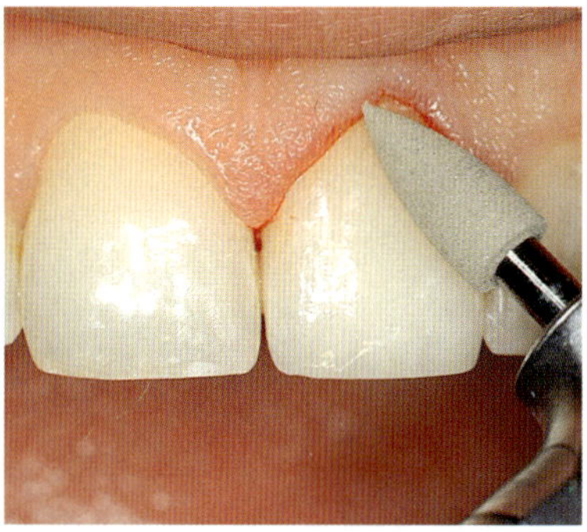

Fig. 6-67hh Polish any areas requiring postcementation contouring.

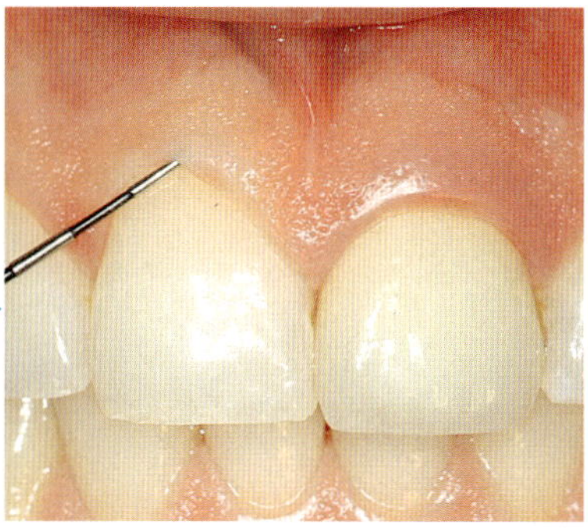

Fig. 6-68a Preoperative view.

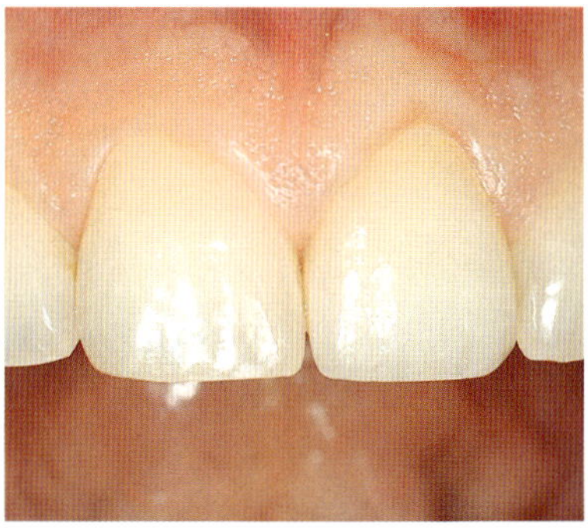

Fig. 6-68b Postoperative view.

postcementation, fine high speed diamonds are used with sufficient water spray. These roughened ceramic surfaces must be smoothed sequentially with extrafine and ultrafine diamonds, 30-fluted carbide burs, rubber ceramic polishing points and finally diamond or an equivalent polishing paste (Fig. 6-67hh). This sequence is the same for ceramic veneers. Generally, the crown margins are of sufficient bulk that they can be contoured prior to cementation and polished or glazed extraorally.

9. Postoperative instructions on home care, hygienist cleaning instructions and precautions for excessive function should be given to the patient. A recall check should be scheduled (Fig. 6-68).

LABORATORY PROCEDURES

Aluminous Oxide Core Strengthened Ceramic Crowns (See, also In-Ceram Core Strengthened)

When an all ceramic crown of higher value and strength is desired or internal block out of discolored supporting structures is necessary, an aluminous oxide core strengthened crown is indicated. Improved strength characteristics are greater than conventional ceramic crowns and the opaque, semitranslucent core provides a good color barrier to discolored substructures (Fig. 6-69a). In addition, the higher temperature core materials provide dimensional stability during

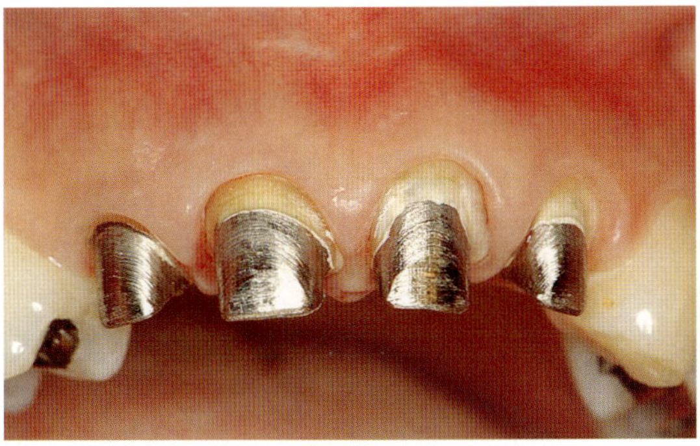

Fig. 6-69a Prepared teeth with dowel cores.

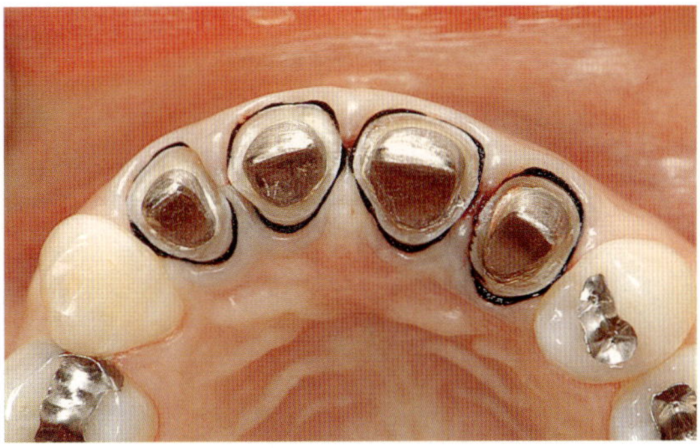

Fig. 6-69b Incisal view of circumferal shoulders.

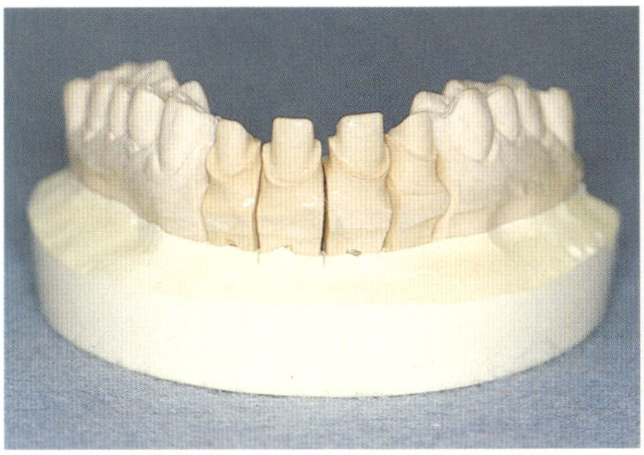

Fig.6-69c Master model with die hardener.

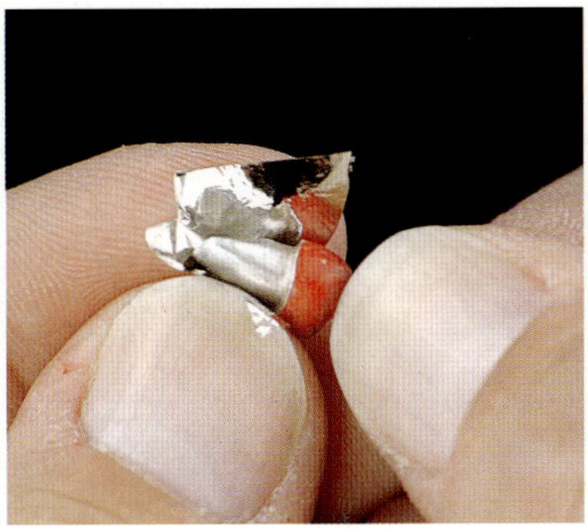

Fig. 6-69d Platinum foil adapted to die.

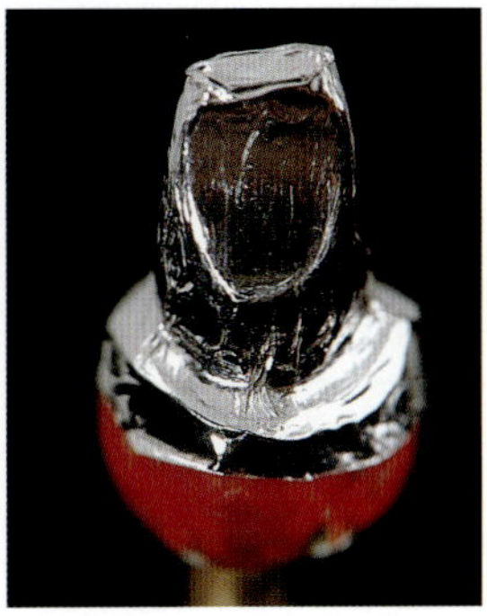

Fig. 6-69e Aluminous oxide core adapted to foil.

extrinsic ceramic staining thermal cycles. As described in the preparation section, adequate preparation depth and a circumferential shoulder finish line are necessary (Fig. 6-69b).

1. Depending upon the type of core material used, the aluminous core is fabricated first using recommended techniques. For a Vitadur aluminous core, the stone dies are made and trimmed. Die spacer and hardener is advisable (Fig. 6-69c). A platinum foil is adapted to the dies and the core material adapted to this foil matrix similar to other ceramic materials (Figs. 6-69d and e). For an In-Ceram core, a special refractory die and a special technique must be used (see the section on In-Ceram fabrication).
2. Internal color modification of the core material is necessary in some instances to achieve the esthetic results desired.
3. Once fabricated the internal aluminous core is seated and checked for marginal accuracy on the original die (Fig. 6-69f). The thickness should be adjusted to about 0.5 mm facially and as thick as possible on the lingual aspect, leaving space for about 0.5 mm of veneering ceramic. The core material must be covered because it does not glaze and polish. The finer particle size of In-Ceram has minimized this problem.
4. The conventional veneering ceramic can now be built up as dictated by esthetic requirements. Dentin, opacious, incisal and ceramic modifiers are used by the skilled ceramist to create the desired results

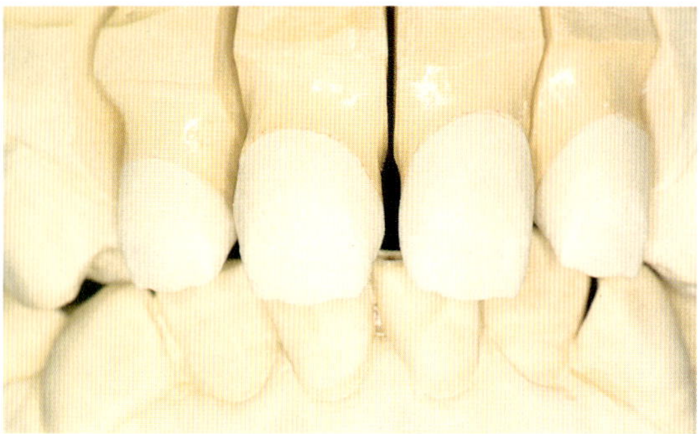

Fig. 6-69f Finished aluminous oxide cores on dies.

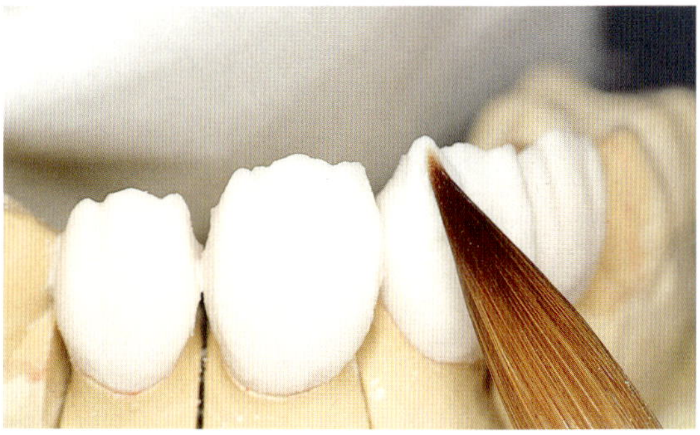

Fig. 6-69g Dentin ceramic additions.

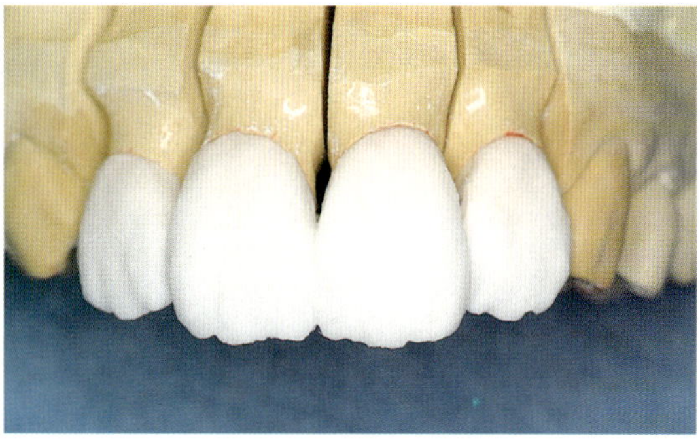

Fig. 6-69h Incisal ceramic additions.

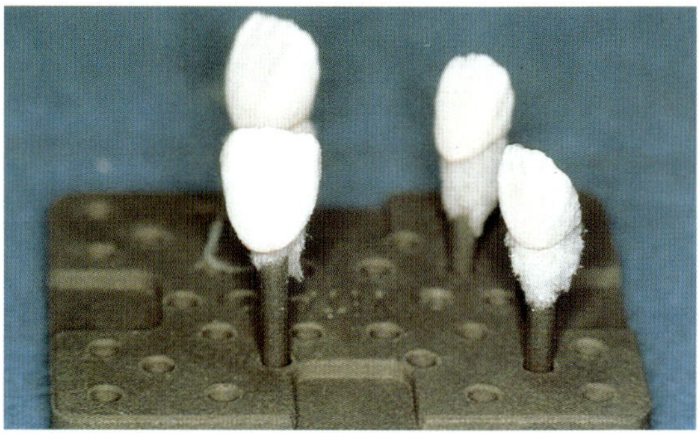

Fig. 6-69i Unsintered crowns on sagar tray.

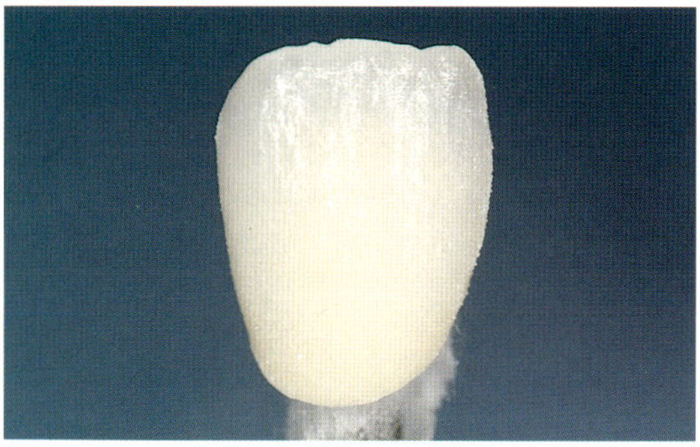

Fig. 6-69j Sintered crown on sagar tray.

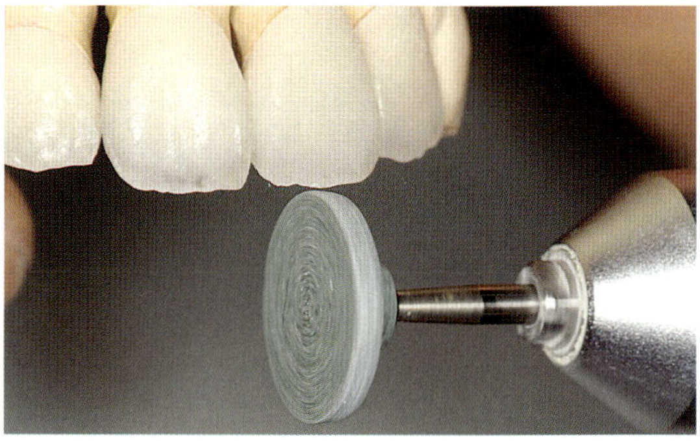

Fig. 6-69k Contouring crowns.

(Figs. 6-69g and h). Opacious dentin is especially useful in minimizing any bright show through of the aluminous core.

5. The crown(s) is now fired as recommended by the manufacturer under vacuum. It can be placed on a fibrous pad, a loosely fitting stand or a combination of the two to avoid core distortion (Figs. 6-69i and j).
6. The fired crown(s) can now be contoured with fine ceramic adjusting stones or fine diamonds. Additional ceramic material is reapplied until the desired esthetic and functional results are achieved. Thorough cleaning prior to new additions is mandatory (Figs. 6-69k to n).
7. Once the crown is complete it can be

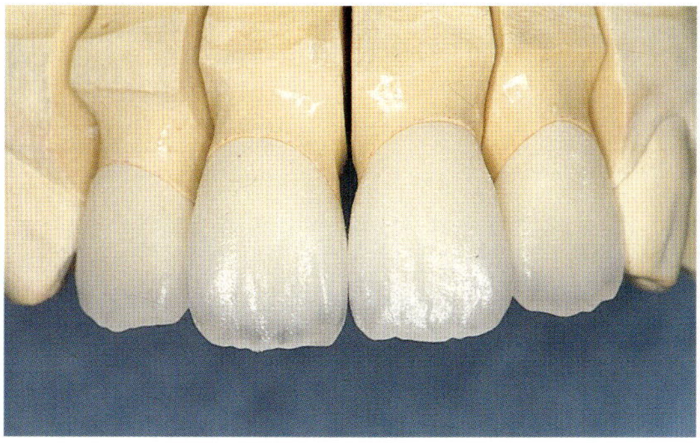

Fig. 6-69l Final surface texture.

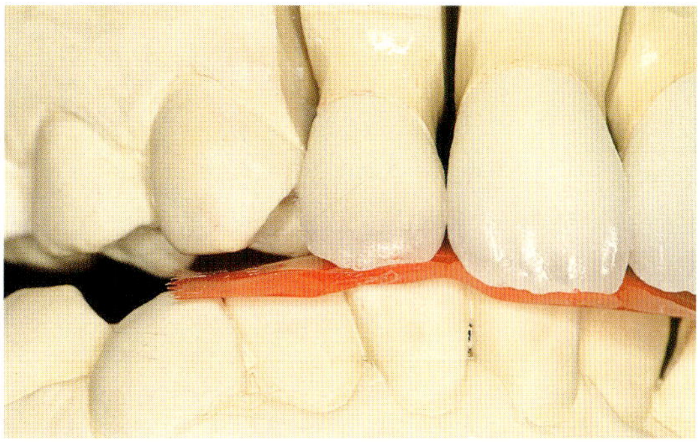

Fig. 6-69m Adjusting occlusion.

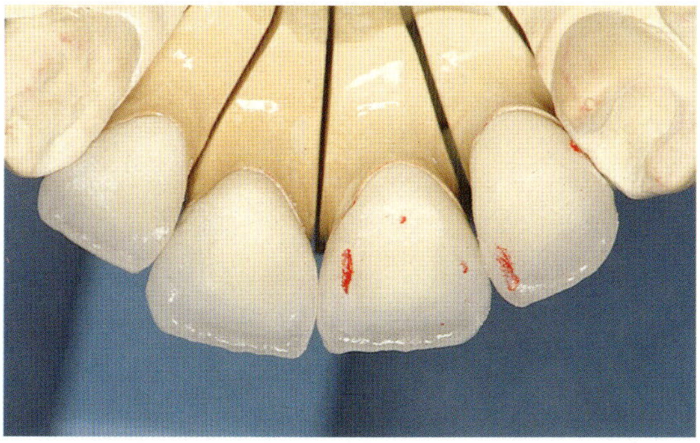

Fig. 6-69n Checking occlusion.

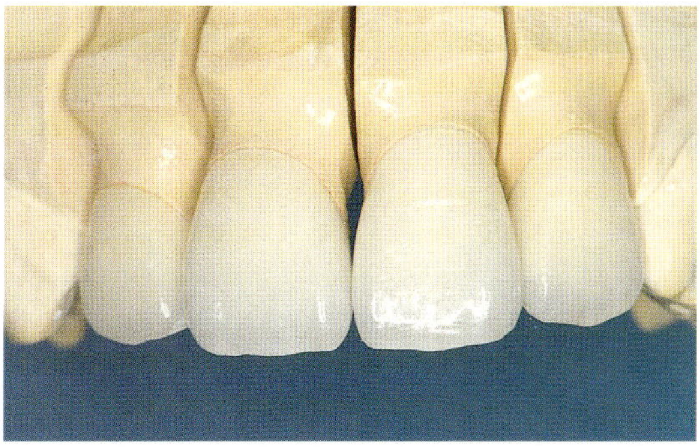

Fig. 6-69o Finished crowns on dies.

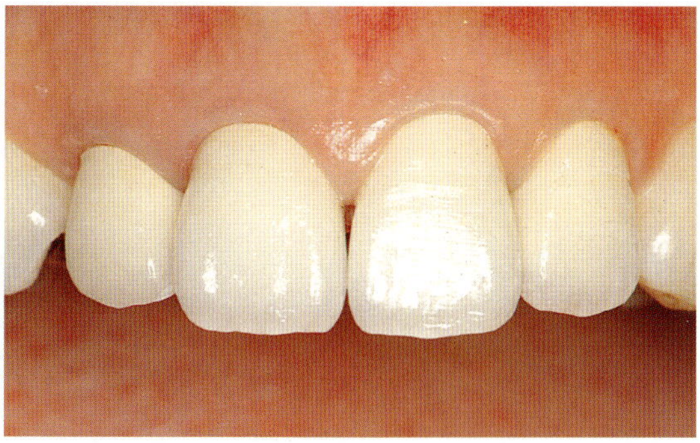

Fig. 6-69p Postcementation (facial view).

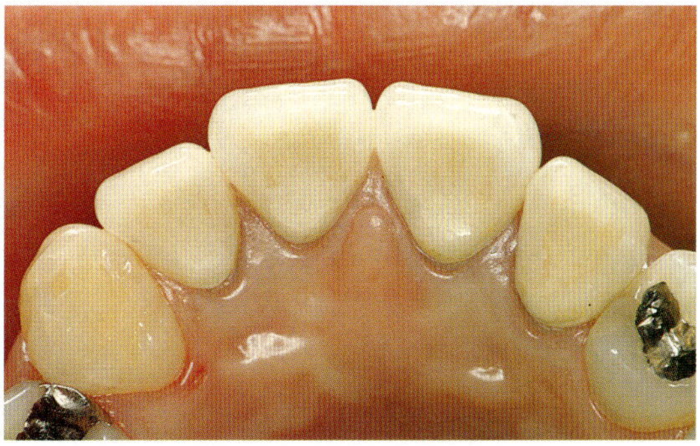

Fig. 6-69q Postcementation (lingual view).

surfaced to achieve the desired texture, steam cleaned and glazed (Fig. 6-69o).

8. The aluminous oxide core strengthened all ceramic crown is now ready for try-in, final esthetic and functional adjustment and cementation (Figs. 6-69p and q).

Strengthened Ceramic Crowns

1. Tooth reduction for a strengthened ceramic crown is similar to that for other all ceramic crowns (Fig. 6-70a). Because no additional room is required for a core, preparation depth may be more conservative in selected instances. Good

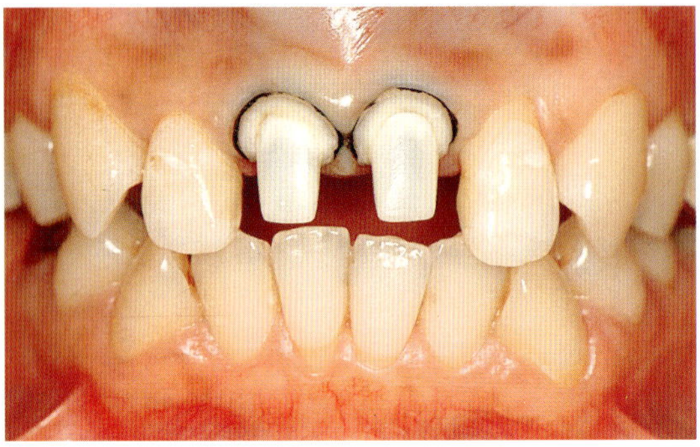

Fig. 6-70a Prepared centrals.

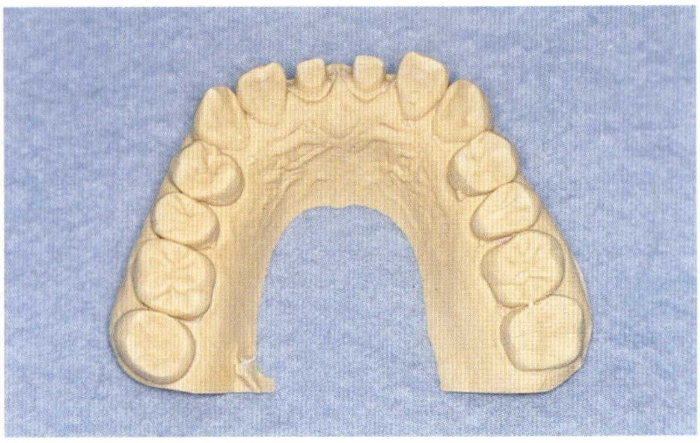

Fig. 6-70b Stone working model.

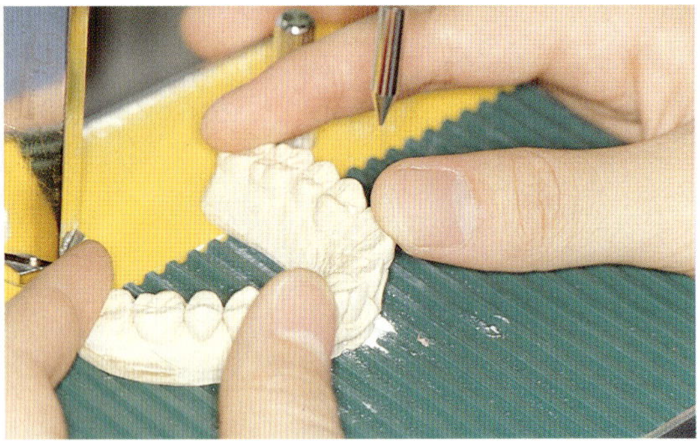

Fig. 6-70c Drilling for die pins.

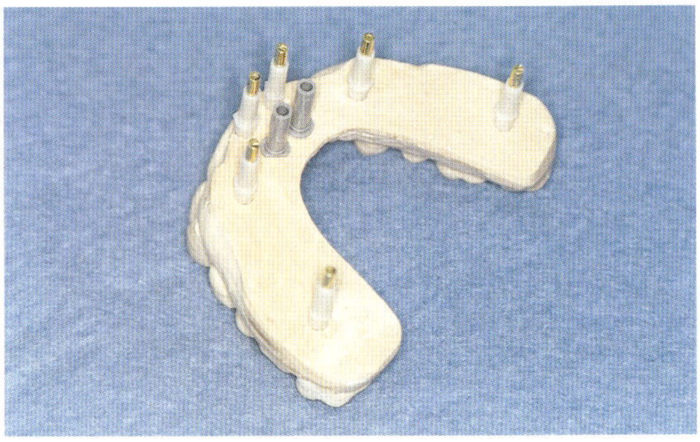

Fig. 6-70d Cement die pins.

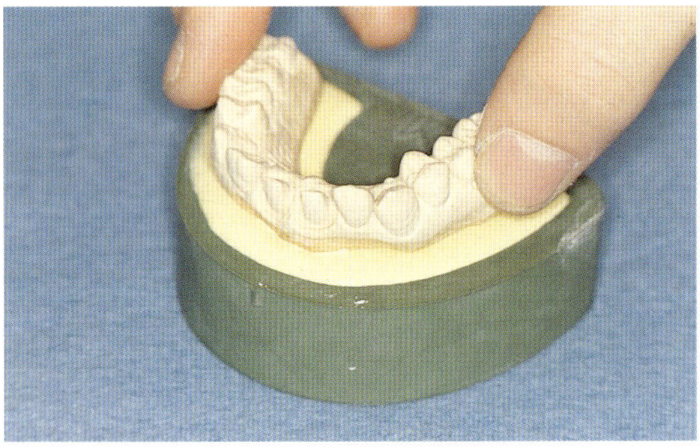

Fig. 6-70e Pour base over pins.

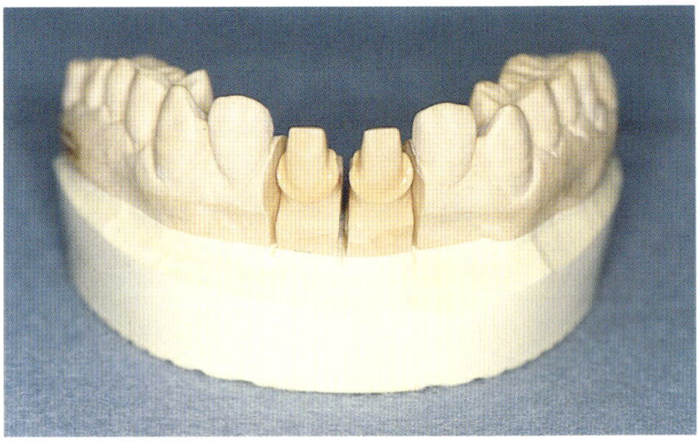

Fig. 6-70f Finished working model.

physical properties are still achieved because the entire ceramic crown is strengthened.

2. The die stone working model is poured from the impression and a removable die master model fabricated (Figs. 6-70b to f).
3. Die spacer should be applied on the die to within about 1.0 mm of the margins in order to provide 25 to 50μ of die relief (Fig. 6-70g).
4. Undercuts around adjacent teeth can now be filled in with wax and an over impression taken of the entire work model

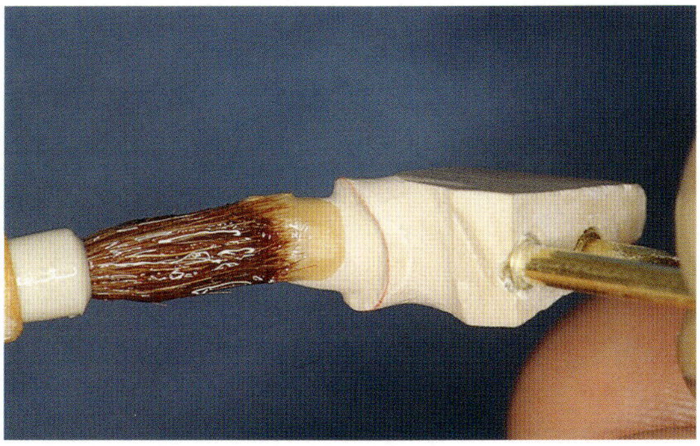

Fig. 6-70g Die spacer application and margins marked.

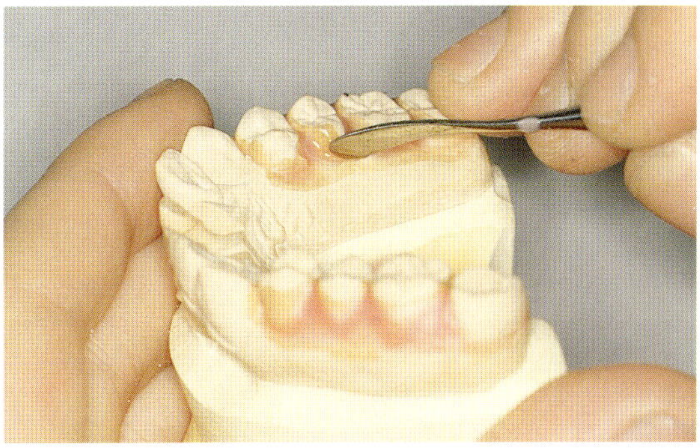

Fig. 6-70h Block out undercuts in working model with wax.

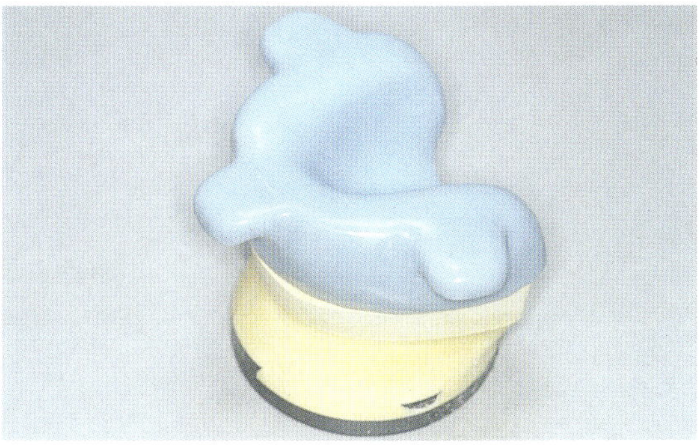

Fig. 6-70i Custom impression tray.

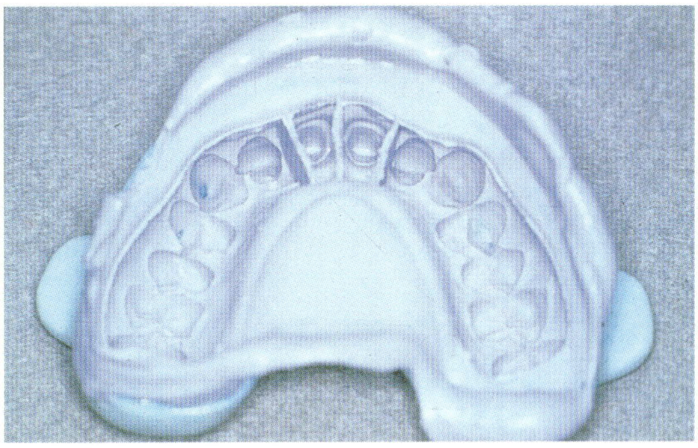

Fig. 6-70j Impression of working model.

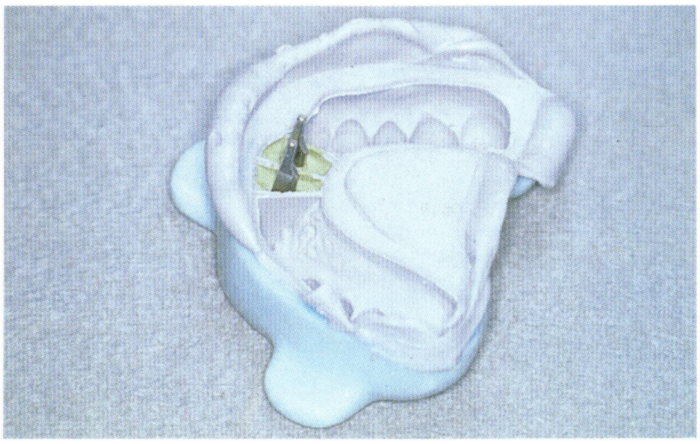

Fig. 6-70k Pour dies in refractory die material and place refractory die pins.

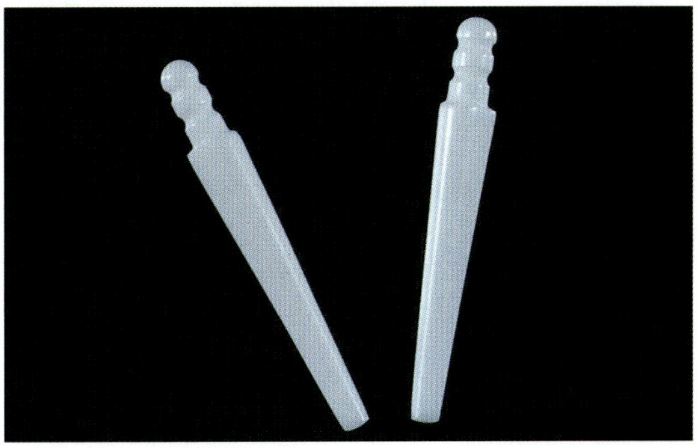

Fig. 6-70l Ceramic die pins.

with a polyvinylsiloxane impression material (Figs. 6-70h to j).

5. The die(s) can be poured in the appropriate refractory die material and metallic (or the new ceramic) refractory dowel pins can be inserted (Figs. 6-70k and l).
6. The remaining portion of the model is poured in improved stone that also covers the lubricated ends of the refractory dies (Fig. 6-70m). The working model is articulated with the opposing model (Fig. 6-70n). Additional refractory dies can be poured as back up dies.
7. The margins of the refractory dies are

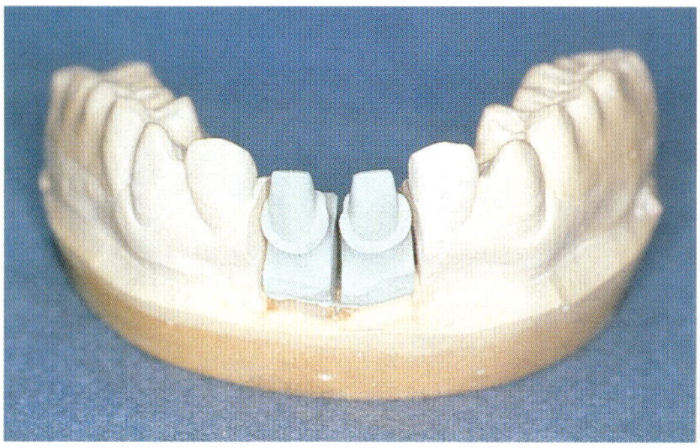

Fig. 6-70m Pour remaining impression in stone.

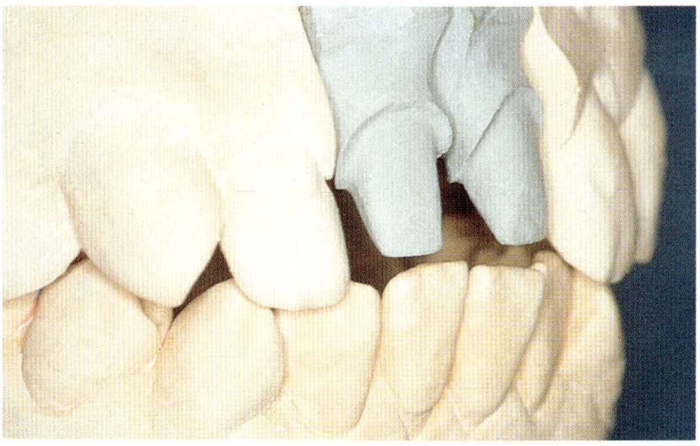

Fig. 6-70n Articulated refractory die models.

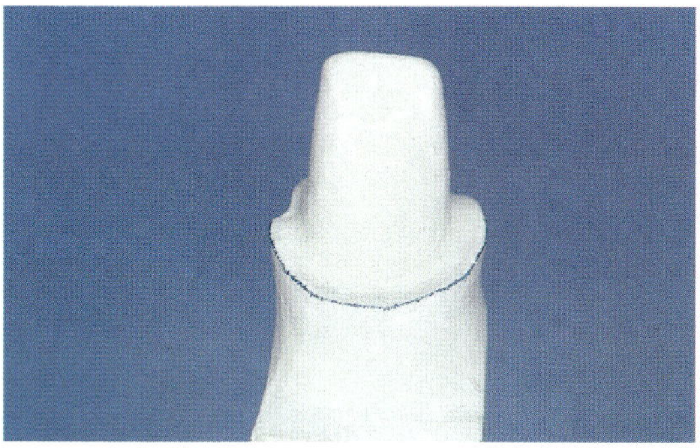

Fig. 6-70o Finished refractory die with margins marked.

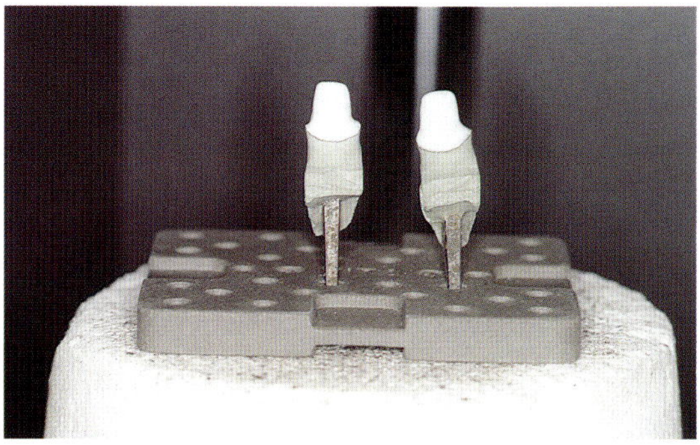

Fig. 6-70p Heat treat refractory dies.

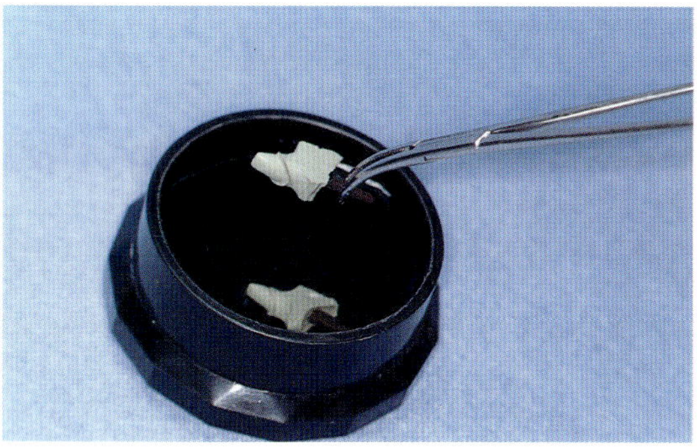

Fig. 6-70q Soak refractory dies in water.

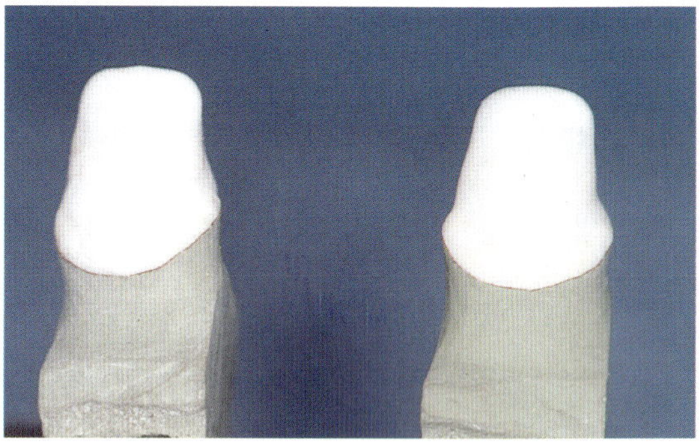

Fig. 6-70r Apply initial ceramic layer and sinter.

marked. The dies are then placed in a room temperature casting oven for initial heat treatment and transferred to a ceramic oven as recommended by the manufacturer of the ceramic material (Figs. 6-70o and p).

8. The cooled die(s) is now immersed in distilled water until no surface bubbles are visible (Fig. 6-70q).
9. The initial ceramic application should be a well condensed layer of body material about 0.5 mm thick covering the entire preparation (Fig. 6-70r). This is fired as recommended. This may be repeated to

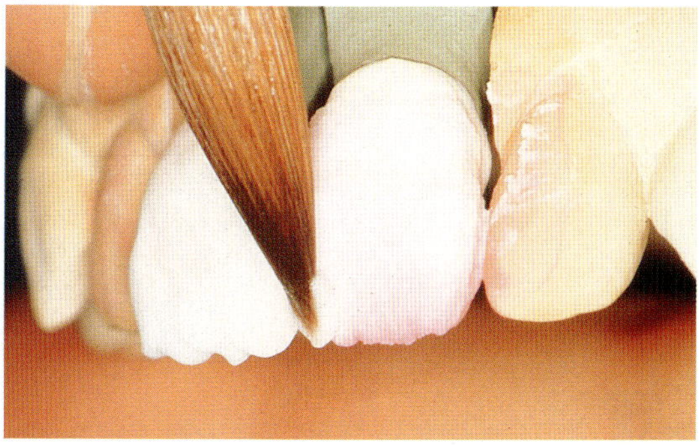

Fig. 6-70s Start bulk ceramic buildup.

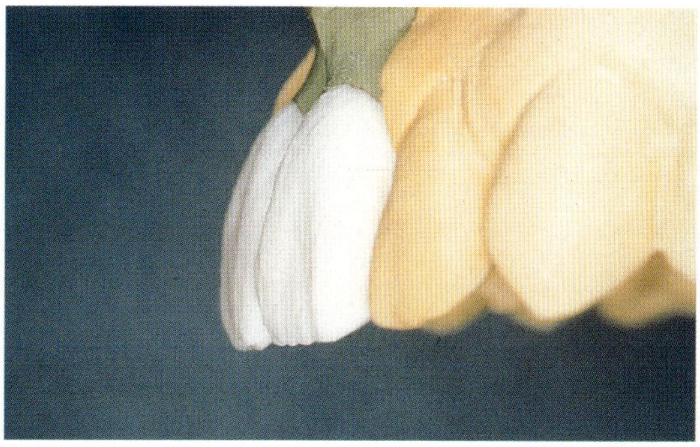

Fig. 6-70t Overcontour finished ceramic buildup.

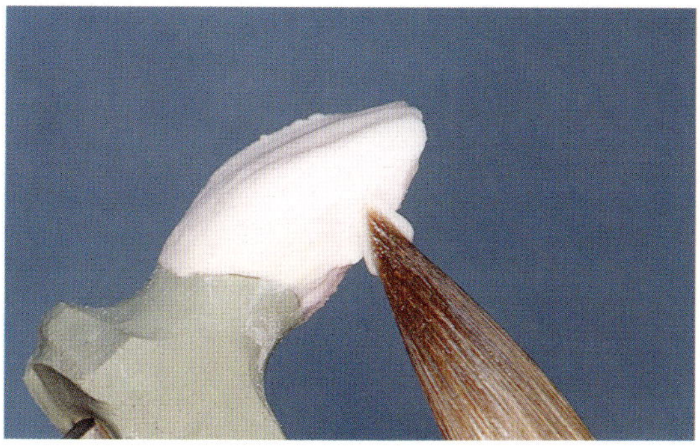

Fig. 6-70u Overcontour proximal contacts.

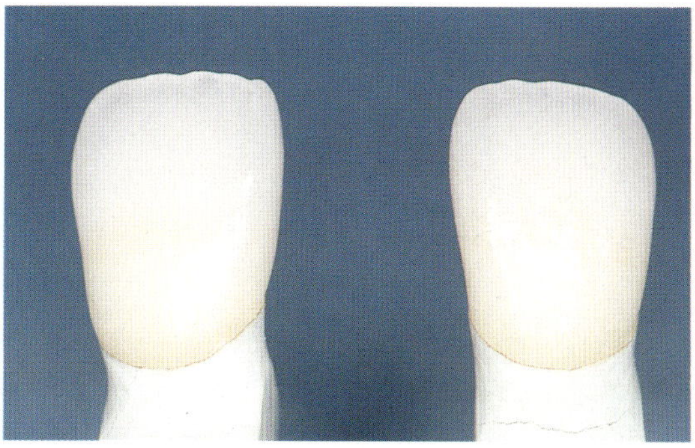

Fig. 6-70v Sintered crowns.

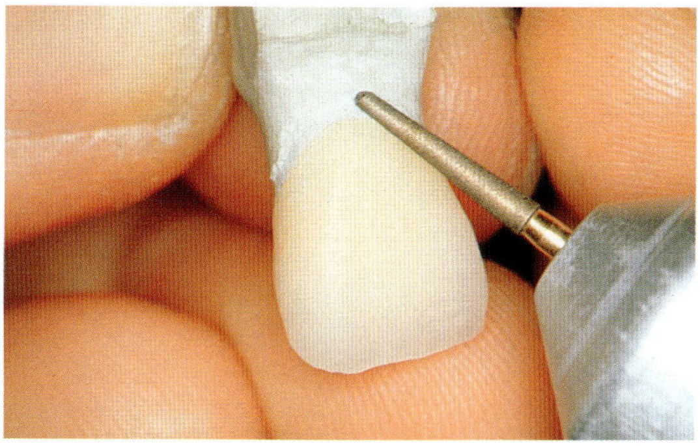

Fig. 6-70w Adjust crowns.

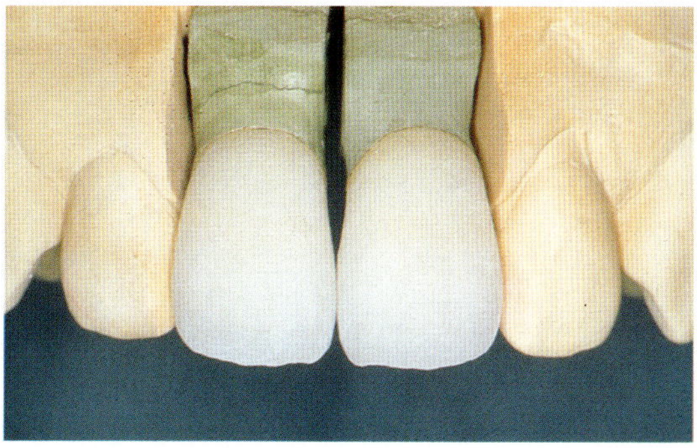

Fig. 6-70x Final contoured crowns.

fill contraction voids.

10. The cooled die is again immersed in distilled water and the bulk build-up begun. Dentin and incisal materials are layered and sculpted as dictated by esthetic demands (Figs. 6-70s to u). The full contour build-up is fired as before (Fig. 6-70v).
11. The fired crown is now contoured both esthetically and functionally with fine diamonds and ceramic adjusting stones. Ceramic additions are repeated as required (Figs. 6-70w and x).
12. The completed crown is steam cleaned

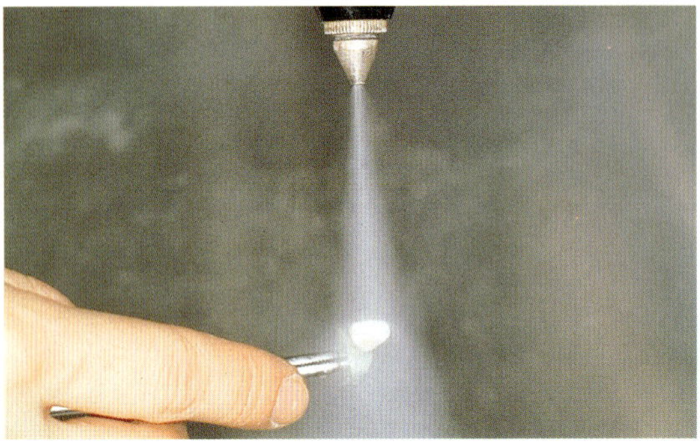

Fig. 6-70y Steam clean and glaze crown.

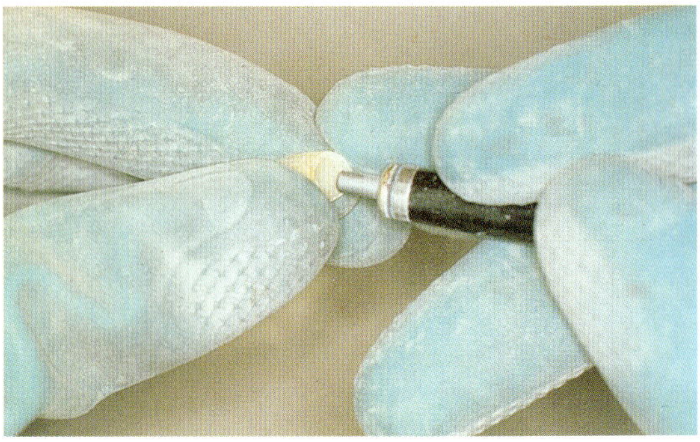

Fig. 6-70z Carefully cut and sandblast away refractory die material.

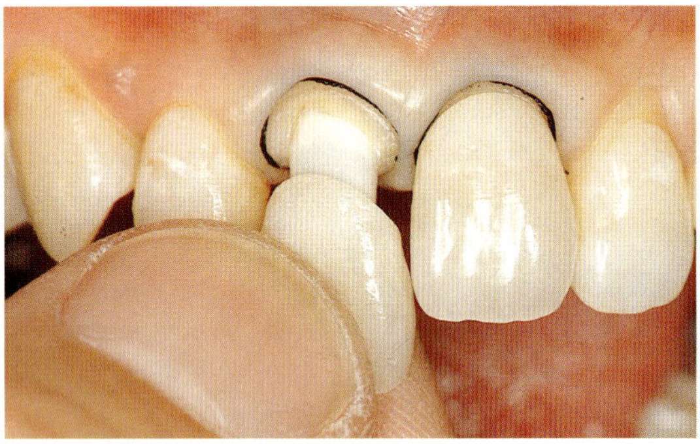

Fig. 6-70aa Try-in and adjust crowns

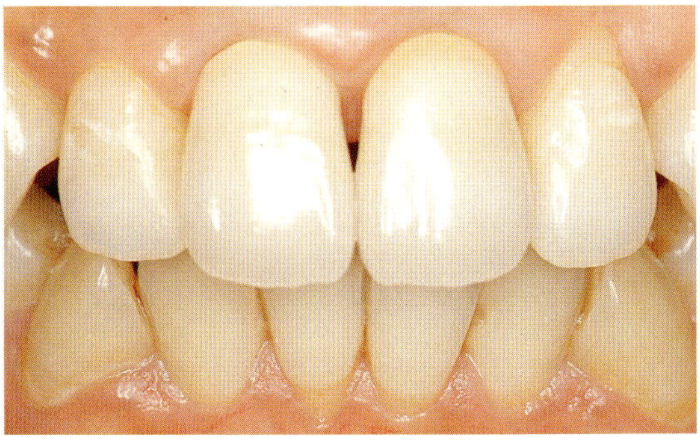

Fig. 6-70bb Postoperative view of cemented crown.

and glazed per manufacturer's instructions and as desired for esthetic surface texture (Fig. 6-70y).

13. The completed crown is divested using rotary instruments to cut away a majority of the refractory die, followed by careful air abrasion with aluminous oxide to avoid excessive marginal contact (Fig. 6-70z).
14. The completed crown is now ready for try-in and delivery as described in previous sections (Figs. 6-70aa and bb).

Cast Ceramic Core Strengthened Crowns

Cast ceramic and cast ceramic core strengthened all ceramic crowns are desirable when maximum translucency is required (Fig. 6-71a).

1. Preparation design is as described previously with a full circumferential shoulder (Fig. 6-71b).
2. Impressions are made and die stone removable dies are fabricated as normal (Fig. 6-71c).

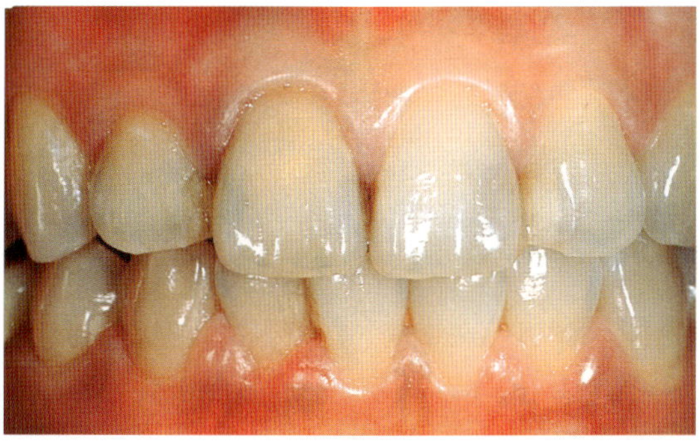

Fig. 6-71a Preoperative view of translucent teeth.

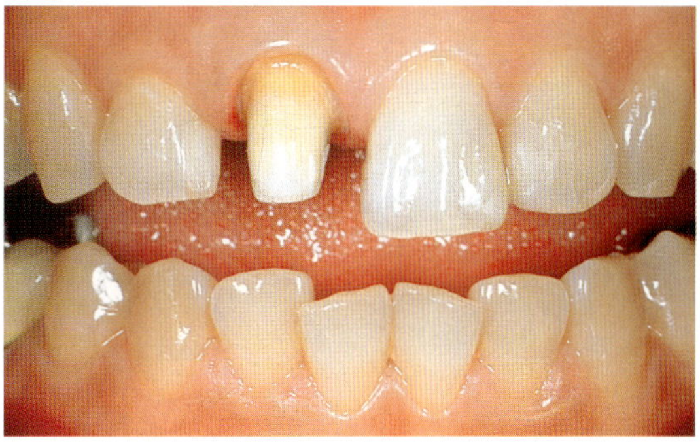

Fig. 6-71b Prepared central for cast ceramic core strengthened crown.

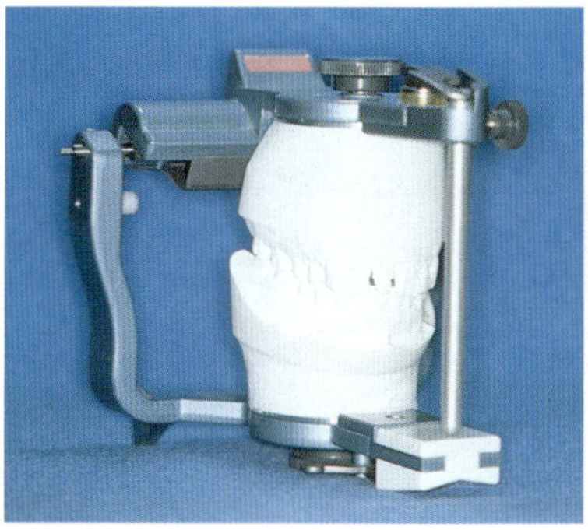

Fig. 6-71c Articulated working model.

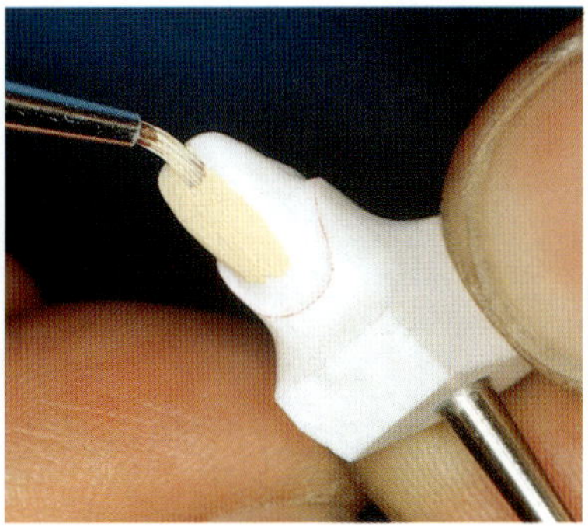

Fig. 6-71d Apply color matched die spacer.

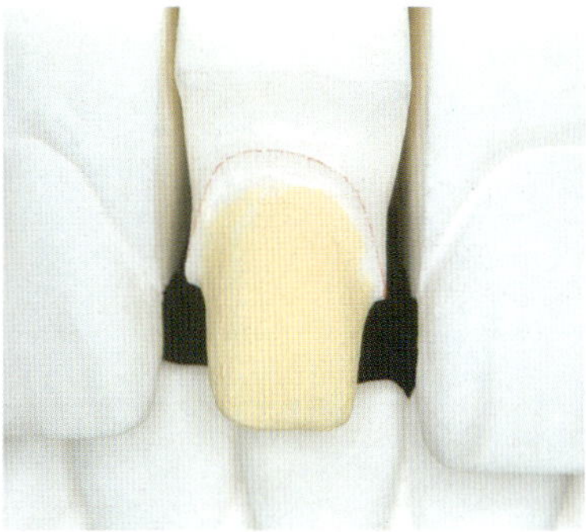

Fig. 6-71e Finished die with die spacer, marked margins and die hardener.

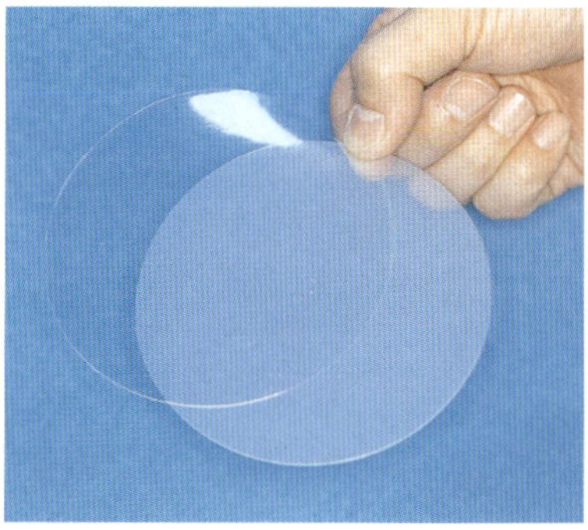

Fig. 6-71f Coping material: 0.025 and 0.7 mm.

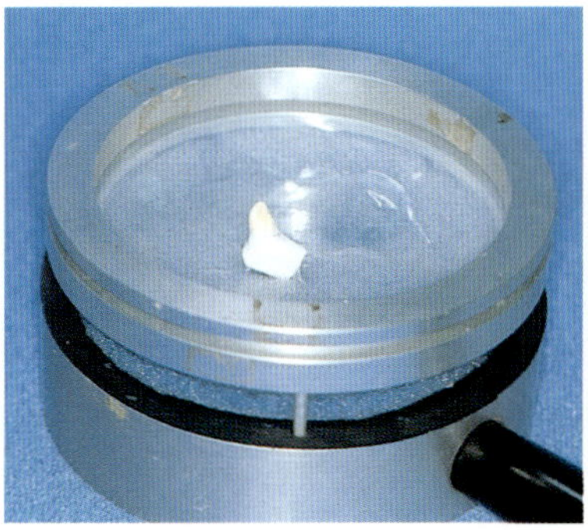

Fig. 6-71g Vacuum form copings.

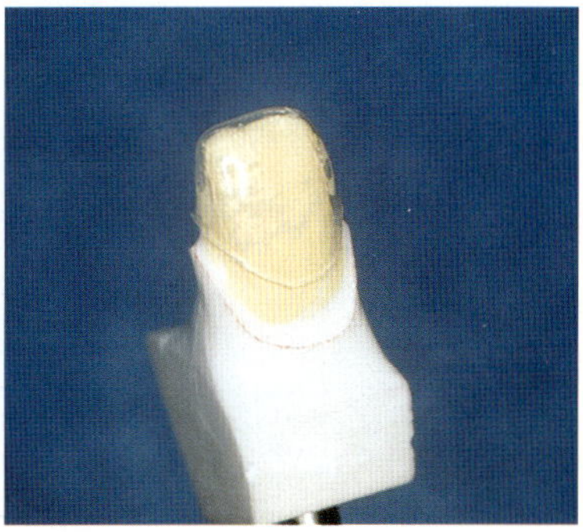

Fig. 6-71h Cut copings 1.5 mm short of margins.

3. Because of the material's translucency, color coordinated die spacers are used to simulate the color of the prepared tooth (Figs. 6-71d and e).
4. The cast ceramic core is now waxed to full contour. A dual plastic coping is useful. An inner coping 0.25 mm thick and an outer coping 0.7 mm thick are vacuum molded against the die (Figs. 6-71f and g).
5. The plastic coping is cut 1.5 mm short of the margins (Fig. 6-71h).
6. Sticky wax is used to lute the coping in place and a full contour waxup is completed on the working model (Figs. 6-71i and j).

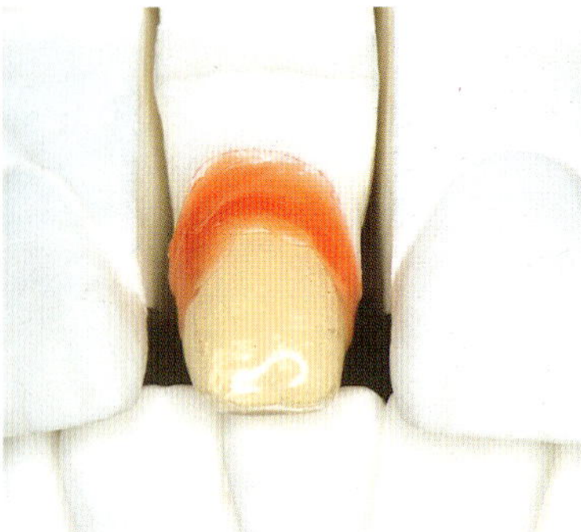

Fig. 6-71i Lute copings to die with sticky wax.

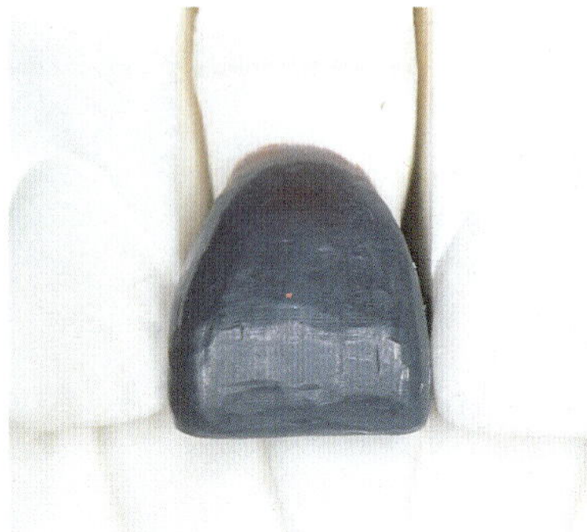

Fig. 6-71j Full contour waxup.

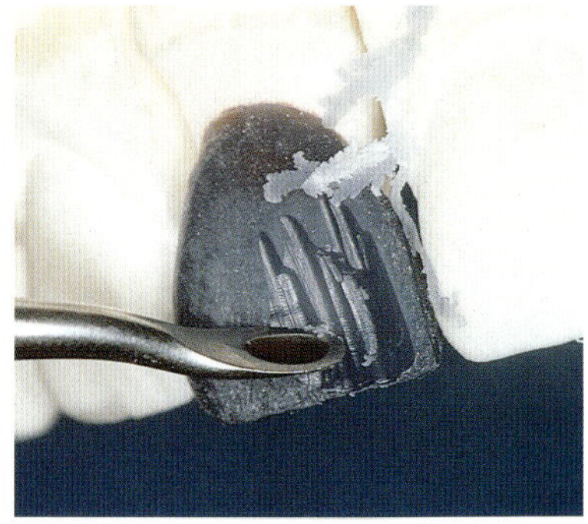

Fig. 6-71k Cut back facial of wax coping.

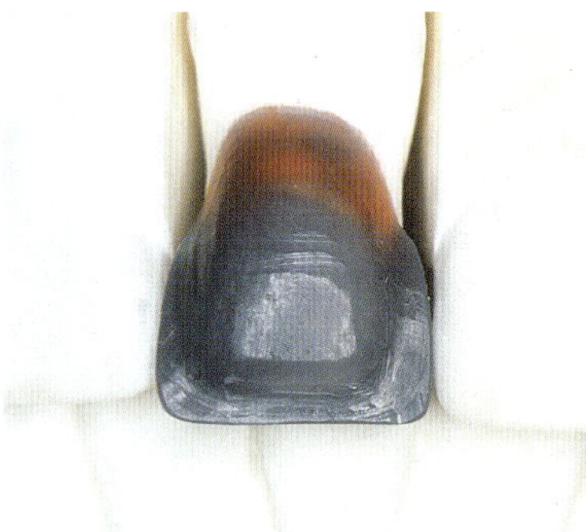

Fig. 6-71l Facial view of final wax pattern.

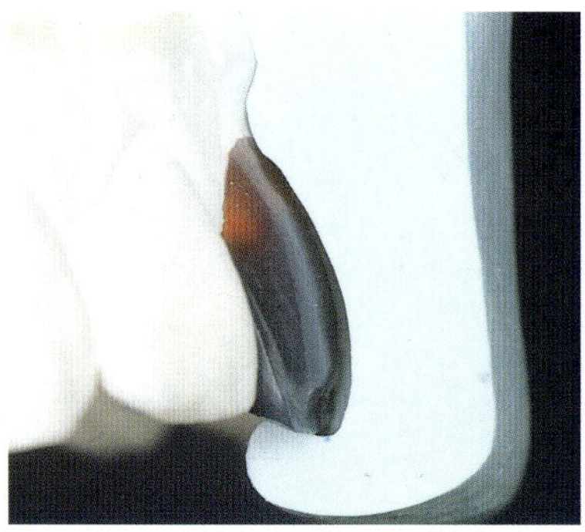

Fig. 6-71m Lateral view of final wax pattern.

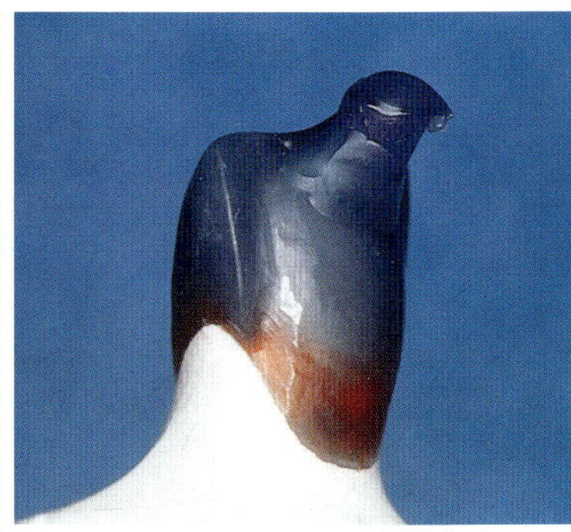

Fig. 6-71n Sprue waxup.

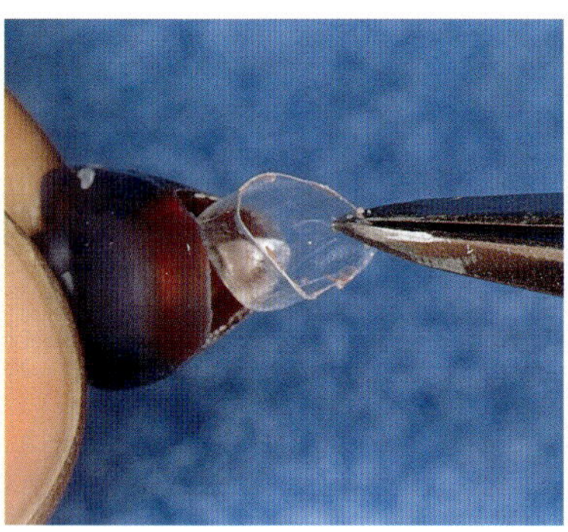

Fig. 6-71o Remove inner 0.25 coping.

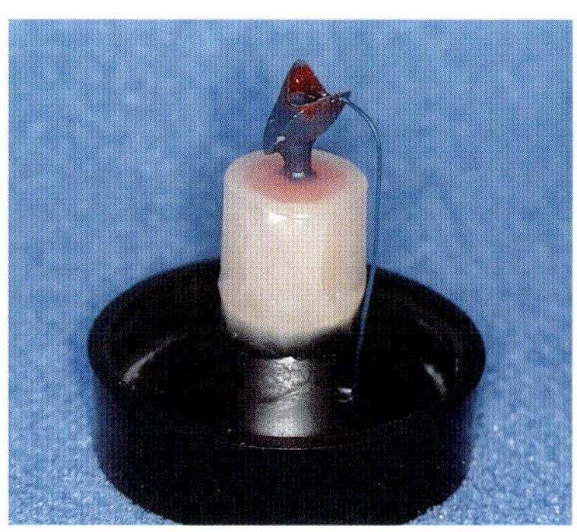

Fig. 6-71p Final sprued was pattern.

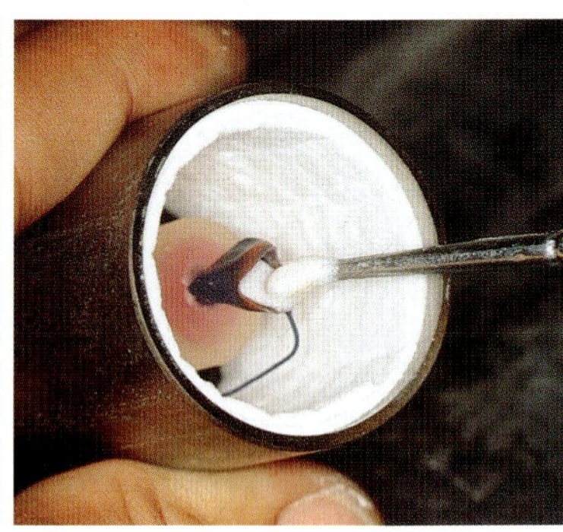

Fig. 6-71q Investing wax pattern.

7. Facial wax is removed saving a 1.0-mm minimal thickness. Proximal contacts are maintained in wax (Figs. 6-71k to m).
8. The wax-plastic pattern is sprued with a 3-mm sprue and the inner plastic coping is removed (Figs. 6-71n and o).
9. Spruing is completed and a small blind vent placed on the facial (Fig. 6-71p). The pattern is invested per manufacturer's instructions (Fig. 6-71q).
10. After a 1-hour setting period, the investment is ground off at the open end of the ring using a model trimmer and placed in a room temperature burn-out oven and run up the recommended burn out temperature (Figs. 6-71r and s).

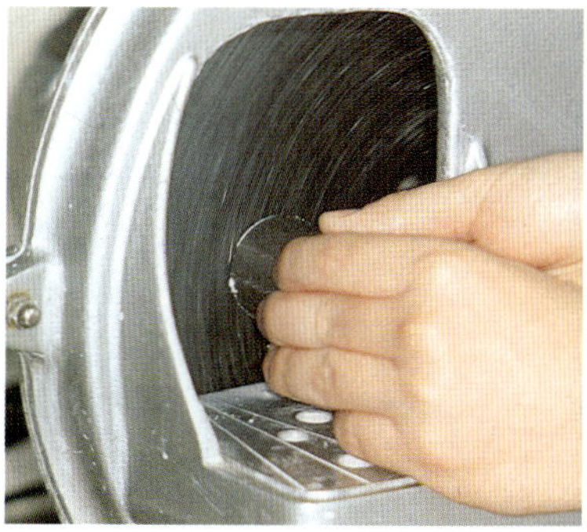

Fig. 6-71r Trim end of set investment.

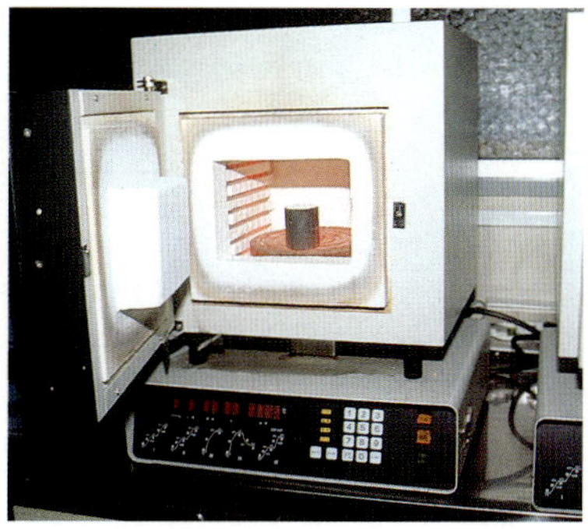

Fig. 6-71s Burn out wash pattern.

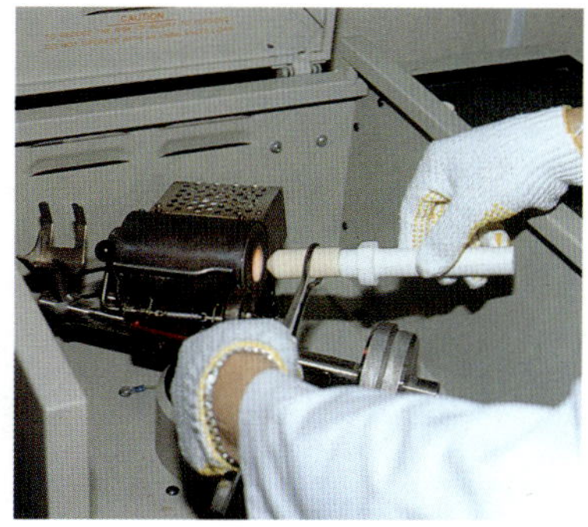

Fig. 6-71t Casting procedure.

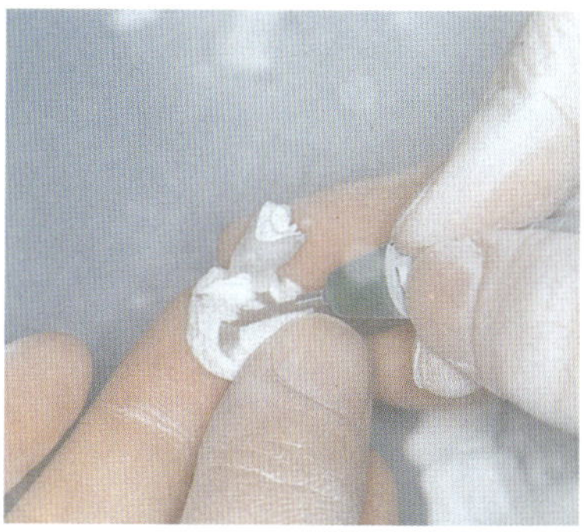

Fig. 6-71u Divest ceramic casting with aluminous oxide air abrasion.

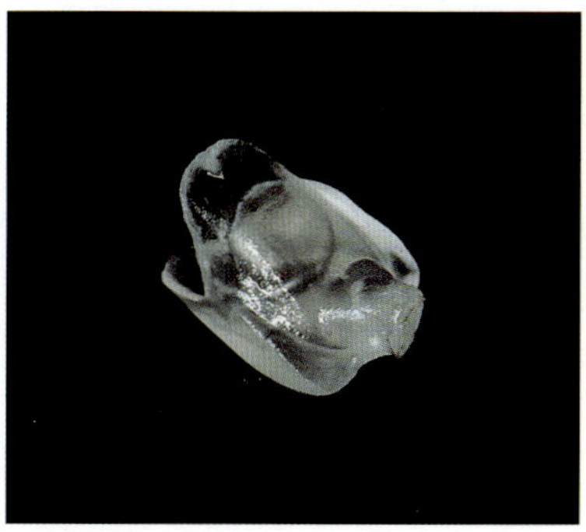

Fig. 6-71v Amorphous as cast ceramic coping.

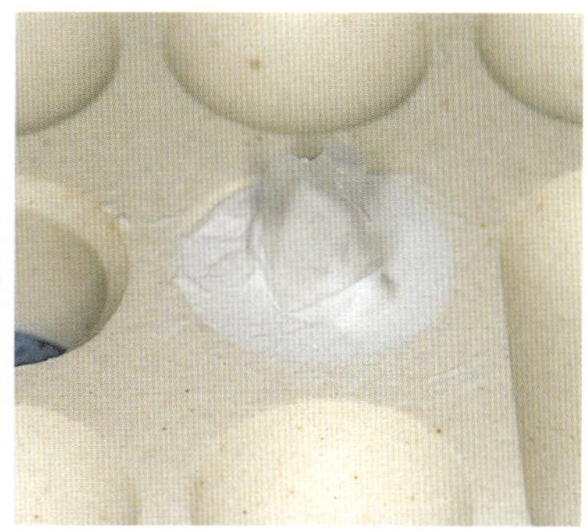

Fig. 6-71w Embedding the cast ceramic coping.

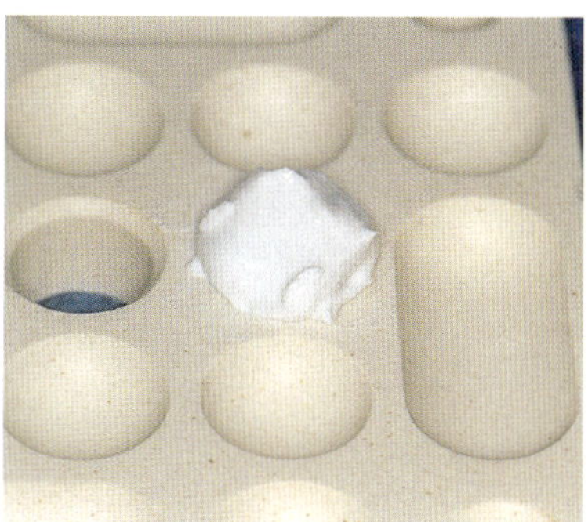

Fig. 6-71x Completely embedded coping.

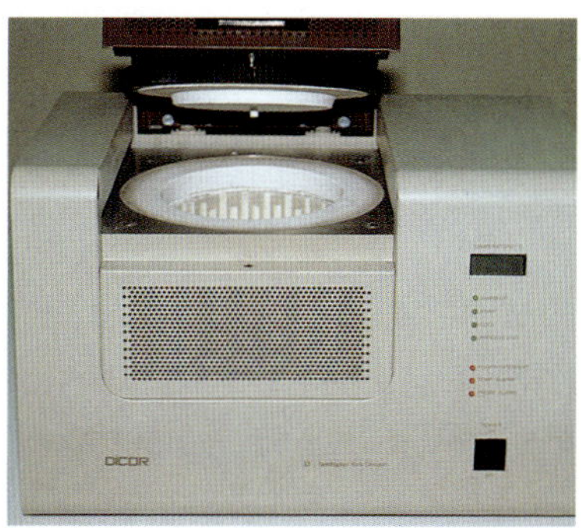

Fig. 6-71y Ceramming oven.

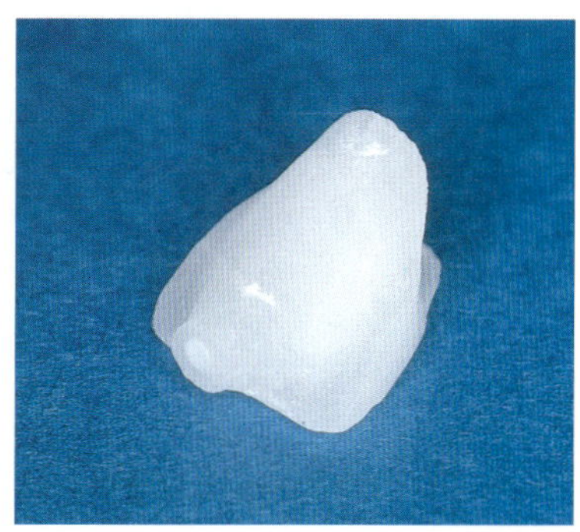

Fig. 6-71z Cerammed "crystallized" glass ceramic coping.

11. The core is cast per manufacturer's instructions (Fig. 6-71t).
12. After bench cooling the investment is pushed out of the metal ring and the core is carefully divested using air abrasion and aluminous oxide. Care must be taken to avoid the fragile margins (Fig. 6-71u).
13. The amorphous glass casting is inspected for bubbles or voids (Fig. 6-71v). In this state the glass is weak and transparent. It must be embedded in a special investment and run through a controlled thermal cycle called "ceramming" (Figs. 6-71w to y). The cerammed crown will now have a crystalline structure that will give it some opacity and a considerable

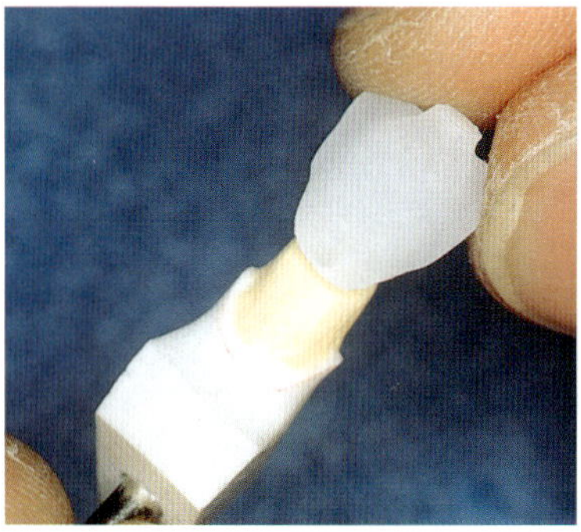

Fig. 6-71aa Seat coping on die.

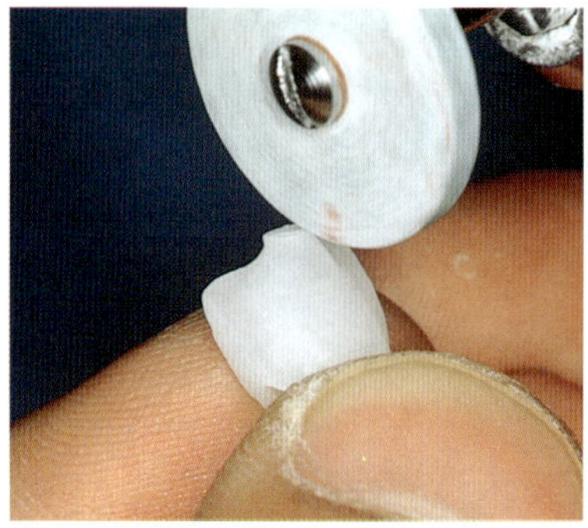

Fig. 6-71bb Adjust contour of coping.

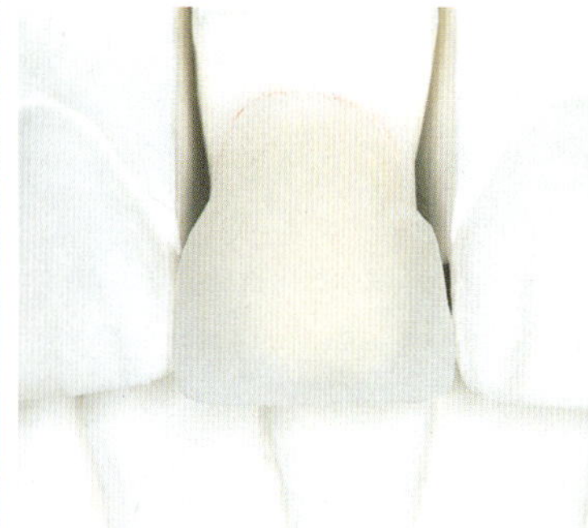

Fig. 6-71cc Final adjusted and seated glass ceramic coping.

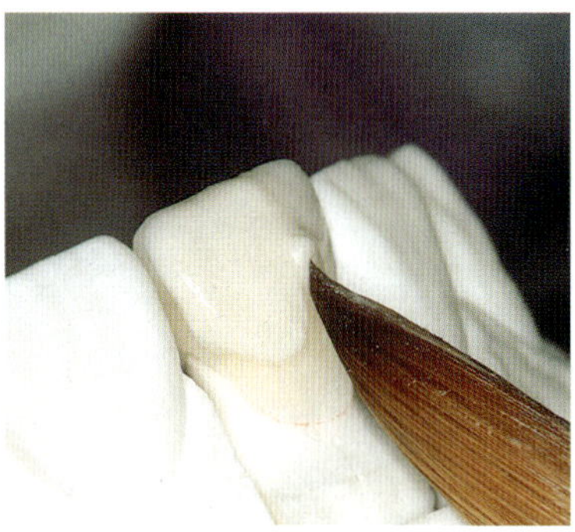

Fig. 6-71dd Apply conventional dentin ceramic materials.

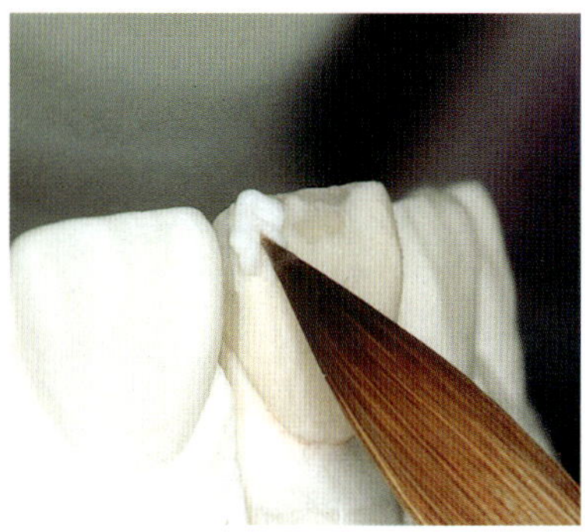

Fig. 6-71ee Apply incisal ceramic materials.

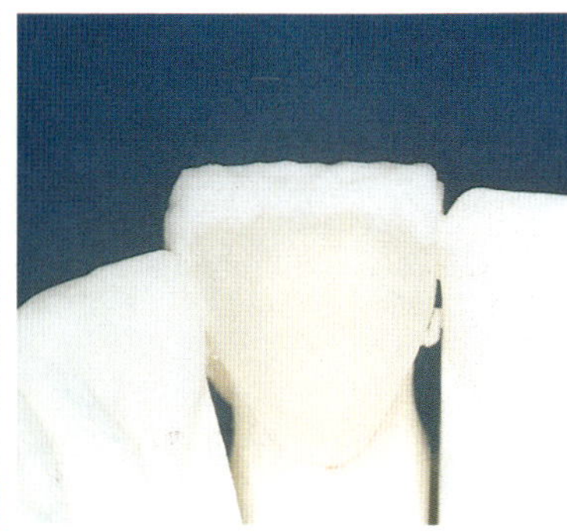

Fig. 6-71ff Overbuild conventional ceramic veneer to compensate for sintering shrinkage.

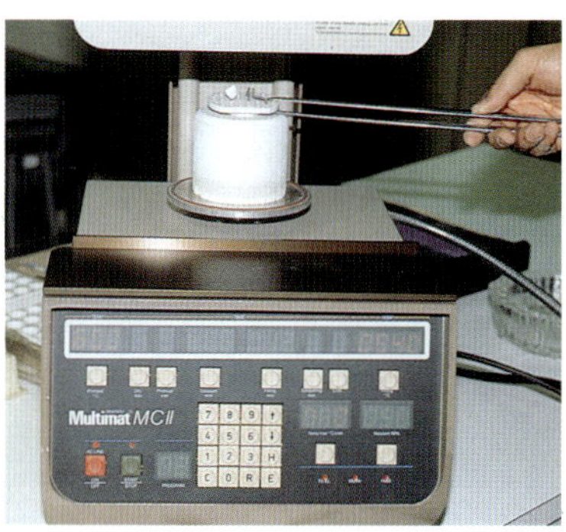

Fig. 6-71gg Sinter conventional ceramic veneer.

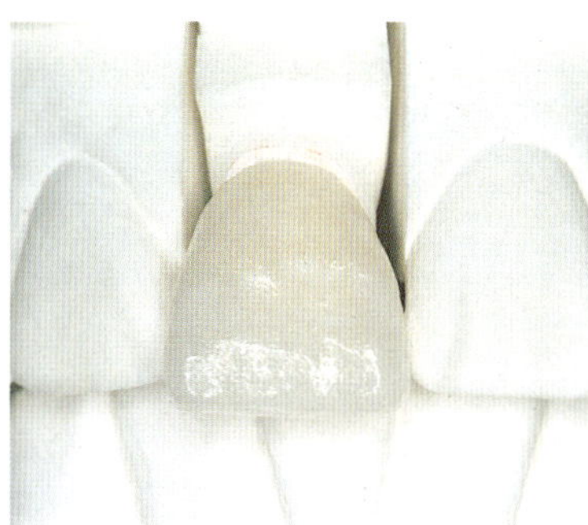

Fig. 6-71hh Contour on working model.

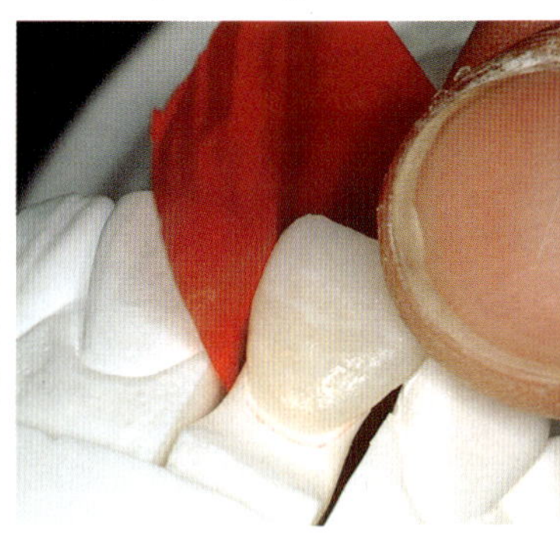

Fig. 6-71ii Mark proximal contacts.

increase in strength (Fig. 6-71z).

14. At this point the cast ceramic core is seated on the die and adjusted on the work model until the desired fit and contour is achieved (Figs. 6-71aa and bb).
15. The facial surface is sandblasted with aluminous oxide and ultrasonically or steam cleaned (Fig. 6-71cc). The facial veneer of conventional esthetic ceramic may now be added. A ceramic must be chosen that has a compatible coefficient of thermal expansion.
16. Body, incisal and modifier ceramic layers are added per esthetic demands (Figs. 6-71dd and ee). The crown should be slightly overcontoured to compensate

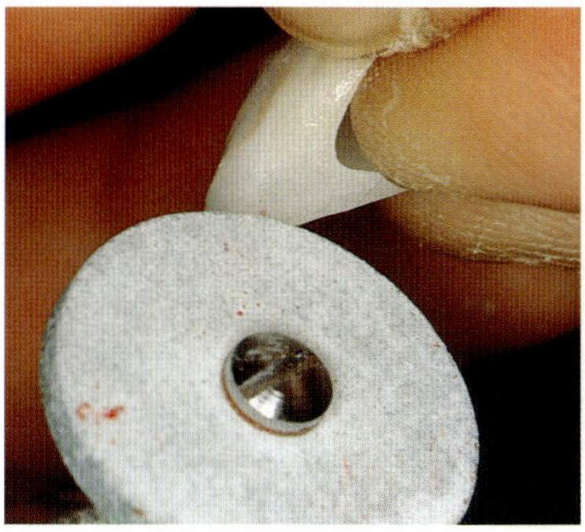

Fig. 6-71jj Adjust proximal contacts.

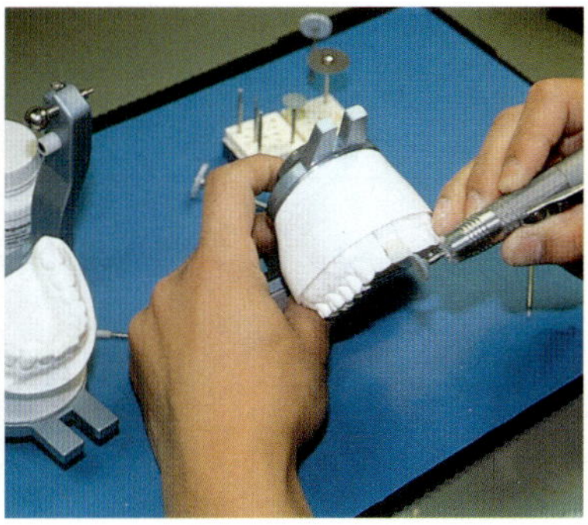

Fig. 6-71kk Finalize contours.

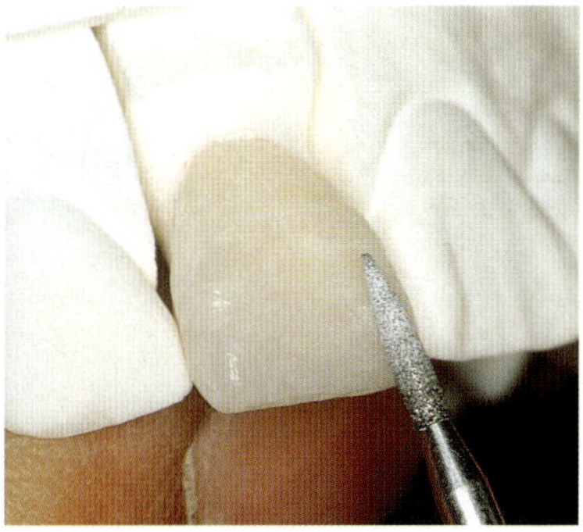

Fig. 6-71ll Finalize surface texture.

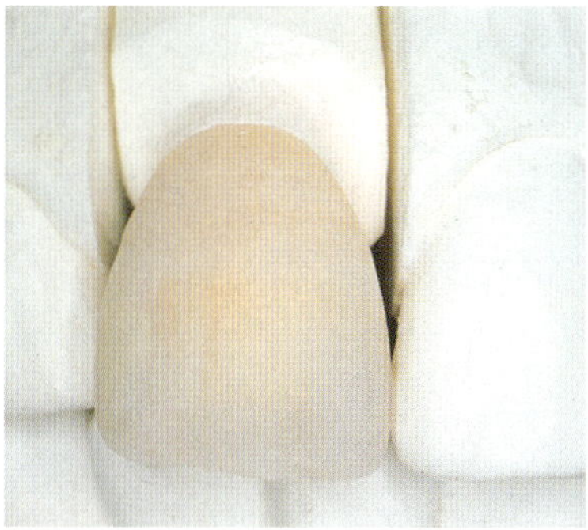

Fig. 6-71mm Clean finished crown.

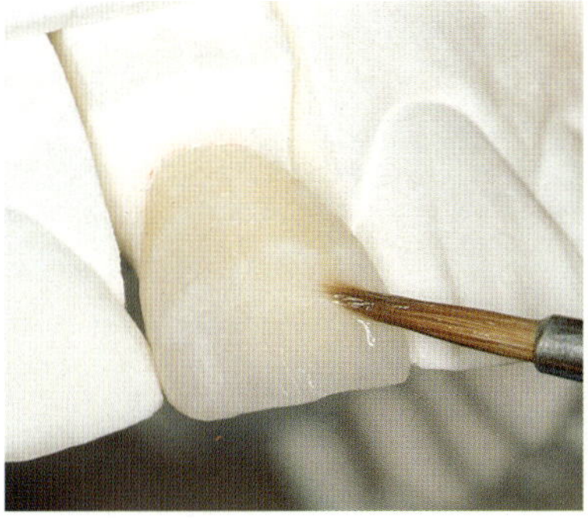

Fig. 6-71nn Apply extrinsic stains as needed for shade match.

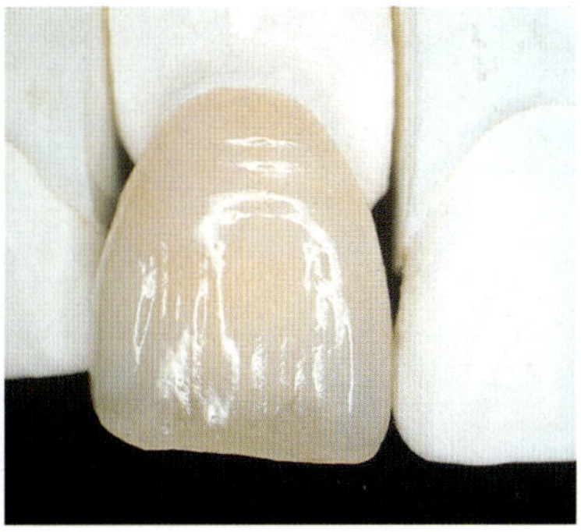

Fig. 6-71oo Finished crown.

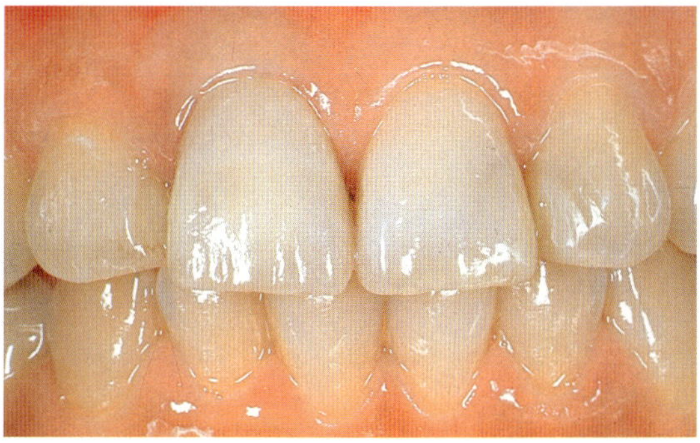

Fig. 6-71pp Glass ceramic core strengthened crown cemented.

for sintering shrinkage (Fig. 6-71ff).

17. The crown is run through the recommended thermal cycle, which is repeated as needed for ceramic additions (Fig. 6-71gg).
18. The full contour crown is first seated on the working model (Figs. 6-71hh and ii).
19. Contour and surface texture are finalized using diamond burs and ceramic stones (Figs. 6-71jj to ll).
20. The contoured crown is again cleaned and external shading ceramic stains may be used to finalize the desired esthetics (Figs. 6-71mm and nn). In situations where only the cast ceramic material is used, the external shading porcelain will provide all the chromatic characterizations.
21. The crown is run through the recommended thermal cycle to glaze the surface and fuse the ceramic colorants (Fig. 6-71oo).
22. The completed crown is delivered and final esthetic and functional adjustments are completed as previously described for a cast ceramic core strengthened all ceramic crown (Fig. 6-71pp).

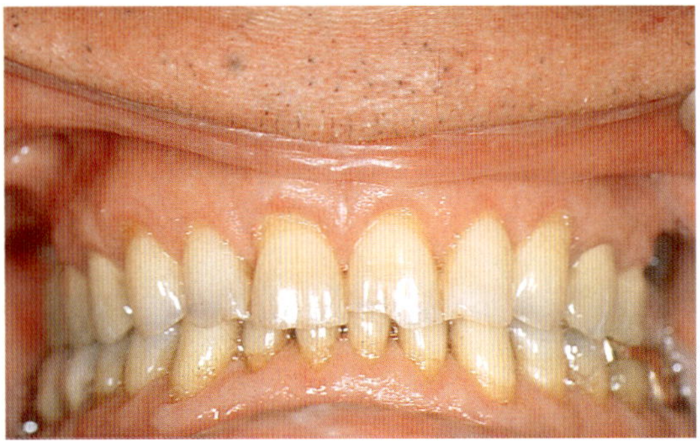

Fig. 6-72a Preoperative view.

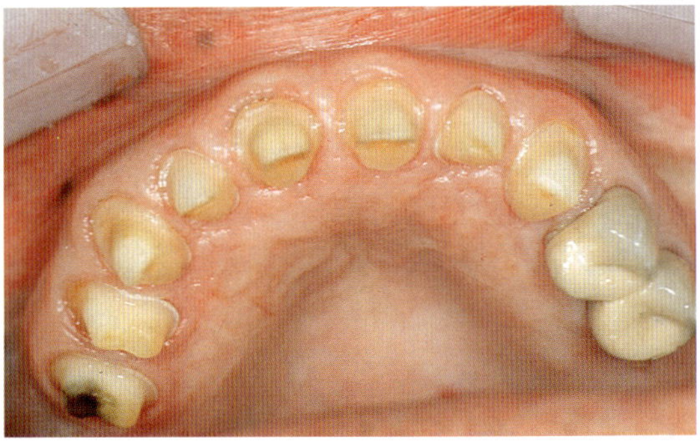

Fig. 6-72b Final preparations.

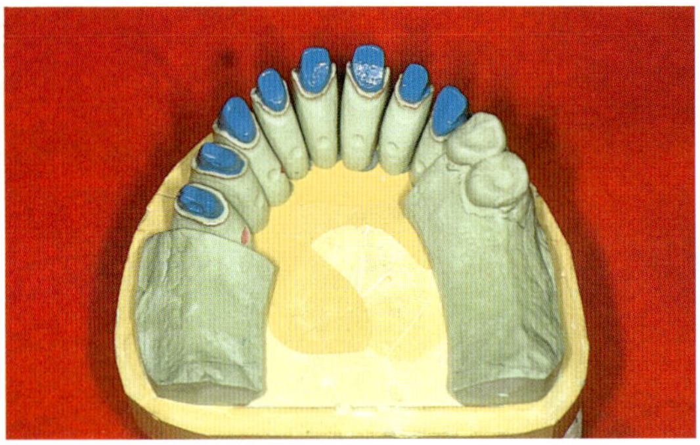

Fig. 6-72c Final stone working model.

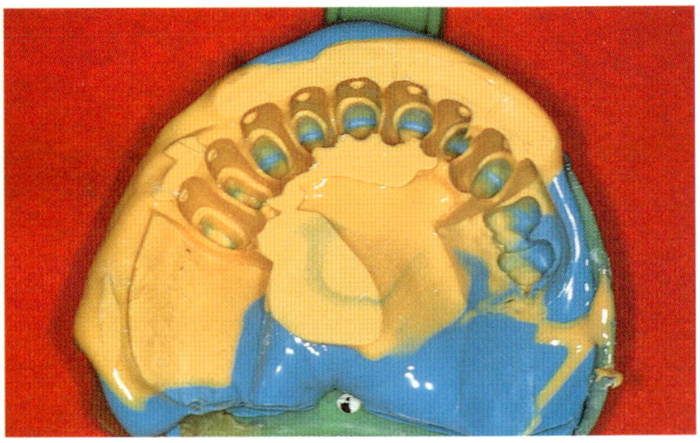

Fig. 6-72d Duplicating impression of working model.

In-Ceram Core Strengthened Crowns

1. Teeth are prepared with a 360° shoulder to the standard depth previously described (Figs. 6-72a and b).
2. Dies are fabricated, trimmed and die spacer is placed (Fig. 6-72c).
3. An impression of the master model is made and poured in the In-Ceram refractory material. The refractory dies are trimmed and finalized (Figs. 6-72d and e).
4. The slip-cast aluminous oxide core material is prepared per manufacturers instructions and adapted to the refractory die, shaped and run through the appropriate thermal cycle using a special In-Ceram oven (Figs. 6-72f to i).
5. The refractory die will shrink away from the sintered core (Figs. 6-72j and k).
6. The core at this point is soft and can be adjusted. Once acceptable the sintered aluminous oxide core is coated with the preselected color of infusion glass and run through a second thermal cycle (Figs. 6-72l and m).
7. The In-Ceram is now at its maximum strength and final seating and adjustment in the die is accomplished (Figs. 6-72n and o).
8. Veneering ceramic is added as previously described (Fig. 6-72p) and the crown is finalized clinically as are other aluminous oxide core strengthened crowns (Figs. 6-72q and r).

(Note: Figs. 6-72a to r are courtesy of Dr. Seung Koo Kang, D.M.D., Seoul, Korea, Former Postgraduate Prosthodontics, UCLA.)

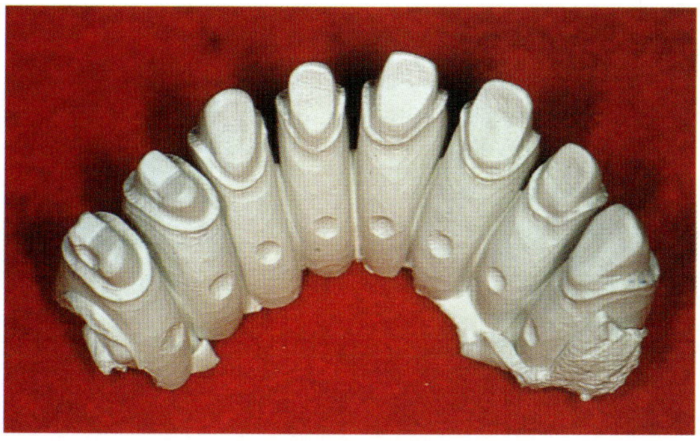

Fig. 6-72e In-Ceram refractory dies made in duplicating impression.

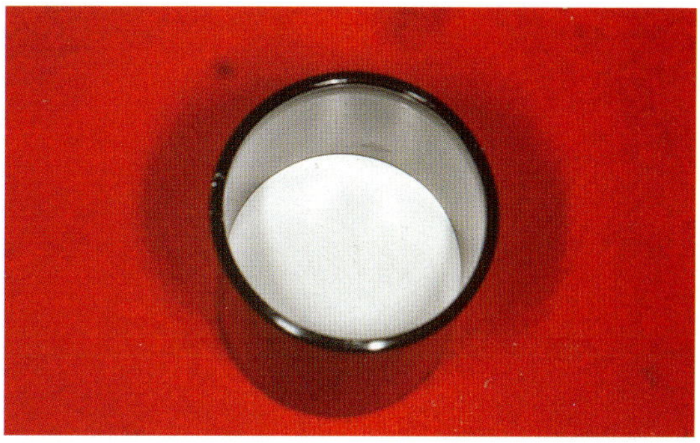

Fig. 6-72f In-Ceram material.

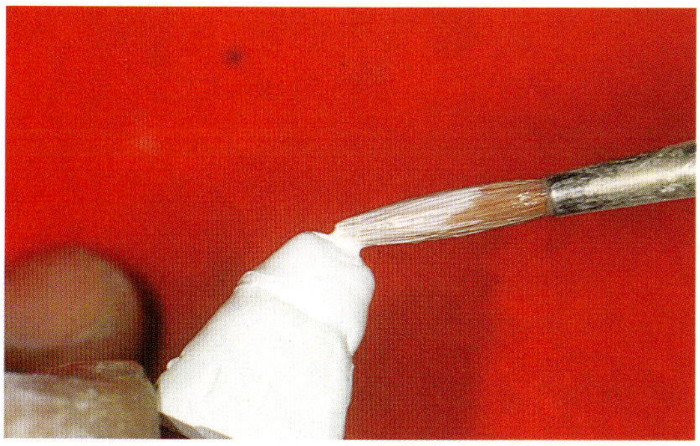

Fig. 6-72g

Fig. 6-72g Apply prepared In-Ceram material to special refractory die(s).

Fig. 6-72h All refractory dies coated with In-Ceram.

Fig. 6-72i Sinter In-Ceram in ceramic oven.

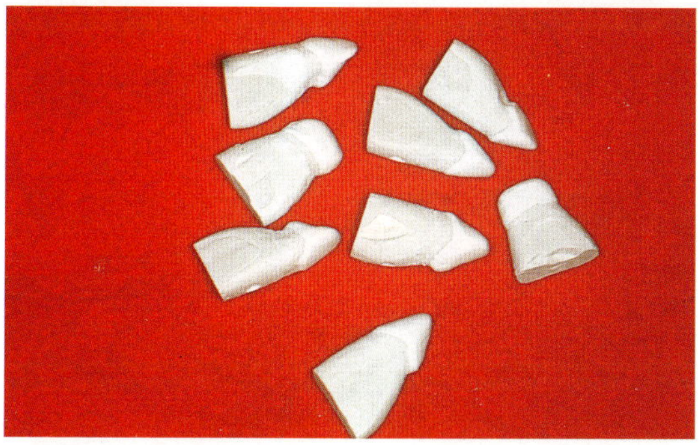

Fig. 6-72h

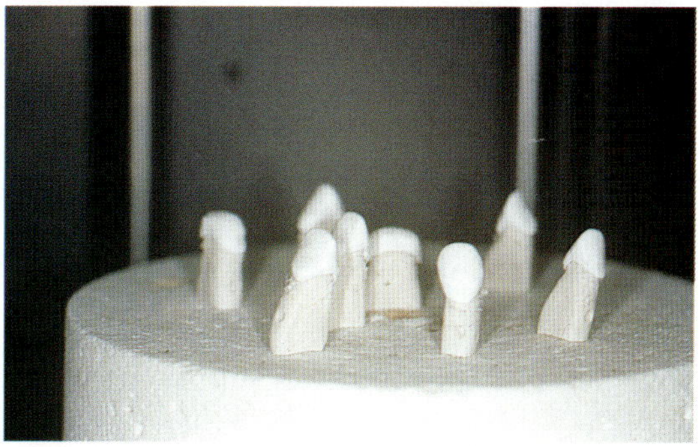

Fig. 6-72i

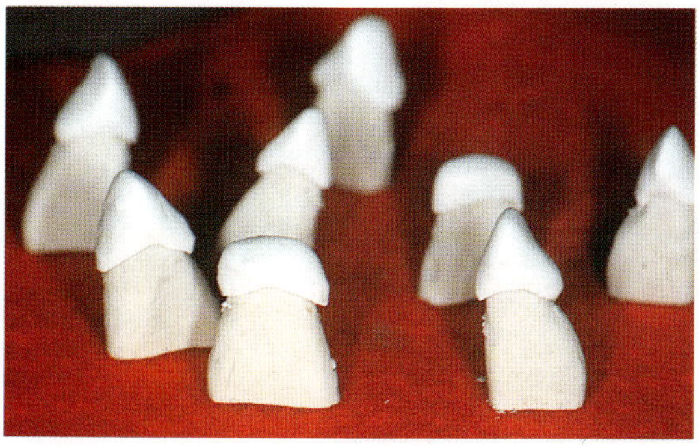

Fig. 6-72j Note how In-Ceram refractory shrinks away from In-Ceram coping.

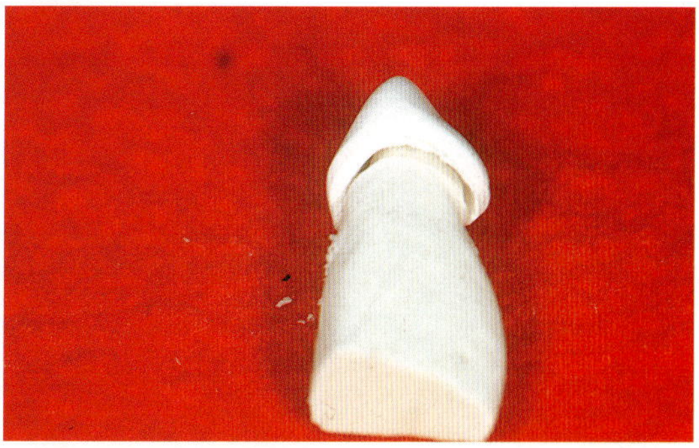

Fig. 6-72k Smaller dies allow for easy removal.

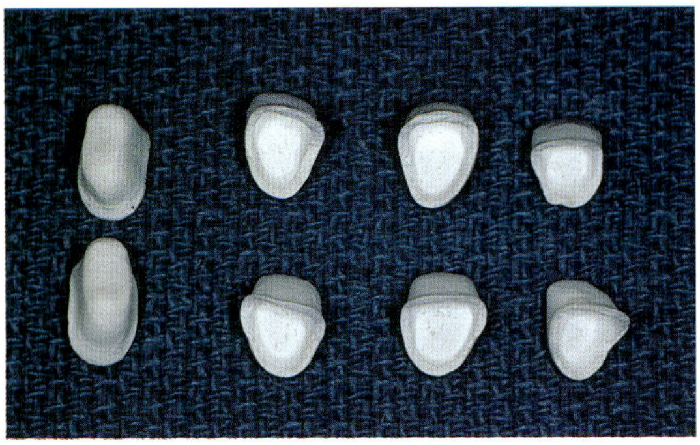

Fig. 6-72l Sintered and adjusted coping.

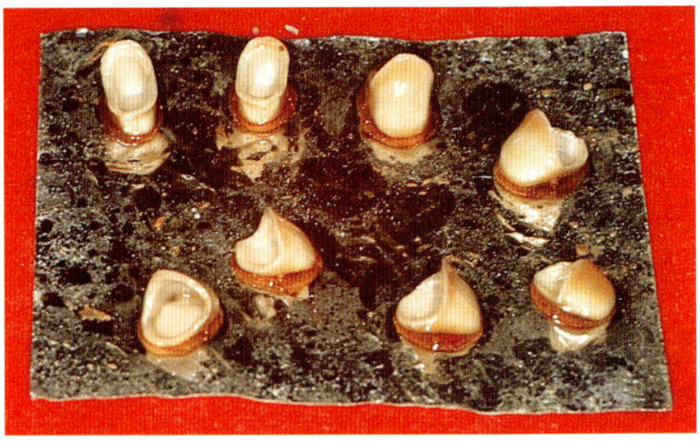

Fig. 6-72m Infusion glass fused to coping.

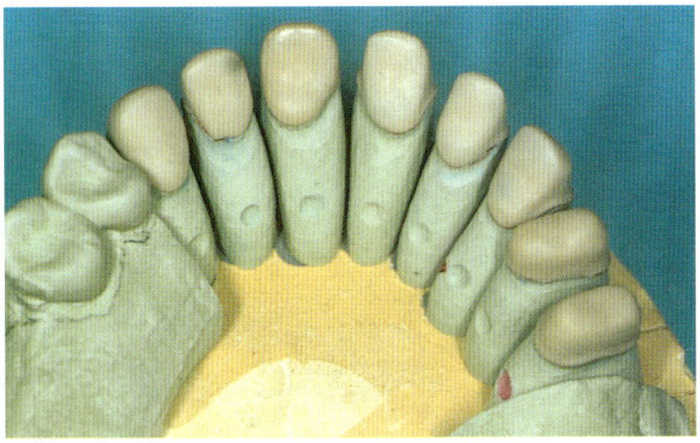

Fig. 6-72n Occlusal view of finished In-Ceram coping.

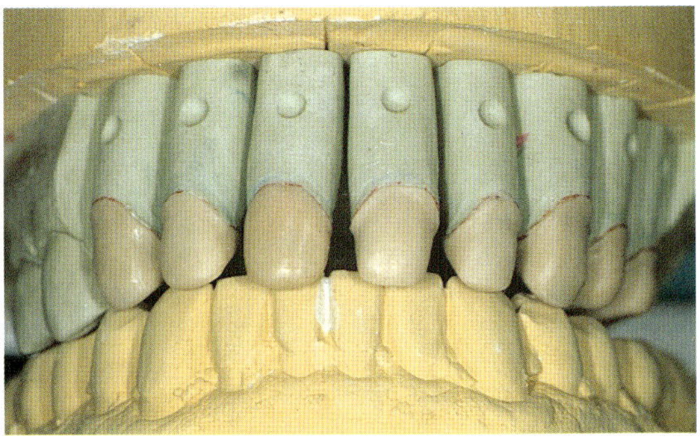

Fig. 6-72o Facial view of adjusted In-Ceram coping.

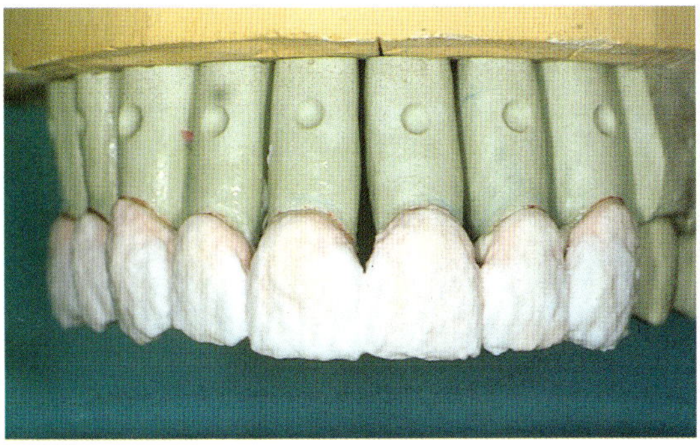

Fig. 6-72p Conventional ceramic veneer application.

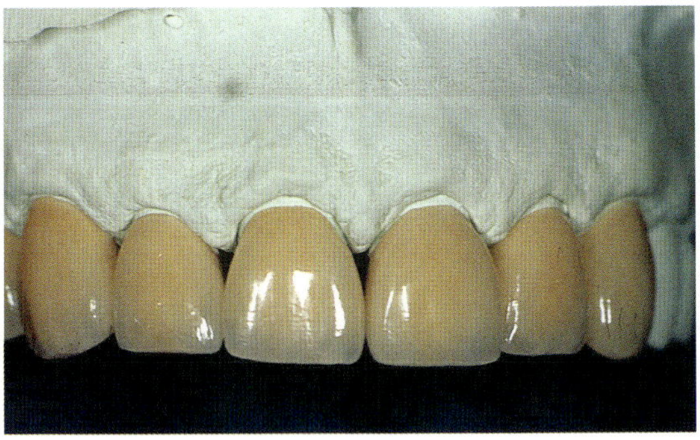

Fig. 6-72q Finished crowns.

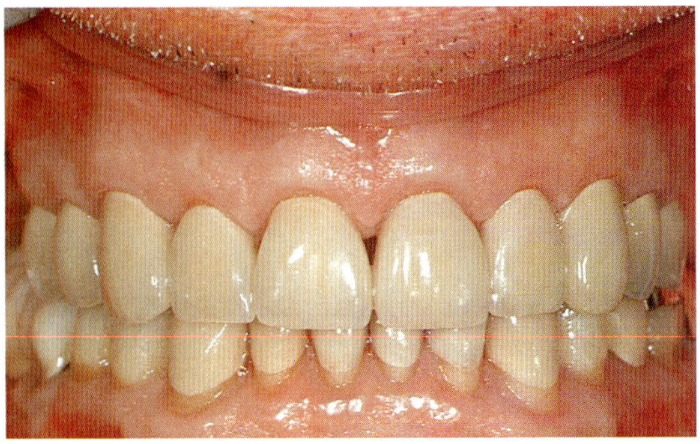

Fig. 6-72r Postoperative view of In-Ceram crowns.

CERAMIC INLAYS AND ONLAYS

INTRODUCTION

The use of ceramic materials for the fabrication of inlays is not new in dentistry. The technology for the fabrication of ceramic inlays using refractory die materials has been available for decades. Early ceramic inlays provided esthetic restorations but the marginal integrity was not comparable to that of cast metallic inlays. Luting cements available at the time, such as zinc phosphate, washed out of these marginal discrepancies relatively quickly and often discolored. In addition, the luting cements did not provide any bond to the tooth or to the inlay so retention was primarily mechanical and thin areas on the inlay were vulnerable to fracture. The clinical results over time were disappointing and ceramic inlays were rarely used.

In the early to mid 1980s, ceramic etching and composite resin bonding techniques provided the key to a predictable bond of ceramic materials to teeth. Retention is significantly enhanced by these techniques and the problem of maintaining marginal seal is significantly reduced using less soluble and more wear resistant composite materials. Laboratory studies have shown that bonded ceramic inlays have the potential to increase the strength of prepared teeth to values similar to those of unprepared teeth. While problems exist and improvements are still needed, ceramic inlays have become a very esthetic and successful addition to the armamentarium of the esthetic restorative dentist.

Margin Controversy

The marginal fit of ceramic inlay/onlay restorations compared to that of cast metallic alternatives is a point of disappointment and controversy among restorative dentists and technicians. For decades the standard of excellence has largely been based upon margins with an approximate marginal discrepancy in the 25- to 50-μm range. Our goals should still include obtaining the most accurate marginal fit possible, but is longitudinal success of bonded ceramic inlays still contingent on achieving this goal?

The need to have closely adapted margins when using luting cements is critical because these cements are vulnerable to washout, staining and microleakage (Fig. 6-73). Most of our traditional margin philosophies are based on the use of this type of cement.

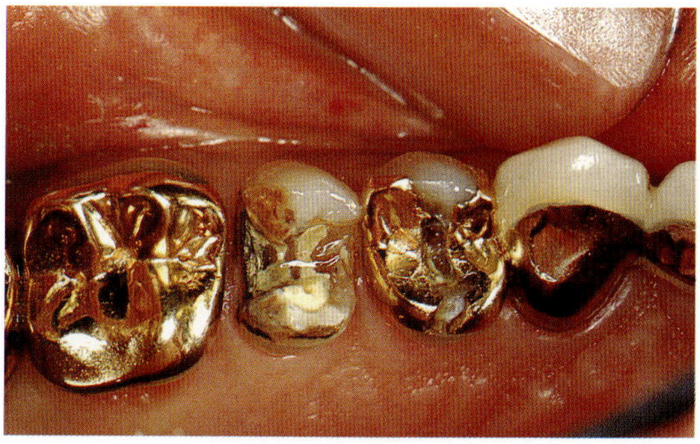

Fig. 6-73 Microleakage under a removed gold onlay.

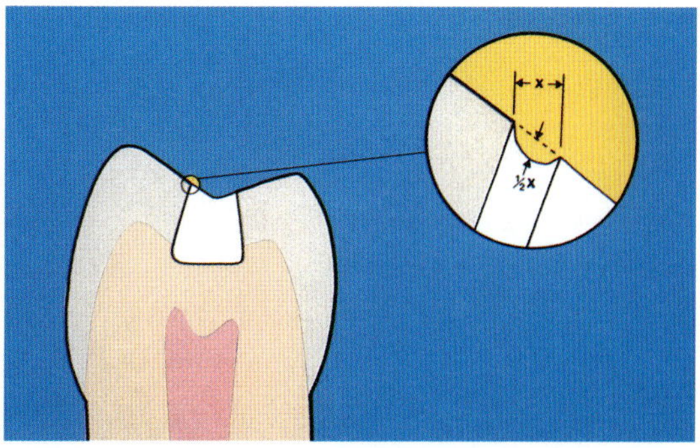

Fig. 6-74 Wear of the marginal composite resin cement forms a self-limiting meniscus about half as deep as the marginal width.

Consequently most practicing dentists today have been educated in this concept of marginal adaptation as a standard of excellence and anything less is considered a clinical compromise. A negative reaction is understandable when one looks at a ceramic inlay or onlay with a marginal void of 100 to 200 μm.

Successful ceramic inlay/onlay restorations require the use of composite resin cements and the application of modern bonding techniques to the various substrates. These cements effectively bond the ceramic/tooth complex together, do not wash out like luting cements, and have a greater potential to minimize marginal microleakage. The tooth is strengthened by the restoration and conversely the restoration is significantly strengthened by bonding to tooth structure. What is the significance of larger marginal discrepancies when using composite resin cement and bonding technologies? In areas of minimal wear or abrasion potential, the loss of resin cement is minimal. In areas of occlusal function, wear occurs more quickly and a concavity between the restoration and the tooth forms as the resin cement wears out. Wear resistance of these composite cements needs to be improved. But what is the consequence of this wear? In a study done at the University of Alabama, it was shown that the depth of the concavity formed as the cement is worn away reached approximately 50% of the width of the marginal discrepancy and seemed to stabilize (Fig. 6-74). While margins become detectable with an explorer and our first reaction is negative, in reality the consequence appears to be minimal. The concavity formed is self-limiting, and microleakage is minimal on enamel and significantly improved on other substrates. The bonds to tooth and restoration appear to be maintained and progressive deterioration of the inlay/onlay appears no greater than that of other restorations.

Additional clinical research is needed to fully substantiate the long term success of bonded ceramic inlays and onlays. Bonded ceramic inlays and onlays provide conservative esthetic restorations that restore structural strength to the tooth. Marginal adaptation alone should not totally eliminate this treatment alternative from our list of procedures.

ANALYZING MATERIAL ALTERNATIVES

There are many materials available for the fabrication of posterior esthetic restorations. However, there is no single material that satisfies all criteria and demands made by the dentist and patient. The process of selecting the most appropriate esthetic restorative material involves an analysis of treatment priorities, the patient's attitudes and the dentist's commitment to procedural demands. Through understanding these factors, materials that are optimal for each individual situation can be selected. In this section, a brief analysis of some of the strengths and weaknesses of a variety of esthetic posterior restorative materials will be presented and a comparison made between various composite and ceramic alternatives.

One Appointment Alternatives

1. **Directly Filled Composite Restoration** (See chapter 4).

Strengths
- Lowest initial cost.
- Less abrasion potential to opposing teeth than ceramic.
- Esthetic results excellent.
- Easier to finish than ceramic.
- Many materials to select from.

Weaknesses
- Wears faster than ceramic.
- Material less stable than ceramic.
- Demanding techniques with significant potential for operator error.
- Not recommended for large occlusion supporting restorations.

2. Direct or Direct/Indirect Composite Inlays (See chapter 5)

Strengths
- Lower cost than indirect restorations.
- Less abrasion potential than ceramic.
- Excellent esthetic results.
- Easier to finish than ceramic.
- Many material options.
- Physical properties of composite enhanced.
- Compensates for composite shrinkage.

Weaknesses
- Wears faster than ceramic.
- Material less stable than ceramic.
- Increased cost over direct filled.
- Requires greater operator skill than indirect restorations.
- Special equipment may be required.

3. CAD-CAM or Copy Milled Ceramic Restorations

Strengths
- Only one appointment ceramic restoration available.
- Potentially can use a greater range of materials.
- Ceramic materials available are superior to laboratory processed ceramics.
- Same advantages of ceramic as outlined in next sections.

Weaknesses
- Training required, varies for each system.
- Cost of equipment high.
- Same disadvantages of ceramic as outlined in next sections.

Two Appointment Alternatives

1. Indirect Composite Restorations

Strengths
- Quality enhanced by skilled technicians.
- Physical properties enhanced over other composites.
- Esthetic results excellent.
- Less abrasive than ceramic.
- Easier to finish intraorally than ceramic.
- Repairable.
- More successful in larger restorations than direct filled composite.
- Many material and technique selections.

Weaknesses
- Indirect restorations require higher costs.
- Requires laboratory procedures.
- Wears faster than ceramic.
- Less stable than ceramic.
- May require special equipment.
- Difficult to modify extrinsic color chairside.

2. Indirect Ceramic Restorations (Conventional ceramic, strengthened ceramic or glass ceramic)

Strengths
- Quality controlled by technician.
- Esthetic.
- More stable than composite.
- Wears slower than composite.
- Can modify esthetics using ceramic stains.
- Many materials and techniques to select from.
- Successful in larger restorations.

Weaknesses
- Indirect restoration require highest cost.
- Requires laboratory procedures.
- More abrasive to opposing teeth than composite.
- Harder to finish and polish intraorally than composite.
- Requires more meticulous finishing than composite if roughened.
- Requires special equipment.

ANALYZING CERAMIC ALTERNATIVES

While ceramic inlays/onlays as a group have many common advantages and disadvantages, specific ceramic types have individual advantages and disadvantages. This section will analyze the main ceramic alternatives individually and present their strengths and weaknesses.

Four main ceramic groups will be analyzed: (1) conventional ceramic, (2) strengthened ceramic, (3) core strengthened ceramic and finally (4) glass ceramic alternatives.

1. **Conventional ceramic** is defined as that group of ceramic materials used to veneer metal substructures or strengthened ceramic cores. This group is often used to fabricate porcelain veneers, inlays or onlays. This group of ceramic materials has the lowest fracture strength and generally would require some means to increase its strength to provide a predictable intraoral restoration.

Strengths
- Very esthetic.
- Many ceramic choices.
- Easily fabricated on refractory dies.
- Readily available in most dental labs.

Weaknesses
- Weakest ceramic.
- Requires low temperature stains for extrinsic shade alteration.
- Abrasive to opposing teeth.
- Requires meticulous intraoral finishing techniques to smooth.

2. **Strengthened ceramic** materials are those that claim to have increased strength over conventional ceramic materials and are strengthened throughout the entire restorations.

Strengths
- Stronger than conventional ceramics.
- Good esthetics.
- Fabrication similar to conventional ceramics.
- No special equipment.

Weaknesses
- Esthetic range and material availability limited compared to conventional ceramics.
- Requires low temperature stains for extrinsic shade alteration.
- Abrasive to opposing teeth.
- Requires meticulous intraoral finishing techniques to smooth.

3. **Core strengthened ceramic** restorations require a high strength core made from a ceramic containing a high concentration of aluminous oxide or magnesium oxide. These core materials provide additional strength to the conventional ceramic veneer that is used as the esthetic component.

Strengths
- Potentially stronger than conventional ceramic.
- Good esthetics.
- Higher temperature stains may be used if the core extends to the margins (often not the case with inlays).

Weaknesses
- Limited space for core material in many inlays and onlays.
- Requires additional fabrication steps.
- Core materials cannot be etched.
- Opaque cores may limit translucency.
- Core abrasive to opposing teeth if exposed.
- Requires meticulous intraoral finishing.

4. **Glass ceramic** alternatives are available using five fabrication techniques. These are cast, injection molding, CAD-CAM, copy milling and prefabricated glass ceramic insets or macrofillers. While these five technique-material combinations produce restorations technically in the classification of glass ceramics, they are quite different in many ways and will be analyzed separately.

A. **Cast glass ceramic** (Dicor) is probably the best known glass ceramic and its unique fabrication technique has not been commercially duplicated. It has special characteristics and physical properties that make this material different from most other ceramic alternatives used for inlay/onlay restorations.

Strengths
- Lost wax-casting fabrication techniques allow for easy morphology control.
- The material wears opposing dentition less than most other ceramic materials.
- Easier to polish than conventional and strengthened ceramic.
- Glazed proximal surfaces are very smooth and resistant to plaque accumulation.
- Good esthetics and translucency allow surrounding tooth color to penetrate the restoration.
- Stronger than conventional ceramics.
- Can use high temperature ceramic stains without investing.

Weaknesses
- Equipment expensive.
- Requires staining or veneering with a conventional ceramic for color modification of the ceramic.
- Superficial colorants are not advised for occlusal surfaces of inlays due to the need for postcementation adjustment of the margins and increased abrasion potential.
- Greater bulk of restorative material in some restorations decreases the chameleon effect and esthetic result.
- Etched surfaces may have slightly lower bond strength to composite cements than other ceramics.
- Available in only one shade.

B. **Injection molded glass ceramic** (IPS Empress) is a new and unique material and technique for the fabrication of single unit all ceramic restorations. This system also uses a lost wax process but the ceramic is forced into the investment mold using a ceramic plunger in a temperature controlled oven.

Strengths
- Lost wax fabrication process allows for easy control of morphology.
- Precerammed (eliminates crystallization step).
- Available in a range of colors.
- Stronger than conventional ceramics.
- Good esthetic potential.
- Can use high temperature ceramic stains.
- Less wear potential than conventional and strengthened ceramics.

Weaknesses
- New with minimal testing.
- Color modification of the injection molded restoration require extrinsic staining or veneering with conventional ceramic.
- Requires expensive equipment.

C, D. **CAD-CAM and copy milled materials** have been developed as a result of new fabrication methods for making ceramic restorations. Because the restoration is milled out of a piece of ceramic that is premanufactured, there is the elimination of many laboratory technique variables and handling modifications. Ceramic manufacturers have been able to produce ceramic materials that have improved properties.

Dicor MGC® (Caulk, Milford, Delaware) is an improved Dicor glass ceramic that has greater strength, comes in colors and has less porosity compared to cast Dicor.

Vita Mark II® and Celay Ceramic Blanks (Vident, Baldwin Park) are an improvement over other conventional ceramic materials. Its controlled manufacturing techniques provide a dense material and its fine particle size produces a ceramic material that has a wear potential similar to glass ceramic.

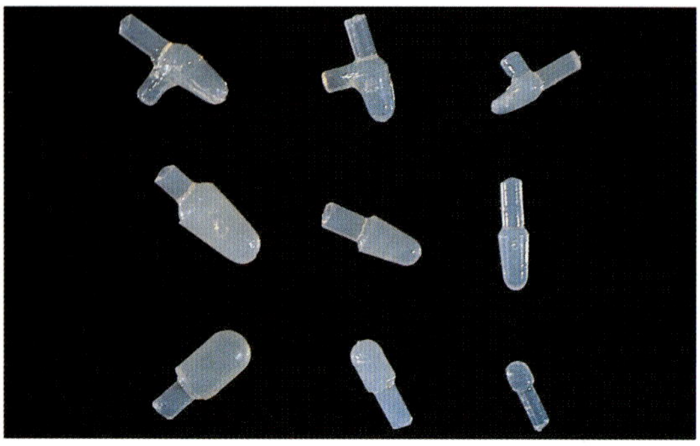

Fig. 6-75 Ceramic inserts.

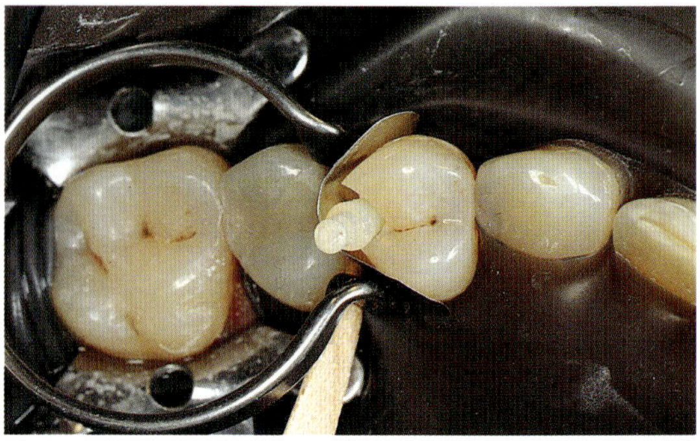

Fig. 6-76a Ceramic insert positioned in preparation.

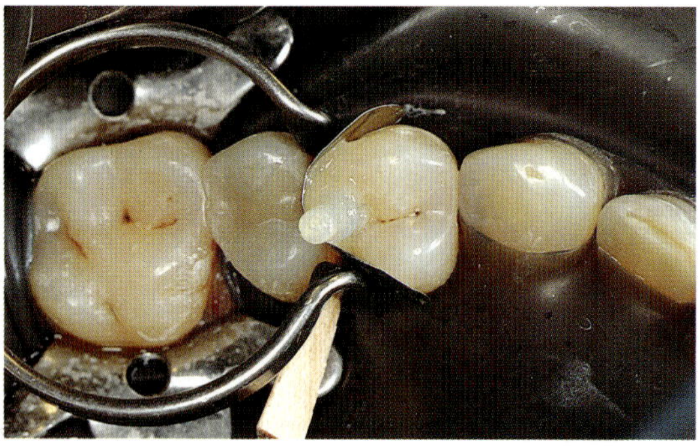

Fig. 6-76b Ceramic insert incorporated into posterior composite restoration.

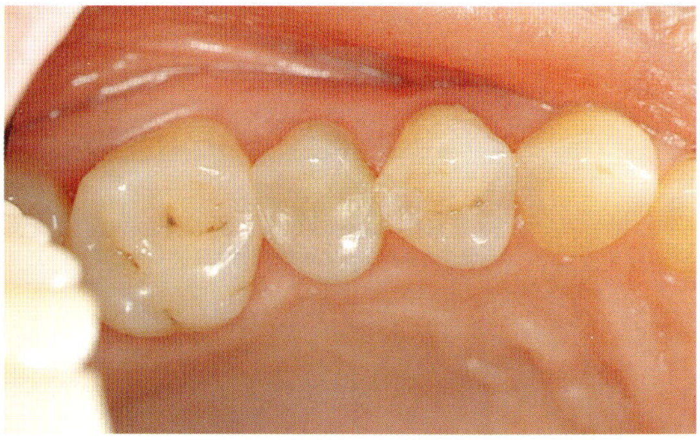

Fig. 6-76c Final restoration.

Disadvantages of these materials are that their utilization requires a special CAD-CAM or copy milling system.

E. **Glass ceramic inserts** or "mega fillers" Beta quarts inserts (Lee Pharmaceuticals, El Monte, CA.) have been developed to provide an intermediate type of restoration between a pure composite and ceramic. Various sized presilanated glass ceramic inserts can be inserted into the composite mass during placement and they become a part of the restoration (Figs. 6-75 and 6-76).

Advantages
- Displaces composite resin volume so there is less cumulative polymerization shrinkage.
- Improves overall properties of restoration.
- Minimizes curing increments.
- Translucency conducts light to deep areas during curing.
- Condenses adjacent composite materials.

Disadvantages
- New with minimal testing.
- Finishing different substrates requires technique modifications.

CLINICAL TECHNIQUES

Preparation

The preparation designs for many ceramic inlays/onlays are based upon the classic amalgam or gold inlay/onlay preparations originally developed by G.V. Black because in many instances, we are replacing traditionally prepared metallic restorations. Classical preparation designs are used in many instances. Contemporary preparations are possible when no previous restoration exist.

Design factors for ceramic inlays/onlays should be dictated by factors that will minimize potential problems. For instance, cavosurface bevels are generally not recommended for ceramic inlays because they are more difficult to fabricate and if successfully fabricated would be vulnerable to fracture during the seating and cementation process. Depth and width of the occlusal isthmus are usually determined by the bulk of ceramic needed to allow for easy fabrication and cementation with minimal fractures.

Studies have shown that ceramic restorations without adequate bulk are more prone to fracture functional areas. The preparation for a ceramic inlay/onlay must (1) remove diseased tooth structure and replace deficient or missing areas, (2) provide adequate retentive surfaces and (3) provide for adequate bulk of material for fabrication, cementation and to resist functional stresses. A variety of preparation designs that have worked successfully will be discussed in the following section.

Occlusal Isthmus Design

Armamentarium:

(1) Tapered fissure carbide bur or diamond

(2) End cutting diamond (Fig. 6-77)

The occlusal surface should be prepared to provide a cavosurface margin in sound enamel. The sound enamel width will vary but should be at least 1 mm in width. The pulpal floor should be 1.5 to 2 mm deep to provide adequate bulk for fabrication (Fig. 6-78). At the inlay cementation appointment any remaining caries or old filling material should be removed and is filled in with cement (Fig. 6-79). This will minimize unnecessary overextension. In situations where caries is extensive and/or an old restoration falls out, deep pulpal areas or undercuts in the occlusal walls may exist (Fig. 6-80). In these situations the deep caries or questionable existing restoration should be removed to ensure that an adequate amount of sound tooth structure exists. Placing a fluoride-releasing base is advisable (Fig. 6-81). This will block out undercuts, minimize die irregularities and simplify the inlay fabrication. During the cementation procedure several options exist. It is advisable to leave the fluoride-releasing base material in areas closest to the pulp. This will ensure a second line of defense against bacterial invasion should microleakage occur in the future. The fluoride-releasing base material should be removed from the undercuts in the occlusal walls if it is not as strong as the material used to bond in the ceramic inlay (Fig. 6-82).

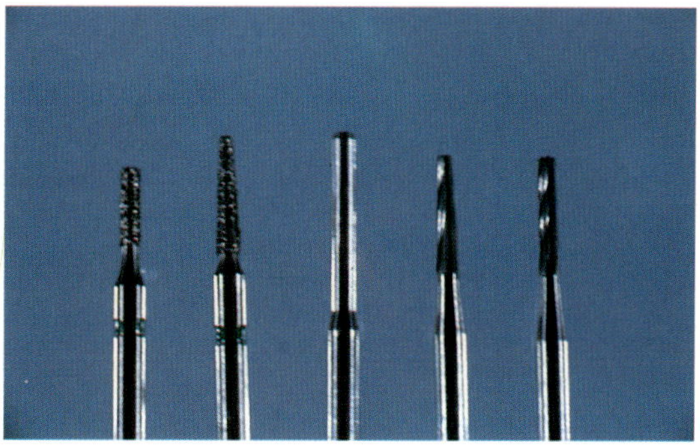

Fig. 6-77 Burs used for inlay/onlay preparation (end cutting diamond center).

Another option would be to simply block out deep areas or undercuts on the die. The use of bonding agents and cement alone may seal the tooth-restoration margins adequately to resist microleakage. This may

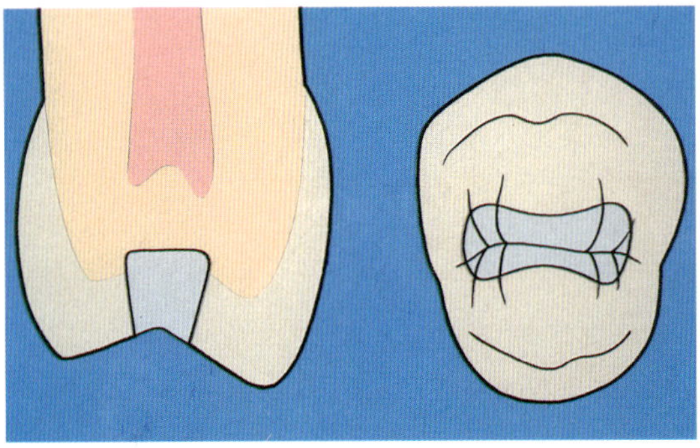

Fig. 6-78a Preoperative view.

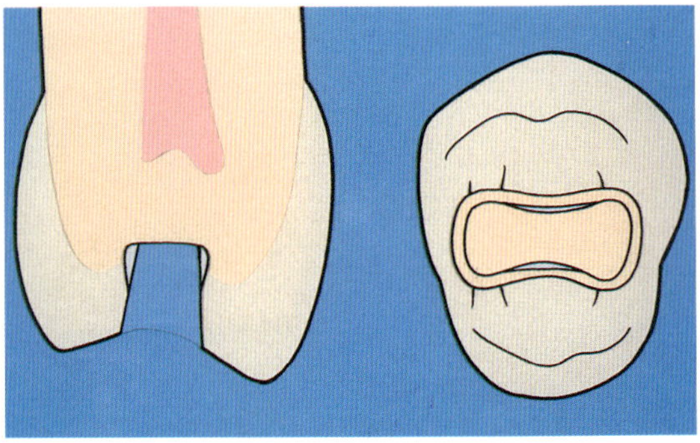

Fig. 6-78b Occlusal isthmus preparation; small amounts of the previous restoration can be left.

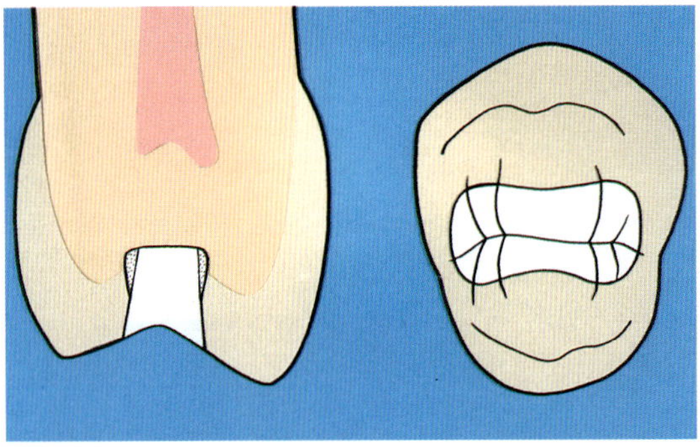

Fig. 6-79 Small amounts of the old restoration are removed before inlay cementation and filled with cement.

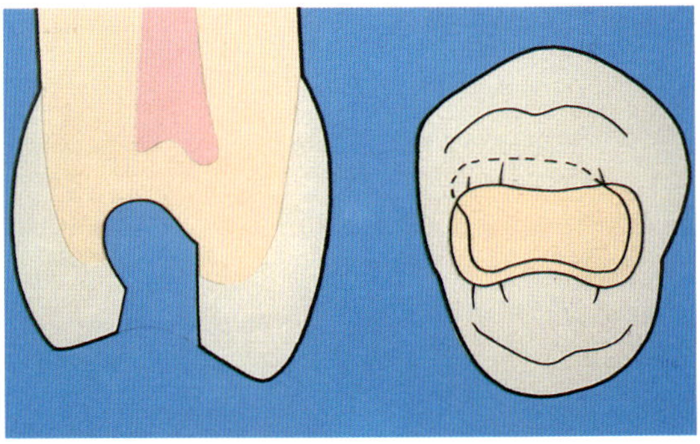

Fig. 6-80 Deep caries removal.

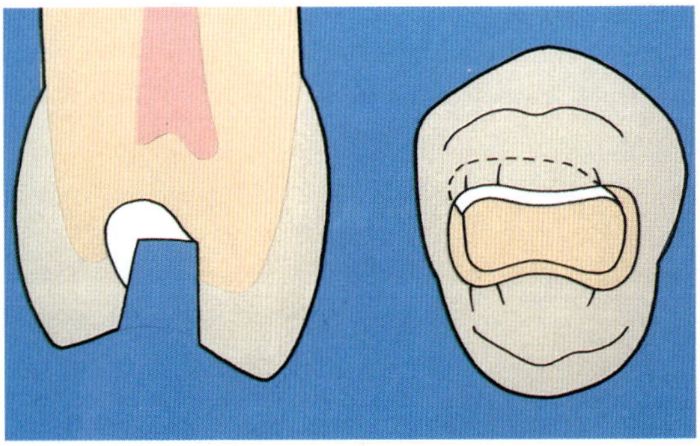

Fig. 6-81 Fill with fluoride-releasing base.

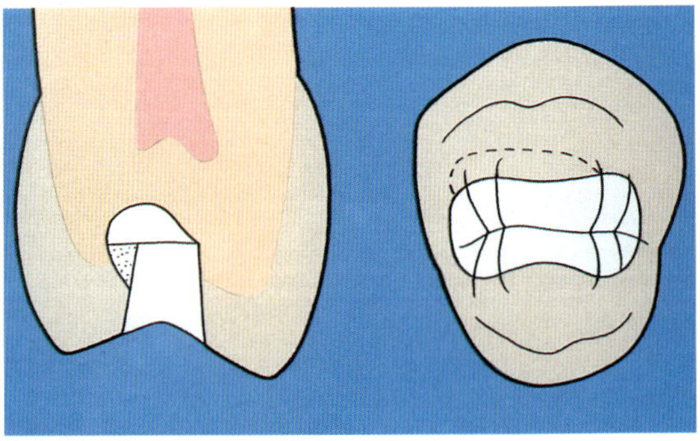

Fig. 6-82 Prior to inlay cementation, remove base and fill with the stronger composite cement.

prove sufficient in occlusal inlays or other preparations with enamel on all the cavosurface margins. Whenever there is a possibility of microleakage, use of a fluoride-releasing base to protect deep areas near a vital pulp is advisable.

The final step in finishing the occlusal portion of the preparation is to use an end cutting diamond to smooth the pulpal floor. This step simplifies fabrication by minimizing the need to block out rough dies and reduces the potential need to adjust irregular inlays during the delivery appointment. Smooth, well finished preparations are advisable for all ceramic inlays.

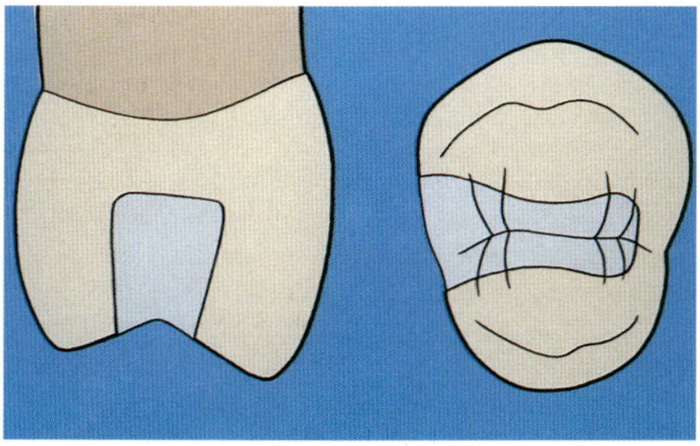

Fig. 6-83 Preoperative view.

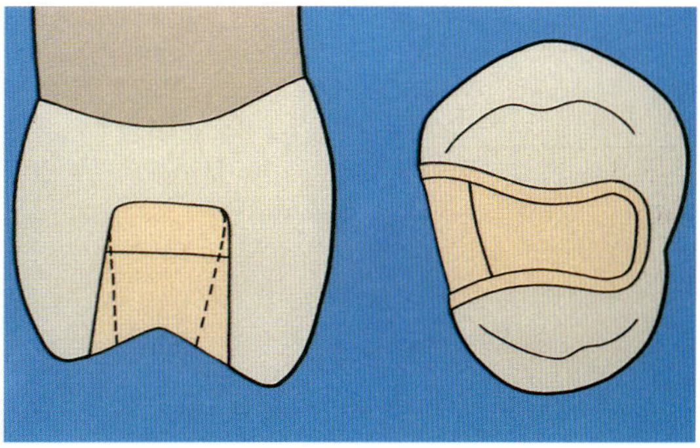

Fig. 6-84 Proximal walls are flared and symmetrical with small restorations.

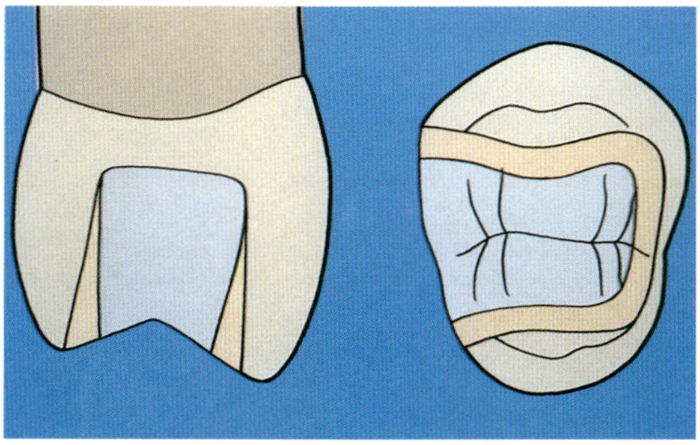

Fig. 6-85 Larger restorations would require excessive reduction if proximal walls were flared symmetrically. (not recommended.)

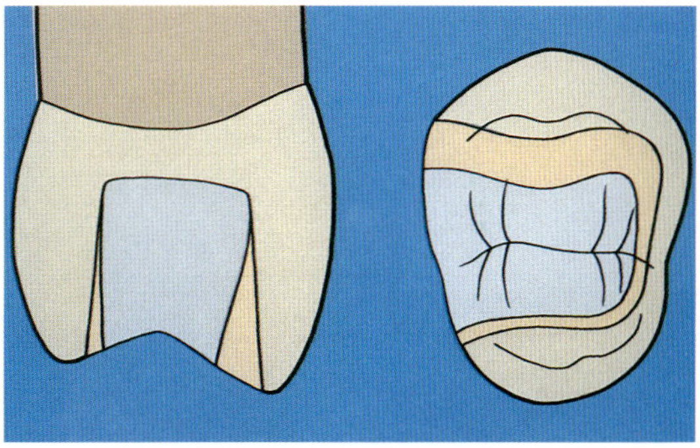

Fig. 6-86 Asymmetrical reduction preserving more of the functional maxillary lingual cusp.

Proximal Design

The proximal portion of a ceramic inlay often requires the removal of a previous restoration, which predetermines the size and extension. Direct filled restorations often have proximal walls that converge occlusally (Fig. 6-83). The proximal wall of inlay preparations must diverge occlusally, which requires additional tooth reduction. Three options exist. The first is to reduce equivalent amounts of the buccal and lingual proximal walls (Fig. 6-84). In minimal size preparations this design is appropriate. In situations where greater tooth loss already exists, this approach may result in excessive tooth removal (Fig. 6-85). In these situations, proximal extension should be more extensive at the expense of the nonfunctional cusp, thus minimizing tooth loss next to the functional cusp (Figs. 6-86 and 6-87).

The gingival cavosurface margin should be maintained in enamel whenever possible (Fig. 6-88). When sound gingival enamel is undermined by caries or a previous restoration, these should be removed and treated similar to the deep occlusal areas. The area immediately adjacent to the undermined external enamel should be filled in with the strongest material, which is usually the bonding cement during cementation (Fig. 6-89). Thin dentin adjacent to a vital pulp should be covered with a fluoride-releasing restorative base or liner (Fig. 6-90). This will provide a secondary defense mechanism should gingival microleakage occur in the future. If no gingival enamel exists, a thin gingival-axial layer of a fluoride-releasing base is recommended until predictable long term dentinal bonding that eliminates microleakage is available (Fig. 6-91).

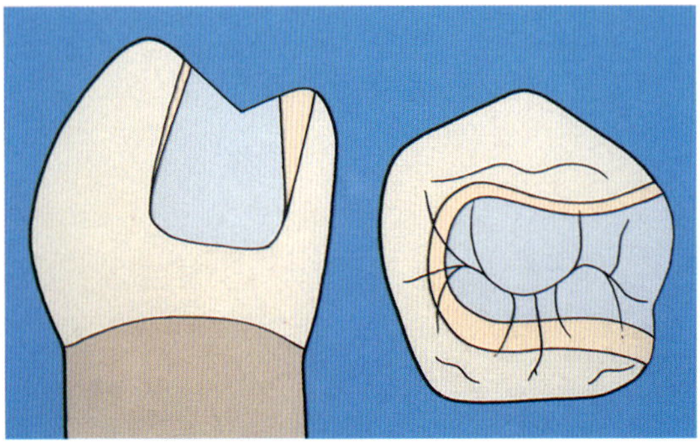

Fig. 6-87 Asymmetrical reduction preserving more of the functional mandibular buccal cusp.

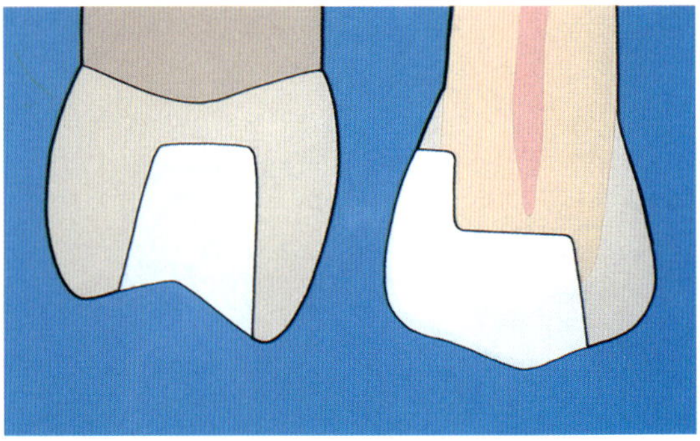

Fig. 6-88 Gingival cavosurface margin in enamel.

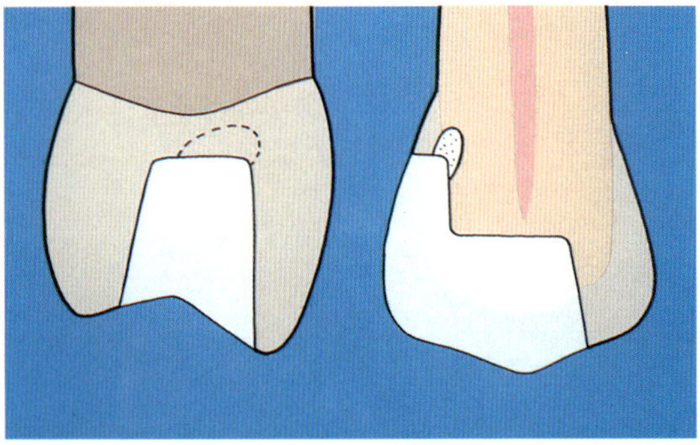

Fig. 6-89 Undermined gingival enamel filled with composite cement during cementation.

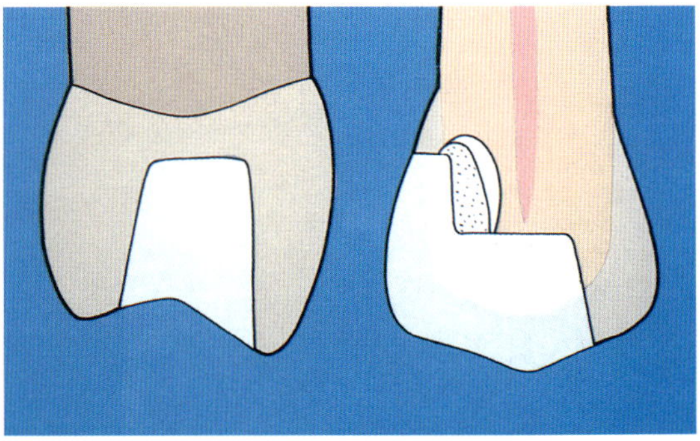

Fig. 6-90 Deep axial wall filled with a fluoride base adjacent to the pulp, composite cement (dotted) and ceramic inlay.

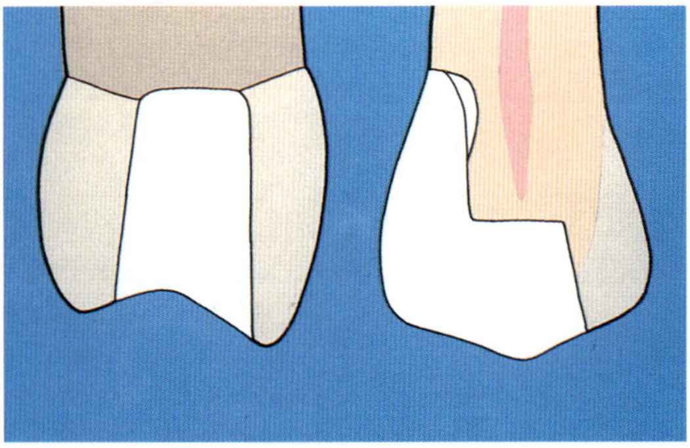

Fig. 6-91 When the gingival cavosurface margin is in dentin, place a fluoride-releasing liner at the gingivo-axial line angle.

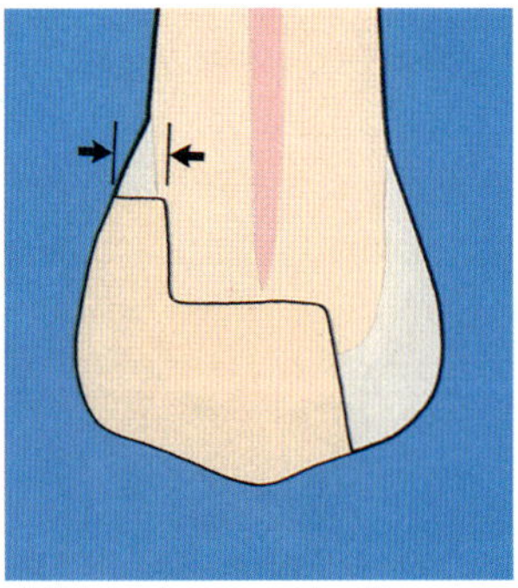

Fig. 6-92 Gingival floor depth should be 1.0 to 1.5 mm.

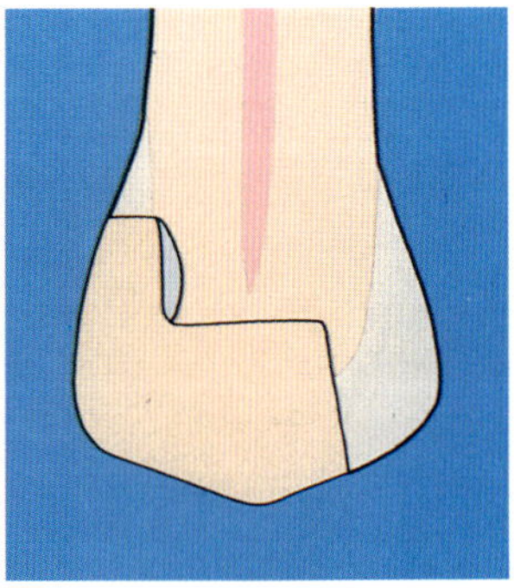

Fig. 6-93 Previous restorations can be left as block out and removed during final cementation.

Axial wall depth should be 1.0 to 1.5 mm (Fig. 6-92). The axial wall depth and width must provide enough ceramic bulk in the proximal region for strength and to eliminate unwanted tooth structure or previous restorations. During the preparation and impression appointment, remnants of old restorations may be left and removed prior to cementation (Fig. 6-93). When doubt exists as to the possibility of pulpal involvement, previous restorations or carious tooth structure should be removed and pulpal

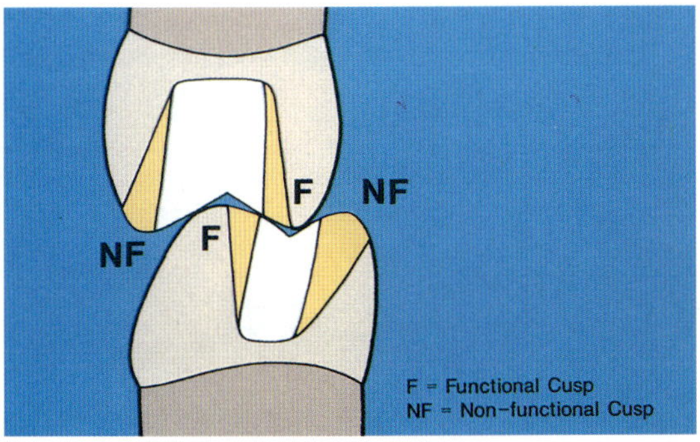

Fig. 6-94 Yellow zone designates area where clinical judgment dictates acceptable margin extension.

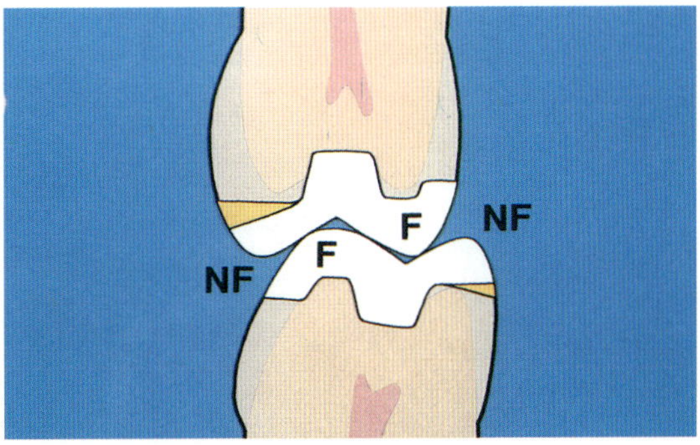

Fig. 6-95 Wrapping of cusps is necessary for functional cusps (F) but not for nonfunctional cusps (NF).

health determined.

Cuspal Protection or Replacement

When a cusp is missing or too thin to be retained, it must be covered occlusally or totally replaced with the ceramic material. The decision to retain or cover a cusp is a clinical judgment decision. Bonded ceramic inlays have been shown to strengthen the tooth in laboratory studies. Cuspal areas generally have thick enamel and enamel bonding has been shown to provide good long term bonds clinically. It is reasonable to assume that the bond between the ceramic inlay and the occlusal enamel of the weakened cusps should provide additional resistance to cusp fracture. It should not be necessary to cover weakened or unsupported cuspal enamel as often as is required, with metallic inlays that are luted but not bonded to the tooth. The required amount of preparation extension is somewhat speculative and clinical research will prove or disprove working theories. We must have a working hypothesis and apply clinical judgment and experience to preparation design when deciding on when to cover cusps with the restorations. Figure 6-94 demonstrates the questionable area where clinical judgment must be applied to each clinical situation. The questionable area of extension for nonfunctional cusps extends from just short of the cusp tip occlusally to slightly beyond it axially. The extension on the functional cusp should be more conservative. Here the questionable area for cuspal protection extends from just short of the cusp tip occlusally to a point about 1 mm closer to the central groove. The final determination of when to cover a cusp with the ceramic inlay must be modified in each clinical situation and based upon many factors. These include (1) amount of enamel, (2) functional occlusal forces, (3) size of the occlusal functional contact, (4) esthetics, (5) mesial-distal length of the questionable area, (6) desire for a more traditional approach and prognosis (rather than maintaining tooth structure), (7) dentist's individual experience and finally (8) insurance coverage, which unfortunately often dictates dental approaches—onlays often are easier to receive payment for.

Once the decision is made to cover a cusp, adequate ceramic bulk must be provided to resist fractures during fabrication, cementation and function. A thickness of 1.5 to 2 mm is often recommended to ensure a favorable prognosis. It is not known if this amount of reduction is necessary with today's bonding technology. This amount of reduction would result in dentin exposure in most preparations. Maintenance of enamel would provide a more predictable bond. For that reason, ceramic margin extension in the occlusal one

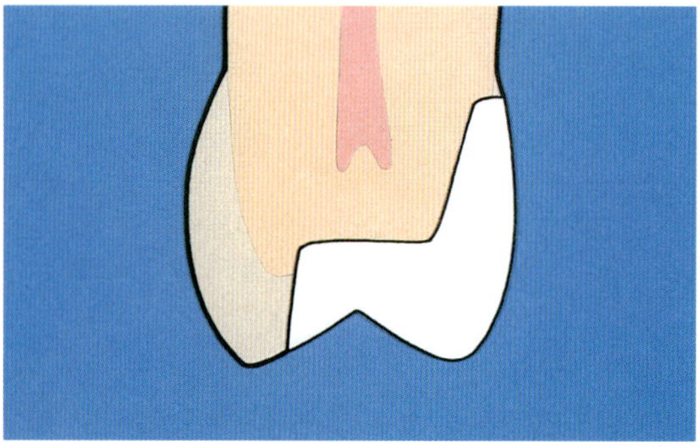

Fig. 6-96 Cross section of lingual cusp replacement.

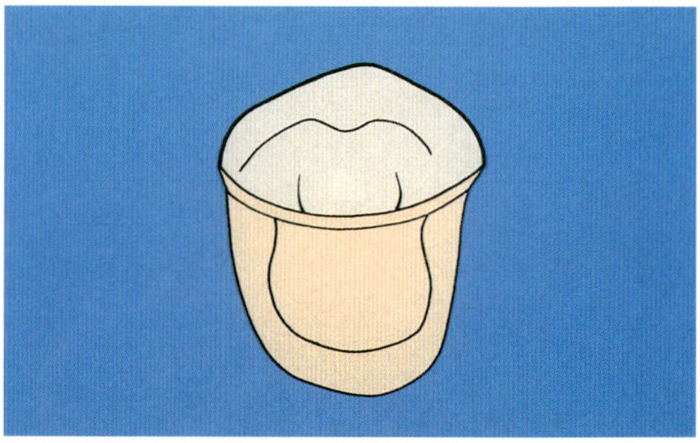

Fig. 6-97 Occlusal view of lingual cusp replacement. Note mesial and distal resistance form; boxes not necessary.

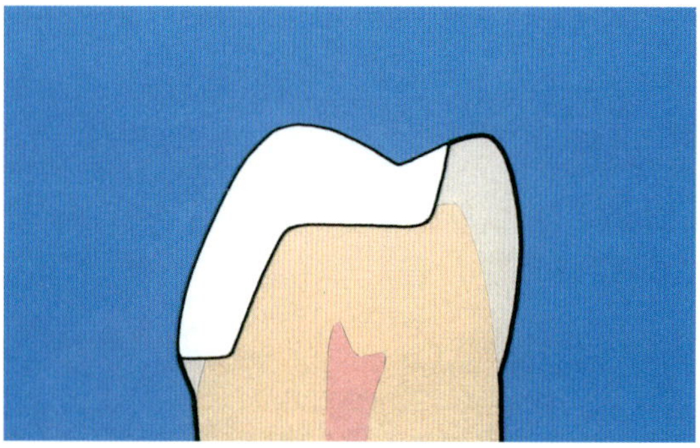

Fig. 6-98 Cross section of buccal cusp replacement.

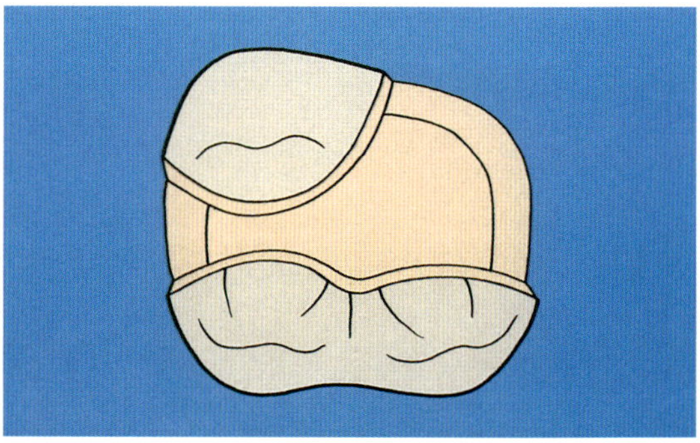

Fig. 6-99 Occlusal view of buccal cusp replacement.

third should be only 1 to 1.5 mm deep. It is advisable to wrap the ceramic over functional cusps to create a step or shoulder. Nonfunctional cusps may often be reduced flat or with a slight bevel-like angulation (Fig. 6-95). Because the bonding materials and techniques used will provide a significant amount of the restorations retention, traditional retention designs such as minimal wall taper and other mechanical retentive features are less necessary.

When a cusp needs total replacement, the preparation design for that portion of the onlay will closely resemble the margin and extension design used for a full ceramic crown (Figs. 6-96 to 6-99). Sound tooth structures should be maintained and defective tooth structure replaced with the ceramic inlay/onlay.

Contemporary Designs for Posterior Ceramic Inlay/Onlays

As bonded inlay/onlay restorations gain in acceptance and become more widely used, preparations in teeth not previously restored can be of a more conservative design. Preparation extensions may be limited to affected areas of the tooth. Retentive design features will be minimized as bonding techniques improve and their longevity is substantiated by longitudinal clinical research. Standardized preparation designs will become less routine as bonded ceramic preparation will only remove whatever tooth structure needs to be replaced and a restorative material is bonded into place. New materials and bonding techniques will significantly change in the next decade. For that reason, conservative tooth reduction should be a common goal today in

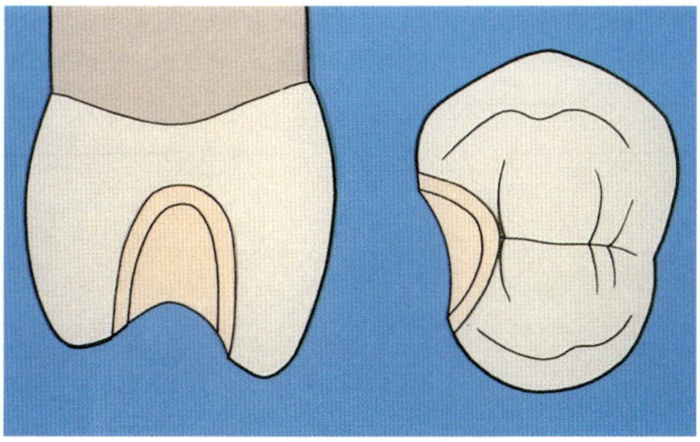

Fig. 6-100a Conservative box design.

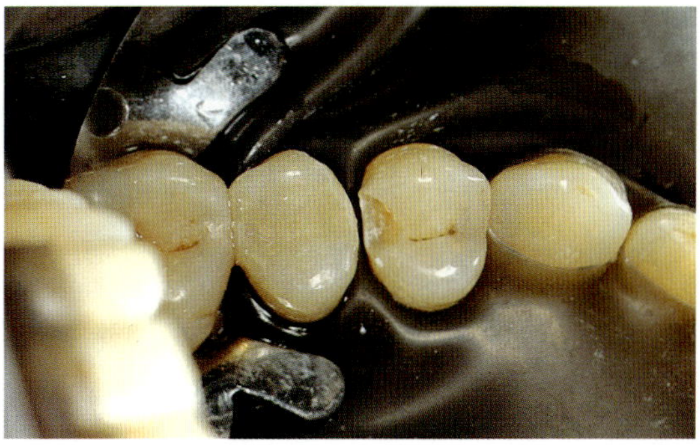

Fig. 6-100b Clinical case.

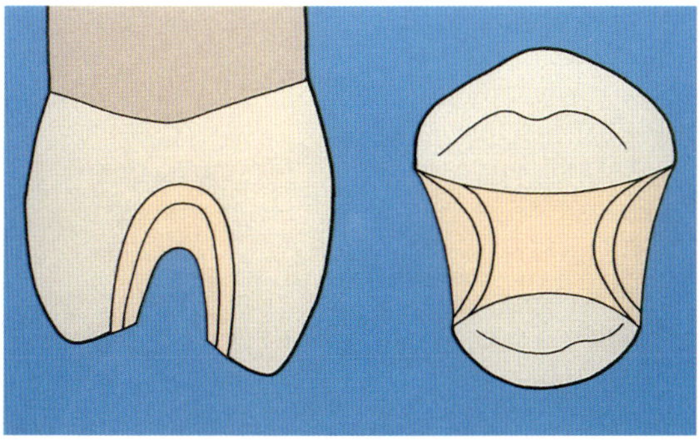

Fig. 6-101 Conservative MOD design.

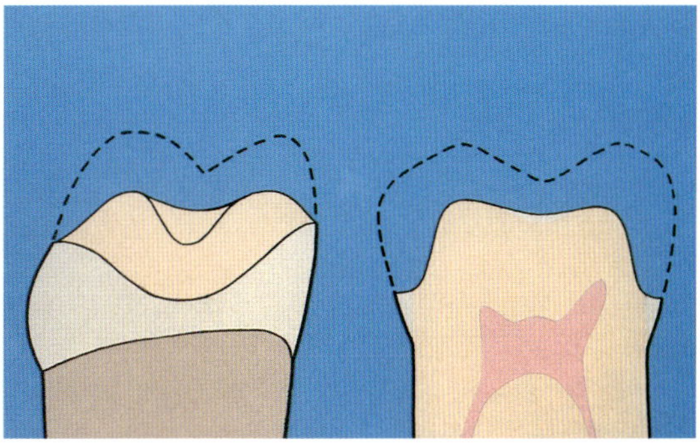

Fig. 6-102a Contemporary onlay design requiring bonding for retention.

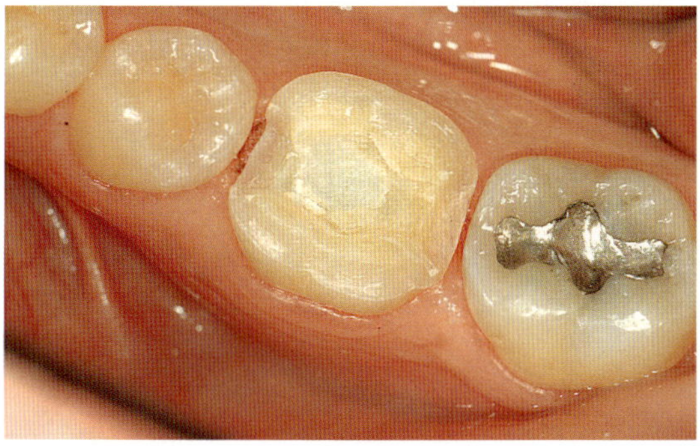

Fig. 6-102b Conservative bonded onlay.

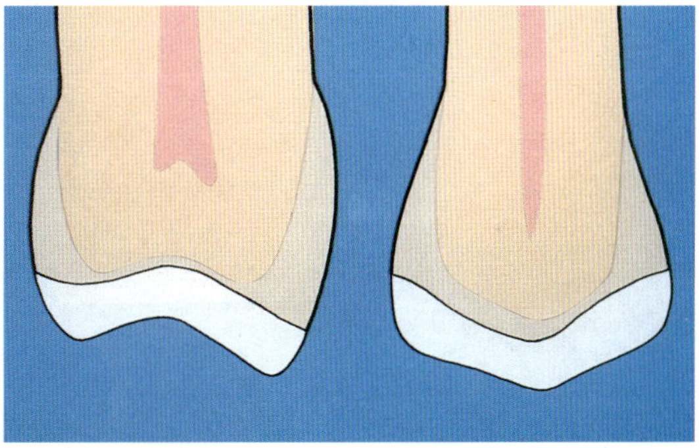

Fig. 6-103 Occlusal ceramic veneer (onlay) bonded to enamel.

order to preserve as much tooth structure as possible for tomorrow's technology. Current technology is allowing restorative dentists to successfully pursue this goal. Even if failures occur, maintenance of tooth structure will allow the use of future technology.

When designing a preparation on a previously unrestored tooth, simply remove diseased tooth structure, finish the margins or fractured areas and evaluate functional demands on the area. Routinely placing conventional retentive features such as boxes, isthmuses and shoulders is not always necessary. Maintaining a maximum amount of enamel for bonding will allow the most predictable long term bond. Select the restorative material of choice and use the best bonding techniques available. Predicting preparation designs that will be successful is premature and speculative at this time. The following preparations are a deviation from the traditional and have been used with good short term success. Use of these designs should only occur with an understanding that long term clinical research may or may not prove them successful. Figures 6-100 to 6-103 demonstrate a few basic approaches. Development of new preparation designs will be necessary as materials and techniques develop.

Provisional Restoration

There are many ways to fabricate provisional restorations. Techniques include the use of cement fillings, gutta percha, light cured resins and conventional crown and bridge provisional resins. It is the author's opinion that the use of a hard-setting resin, cemented in place, provides the fewest problems overall and if done properly, can be very time efficient. A simplified inlay fabrication technique will be presented.

Technique:

- The provisional restoration should be made before the final impression is made. It can be trimmed while the impression is in the mouth and be ready to cement shortly after removal of the impression.
- The prepared tooth is moistened with saliva.
- Mix the provisional resin, pick up the appropriate amount with a hand instrument and dip in warm water to accelerate the set to a doughy, nonsticky stage (Figs. 6-104a and b). (vinylethyl methacrylates recommended.)
- Roll it into a ball or cylinder and press into the inlay preparation with a finger, pushing away occlusal excess (Figs. 6-104c to e).
- The patient should now bite together and chew for 5 seconds.
- Using a carver or explorer, remove excess materials and carve axial contours (Fig. 6-104f).
- While the resin is still in a heavy doughy stage, insert the explorer into a bulky area, pull out the restoration and place it in warm water (Figs. 6-104g and h). (take impression.)
- When the resin is set, trim away flash, undercuts and rough contour. After the impression is removed the fit is verified and the occlusion adjusted (Figs. 6-104i and j).
- Areas near the gingival tissues should be smoothed with paint on glaze or polished with fine pumice .
- Cement with a eugenol free cement. These

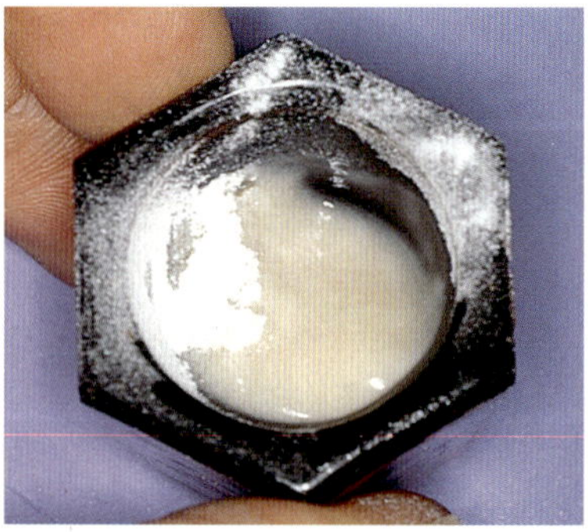

Fig. 6-104a Mix acrylic resin.

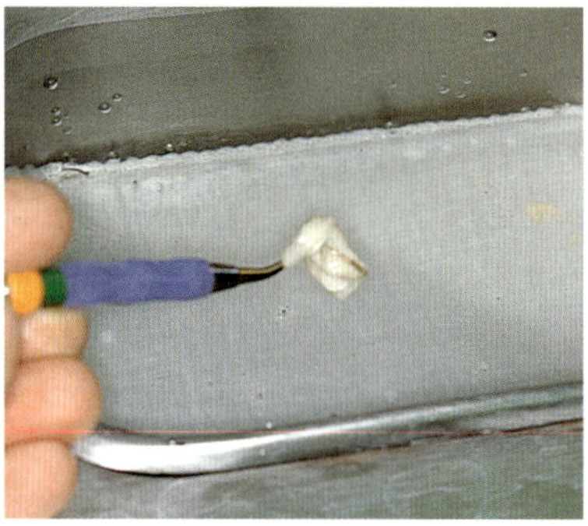

Fig. 6-104b Warm water will accelerate the polymerization.

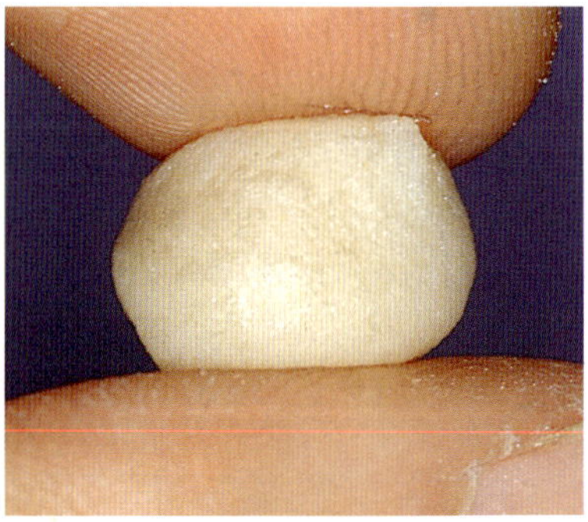

Fig. 6-104c Form a doughy ball.

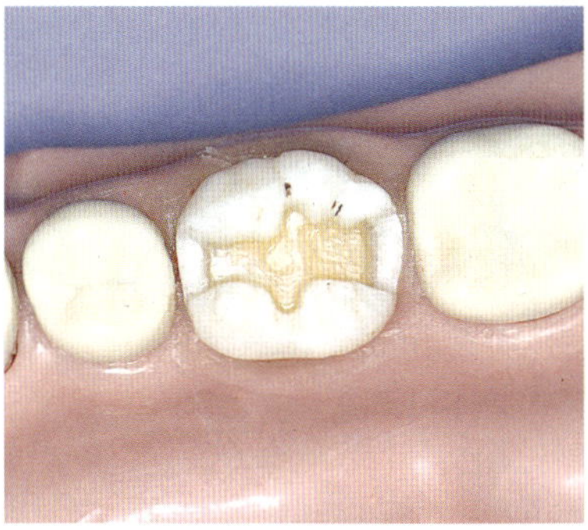

Fig. 6-104d Prepared inlay on model.

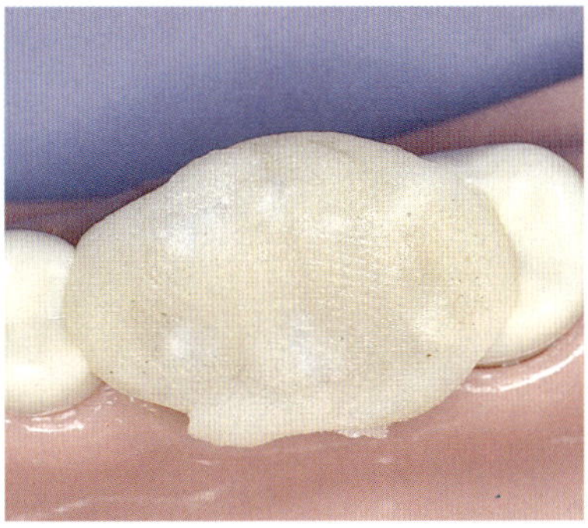

Fig. 6-104e Press acrylic resin into lubricated inlay.

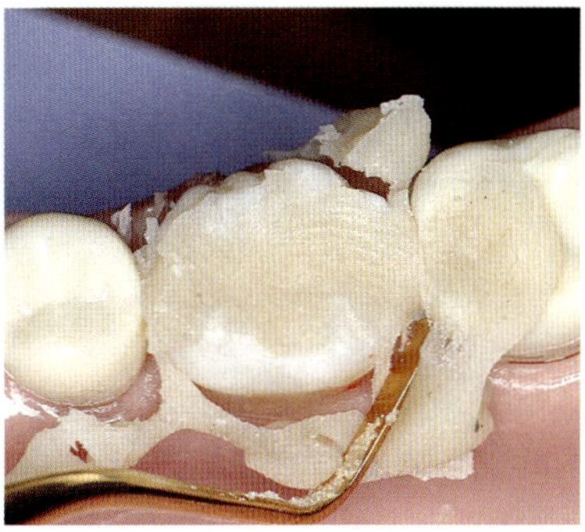

Fig. 6-104f Carve away excess.

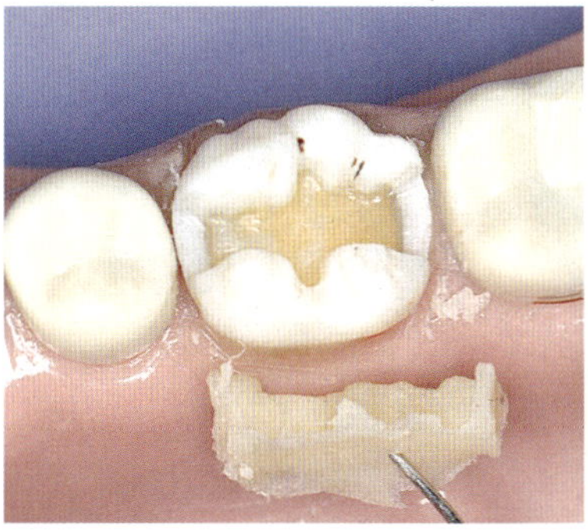

Fig. 6-104g Pull out with explorer.

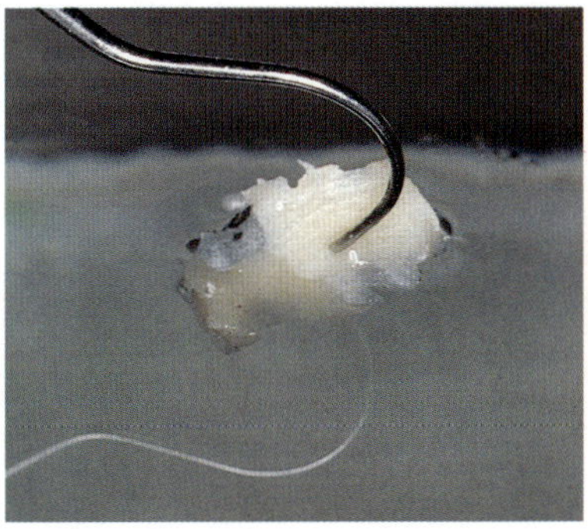

Fig. 6-104h Place in warm water to accelerate final polymerization.

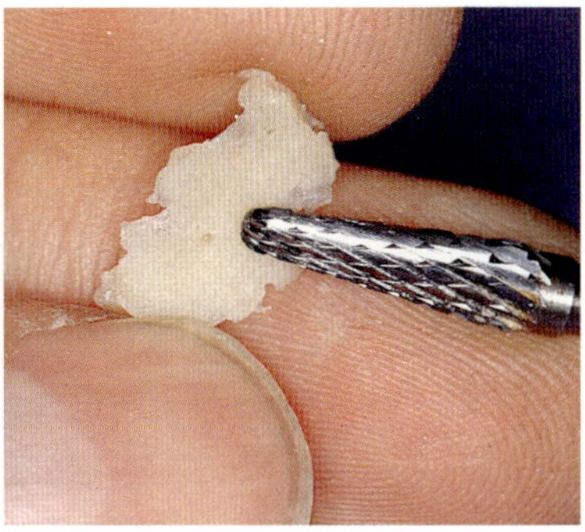

Fig. 6-104i Trim the provisional with carbide burs.

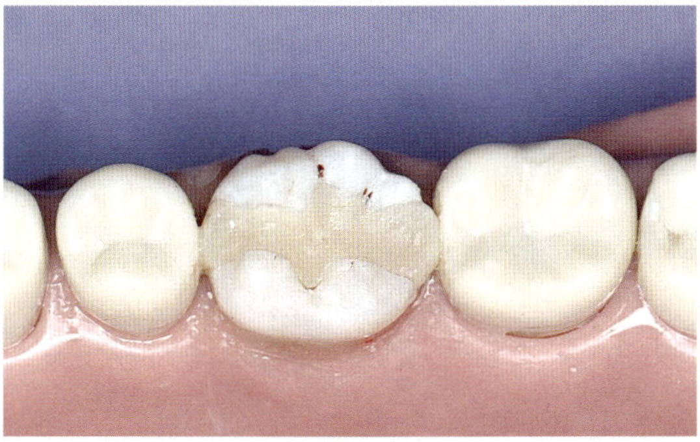

Fig. 6-104j Check the fit.

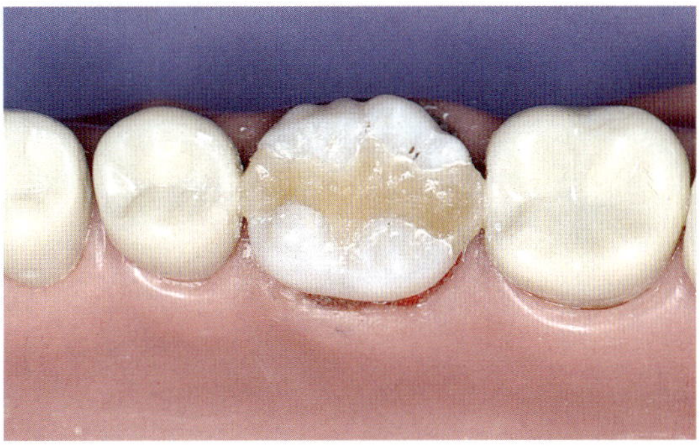

Fig. 6-104k Cement provisional with noneugenol cement.

cements are quite weak and polycarboxylate cements may be used when mechanical retention is minimal. Provisional resin cements may also be useful (Fig. 6-104k).

- Removal of the resin provisional at the delivery appointment is easily accomplished by auxiliaries. Should the restoration fall out prematurely, these durable restorations rarely break and can easily and quickly be recemented. These resin provisional restorations are durable, time saving and cost effective due to minimal overall chair time.

Precementation Evaluation

- The restoration should be examined on the die prior to the cementation appointment.
- Verify marginal accuracy, contour, occlusion, finish and overall acceptability.
- Check the inner surfaces of the restoration to verify a clean and etched surface, which will have an even frosty appearance.

Try-in and Cementation

- Isolate the tooth using a rubber dam or other means to ensure a clean, dry field during cementation. (Figs. 6-105a and b).
- Remove the provisional restoration and clean off all visible cement from the preparation.
- Clean the inner surfaces of the preparation by scrubbing it with a pumice impregnated cotton pledget (Fig. 6-105c).
- Rinse and dry the cleaned preparation. (Fig. 6-105d).
- Anesthesia is often unnecessary, but may be used if necessary.
- Gently seat the restoration with a light seating pressure. Avoid excessive force that may chip the restoration or wedge it in place (Fig. 6-105e).
- Mark proximal high spots with carbon paper (Fig. 6-105f).
- Tight proximal contacts most often cause incomplete seating. While holding the restoration in place with a hand instrument, check for excessive contact with dental floss (Fig. 6-105g).
- Adjust the proximal contact using a fine grit ceramic adjusting wheel or fine diamond

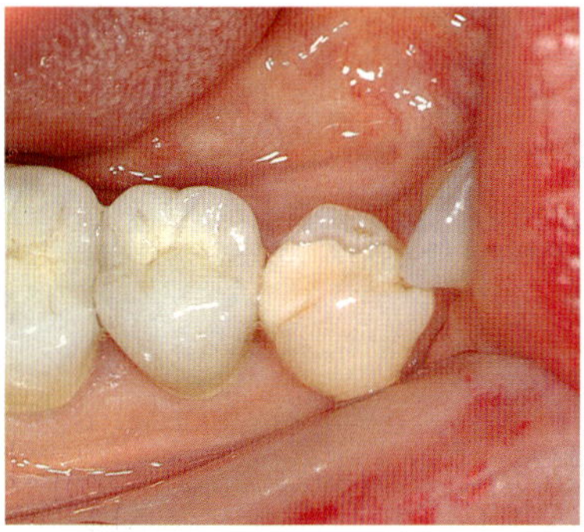

Fig. 6-105a Remove provisional.

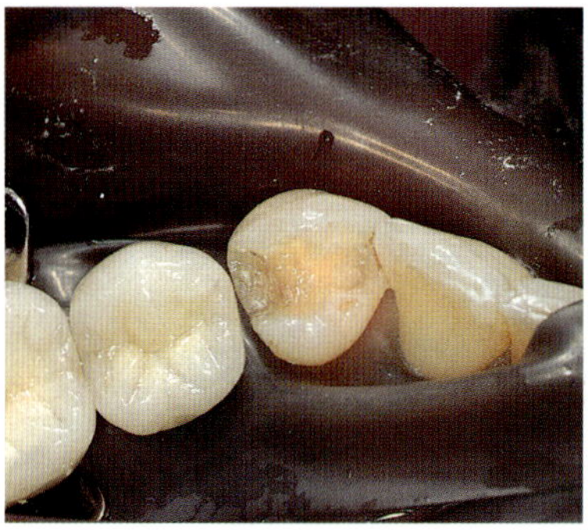

Fig. 6-105b Isolate prepared tooth.

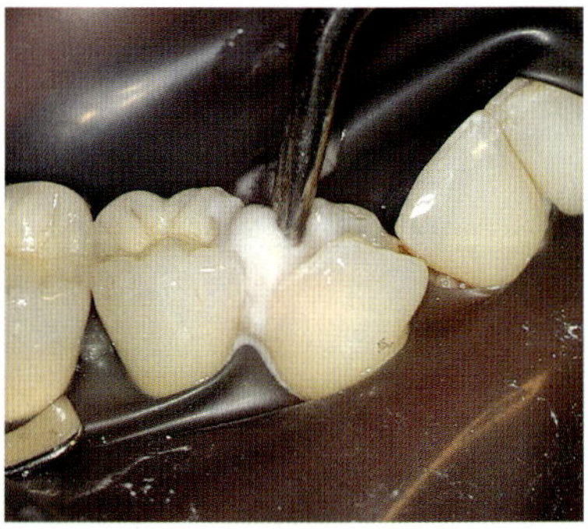

Fig. 6-105c Clean preparation with cotton and pumice.

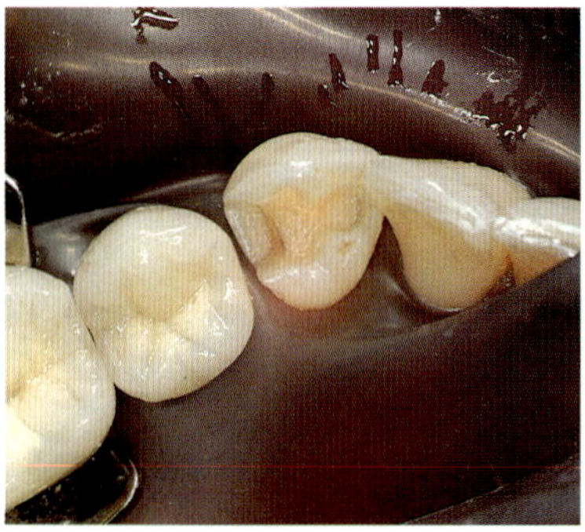

Fig. 6-105d Cleaned inlay preparation.

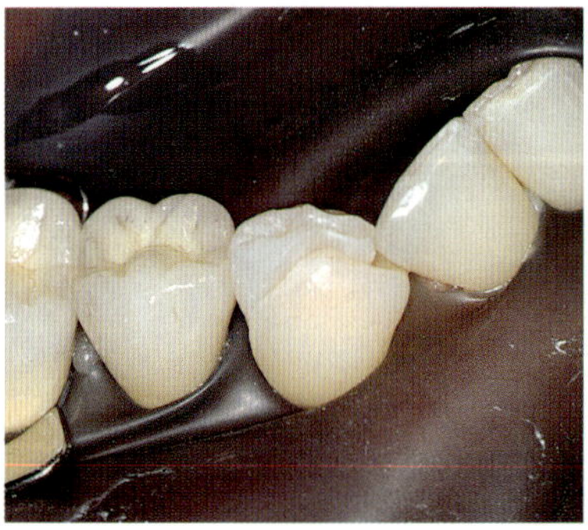

Fig. 6-105e Gently seat inlay (do not force).

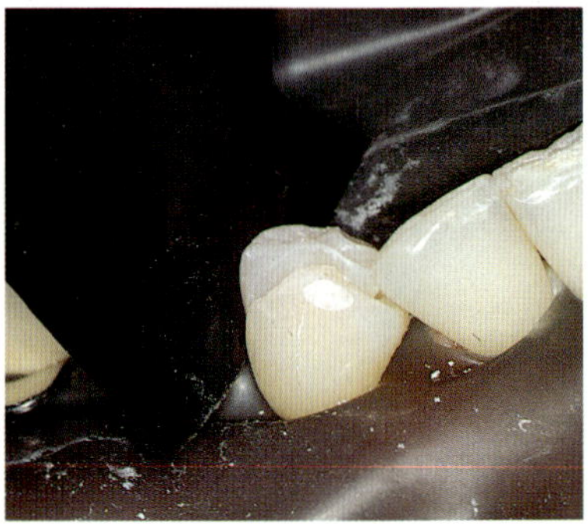

Fig. 6-105f Mark high spots with carbon paper.

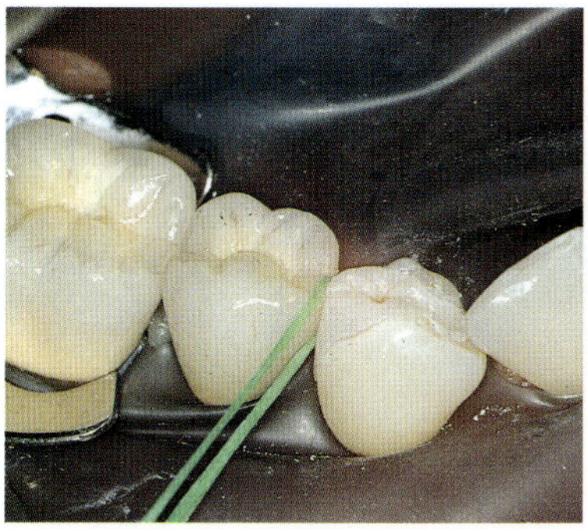

Fig. 6-105g Use floss to check proximal contact.

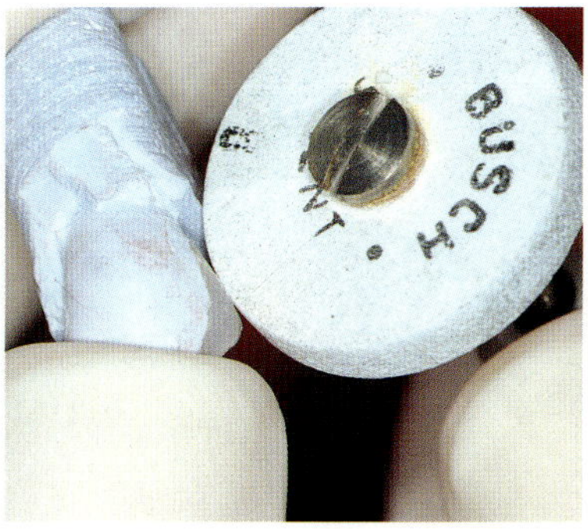

Fig. 6-105h Adjust proximal contact with fine ceramic adjusting stone.

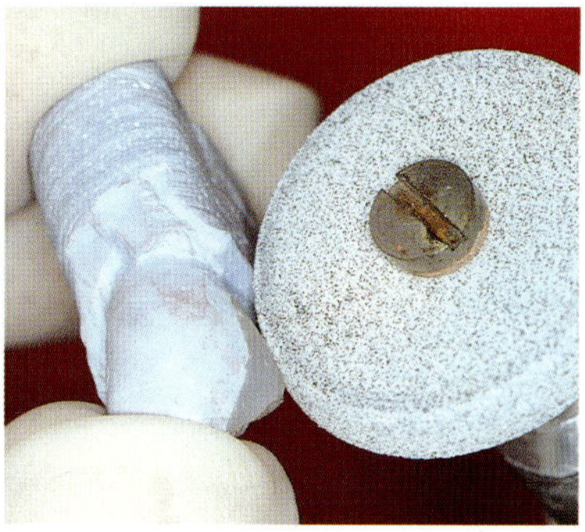

Fig. 6-105i Polish proximal contact with a rubber wheel.

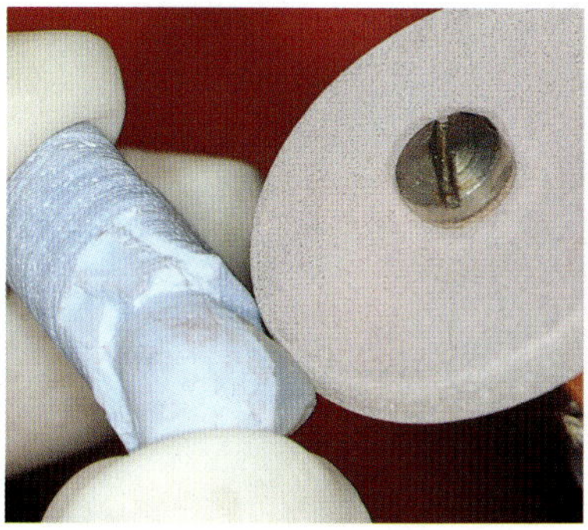

Fig. 6-105j Final polish with extra-fine rubber wheel.

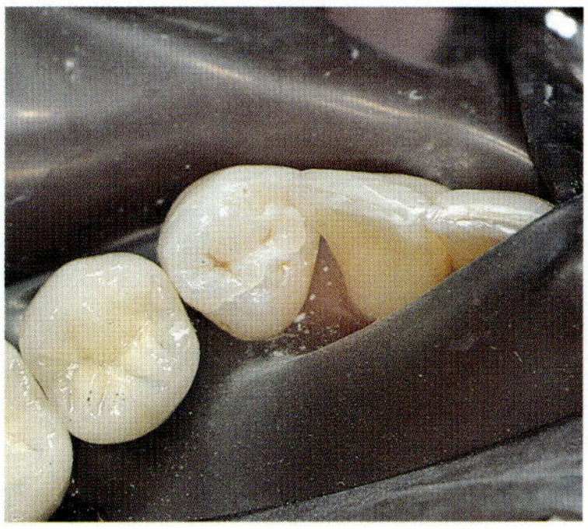

Fig. 6-105k Ceramic inlay ready to cement.

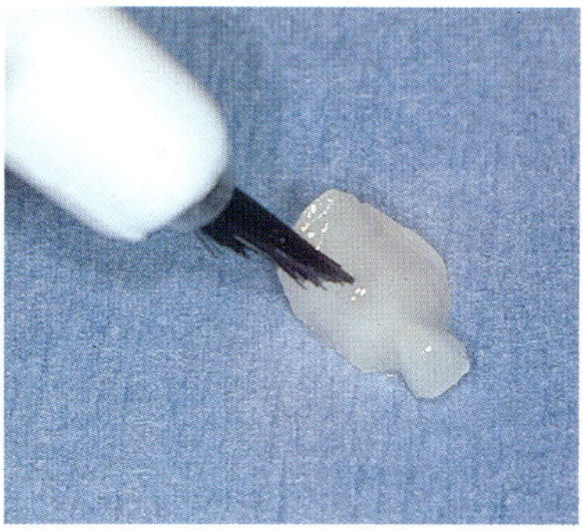

Fig. 6-105l Coat cleaned bonding surfaces with silane and multipurpose bonding agents.

(Fig. 6-105h).

- Polish the contact with ceramic polishing abrasive rubber wheels (Figs. 6-105i and j).
- If the ceramic inlay/onlay still does not seat, check for marginal overextensions or areas of internal binding. Tight spots may be localized by checking the die for abraded areas.
- Small interior adjustments should be done on the tooth. This will eliminate the necessity to re-etch the ceramic inlay.
- If the inlay still does not seat, look for a rocking motion and fulcrum to localize the binding spot.
- The use of quick-setting silicone impression materials to detect tight internal contacting areas must be used with caution. Studies have shown that the silicone may penetrate the etched ceramic surface and reduce potential bonding sites.
- If these silicone materials are used to check fit, a layer of unfilled resin should be placed on the etched ceramic surface first.
- If ceramic restorations routinely require excessive time and adjustment to seat, thought should be given to selecting another ceramist or the laboratory techniques should be reviewed.
- Esthetic modifications are not often required. If needed, procedures are as described in Ceramic Crown section.
- After the ceramic restoration is completely seated and acceptable, it should be ultrasonically cleaned in a solvent such as acetone and dried. Steam cleaning is advisable if available (Fig. 6-105k).
- A layer of silane should be painted on the etched ceramic surfaces and the restora-

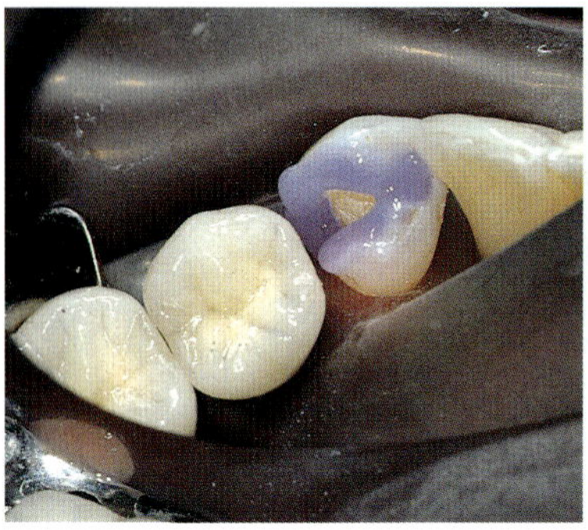

Fig. 6-105m Etch enamel.

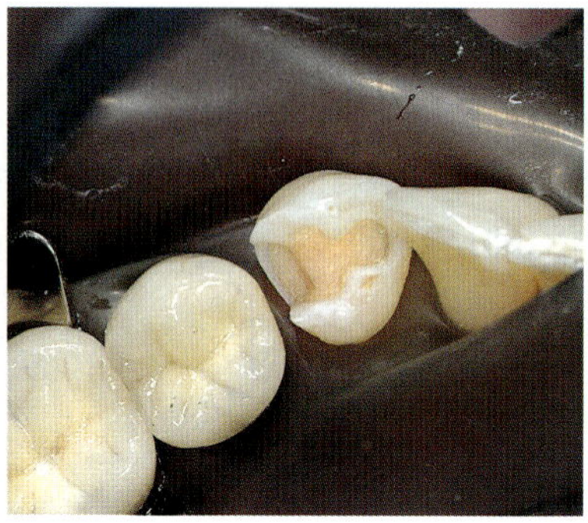

Fig. 6-105n Dried etched enamel appears frosty.

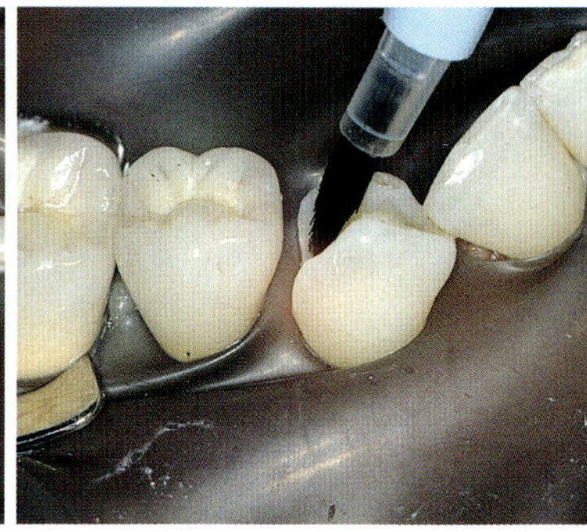

Fig. 6-105o Apply multipurpose bonding agents.

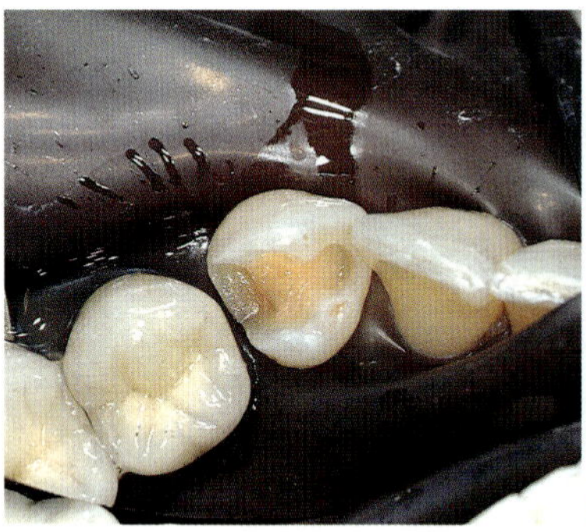

Fig. 6-105p Surface now appears shiny.

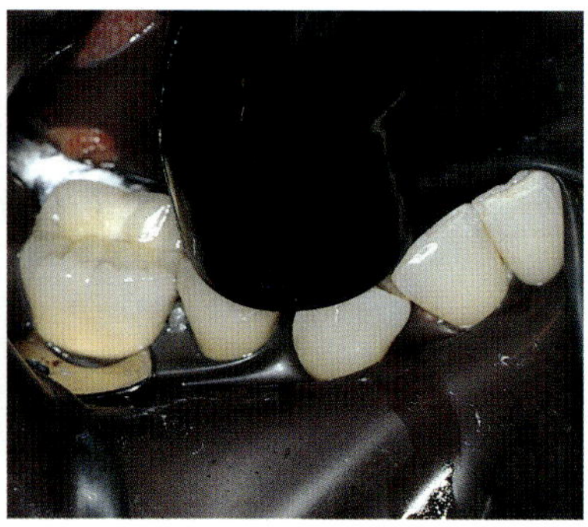

Fig. 6-105q A dry air source such as an electric dryer must be used.

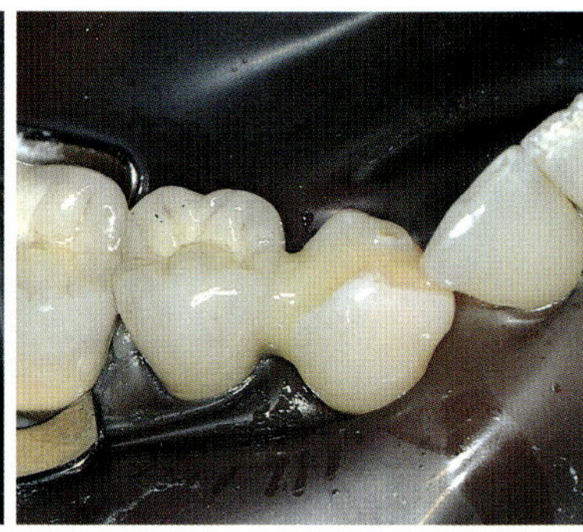

Fig. 6-105r Inject the cement into the preparation.

tion placed in a safe clean location (Fig. 6-105l).

- The prepared tooth may now be ready for cementation.
- All enamel on the internal prepared surfaces and slightly beyond the external cavosurface margins should be etched with 37% phosphoric acid gel for 15 seconds, rinsed thoroughly with water and dried until frosty (Figs. 6-105m and n). A matrix band should be used to avoid etching adjacent teeth. This will expedite removal of excess cured set cement. It is the author's opinion at this time that "total etch" techniques with 37% phosphoric acid are primarily an attempt at technique oversimplification. Because enamel and dentin are very different substrates, whenever possible etch the enamel with 37% phosphoric as suggested and etch or treat the dentin separately with the selected multipurpose bonding system. The additional steps and the demands are not significant. When "total etch" with phosphoric acid is unavoidable, as in small preparations, limit the etching time to 15 seconds and seal immediately.
- Exposed dentin should be treated with the dentinal bonding system of choice. A dentinal bonding system should be utilized that will seal the dentinal tubules, enhance the bond to the ceramic restoration and not interfere with complete seating of the restoration (Figs. 6-105o and p). Most newer dentinal bonding materials are multipurpose and should be used on all surfaces to be bonded; including enamel, dentin and the etched ceramic surfaces. A dry air

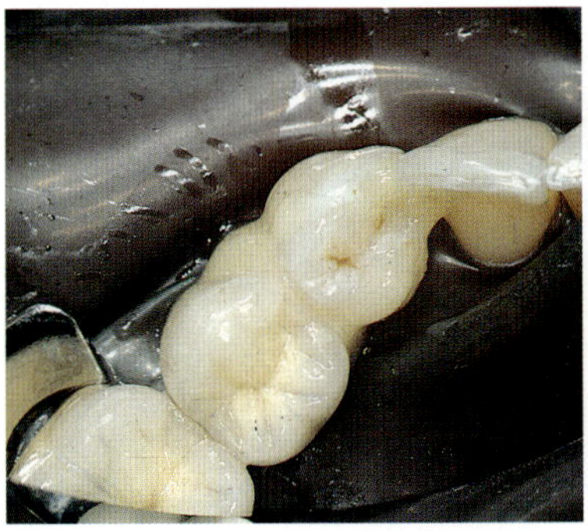

Fig. 6-105s Seat the ceramic inlay and look for marginal excess at all margins.

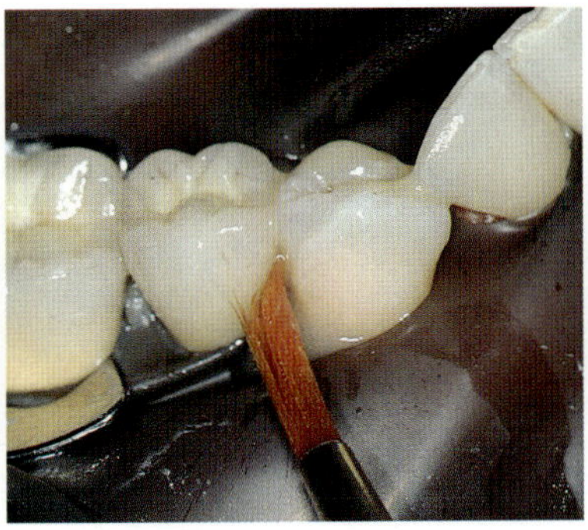

Fig. 6-105t Use a fine brush to remove excess.

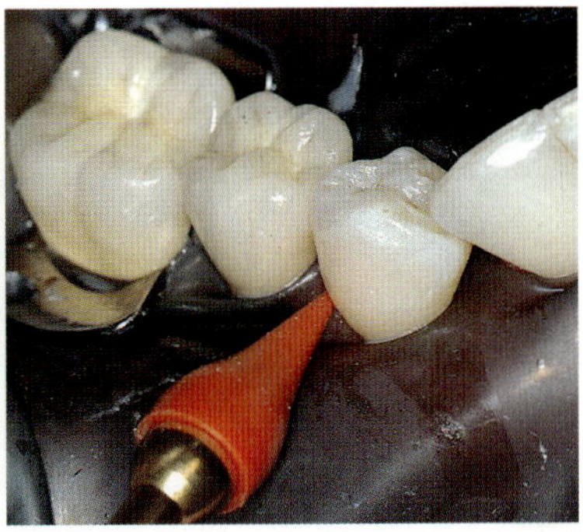

Fig. 6-105u A rubber tip is useful for cement removal.

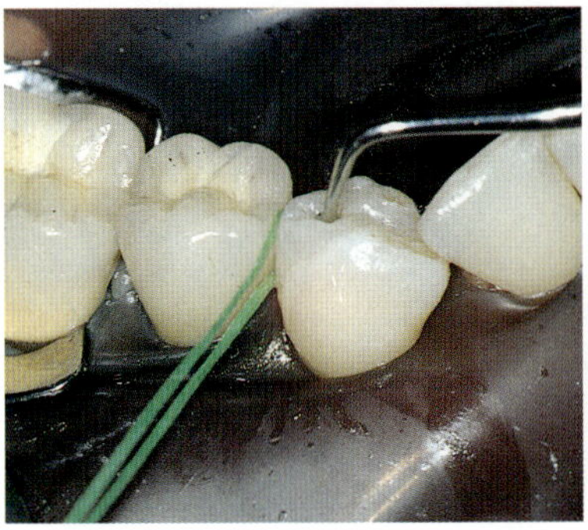

Fig. 6-105v Use floss to remove excess around the contact while holding it in place.

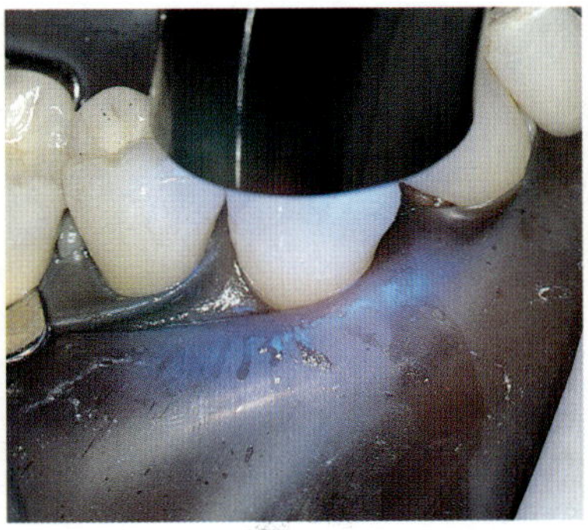

Fig. 6-105w Light cure thoroughly.

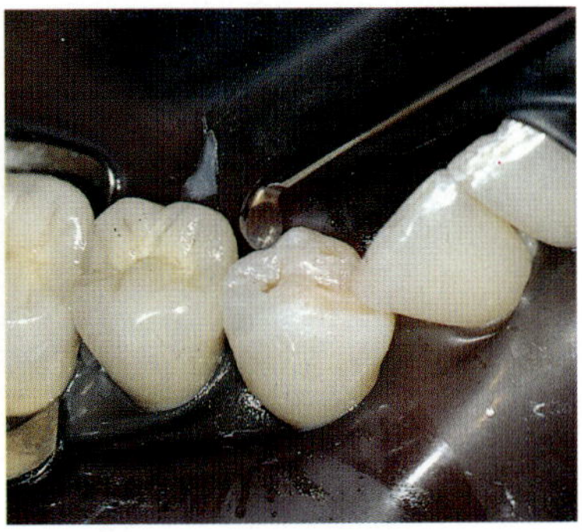

Fig. 6-105x Use a tungsten carbide discoid carver to remove occlusal excess.

source should be used at this point to avoid moisture (Fig. 6-105q).

- Once all surfaces are pretreated with the bonding agent sequence, mix a dual cure composite cement and for small inlay/onlays, inject it into the preparation (Fig. 6-105r). Seat the restoration, making sure that excess cement is evident at all margins (Fig. 6-105s). For larger onlays, the cement may be placed directly into the inner surface of the restoration prior to seating.
- Cement excess should be removed with a fine brush and hand instruments (Fig. 6-105t). A rubber tip used for oral hygiene also works well (Fig. 6-105u). Proximal excess should be removed with dental floss (Fig. 6-105v). A little excess should be left at the margins to compensate for polymerization shrinkage; it is far easier to remove excess than fill voids.
- Cure the restoration for 30 to 60 seconds adjacent to each surface and margin (Fig. 6-105w).
- After completely polymerizing the cement, a thin, often transparent film will remain. A discoid tungsten carbide carver can be used to remove this occlusal excess from the tooth and restoration prior to adjusting the occlusion (Fig. 6-105x). This will minimize unnecessary occlusal adjustment.
- Interproximal excess should be thinned at the margins with a fine pointed 30-fluted carbide bur. The use of a 30-fluted carbide bur will amputate excess cement flush with the ceramic/enamel margin and avoid excessive roughening caused by diamonds. The use of hand instruments to chip out excess interproximal cement should be

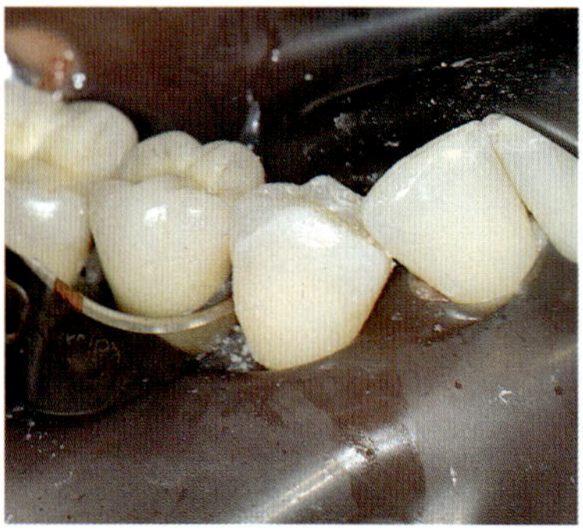

Fig. 6-105y Use a #12 bladed scalpel for interproximal cement removal.

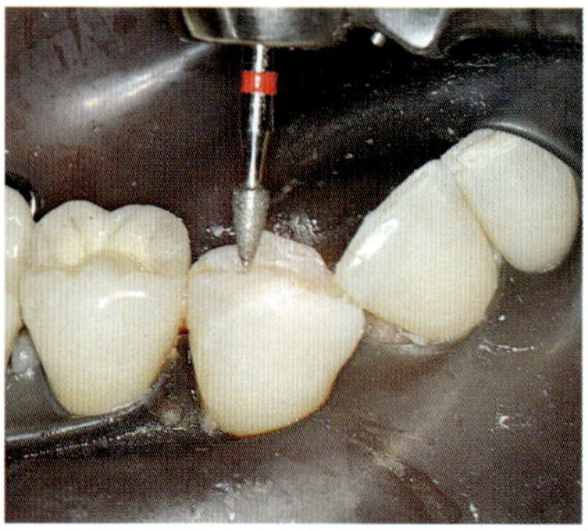

Fig. 6-105z Contour the occlusal with fine diamonds and water.

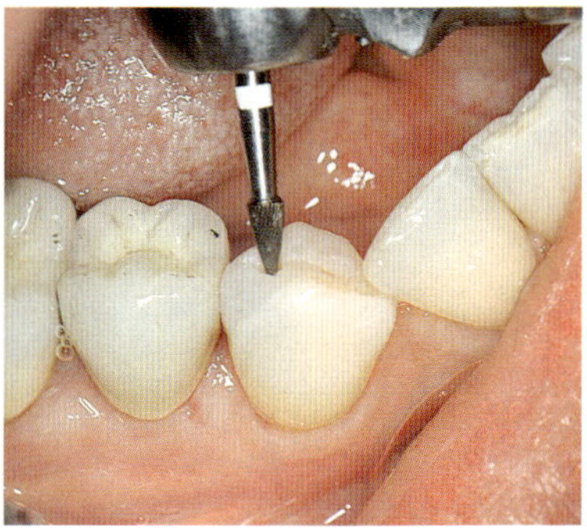

Fig. 6-105aa After the extrafine diamond series, a 30-fluted carbide is used.

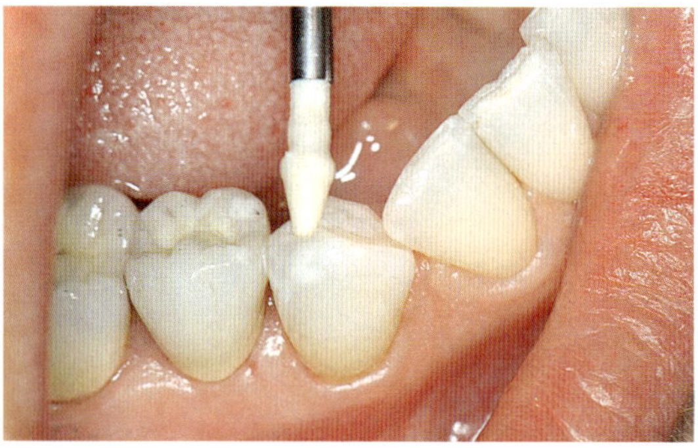

Fig. 6-105bb Final polishing with diamond polishing paste.

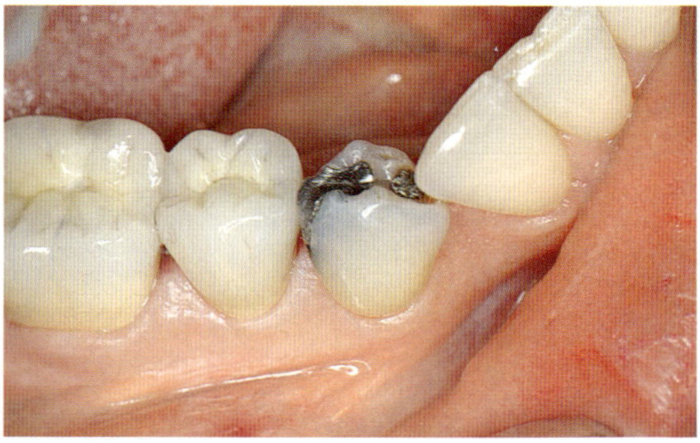

Fig. 6-106a Preoperative view.

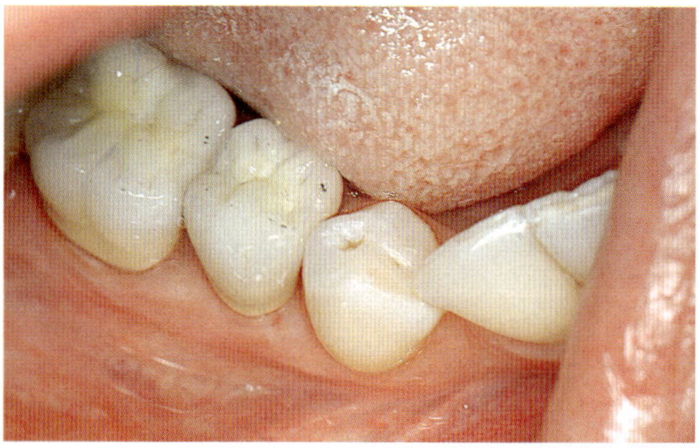

Fig. 6-106b Postoperative view.

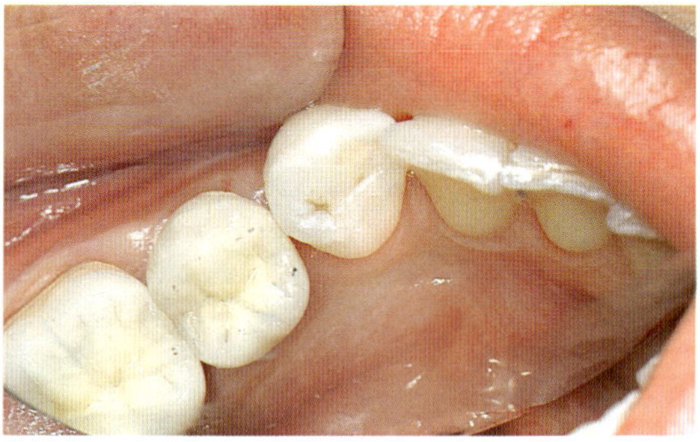

Fig. 6-106c Postoperative occlusal view.

avoided if possible. They may pull the cement out of a margin creating a void. Poor access often limits repair or finishing procedures. A scalpel with a #13 blade is used to remove deep gingival excess or excess around the contact (Fig. 6-105y). Cleanup is usually easy if the adjacent teeth are not etched and the proximal ceramic surface is adequately polished.

- The need for interproximal adjusting should be limited if precementation adjustment was adequate.
- Occlusally any gross contour and margin adjustments are completed and the rubber dam is removed (Fig. 6-105z). Final occlusal adjustment is completed using a

medium to fine diamond.

- The final finishing sequence should consist of medium to extrafine diamonds, 30-fluted carbide finishing burs and diamond polishing pastes (Figs. 6-105aa and bb). Abrasive rubber ceramic polishing points may also be useful. Unfortunately these points constantly change shape as they wear.
- Care must be taken to adequately finish ceramic restorations to prevent excessive wear or plaque accumulation (Fig. 6-106).
- Patients should be instructed in home care and counseled on possible postoperative symptoms.
- With use of appropriate enamel and dentin multipurpose bonding techniques, postoperative problems are minimal. A small number of patients will experience postcementation sensitivity upon chewing. This is a concern to patients and they should be made aware of the potential problem before being dismissed and assured that it usually goes away in a few weeks.
- Any persistent symptoms or symptoms that are increasing in severity should be reported immediately to the treating dentist.

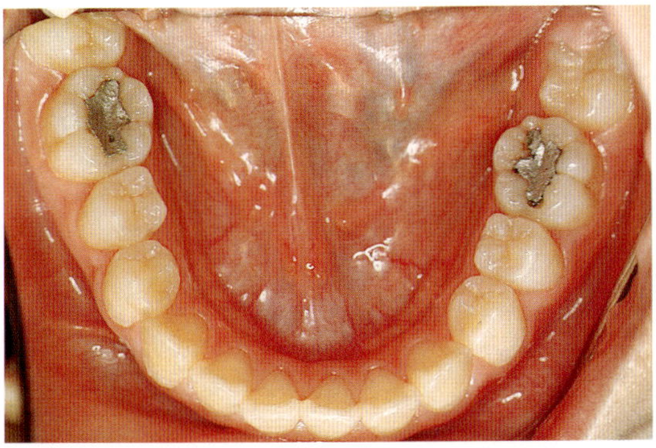

Fig. 6-107a Preoperative view.

LABORATORY PROCEDURES

Strengthened Ceramic

- Prepare the inlays as previously described (Figs. 6-107a to c).
- Make an accurate impression and fabricate die stone models of the prepared teeth and opposing dentition (Fig. 6-107d).
- The die model is trimmed to fit into an Accutrak® tray. Horizontal retention grooves are ground into the lateral surface to provide die retention (Fig. 6-107e).
- Stone is poured into the Accutrak tray and the trimmed model is seated into it (Fig. 6-107f).
- Once set the model is removed and the dies are sectioned and trimmed (Figs. 6-107g and h).
- Block out the die areas and fabricate custom trays (Figs. 6-107i and j).
- Make a polyvinylsiloxane impression of the die model and dies (Figs. 6-107k and l).

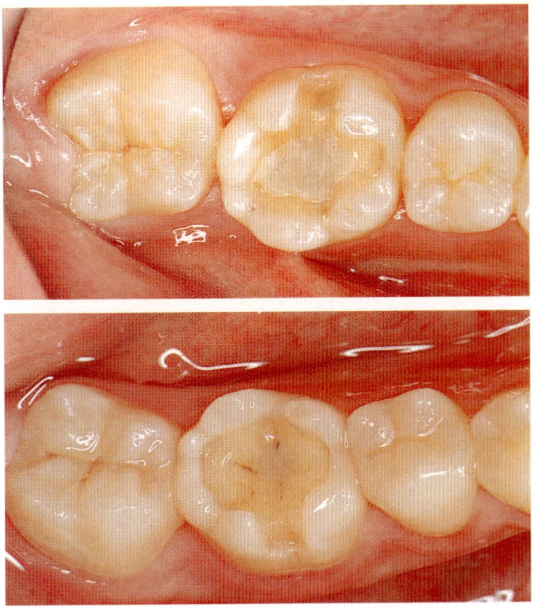

Fig. 6-107b (upper) and c (lower) Inlay preparations.

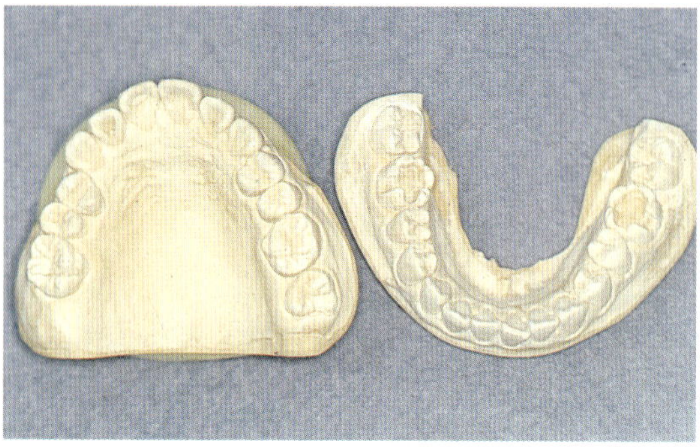

Fig. 6-107d Die stone models.

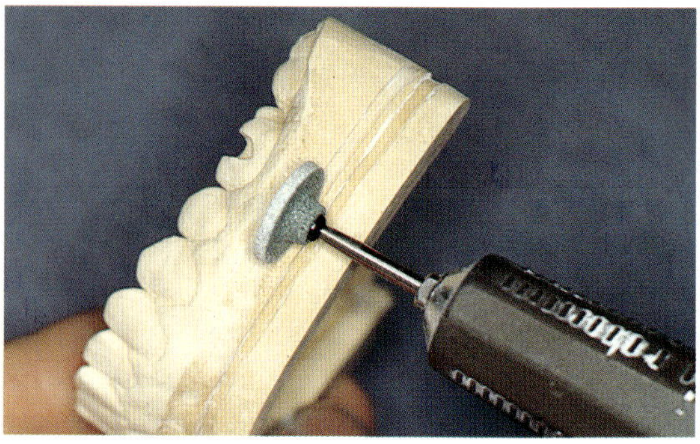

Fig. 6-107e Grind horizontal retentive grooves in model.

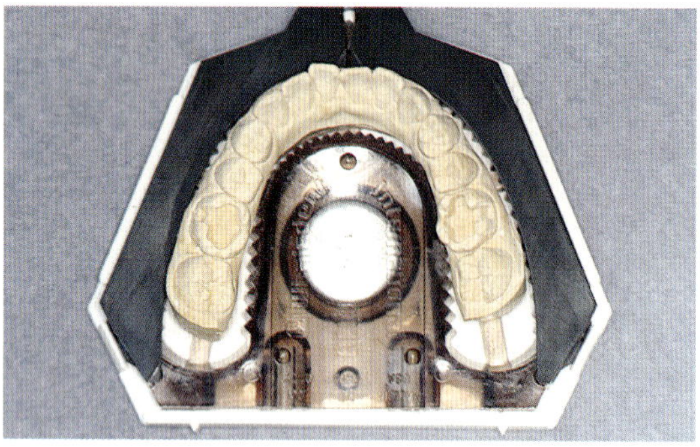

Fig. 6-107f Seat model into Accutrak assembly.

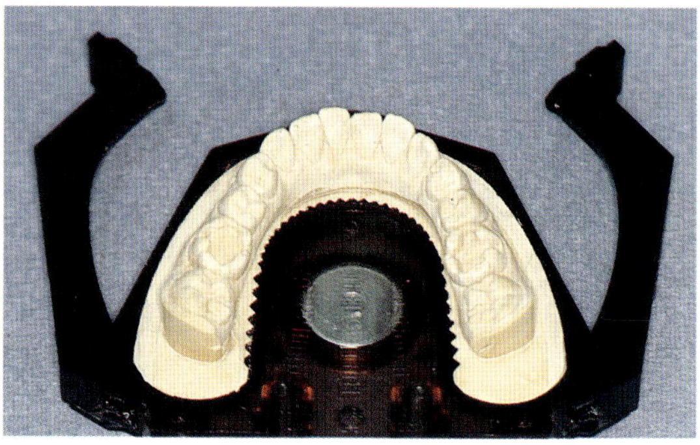

Fig. 6-107g Remove model.

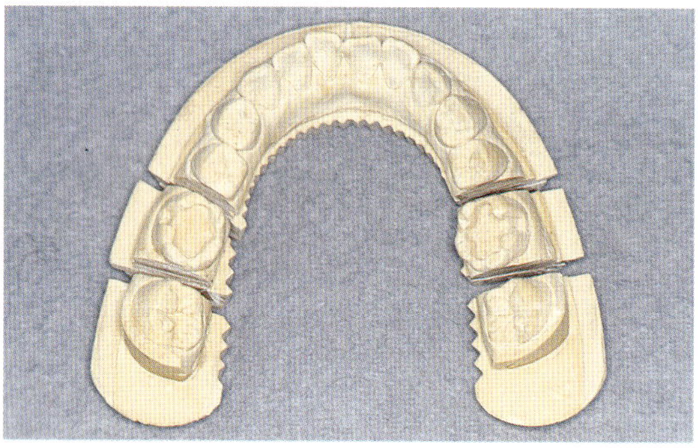

Fig. 6-107h Cut and trim dies.

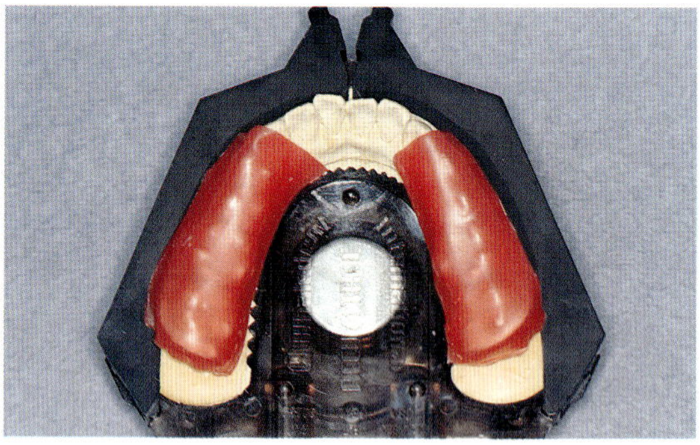

Fig. 6-107i Block out die areas.

- Remove the stone dies and seat the impression over the die model. Pour the die area with the appropriate refractory material that matches the thermal expansion properties of the ceramic to be used (Figs. 6-107m to o). Follow manufacturer's instructions for mixing and handling procedures. A removable refractory die is now positioned on the work model and ceramic inlay fabrication may begin. Retain stone dies for finalizing the inlay.
- Refractory die margins should be marked with a refractory die marking pencil and run through the appropriate thermal cycle. The die is then immersed in distilled water until air bubbles stop surfacing on the die (Figs.

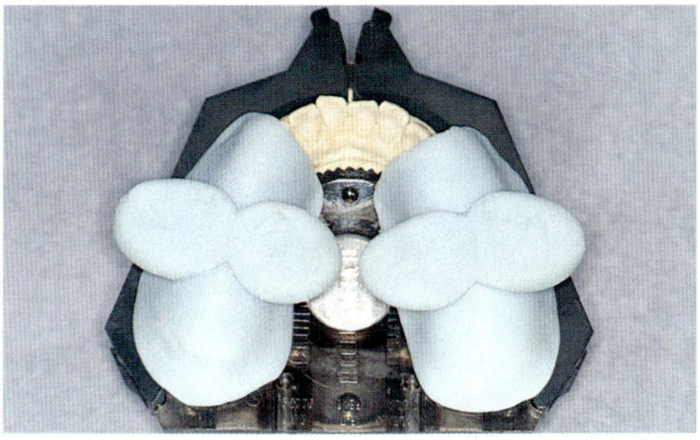

Fig. 6-107j Fabricate impression trays.

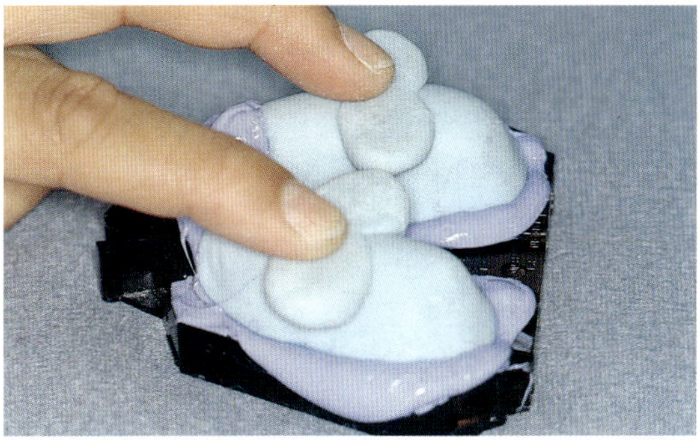

Fig. 6-107k Make impressions of dies and working model.

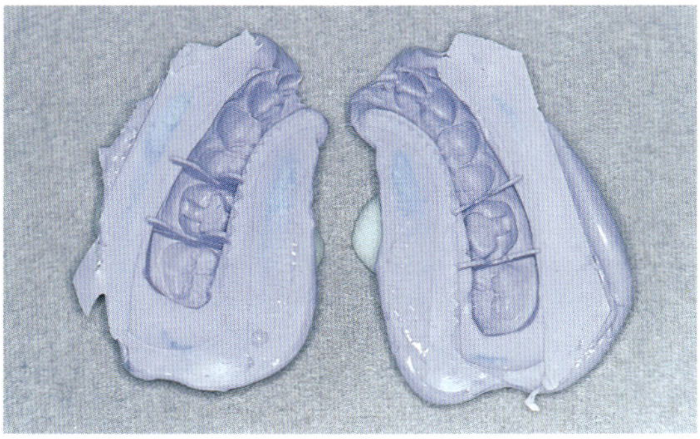

Fig. 6-107l Impressions of working model.

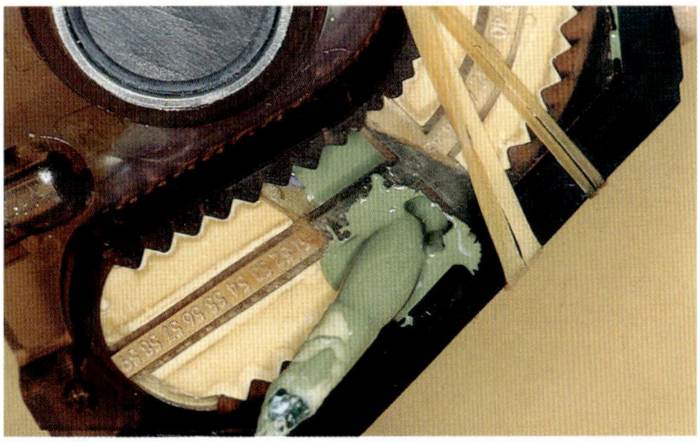

Fig. 6-107m Remove dies, seat in impressions and repour dies in refractory die material.

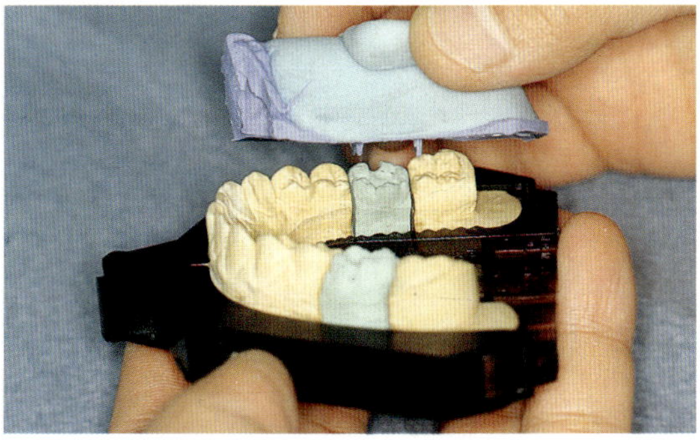

Fig. 6-107n Working model with refractory dies.

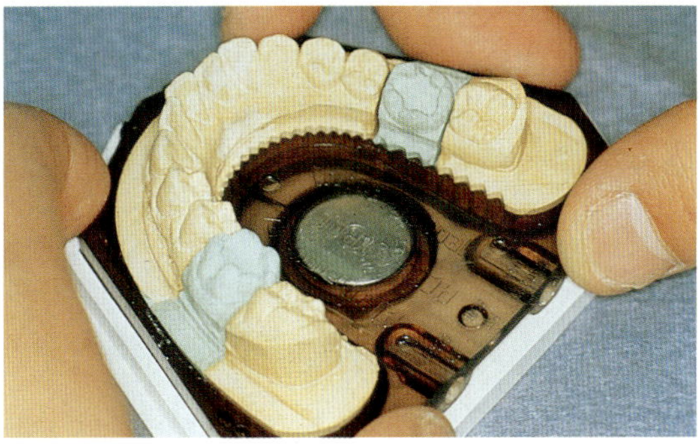

Fig. 6-107o Occlusal view of working model with refractory dies.

6-107p and q). The die is ready to begin ceramic addition. Each ceramic system will have slightly different firing temperatures and techniques that must be carefully followed.

- An incremental addition of the various esthetic ceramic components is required. This will compensate for shrinkage during the sintering process and allow for an esthetic buildup using layered ceramics. The first layer should cover the pulpal-axial walls with about 0.3 mm of dentin ceramic (Figs. 6-107r to t). Immerse the die in distilled water prior to each additional ceramic addition.
- The second ceramic increment should

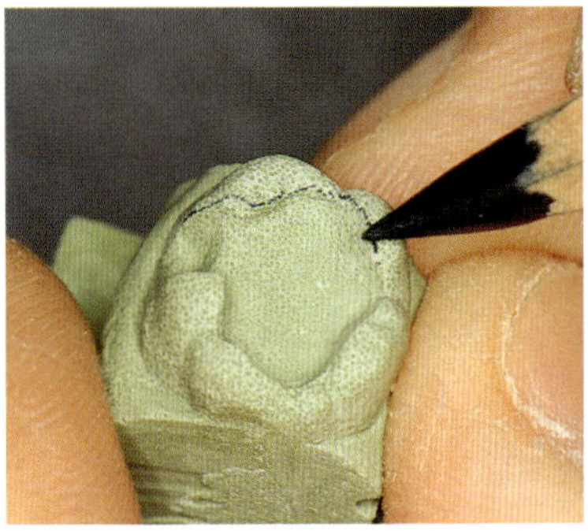

Fig. 6-107p Mark margins on the die.

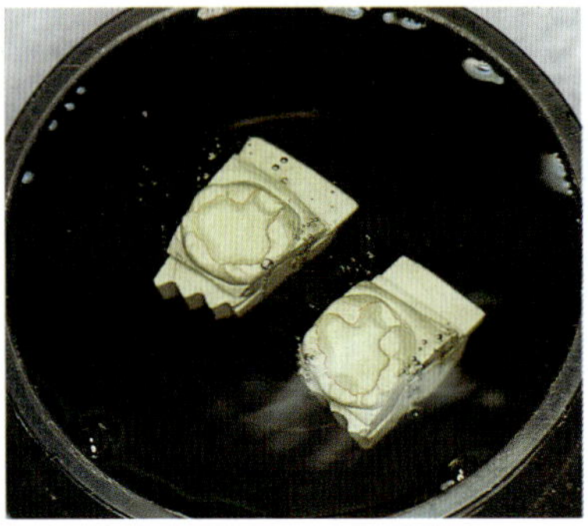

Fig. 6-107q Place refractory dies in water until bubbling stops.

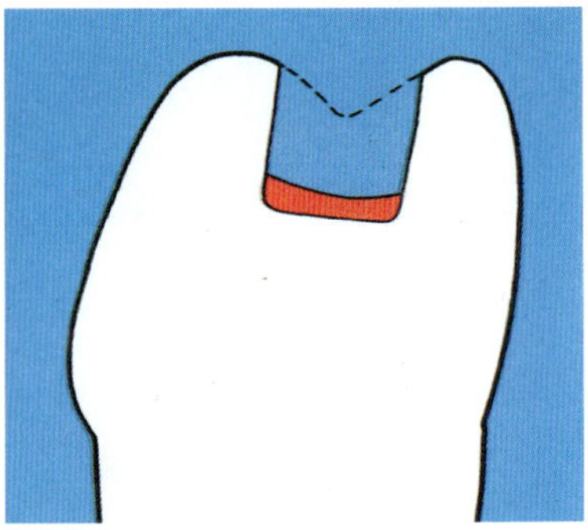

Fig. 6-107r Diagram of first ceramic increment on pulpal and axial walls.

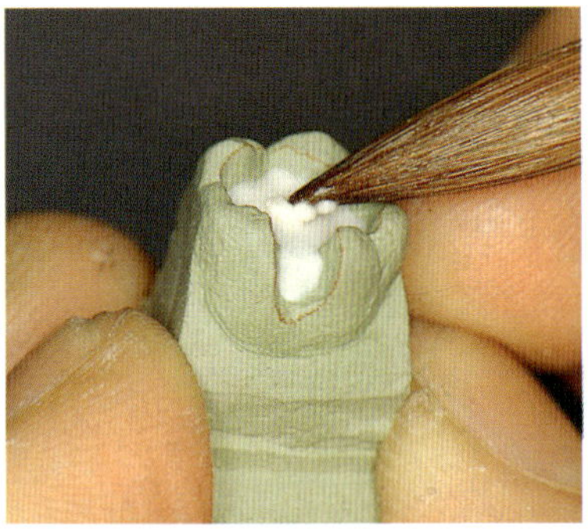

Fig. 6-107s First ceramic application on die.

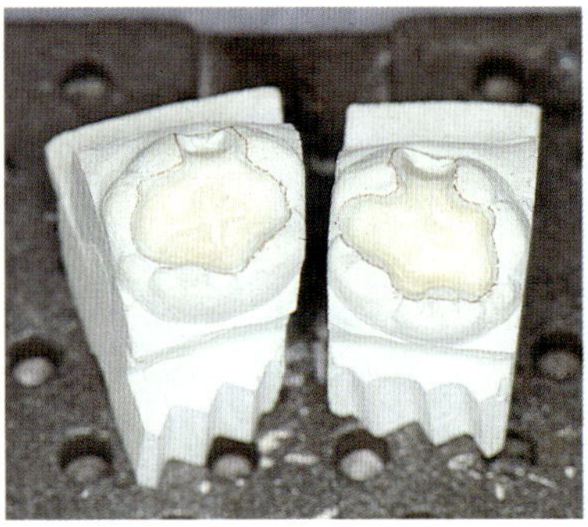

Fig. 6-107t Place dies in an oven and sinter first ceramic increment.

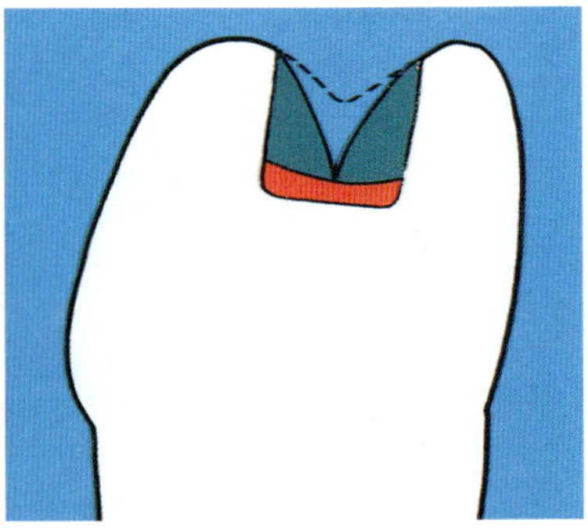

Fig. 6-107u Diagram of second ceramic increment covering walls.

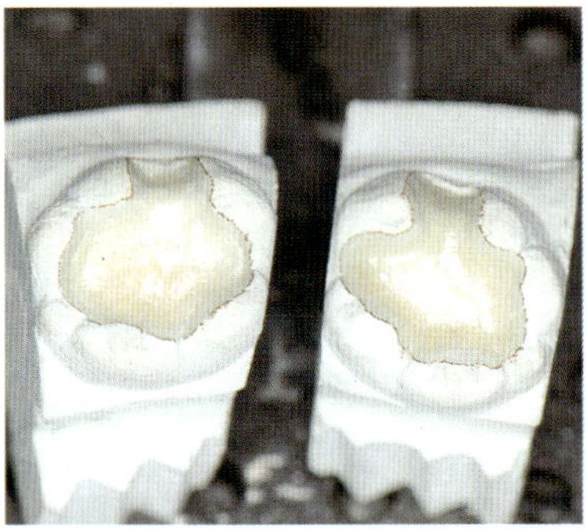

Fig. 6-107v Second ceramic increment sintered on die.

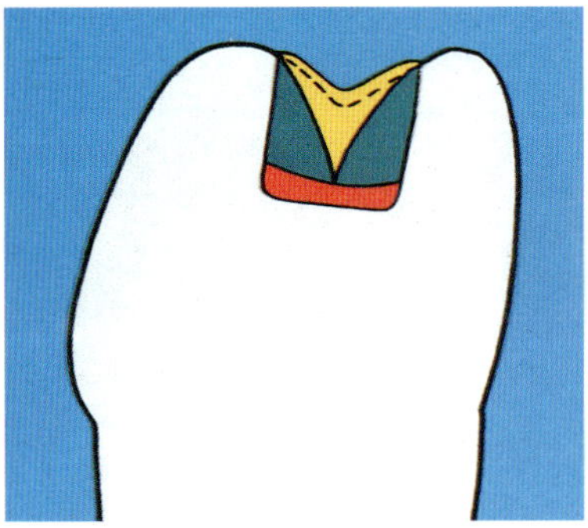

Fig. 6-107w Diagram of final ceramic increment.

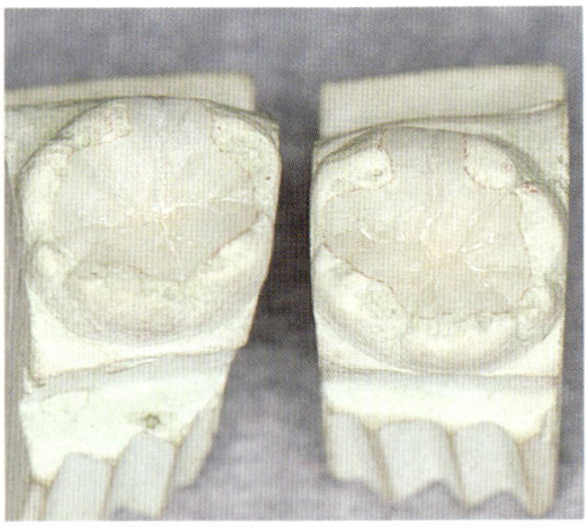

Fig. 6-107x Final sintered ceramic increment rough contoured.

cover the walls of the preparation to the cavosurface margins. Note that opposing walls are not joined during this step (Figs. 6-107u and v).

- The third ceramic addition will fill the remaining central portion of the occlusal and lateral surfaces. Final morphology plus functional occlusion and proximal contacts should be developed (Figs. 6-107w and x). Place the die back on the model for final adjustments.
- Once the ceramic additions are complete, exposed surfaces are contoured and smoothed with fine diamonds, steam cleaned, stained as necessary and glazed in a ceramic oven without vacuum. Inspect

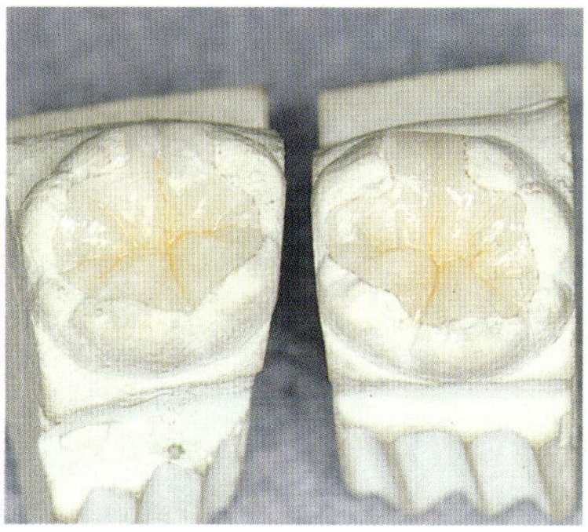

Fig. 6-107y Final stained and glazed inlays.

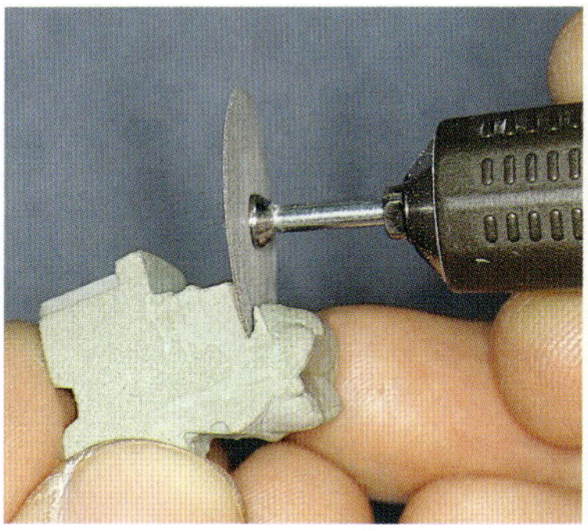

Fig. 6-107z Cut away excess die material.

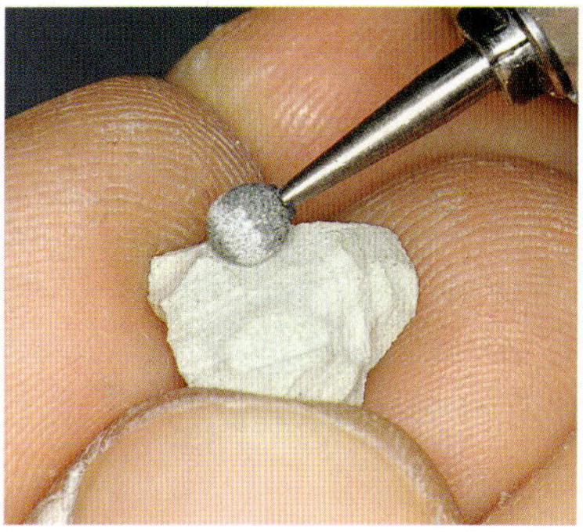

Fig. 6-107aa Use stone to remove die material excess near inlay.

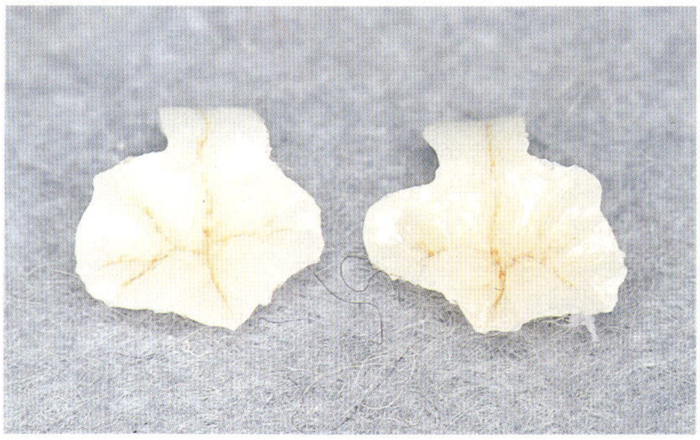

Fig. 6-107bb Divested inlays.

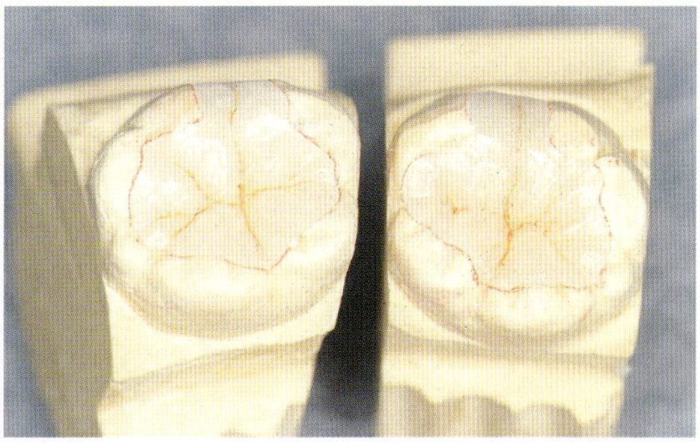

Fig. 6-107cc Inlays seated on stone dies.

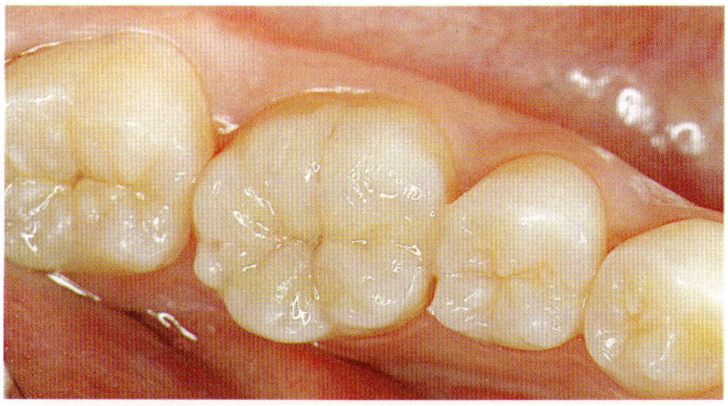

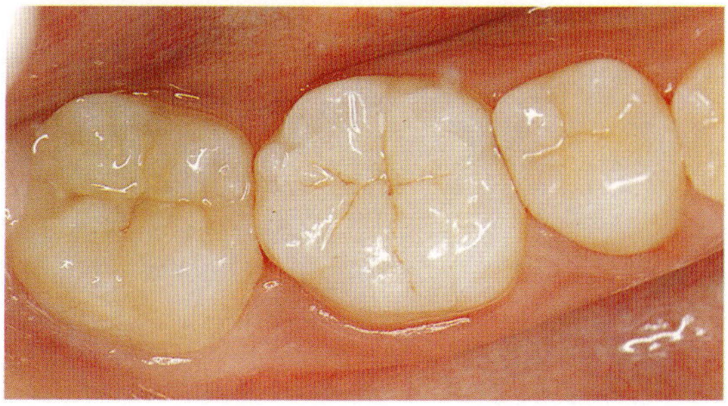

Figs. 6-107dd and ee Close up postcementation views.

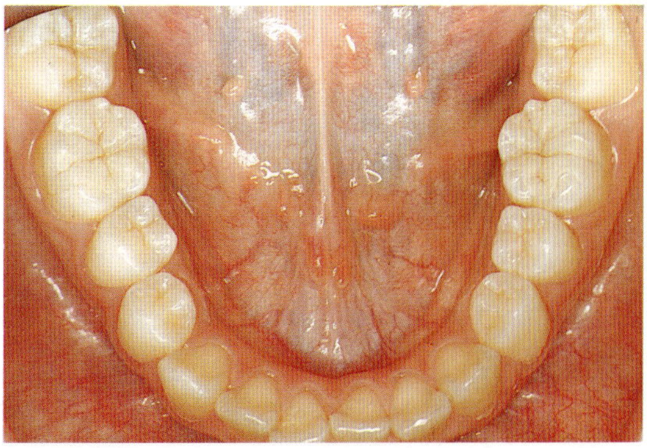

Fig. 6-107ff Postoperative occlusal view.

the completed inlay on the work model once more before divesting (Fig. 6-107y).

- To divest the completed inlay, cut away the majority of the refractory die with a disk and rotary points until only a small amount remains (Figs. 6-107z and aa). Carefully use air abrasive equipment and 25 to 50 μm aluminous oxide to remove the remaining refractory. Care must be taken not to damage the fine margins of the completed ceramic inlay (Fig. 6-107bb).
- The inlay is now carefully seated on the stone die and evaluated. Minimal seating pressure must be used to prevent die abrasion and/or fracture of the fragile inlay. Heat and vibration will lead to ceramic fracture. Internal adjustments should be done with fine high speed diamonds using a water spray. The inlay is adjusted until an acceptable fit is achieved (Fig. 6-107cc). All internal surfaces are once again carefully air abraded and steam or ultrasonically cleaned. If acid etching of the bonding surface is required, glazed surfaces should be covered with wax and the exposed surfaces etched with hydrofluoric acid for the recommended time. Extreme care must be taken when using hydrofluoric acid. Rinse off the acid and neutralize in a basic solution (sodium bicarbonate). Steam or ultrasonically clean the ceramic inlay and place in a safe container until the delivery appointment (Figs. 6-107dd to ff).

Cast Ceramic

- The fabrication of a cast glass ceramic inlay is very similar to the technique described for the all ceramic crowns.
- A stone die is fabricated and die spaced and the inlay wax pattern is fabricated as with metallic inlays.
- The inlay pattern is invested, cast and cerammed (Figs. 6-108a and b).
- Using fine diamonds and water spray the inlay is seated and checked on the die. The occlusion and proximal contacts are finalized (Figs. 6-108c to e).
- The procedures used to finalize a cast glass ceramic inlay are unique and should be noted. Occlusal functional surfaces should be polished with fine diamonds, 30-fluted carbide burs, porcelain polishing abrasive, rubber points and a diamond polishing paste. Occlusal glaze is avoided because it is more abrasive than pure glass ceramic. Stain and glaze may be added to nonfunctional grooves that are difficult to polish (Fig. 6-108g).
- Proximal surfaces are polished with porcelain polishing wheels and glazed with clear ceramic glaze. This will create an extremely smooth surface that is plaque resistant.
- The internal bonding surfaces are etched with ammonium bifluoride (not hydrofluoric acid) for 1 minute (Fig. 6-108h).
- Finally, it is recommended that cast glass

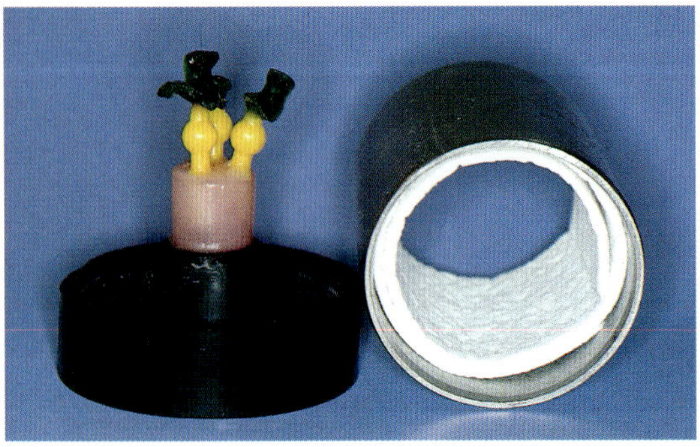

Fig. 6-108a Waxed inlays ready to invest.

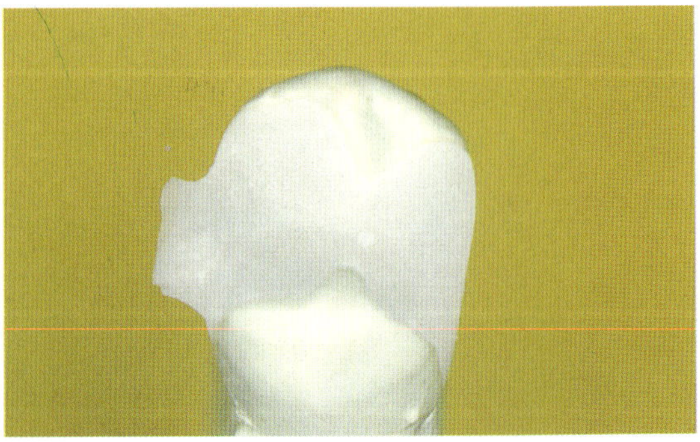

Fig. 6-108b Cast and cerammed inlay on die.

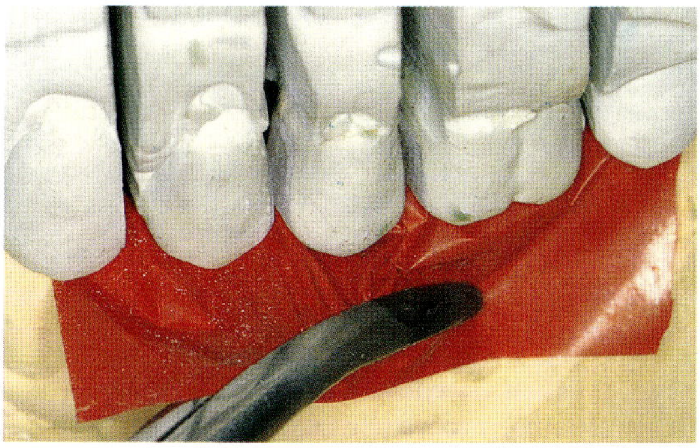

Fig. 6-108c Marking occlusal contacts.

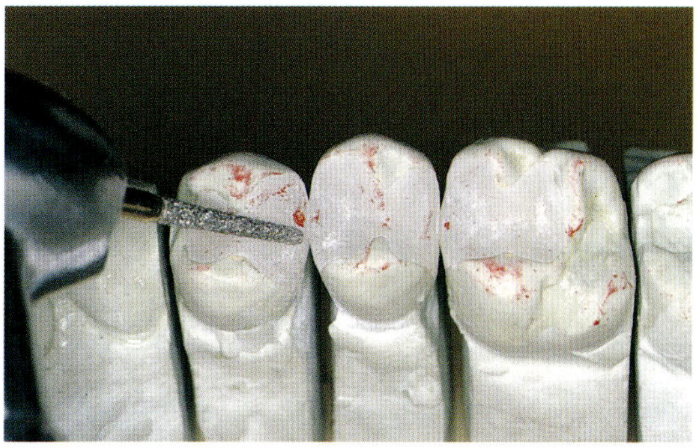

Fig. 6-108d Adjusting occlusal contacts.

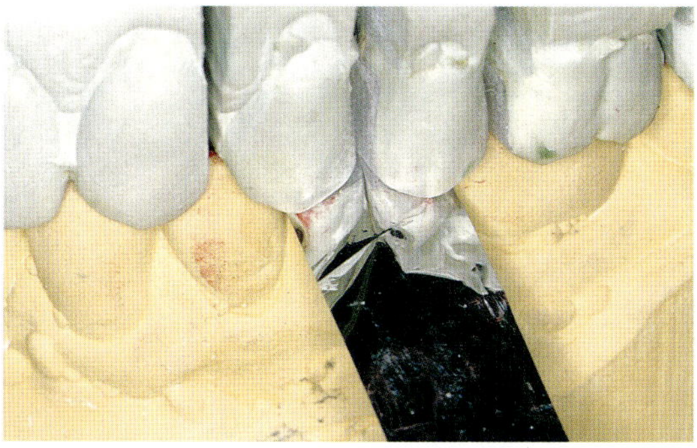

Fig. 6-108e Check occlusal contacts with thin mylar.

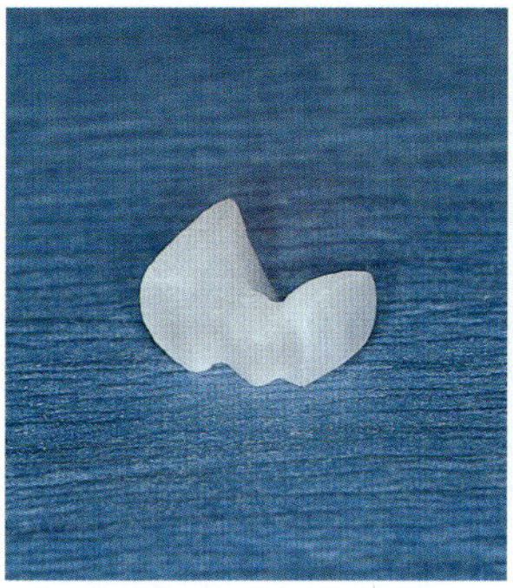

Fig. 6-108f

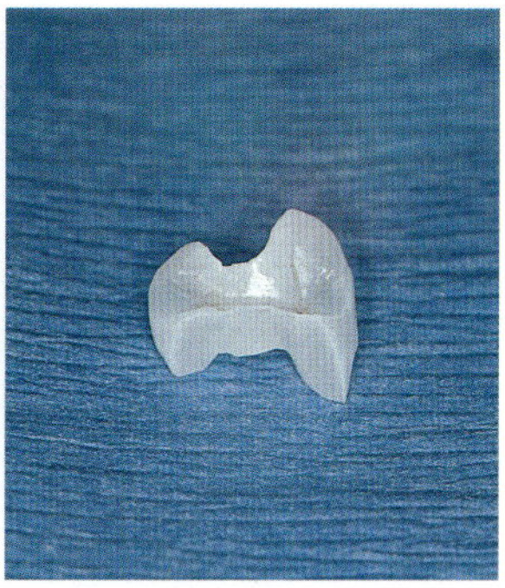

Fig. 6-108g

Fig. 6-108f Finished Dicor inlay with polished and glazed proximal surface.

Fig. 6-108g Finished Dicor inlay with polished occlusal surface, stain in grooves.

Fig. 6-108h Etching bonding surfaces with ammonium bifluoride.

Fig. 6-108i Apply silane to bonding surfaces 24 hours before cementation.

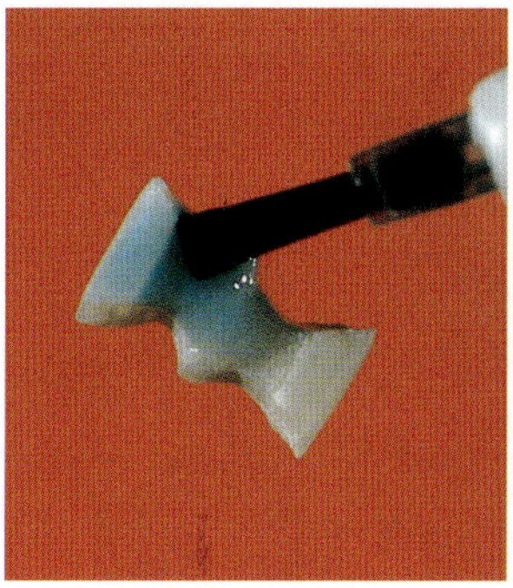

Fig. 6-108h

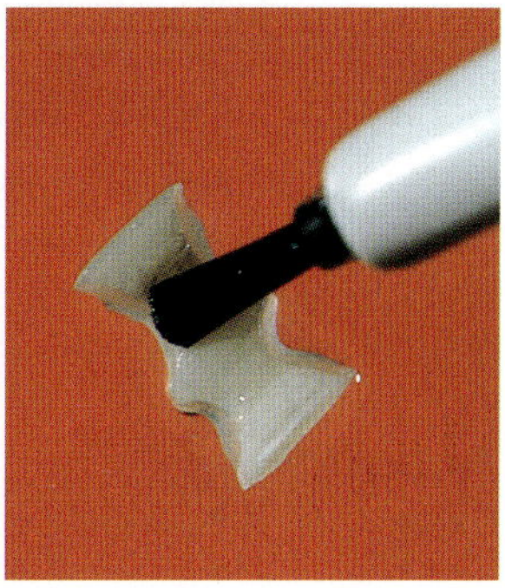

Fig. 6-108i

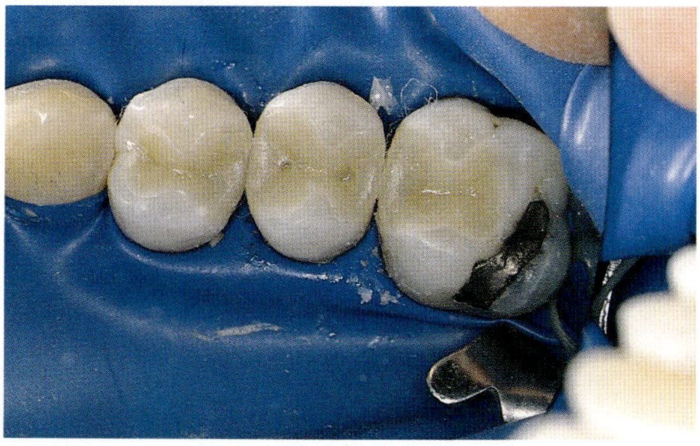

Fig. 6-108j Post-cementation occlusal view.

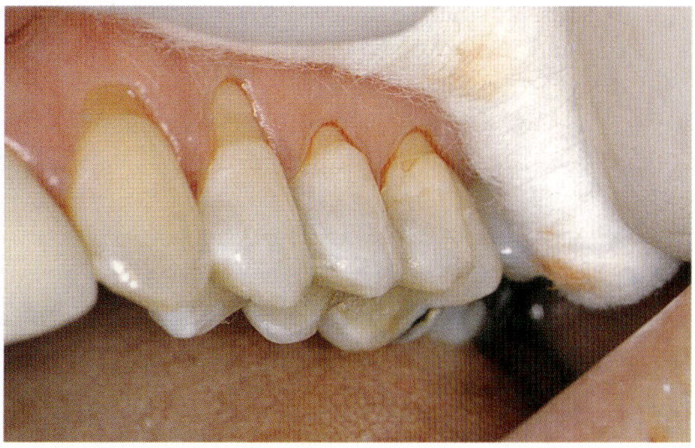

Fig. 6-108k Post-cementation facial view.

ceramic inlays be silanted 24 hours prior to cementation to optimize bond strengths (Fig. 6-108i).

- The completed cast glass ceramic inlay, once cemented, provides a reasonably esthetic restoration that potentially is more functionally compatible than many other ceramic alternatives (Figs. 6-108j and k).

CAD-CAM (Cerec)

Introduction

Most composite resin or ceramic materials used today are limited to fabrication techniques on the actual tooth or indirect models. Multiple fabrication steps by technicians result in a range of variability and limit the quality control of the final material used. Ceramic restorations require indirect fabrication, time consuming procedures and a skilled laboratory technician.

CAD-CAM technology such as the Cerec System (Siemens, Charlotte, NC) in particular has allowed for significant improvements in both of these important areas. First, the ceramic materials used for restoration fabrication are manufactured with a high level of quality control and provided in block form. Both the glass ceramic (Dicor MGC, Caulk, Milford, DE) and the conventional ceramic (Vita Mark II, Vident, Baldwin Park, CA) are significantly improved over the comparable laboratory fabricated alternative from each manufacturer. Because the final restoration is milled and not adapted to a tooth form, there is no laboratory alteration or modification of physical properties. CAD-CAM and other milling technologies used for the fabrication of inlay/onlay restorations have made possible this development of significantly improved materials that are more compatible to the oral environment.

Secondly there is no need for a trained ceramist. The computer software used to fabricate Cerec restorations is easily learned by the dentist or office auxiliary. Consequently, a high quality one appointment ceramic restoration is now a reality.

The Cerec System

The Cerec System is a very portable unit that can be moved easily from one location in the practice to another (Fig. 6-109). The components (Fig. 6-110) are a three-dimensional video camera (scan head), an electronic image processor (video processing) and memory unit (contour memory), and a processor (computer), which is connected to a miniature milling machine (three-axis milling machine). The recorded three-dimensional

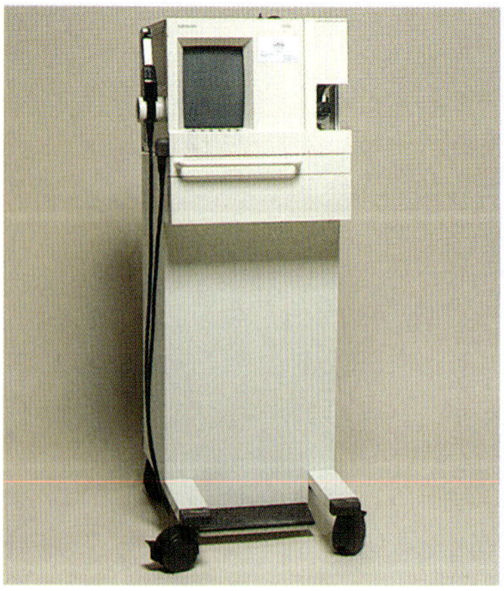

Fig. 6-109 A Cerec unit.

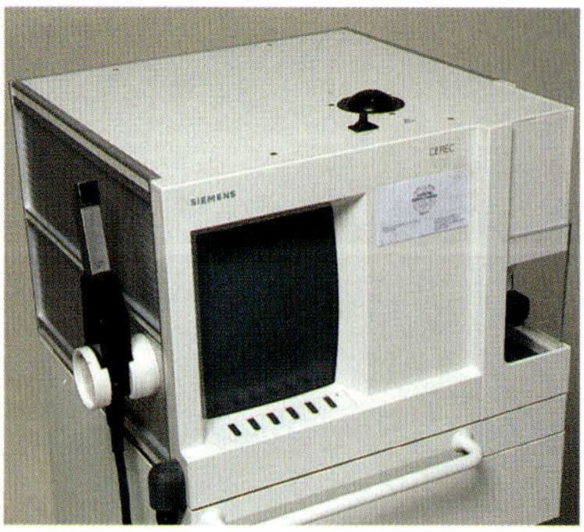

Fig. 6-110 Close up view showing (left to right) camera, monitor and milling chamber.

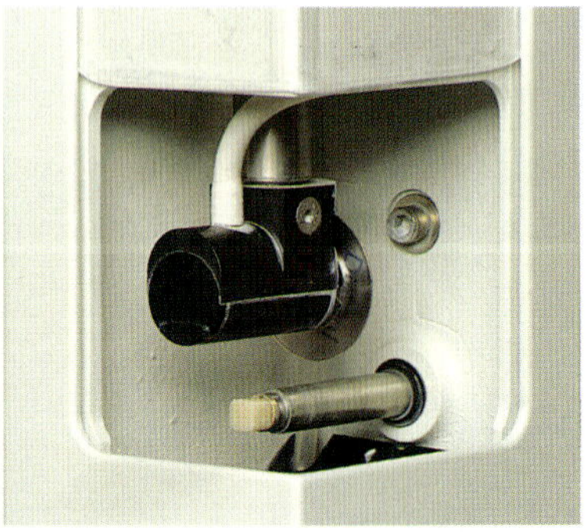

Fig. 6-111 Milling chamber with electric motor and 40-mm diamond disc.

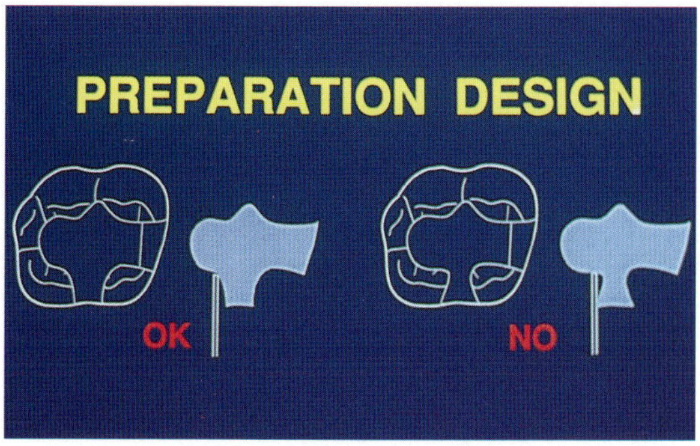

Fig. 6-112 Preparation designs limited by disc access.

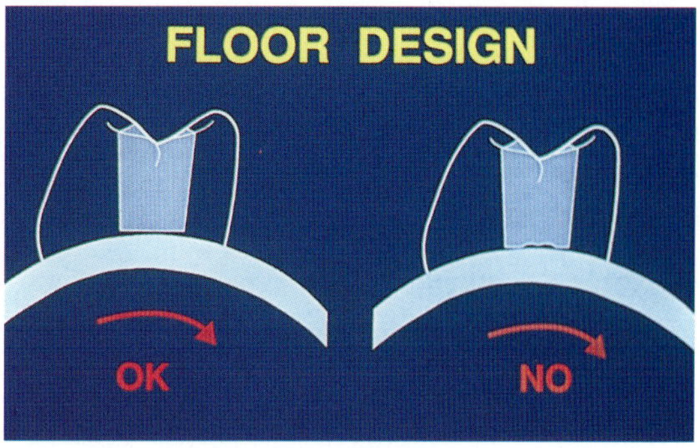

Fig. 6-113 All floors should be flat.

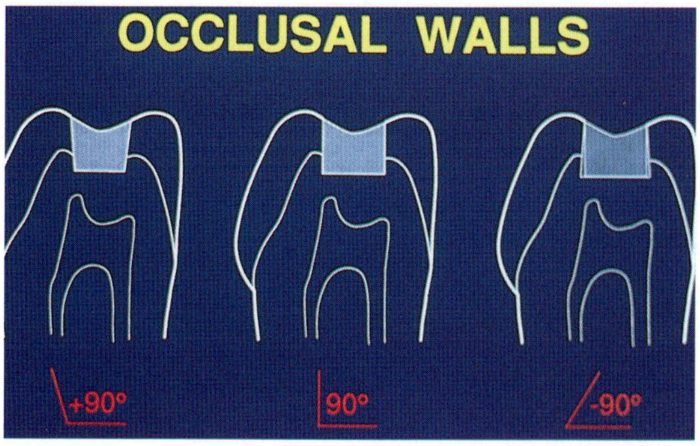

Fig. 6-114 Occlusal walls may be divergent, parallel or convergent.

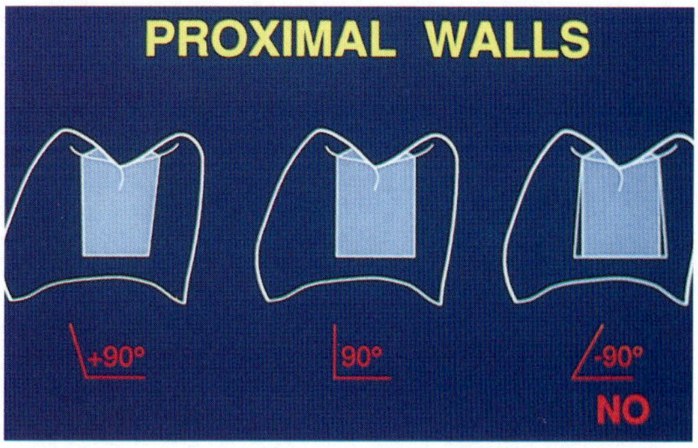

Fig. 6-115 Proximal walls must diverge slightly from gingival to occlusal.

data of a preparation are immediately displayed as a freeze-frame video image on the monitor. The preparation image on the monitor can be revised easily and any necessary modifications made prior to inlay fabrication. The milling component utilizes a 40-mm-diameter diamond disc (Fig. 6-111). This disc configuration limits the contours that can be milled and requires the application of certain preparation design criteria.

The final inlay/onlay fabricated by the Cerec System is milled to fit the internal aspects of the preparation and proximal contracts but requires the dentist to finalize occlusal morphology and proximal contacts.

Technique Overview (Preparation Modification)

Design of the preparation is limited to configurations that can be milled with a diamond disc that functions much like a wood lathe. The inlay rotates as the diamond disc cuts circumferential slices as programmed by the computer. Any sharp or deep contours perpendicular to the disc rotation are impossible to mill (Fig. 6-112). Any contour irregularities on the pulpal or gingival floors cannot be milled. Pulpal and gingival floors must be as flat as possible (Fig. 6-113). As with any ceramic inlay, the margins must be smooth and distinct. Indistinct margins are more difficult for the computer and operator to detect and result in a poorly fitting inlay.

The occlusal walls need not be divergent occlusally, as with traditional inlay preparations (Fig. 6-114). The optical impression cannot read undercuts, and minimal taper can be programmed into the restoration. This allows for a potentially more conservative preparation when old undercut restorations

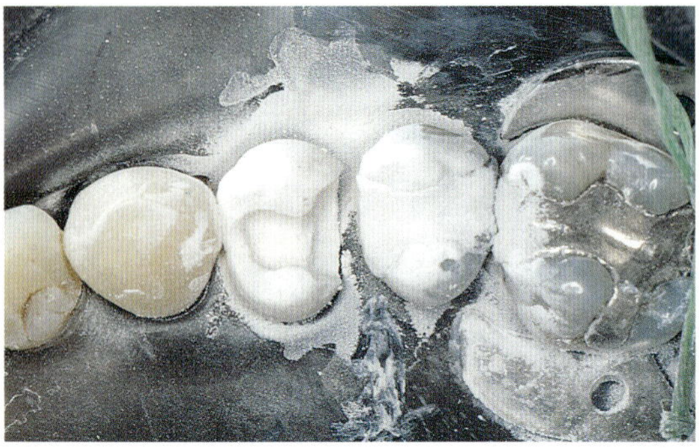

Fig. 6-116a The preparation is coated with titanium dioxide contrast powder.

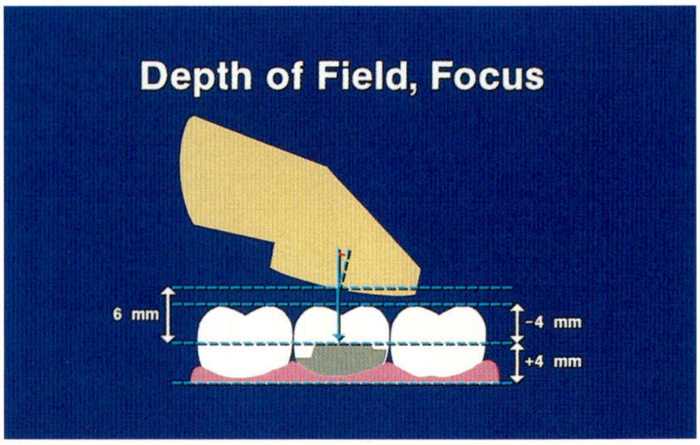

Fig. 6-116b Optical impression is taken intraorally (courtesy of Siemens).

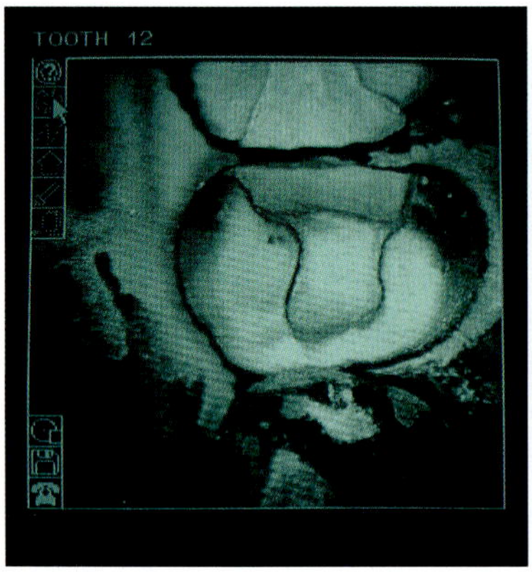

Fig. 6-116c

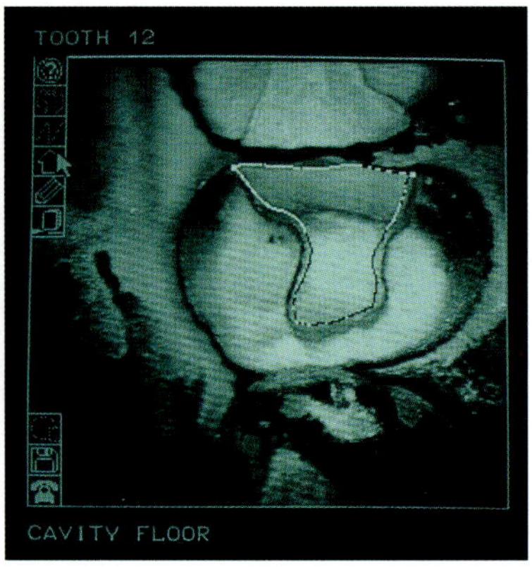

Fig. 6-116d

Fig. 6-116c View of preparation on monitor.

Fig. 6-116d Draw the "bottom line" boundaries first.

are removed. The proximal box must be parallel to slightly divergent occlusally. The latter is recommended, whereas excessive divergence or undercuts should be avoided (Fig. 6-115).

Optical Impression

Once the preparation is completed, an optical impression can be made. Teeth lack sufficient uniform reflectivity so the preparation and approximating structures are coated with a contrast powder (Fig. 6-116a). The scanning camera head lens is positioned over the prepared tooth and the preparation can be seen on the monitor (Fig. 6-116b). An optimal scanning direction is determined that is perpendicular to the pulpal floor and visualizes all critical areas (Fig. 6-116c). Once obtained, the optical impression is saved. Up to three impressions can be saved on each 3.5-inch computer storage disc.

Inlay Fabrication

Inlay fabrication can now be completed by the dentist or auxiliary. The first step is to draw in all pulpal and cervical borders, now called "bottom line" (Fig. 6-116d). Next, the proximal contact contour is programmed (Fig. 6-116e). Finally, the computer determines the occlusal and proximal cavosurface margins and the marginal ridge position (Figs. 6-116f and g).

Milling

Once the computer is programmed, the inlay is milled. The computer determines the size of the block to use and the operator selects the desired shade. Currently, two

Fig. 6-116e Draw proximal contour.

Fig. 6-116f The computer draws the occlusal cavosurface margins.

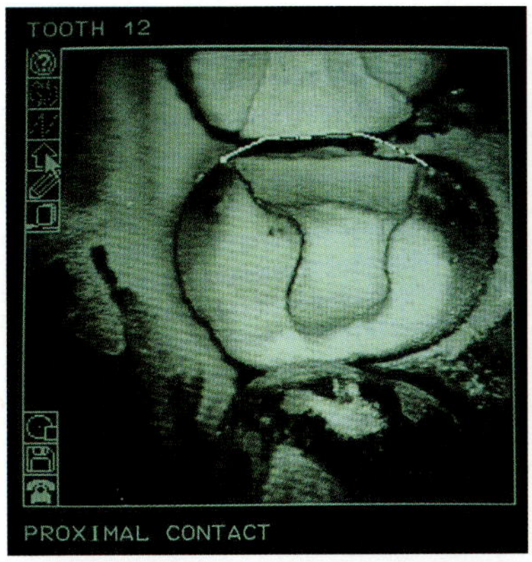

Fig. 6-116e

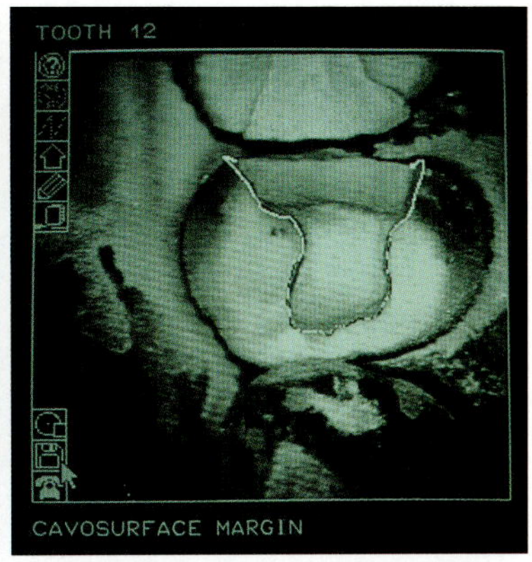

Fig. 6-116f

Fig. 6-116g The computer determines the marginal ridge contour.

Fig. 6-116h Several editing options exist, such as this window showing horizontal profiles.

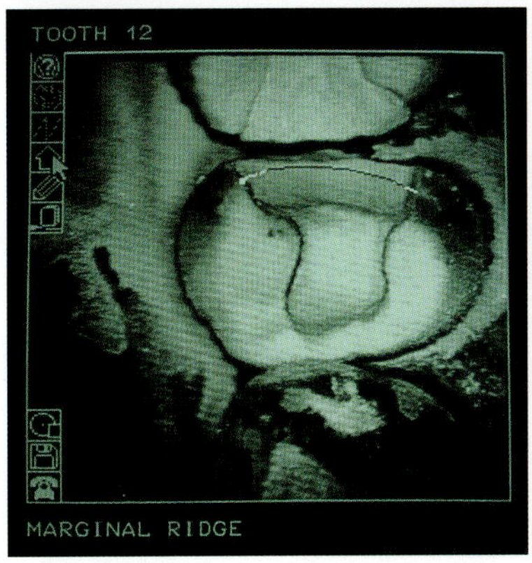

Fig. 6-116g

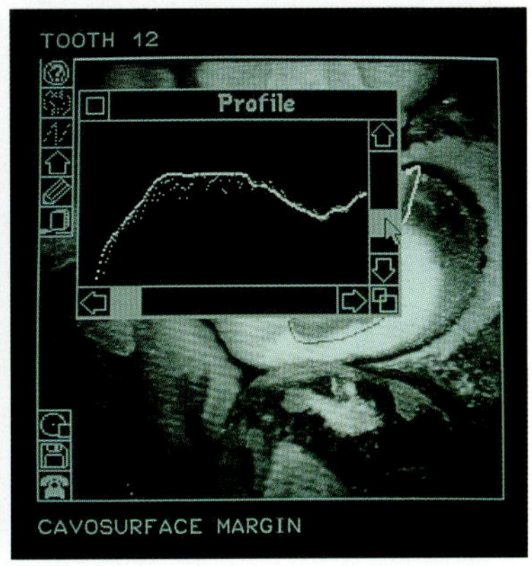

Fig. 6-116h

glass ceramic and several conventional ceramic shades are available and these are adequate for most posterior inlays/onlays.

Try-in and Cementation

The ceramic inlay is tried in, the contact is adjusted with a fine ceramic adjusting stone and the fit is analyzed. If the marginal fit is adequate, the proximal surface is polished with ceramic polishing wheels and the cementation process begins. In the event that the design is not acceptable, reentry into the stored data is possible. Margins can be repositioned and contours can be modified by using the edit mode (Fig. 6-116h).

An alternative technique involves fabricating a quick-setting hard or flexible model that can be used by the individual fabricating the inlay to make a majority of the adjustments as well as analyze fit prior to returning to the patient for try-in. This technique allows for delegation of the inlay fabrication to an auxiliary and will minimize chair time and utilization time required by the dentist.

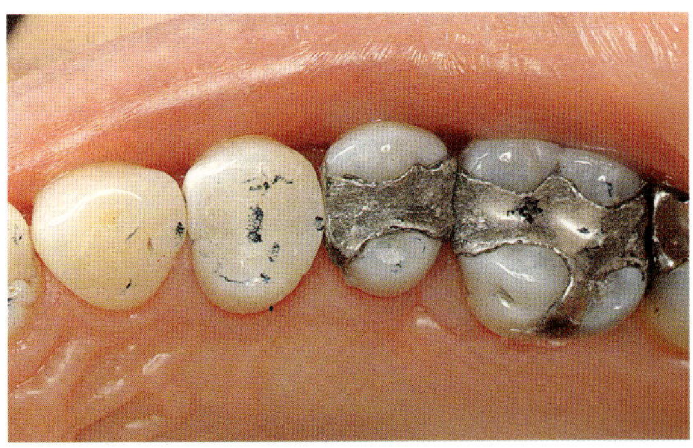

Fig. 6-116i Final occlusal adjustment and contouring after cementation.

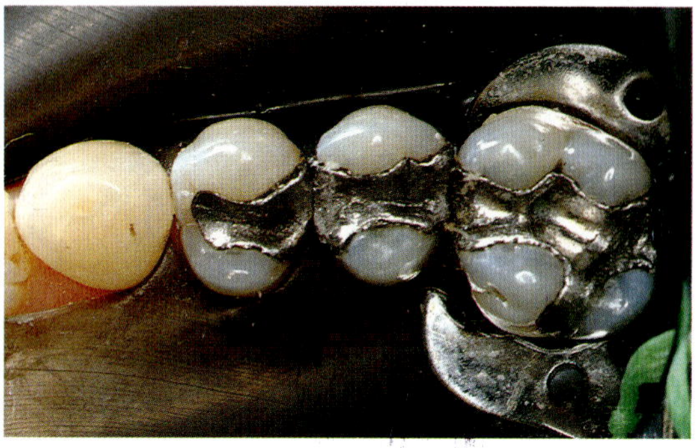

Fig. 6-117a Preoperative view.

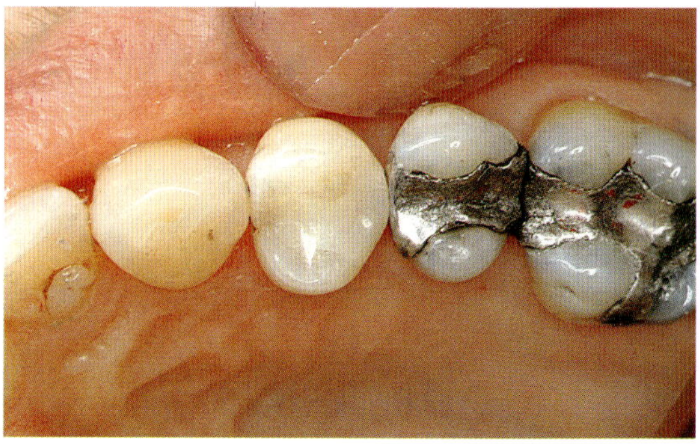

Fig. 6-117b Postoperative view.

The completed inlay with polished proximal surfaces is now ready to cement. The cementation procedures are similar to laboratory fabricated inlays. The inlay is etched internally and coated with silane. The preparation is etched and treated with the desired dental multipurpose bonding agent. A dual cure composite cement is placed in the preparation and the inlay is seated. Excess cement is removed and the cement is cured.

Because the Cerec System does not completely contour the occlusal surface, the dentist must now finalize the occlusal morphology using small flame shaped diamonds of course to medium grit. This generally requires a minimum of time, but optical magnification is recommended to decrease the potential for excess tooth reduction. Once this is accomplished, the rubber dam is removed and the final occlusion is checked and adjusted (Fig. 6-116i). Final finishing should include the use of fine and extrafine diamonds, 30-fluted finishing burs, abrasive rubber ceramic polishing points and/or diamond polishing paste.

The completed restorations are well within the range of acceptable esthetics for posterior restorations and provide a restoration in one appointment that has the potential to be made from a wide range of materials (Fig. 6-117)

Copy-Milling (Celay®)

Introduction

Another unique manufacturing system that will produce esthetic inlay/onlay restorations from the improved ceramic materials mentioned in the CAD-CAM section is called Celay (Mikrona Technologie AG, Spreitenbach, Switzerland). The Celay system does not use a CAD-CAM approach but uses copy-milling techniques. A hard composite resin pattern of the restoration must be made in the mouth or on a model and these patterns are duplicated.

Technique

The inlay/onlay is prepared as recommended in the previous preparation section. Most designs can be duplicated. On the tooth or on a model a pattern is fabricated out of a rigid material (Fig. 6-118). This pattern is mounted on the copying side of the Celay unit (Fig. 6-119). A block of esthetic material is mounted on the milling side (Fig. 6-120). (see materials supplement.) Various sized probes that represent the sizes of the different milling burs are run over the surface of the rigid pattern. At the same time, the matched rotary instrument mills the same shape out of the restorative block (Fig. 6-121). Using a series of rotary instruments, an exact duplicate of the pattern is copy-

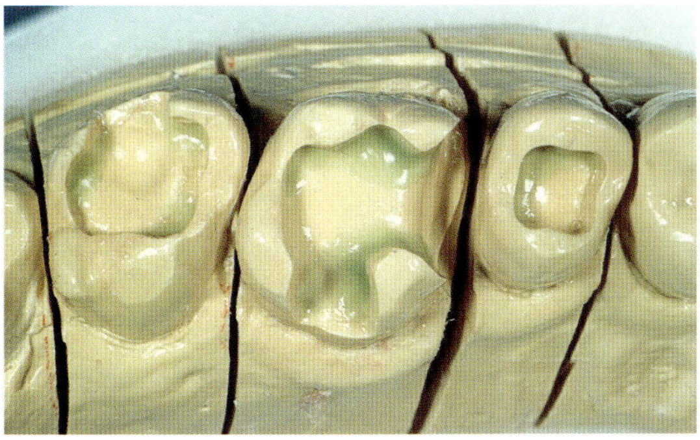

Fig. 6-118a Working model of prepared inlays.

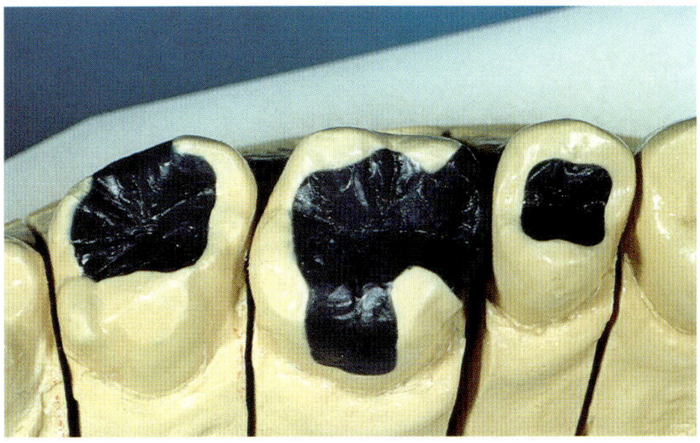

Fig. 6-118b Hard composite inlay patterns.

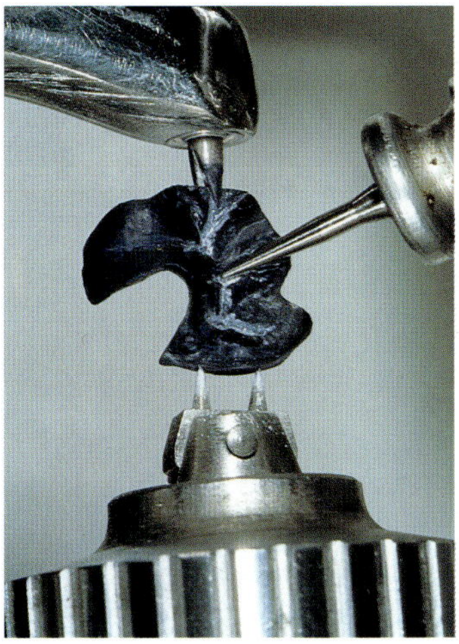

Fig. 6-119 Inlay pattern mounted in the Celay unit (copy side).

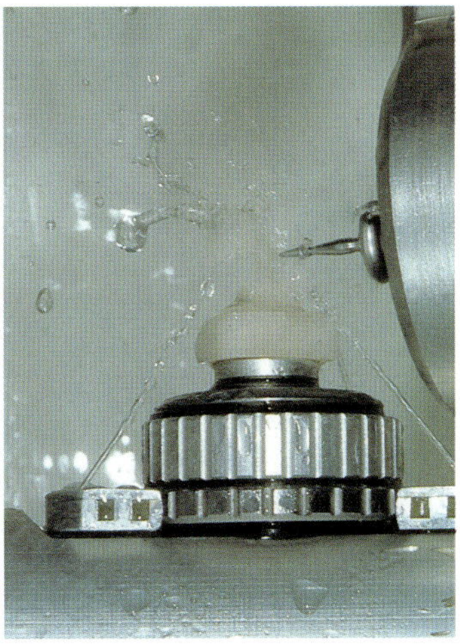

Fig. 6-120 Celay unit (milling side) copy-milling pattern out of a ceramic material.

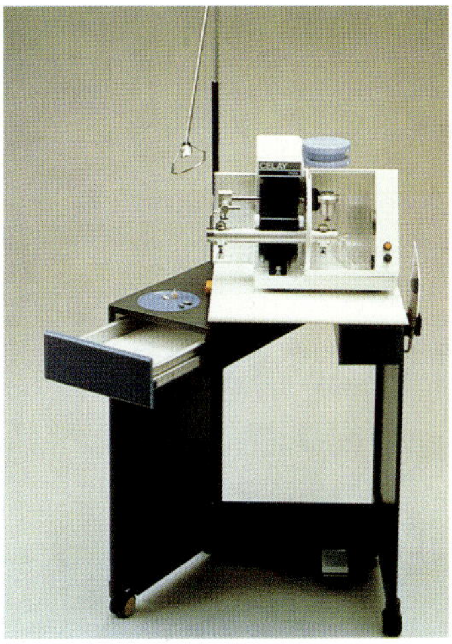

Fig. 6-121 Celay unit.

milled. This rough pattern can now be seated on the die or back in the mouth, checked for accuracy and the proximal adjusted and polished. Depending upon the material used the bonding surfaces are etched and silane applied.

Finally, the inlay/onlay is cemented as outlined previously using dual cured composite resin cement and all purpose bonding materials. Occlusal and accessible areas are adjusted and polished (Fig. 6-122).

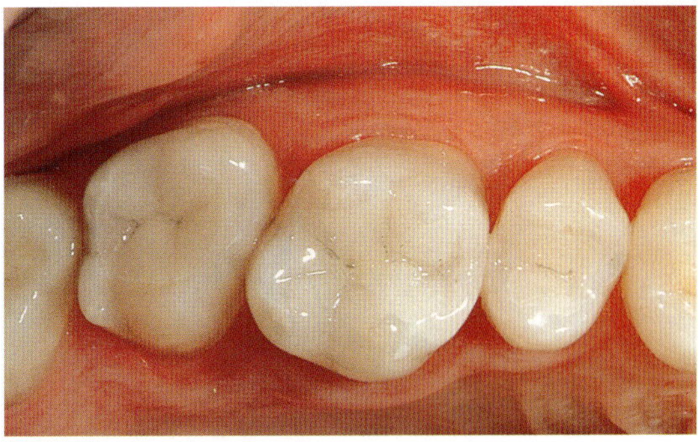

Fig. 6-122 Finished ceramic inlays.

Speculation

This system is too new to speculate on exactly how it will be applied but it appears to be more laboratory oriented than clinically

(Note: Figs. 6-118 to 6-122 are courtesy of Mikrona Technologie, AG Spreitenbach, Switzerland.)

oriented. While a one appointment inlay/onlay may be possible, fabricating patterns intraorally is time consuming and requires a special aptitude and desire to accomplish. In contrast, pattern fabrication on an indirect model in a laboratory appears to be a cost affective approach to esthetic inlay/onlay fabrication. Time will tell how this system will be applied and if its versatility and simplicity are an advantage.

Injection Molded Glass Ceramic (IPS Empress)

Injection molded glass ceramic IPS Empress® (Williams, Ivoclar, Buffalo, NY) is similar to cast glass ceramic but with some distinct differences. While using a glass ceramic material, it is precrystallized and supplied in different colored ingots (Fig. 6-123). The crystals are lucite and appear to have strength and wear properties superior to those of conventional ceramics and possibly many of the various strengthened groups. However, it is not as strong as In-Ceram.

- A lost wax process is utilized in fabrication (Fig. 6-123). The restoration pattern is sprued and invested (Figs. 6-124a to d).
- Ceramic ingots fit precisely into the sprue former and a ceramic rod is used as a piston type device to push the ceramic into the investment void (Fig. 6-124e). The wax pattern is burned out and the heated ceramic ingot and aluminous oxide ceramic plunger are positioned in the cylindrical sprue former space (Figs. 6-124f and g). The entire assembly is placed in a special pressing oven that heats and applies pressure on the plunger, injecting the molten ceramic into the void created by the wax pattern (Figs. 6-124h and i). This takes about 45 minutes.
- The cooled investment is cut and the injection molded restoration carefully divested (Fig. 6-124j).
- The ceramic inlay is cut off of the sprue and seated on the die (Figs. 6-124k and l).
- Depending upon the treatment goals, the glass ceramic can be polished, stained or veneered with conventional ceramic materials (Figs. 6-124m to o). Custom colored dies aid in accurate color matching.
- This versatile glass ceramic system can be used to fabricate a variety of restorations. Functional and esthetic priorities should dictate techniques utilized for optimal results (Fig. 6-125).

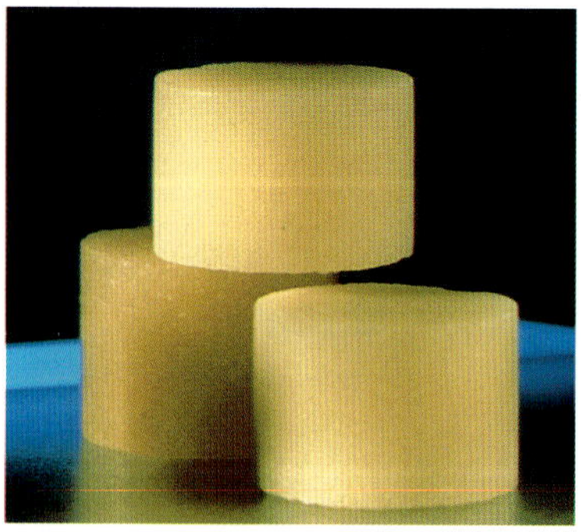

Fig. 6-123 Precrystallized and colored IPS Empress glass ceramic ingots.

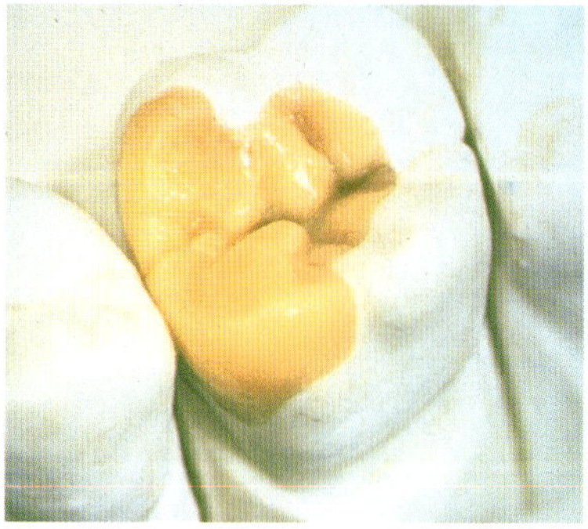

Fig. 6-124a Waxed inlay.

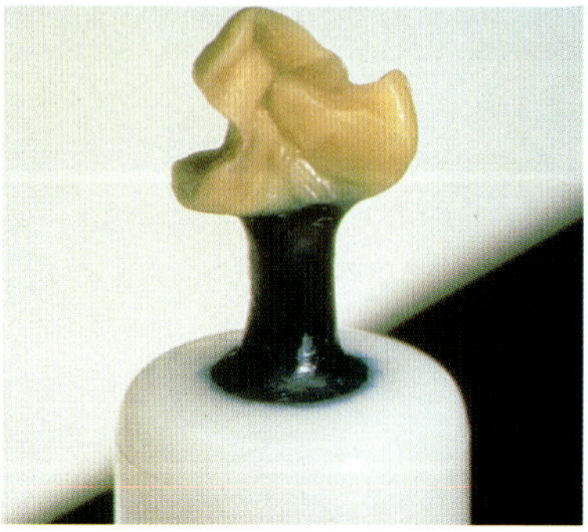

Fig. 6-124b Sprued wax pattern.

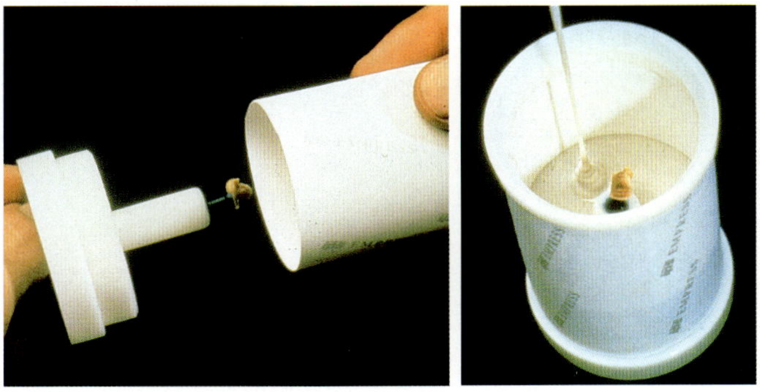

Figs. 6-124c and d Investing the wax pattern.

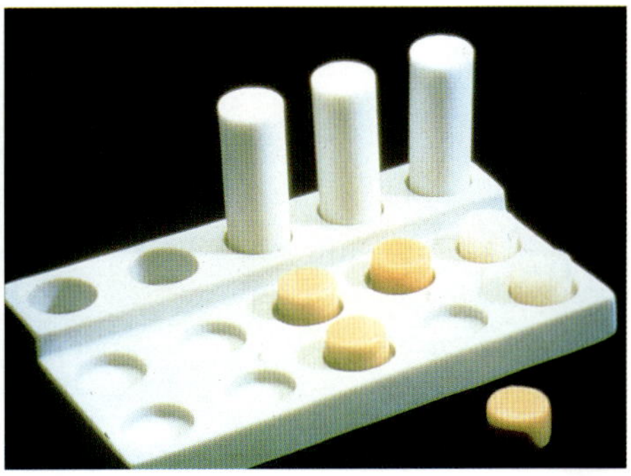

Fig. 6-124e Ceramic ingots and ceramic plunger placed in refractory tray.

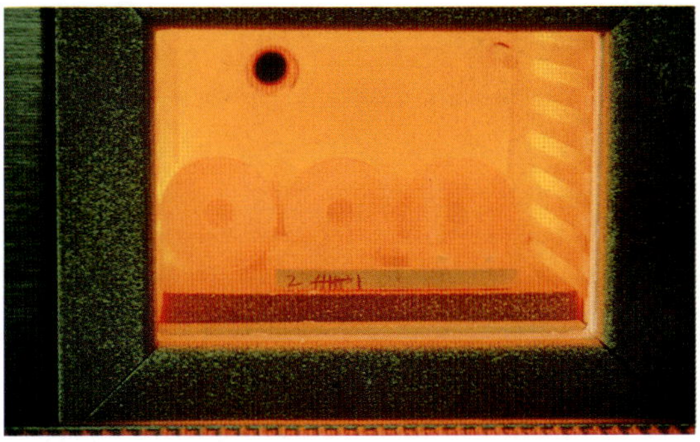

Fig. 6-124f Place all components in burnout oven simultaneously.

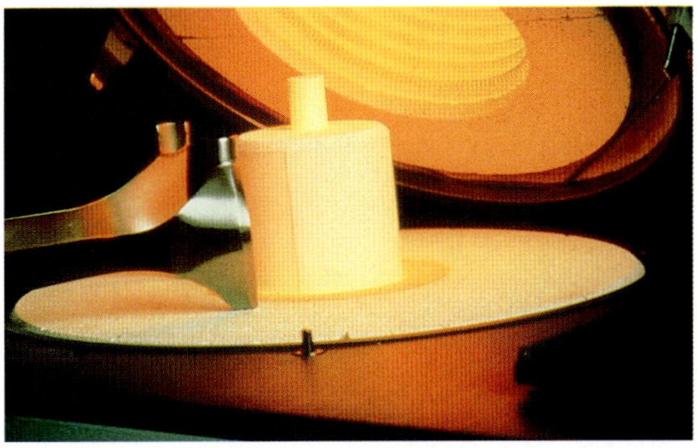

Fig. 6-124g A ceramic ingot and plunger is placed in the burnout investment and positioned in pressing oven.

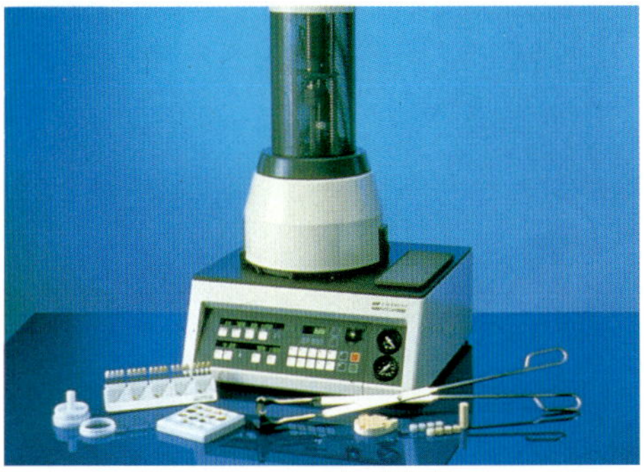

Fig. 6-124h Pressing oven.

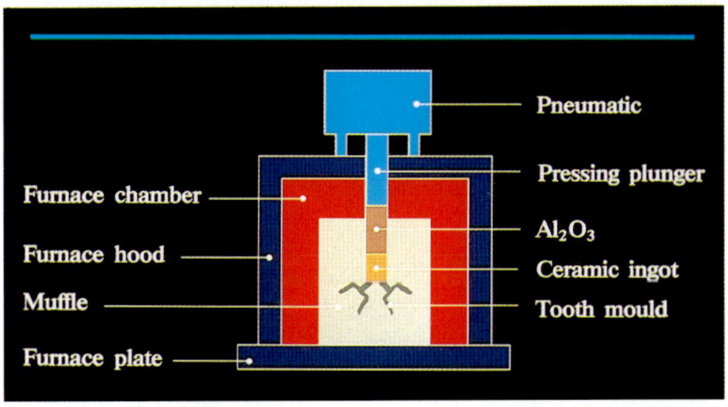

Fig. 6-124i Drawing showing how the ceramic plunger pushes the glass ceramic into the voids created by the burned out wax pattern. All done in the pressing oven.

(Note: Figs. 6-123 to 6-125 are courtesy of Williams Ivoclar, Buffalo, NY.)

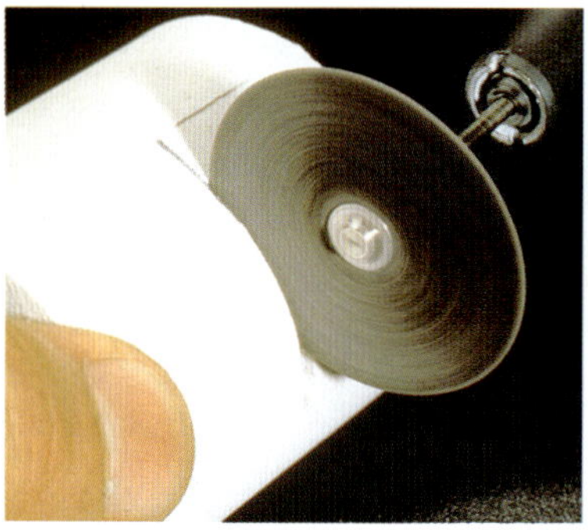

Fig. 6-124j Carefully divest the cooled refractory.

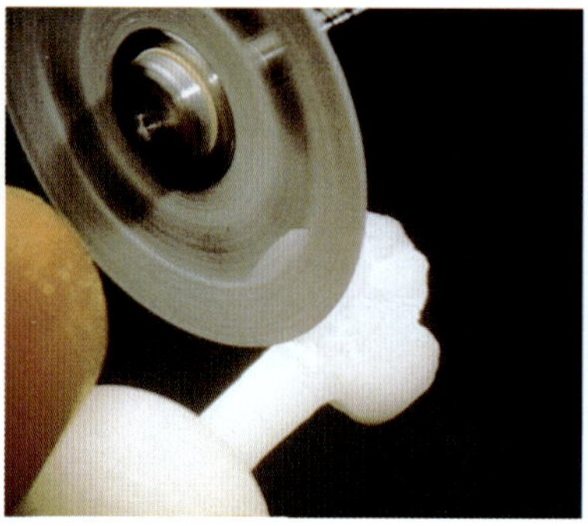

Fig. 6-124k Cut pattern off sprue.

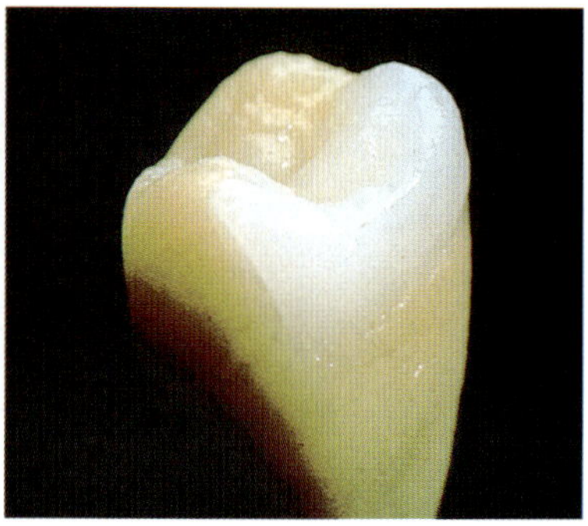

Fig. 6-124l Try the casting onto the die.

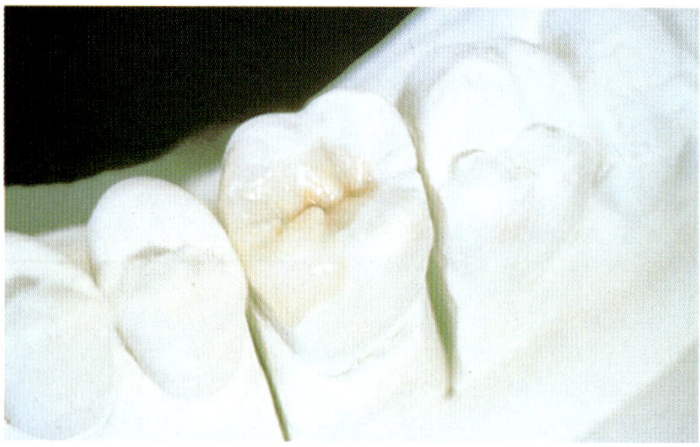

Fig. 6-124m Finished restoration on the die.

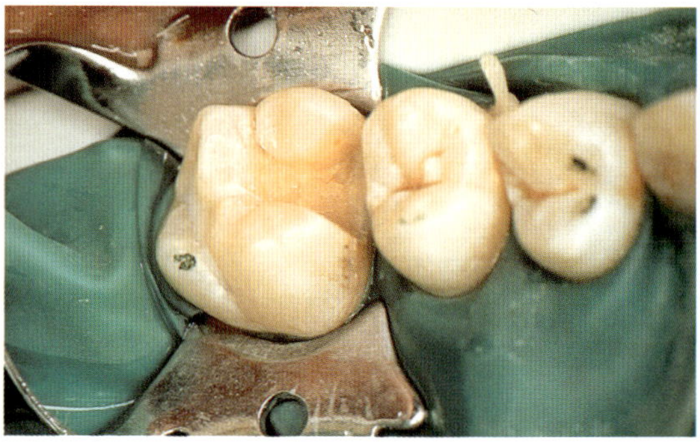

Fig. 6-124n Prepared tooth ready for cementation.

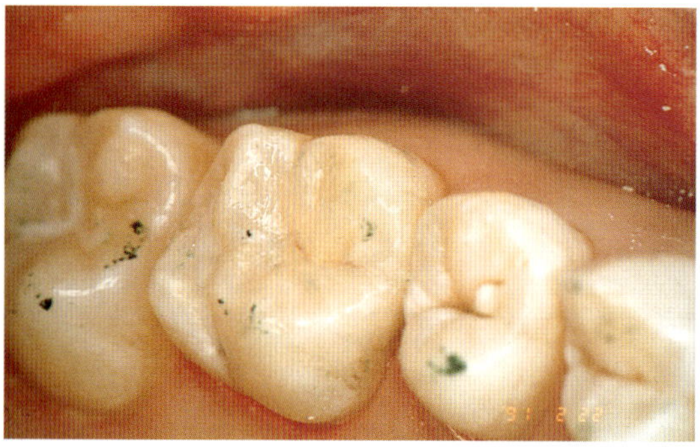

Fig. 6-124o Finished restorations.

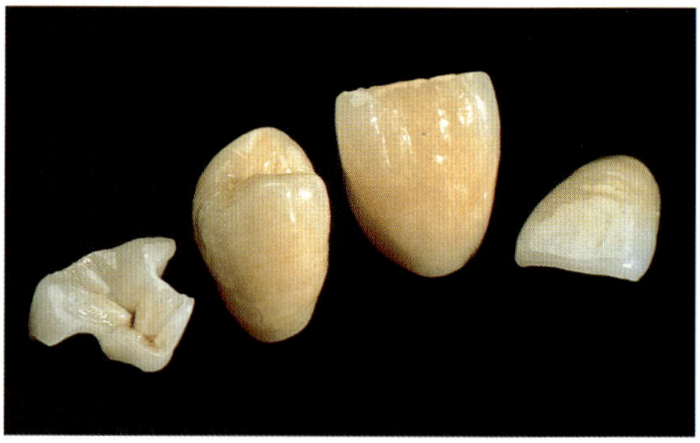

Fig. 6-125 Various IPS Empress restorations.

CERAMIC VENEERS

INTRODUCTION

The procedures used and the success achieved in bonding thin veneers of ceramic to tooth structure must be considered a major milestone for esthetic restorative dentistry. In many instances the need for conventional crowns or short-lasting composite restorations has been eliminated by this esthetic, durable and conservative alternative that is well within the capabilities of the average dentist and technician. While the procedures are technique sensitive, ceramic veneers provide a highly esthetic restoration requiring minimum tooth destruction or periodontal involvement.

In 1983, Horn introduced a method to bake the ceramic laminate veneer on a platinum matrix, then etch the inside of the veneer with hydrofluoric acid. A silane coupling agent was applied onto the veneer then bonded to the tooth using a light cured composite resin cement. Simonsen and Calamia etched ceramic specimens with 7.5% hydrofluoric acid for 20 minutes in an ultrasonic cleaner, then checked the etched surface using SEM. They found that the surface of the ceramic had microscopic pits similar to etched enamel that could be easily bonded with composite resin. The bond strength of the composite resin to unetched ceramic was only 230 psi and the strength was increased to 1670 psi when the ceramic was etched. Calamia and Simonsen also found that by using a silane coupling agent the bond strength between the ceramic and the composite resin increased to 2080 psi. The technique of etching the ceramic veneer surface using a low concentration of hydrofluoric acid made possible the development of ceramic laminate veneers.

In the early 1980s, the combination of enamel and ceramic etching techniques were developed using composite cements to bond ceramic veneers to the facial surfaces of teeth. The excellent success of these early attempts soon led to the development of more sophisticated techniques and materials. Ceramic veneer restorations are now a routine procedure in many esthetic restorative practices throughout the world.

The success of most contemporary indirect esthetic restorations depends upon the ability to predictably bond the tooth and restoration together using a stable interface. The techniques of enamel etching and bonding are well established and predictable. The preparation of the surface of ceramics using hydrofluoric acid, ammonium bifluoride and/or abrasion (microetching) has been shown to provide an extremely retentive surface. The use of silanes and multipurpose bonding agents in conjunction with composite cements result in bond strengths that are adequate for clinical success.

Ceramic veneer procedures and applications are in a state of continued development and evaluation. Long term controlled clinical evaluation of any relatively new procedure, over a 10 to 15 year period, is necessary to establish a new technique as predictably successful. Ceramic veneers are entering into that period of success with positive results. The expanded applications of ceramic veneer procedures to rebuild functional tooth surfaces or correct more complex occlusal alignment problems must be considered short term adaptations requiring additional evaluations. These more advanced bonded ceramic applications will be presented but must be considered speculative and experimental compared to more established techniques of veneering labial surfaces alone with ceramic materials.

The main benefit of the ceramic veneer

procedures is that they provide an extremely esthetic yet conservative alternative to restorative procedures requiring more extensive preparations. These conservative esthetic techniques are less invasive to both hard and soft intraoral tissues. They provide an excellent esthetic result and improved periodontal response that are easier to achieve than with traditional alternatives.

Esthetic restorative dentistry requires the use of bonded ceramic procedures. As technology advances and longitudinal success is verified, many traditional restorative procedures will be replaced by contemporary bonded ceramic alternatives.

INDICATIONS AND LIMITATIONS

The veneering of a tooth with a thin ceramic veneer has many potential applications. Well established procedures include veneering the facial and incisal-occlusal surfaces of maxillary anterior and posterior teeth (Fig. 6-126). The veneering of the facial and incisal surfaces of the mandibular teeth is done routinely but must be considered a more vulnerable procedure due to increased functional stresses on the ceramic veneer (Fig. 6-127). When should ceramic veneering procedures be considered?

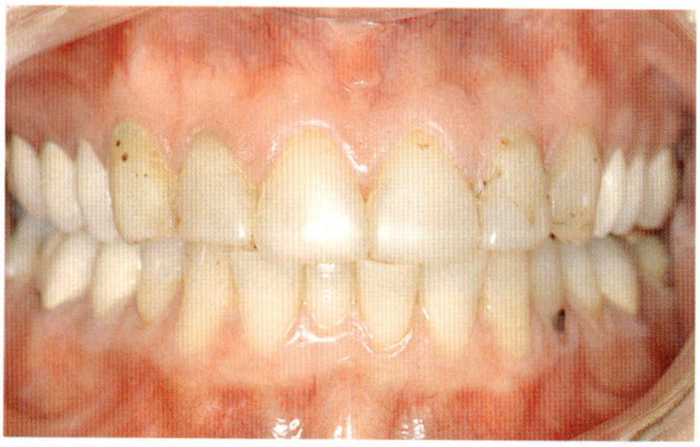

Fig. 6-126a Preoperative view.

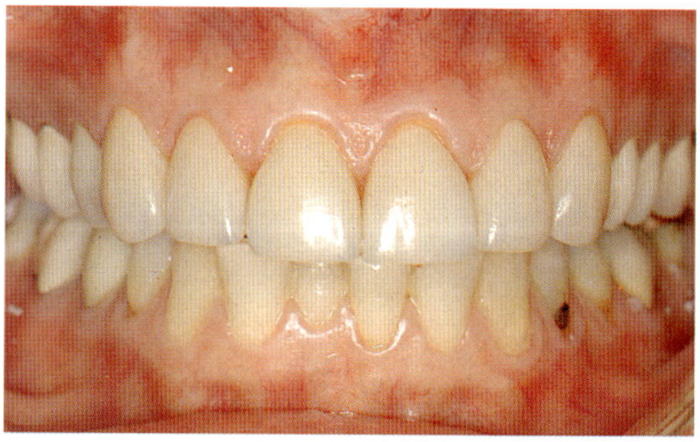

Fig. 6-126b Ceramic veneers on teeth 6 to 11.

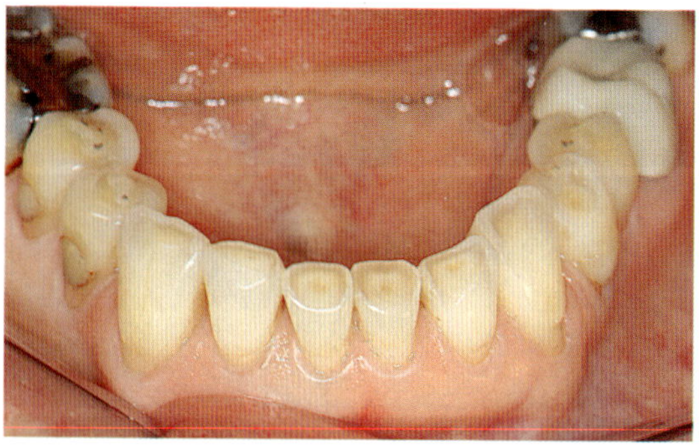

Fig. 6-127a Preoperative view.

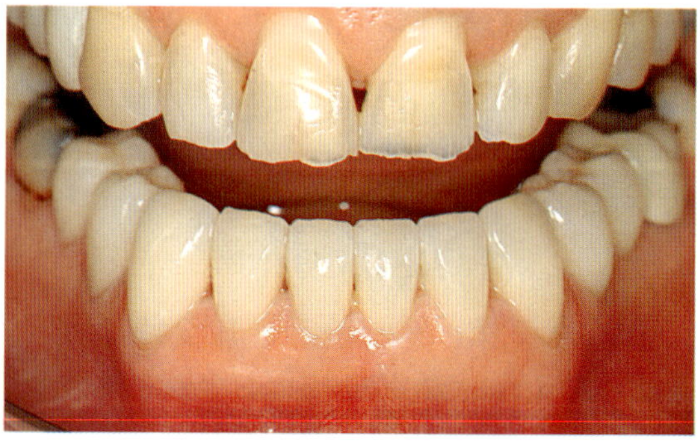

Fig. 6-127b Ceramic veneers on teeth 22 to 27, "full veneers" covering the facial and occlusal surfaces of teeth 20, 21, 28, 29.

Tooth Color Modification

Ceramic veneers are a predictable and stable way to modify tooth color. When a more conservative technique such as tooth bleaching is not successful in providing the desired color modification, ceramic veneers may be indicated (Fig. 6-128). They may also be indicated when a patent desires a predictable and stable long term esthetic result. Bleaching alone may not satisfy the requirement. Ceramic veneers provide a potentially more durable and stable esthetic restoration than direct composite bonding, and they do not require a high degree of operator artistic skill to achieve excellent results. Veneers fabricated by a skilled technician generally will result in better esthetic results than can be achieved with direct composite bonding procedures. While excellent results can be achieved using direct techniques, the average dentist can achieve more predictable results using indirect bonded ceramic techniques.

The ability of a thin veneer of ceramic to modify tooth color is largely controlled by modifying opacity or translucency. The amount of veneer opacification necessary is determined by the difference between the prepared tooth shade and the desired final shade. Some esthetic problems cannot be completely corrected with 0.5- to 1.0-mm ceramic veneers. Necessary compromises must be understood and accepted by the patient prior to treatment (Fig. 6-129).

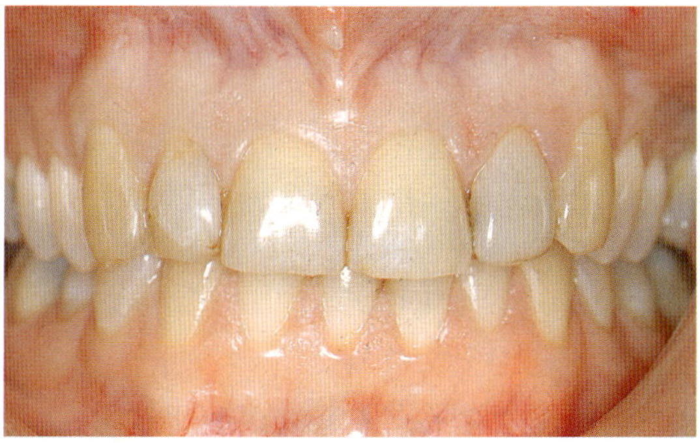

Fig. 6-128a Preoperative view.

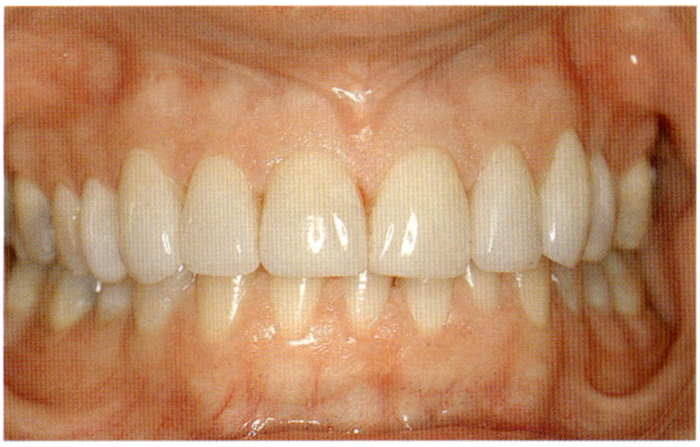

Fig. 6-128b Ceramic veneers placed on maxillary anterior teeth.

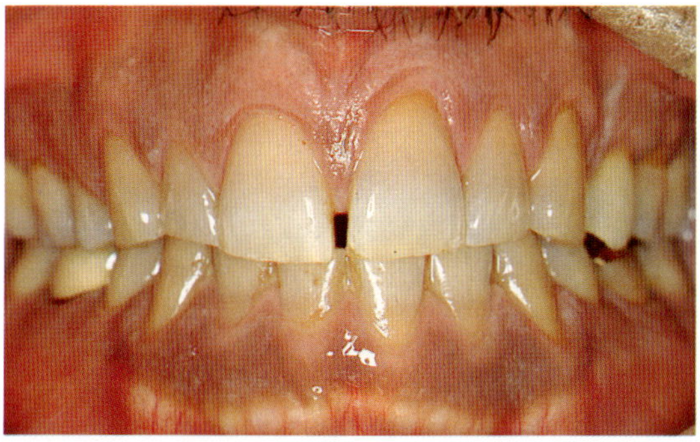

Fig. 6-129a Preoperative view.

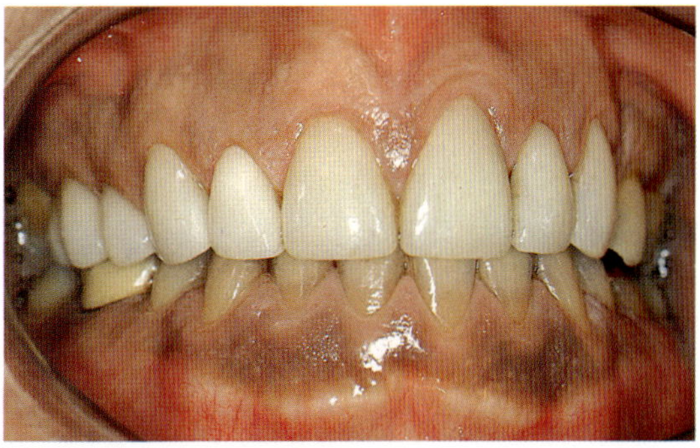

Fig. 6-129b Preoperative view showing opaque-looking veneers when extreme color chage is desired.

Tooth Position And Contour Modifications

Ceramic veneers are an excellent procedure to align teeth or modify undesirable contours. The ability to align malpositioned teeth without orthodontics is highly desirable to many individuals because immediate results can be achieved along with other modifications such as color change (Fig. 6-130). Malformed or broken teeth that have an undesirable contour are also possible

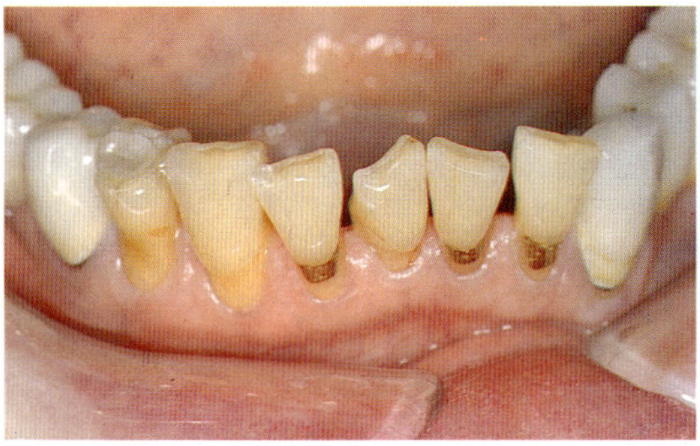

Fig. 6-130a Preoperative view.

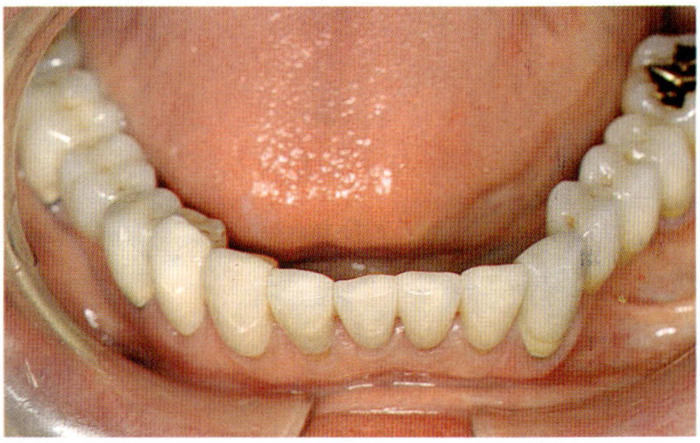

Fig. 6-130b Ceramic veneers used to lighten and align mandibular anterior teeth.

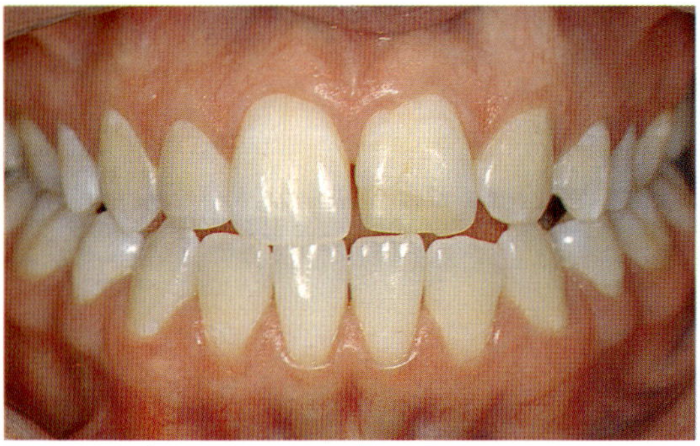

Fig. 6-131a Preoperative view.

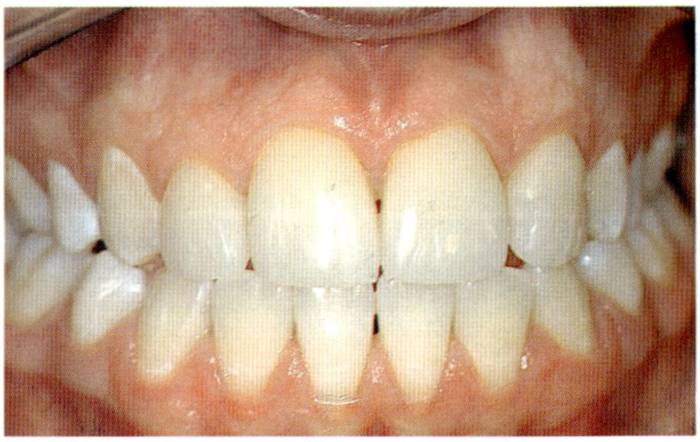

Fig. 6-131b Ceramic veneers used to repair fractured tooth 9, fill spaces and reshape teeth 7 to 10.

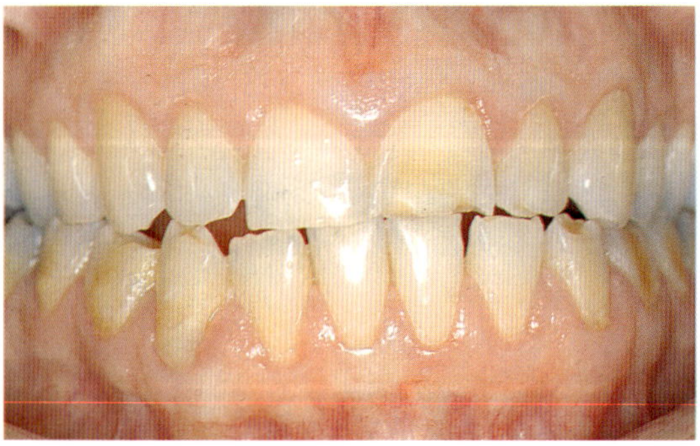

Fig. 6-132a Preoperative view.

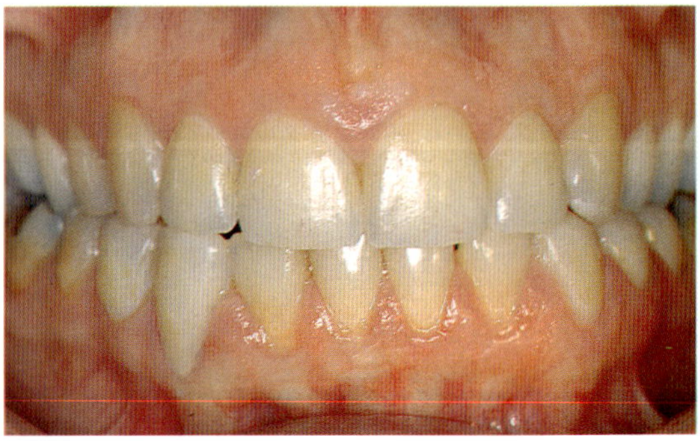

Fig. 6-132b Ceramic veneers used to replace enamel deficiencies on teeth 7 to 10, 20 to 22, 27 and 28; cusp tip added to tooth 11.

indications for ceramic veneers (Fig. 6-131). Ceramic veneers can be equated to replacement or augmented enamel. When the addition of new enamel will provide a desirable esthetic result, ceramic veneers should be considered. Ceramic veneers generally will cover most of the facial enamel for esthetic modifications. Interproximal or lingual extension will be determined by existing tooth conditions and treatment goals. Partial coverage veneers replacing a small portion of a tooth have been used by some dentists, and often involve functional modifications as well (Fig. 6-132).

Functional Indications

Modification of a tooth for functional reasons may also provide an indication for a ceramic veneer. Worn or fractured incisal edges, loss of adequate anterior guidance and open occlusal or interproximal contacts all provide possible indications for ceramic veneers. These veneers may or may not cover facial or esthetic surfaces. Less esthetic lingual or occlusal surfaces may also be veneered with bonded ceramics (Fig. 6-133). These techniques have been adapted as a result of the high level of success achieved with facial veneers. Such applications have less documented longitudinal success and should be considered more experimental. The conservative nature of these applications still makes them viable alternatives in many instances as long as the patients are adequately informed of the risks.

Full Coverage Veneers

Situations often exist where a tooth requires a significant amount of exterior modification but is relatively intact with a significant amount of enamel remaining. A traditional full esthetic crown requires the removal of virtually all coronal enamel. Conservative preparation, with the preservation of a maximum amount of enamel, allows for maximum bond strength and the use of a thin veneer of ceramic to restore all or part of the coronal surface. These restorations can be useful in combination with adjacent ceramic veneers. The term "full veneer" will be used to describe such a restoration (Figs. 6-134 to 6-138). These restorations provide a conservative alternative to traditional full crowns in selective instances but it must be recognized that their longitudinal success has not been verified and many design parameters are not conclusively established. "Full veneers" might be considered by the restorative esthetic dentist with patients who are willing to experiment with restorations requiring minimal

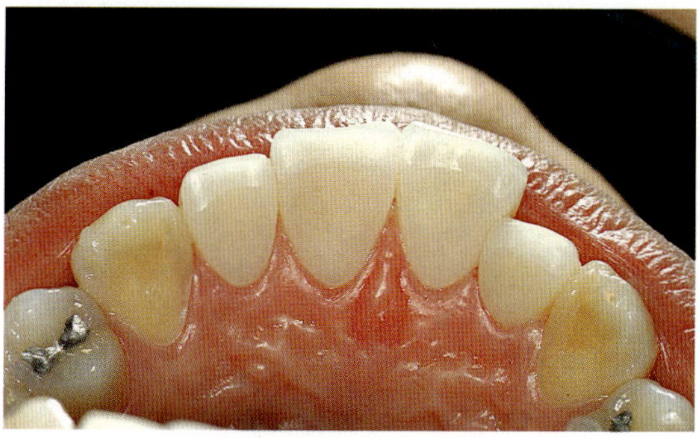

Fig. 6-133 Lingual ceramic veneers on teeth 7 to 10, replacing lost enamel.

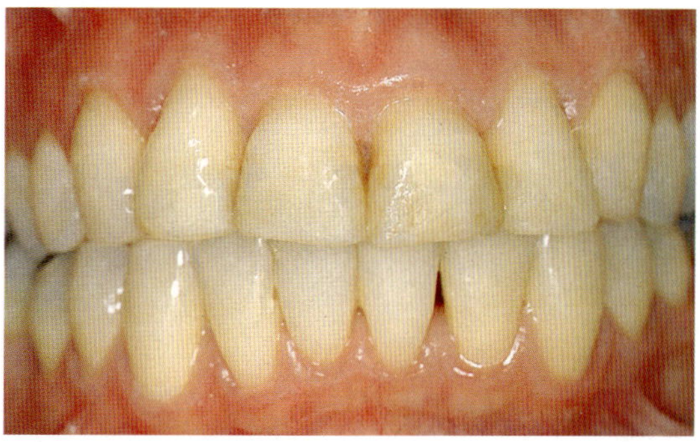

Fig. 6-134a Preoperative view.

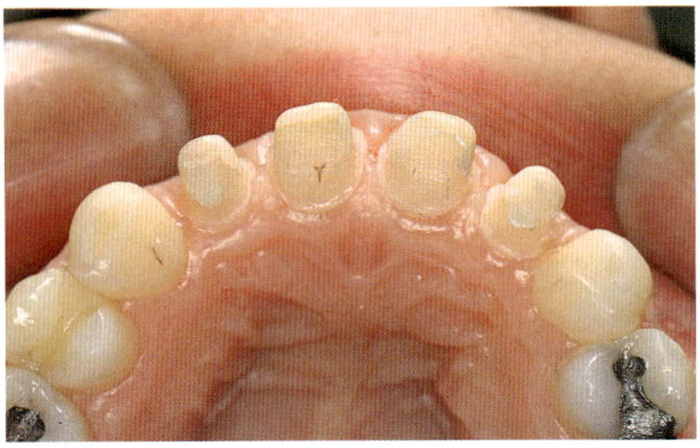

Fig. 6-134b Teeth 6 and 11 prepared for ceramic veneers, teeth 7 to 10 prepared for "full veneers" (note conservative depth).

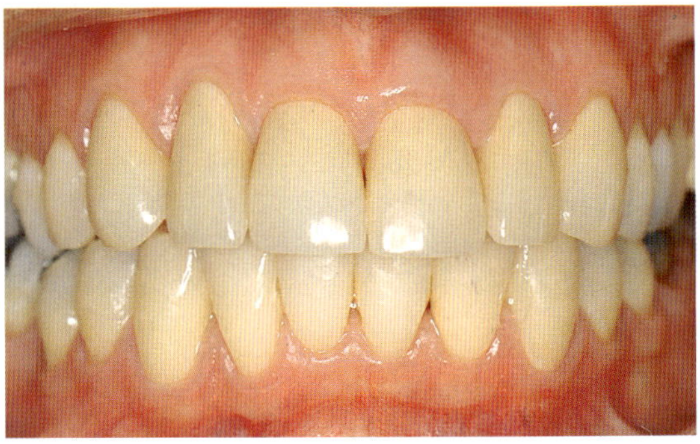

Fig. 6-134c Postoperative facial view. Note how full veneers easily match ceramic veneers due to similar preparation depth and identical materials.

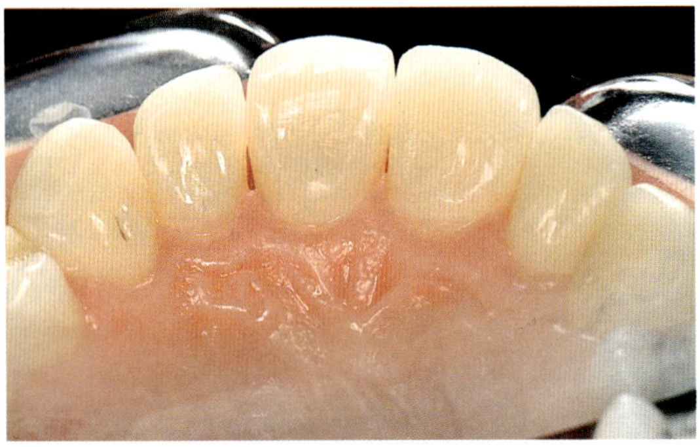

Fig. 6-134d Postoperative lingual view of Fig. 6-134c.

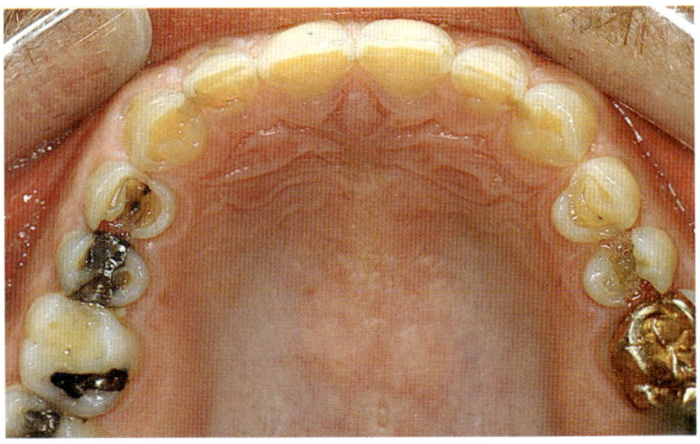

Fig. 6-135a Preoperative view of generalized enamel loss.

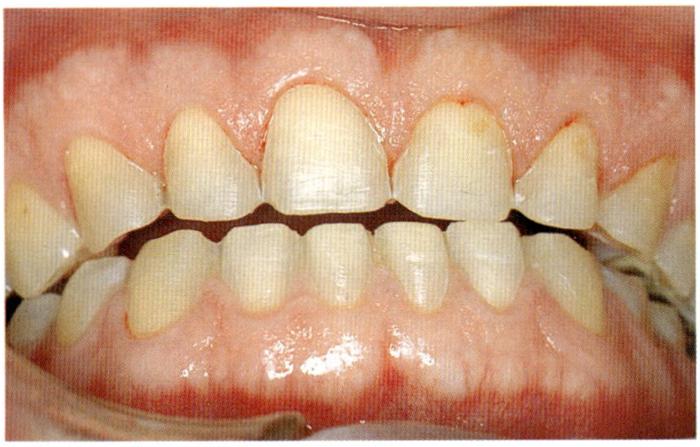

Fig. 6-135b All maxillary anteriors prepared for full veneers. Mandibular anteriors prepared for ceramic veneers.

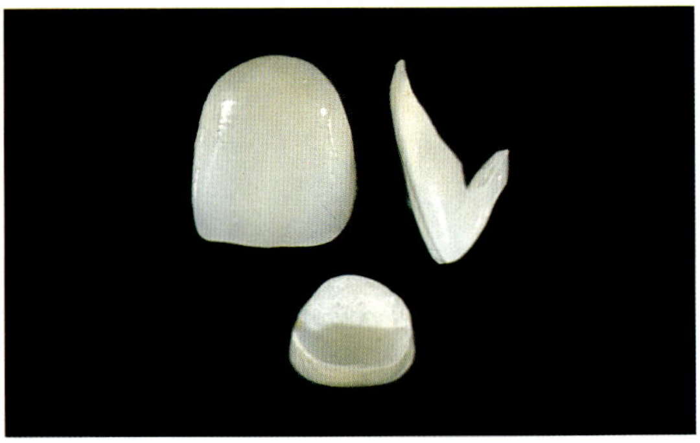

Fig. 6-135c Frontal and lateral views of maxillary full veneer (top); mandibular ceramic veneer (bottom).

tooth reduction. Even moderate success with such conservative restorations will preserve tooth structure and maintain future restorative options as newer materials and techniques are developed.

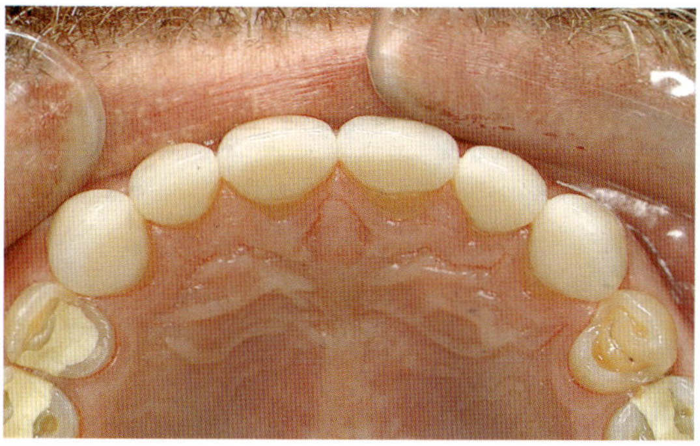

Fig. 6-135d Postoperative occlusal view of full veneers on teeth 6 to 11.

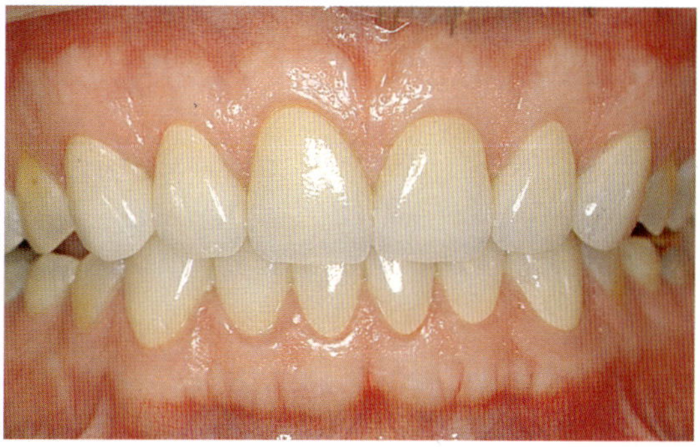

Fig. 6-136 Postoperative view with anterior ceramic veneers in place (note posteriors to be restored with full veneers).

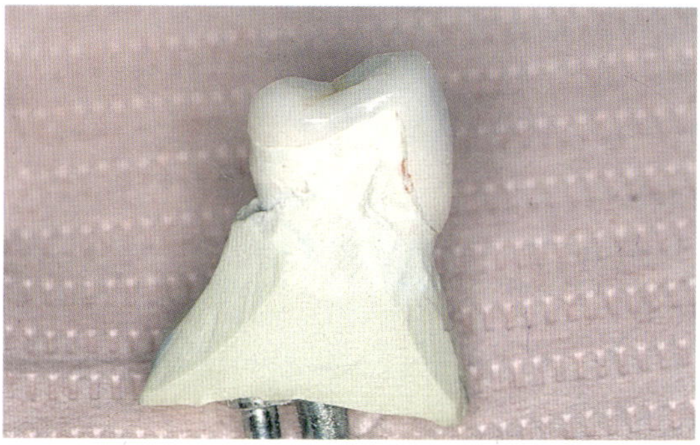

Fig. 6-137 Occlusal-facial full veneer on die.

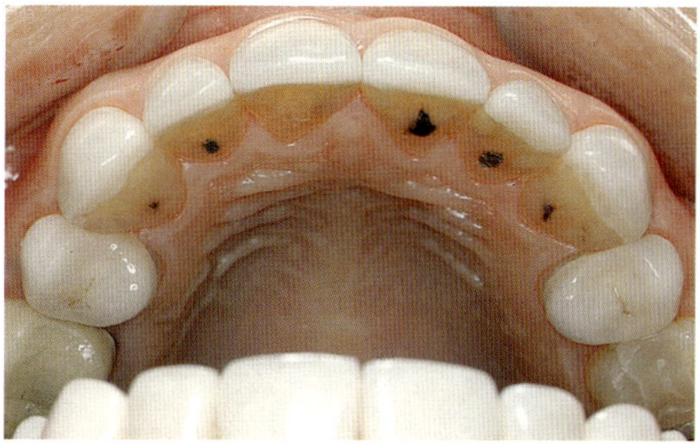

Fig. 6-138 Full (occlusal-facial) veneers on teeth 5 and 12.

Veneering Existing Restorations

In situations where a previous crown or fixed partial denture is intact and functional but esthetically unacceptable, ceramic veneers can be used to provide a conservative alternative to total replacement (Fig. 6-139).

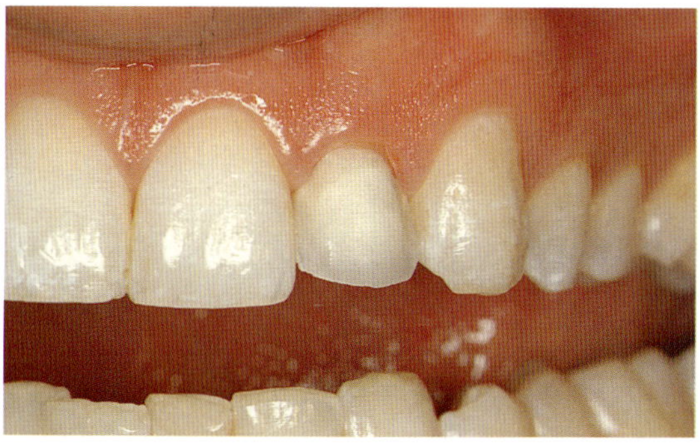

Fig. 6-139a Crown on tooth 10 prepared for ceramic veneer.

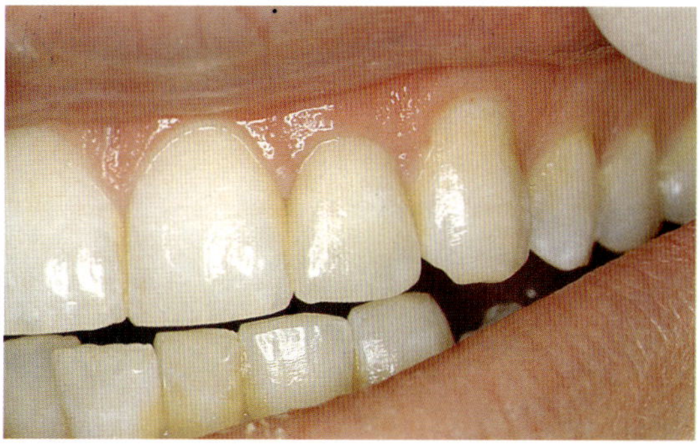

Fig. 6-139b Ceramic veneer bonded to tooth 10 ceramic crown.

PREPARATORY CLINICAL PROCEDURES

Pretreatment Preparation

Because esthetic demands are often difficult to communicate, an understanding of esthetic goals and limitations among the treating dentist, patient and laboratory is difficult to establish. Visualization techniques must be used wherever possible to allow all involved to see a common point of reference. Study models and diagnostic waxups, using tooth colored waxes, are helpful in showing morphologic changes but it may be difficult for patients to visualize such modifications on themselves. Preoperative and postoperative photographs of restorations on other patients instill confidence but may not assist in understanding an individual patient's esthetic requirements. One of the most effective modalities for visualizing a patient's individual needs, desires and limitations is through the use of computer imaging (see chapter 1). Treatment goals for color, form, tissue contours as well as limitations can be clearly visualized by the dentist and patient simultaneously. Color prints of imaged results are sent with the prescription or sent directly to the dental laboratory via a modem. Visual information is helpful to the ceramist as well. Photographic prints or slides may also be used. Clear communication and understanding are the keys that lead to constant and predictable success.

Sufficient preoperative time must be spent with the patient discussing procedures and esthetic desires and establishing treatment goals. Treatment expectations and limitations must be clearly understood or the patient may be disappointed in the result due to unrealistic expectations. Time spent educating the patient and developing a joint understanding of treatment goals preoperatively is a critical component when placing restorations with a significant esthetic impact.

General Preparation Criteria

1. Enamel should be maintained whenever possible for maximum bonding potential. Figures 6-140 and 6-141 show the variability of enamel thickness according to Crispin and Hewlett.
2. Preparations should have distinct margins that provide bulk and clear boundaries for fabricating veneers with minimal overcontouring or overextension (Fig. 6-142). Veneers placed on unprepared teeth require extensive marginal finishing and usually result in overcontouring.
3. Preparation depth must be adequate to provide sufficient room to accomplish

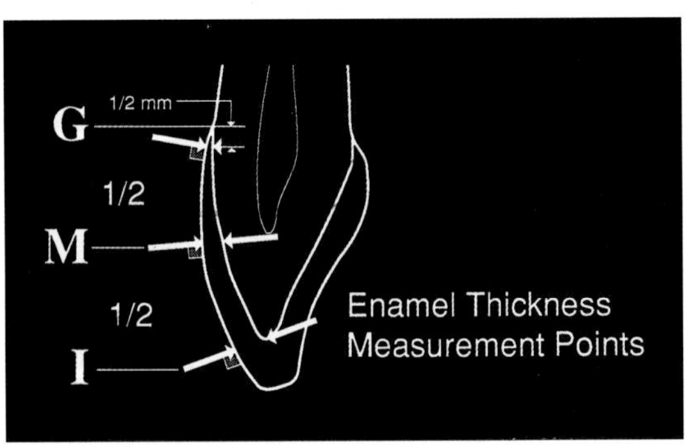

Fig. 6-140 Diagram showing the three points where enamel thickness was measured.

TABLE 1. Enamel Thickness (mm)

	G (Gingival)	M (middle)	I (Incisal)
MAXILLARY			
Centrals	.245 ±.069	.795 ±.115	.863 ±.094
Laterals	.260 ±.082	.920 ±.199	1.018 ±.183
Canines	.236 ±.090	.997 ±.236	1.189 ±.288
Bicuspids	.262 ±.189	1.245 ±.188	1.415 ±.176
MANDIBULAR			
Centrals	.196 ±.080	.660 ±.143	.782 ±.091
Laterals	.178 ±.031	.579 ±.124	.883 ±.135
Canines	.235 ±.055	.943 ±.141	1.114 ±.180
Bicuspids	.258 ±.074	1.298 ±.207	1.400 ±.186

Fig. 6-141 Chart showing average enamel thickness at the three points for various teeth types.

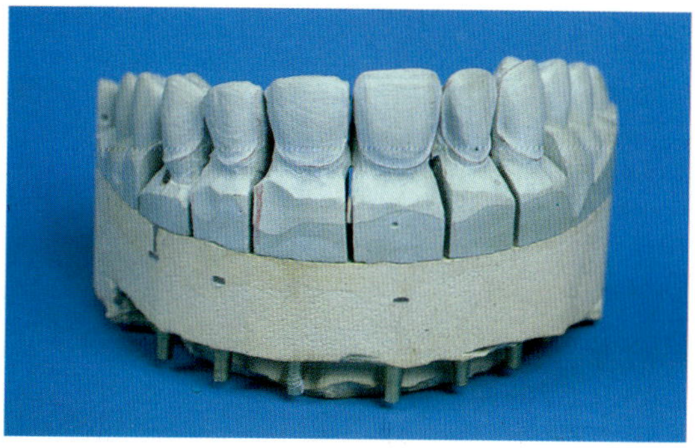

Fig. 6-142 Distinct margins are easy to identify on working model.

treatment goals. For example, extremely dark teeth may require a deeper preparation to allow greater ceramic thickness to block out this color. In contrast, teeth that are facially eroded or already deficient in enamel may require minimum to no reduction, other than defining the margins.

Normal Preparation Sequence

1. Two horizontal depth grooves are prepared on the facial surface of the tooth dividing it into thirds. The depth of the grooves should be determined by the desired depth of the preparation (Figs. 6-143 and 6-144). A variety of depth cutting diamonds is necessary to accommodate these variations (Fig. 6-145). Depth grooves, of the predetermined depths, should be prepared on all teeth simultaneously (Fig. 6-146). Controlled depth grooves are critical to allow for optimal veneer thickness.
2. Prepare a midfacial gingival minichamfer to a depth of approximately 0.2 to 0.3 mm using a chamfer diamond (Fig. 6-147). Deeper preparations near the cemento-enamel junction will generally extend into dentin but may be necessary in order to mask severe discoloration. Gingival extension should be to the free gingival margin and if possible remain in enamel (Fig. 6-148).
3. Extend the gingival margin interproximally and extend to the incisal surface creating the mesial and distal margins (Fig. 6-149). This finish line should extend sufficiently into the gingival interproximal area to cover discolored tooth surface or to allow for necessary contour corrections (Fig.

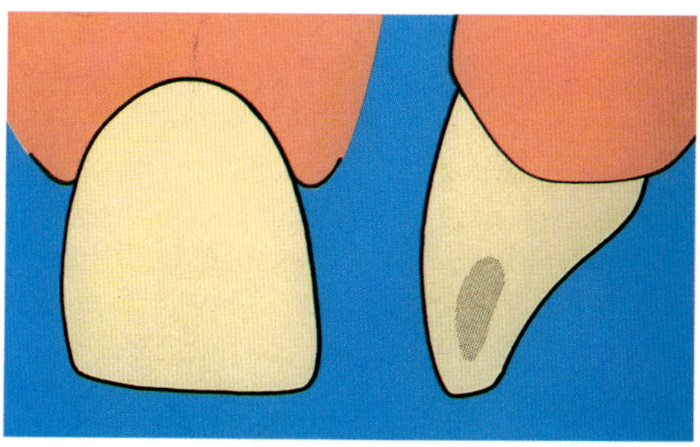

Fig. 6-143 Diagram of unprepared maxillary central incisor.

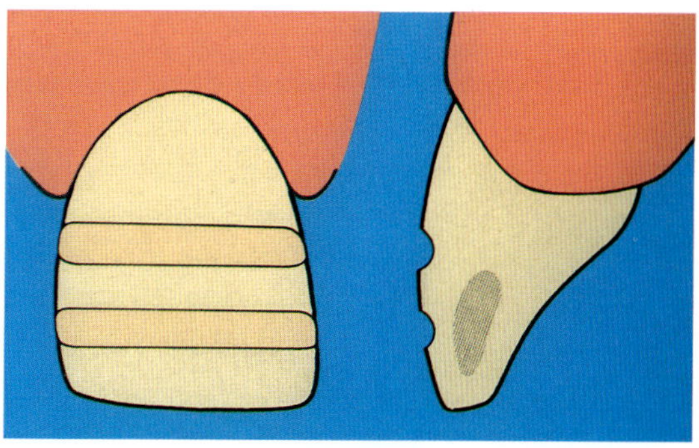

Fig. 6-144 Two horizontal depth grooves establish preparation depth and divide the tooth into thirds.

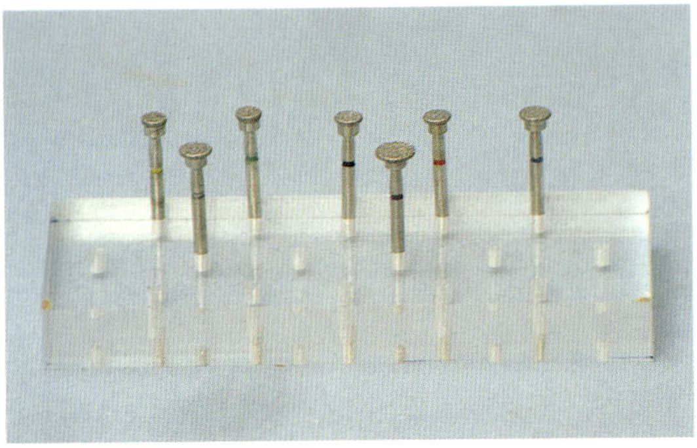

Fig. 6-145a

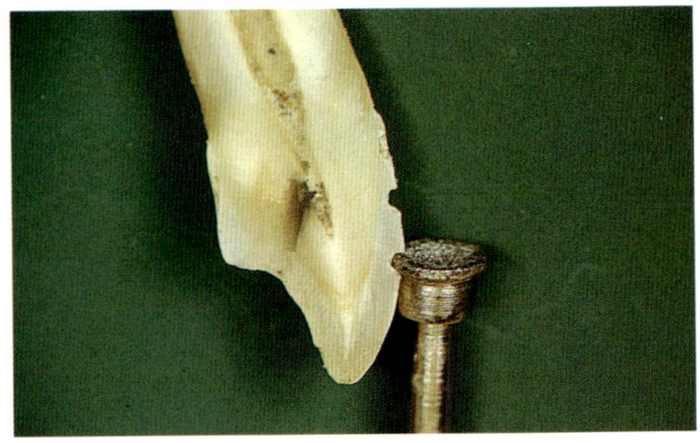

Fig. 6-145b

Fig. 6-145a Example of depth cutting diamond for several possible depths (Lasco, Chatsworth, CA).

Fig. 6-145b Cross section of tooth showing how depth cutting diamond works.

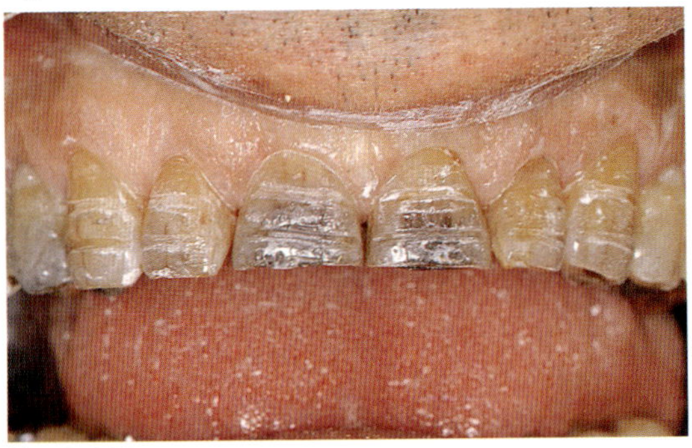

Fig. 6-146

Fig. 6-146 Clinical case with depth grooves placed.

Fig. 6-147 Use a chamfer diamond to prepare the gingival chamfer.

Fig. 6-148 Diagram of gingival margin preparation.

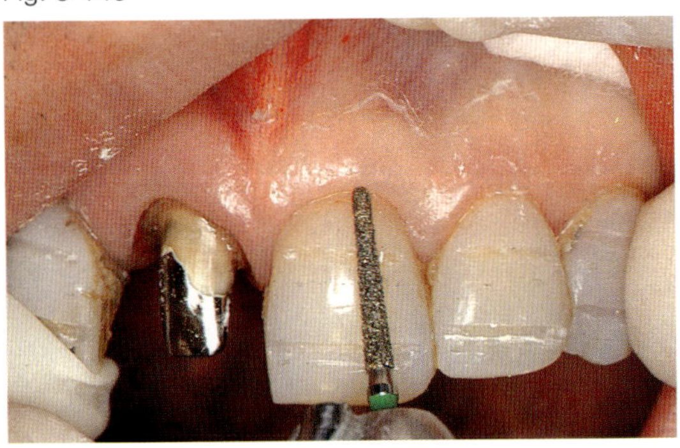

Fig. 6-147

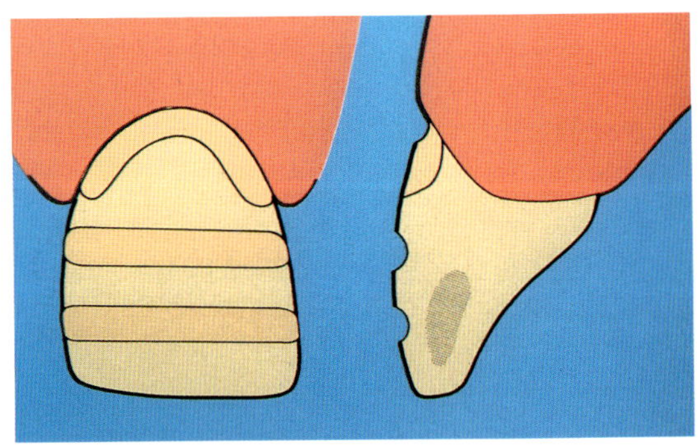

Fig. 6-148

6-150). Gingival interproximal extension may be kept minimal when color change is minimal. Extensive preparation extension into the interproximal area will require a more facial path of veneer insertion that must be allowed for with the remaining preparation design (Fig. 6-151). Unnecessary interproximal extension should be avoided. Interproximal preparation extension into the contact area should include two thirds to three quarters of a normal anterior contact (Fig. 6-152). This will maintain a small lingual portion of the natural tooth contact that will maintain positional relationships and minimize potential lateral tooth migration. While this does complicate die separation somewhat, it minimizes clinical problems. In contrast, if proximal contacts are broken, potential complications are created (Fig. 6-153). First, the teeth must be stabilized to prevent migration and the diastemas created make provisional restorations mandatory. Second, this degree of interproximal exten

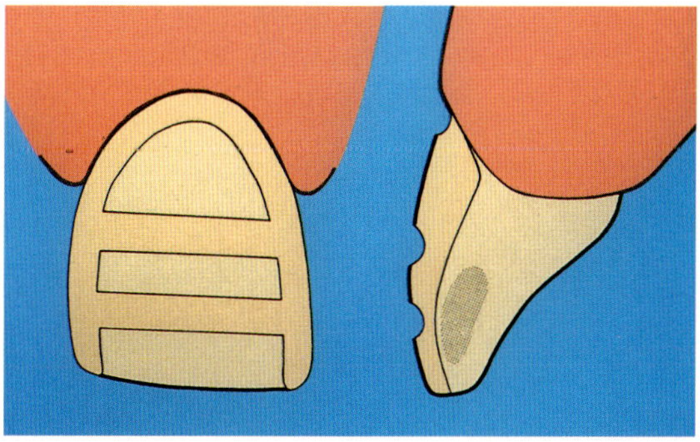

Fig. 6-149

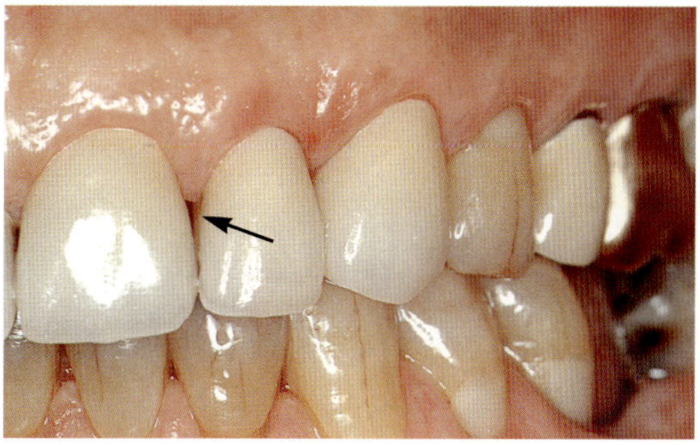

Fig. 6-150

Fig. 6-149 Interproximal margin preparation.

Fig. 6-150 Underextension of interproximals on discolored teeth will result in margin shown as seen on the mesial of tooth 10.

Fig. 6-151 Excessive interproximal extension requires a more facial line of veneer withdrawal.

Fig. 6-152a Preoperative incisal view.

Fig. 6-152b Proximal preparation should extend into two thirds to three quarters of a normal anterior contact.

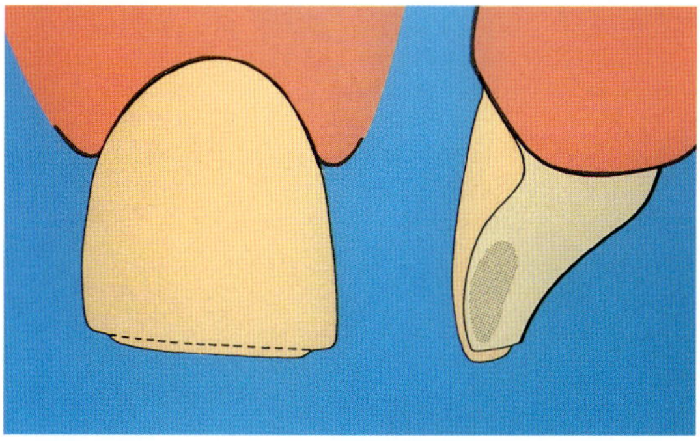

Fig. 6-151

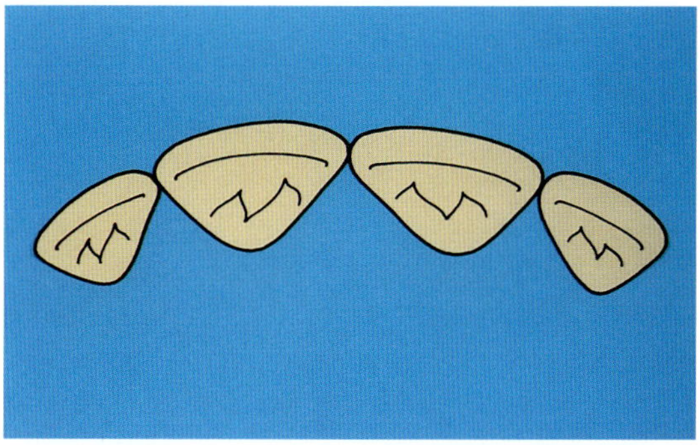

Fig. 6-152a

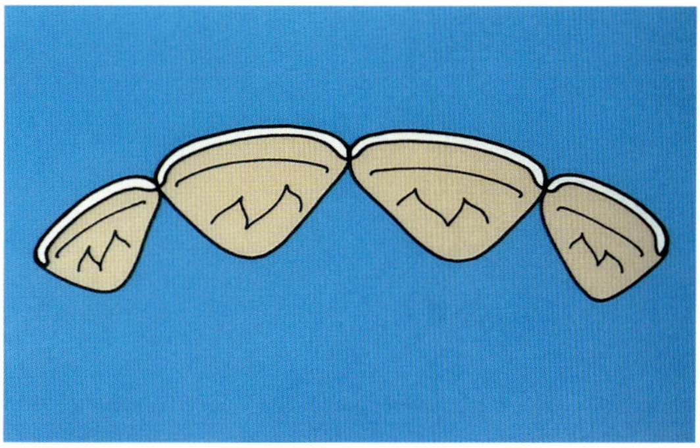

Fig. 6-152b

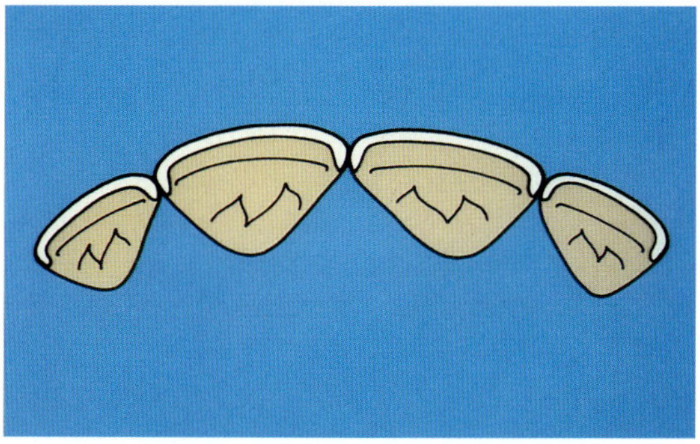

Fig. 6-153 Preparations that completely open proximal contacts are satisfactory but teeth must be stabilized to prevent movement.

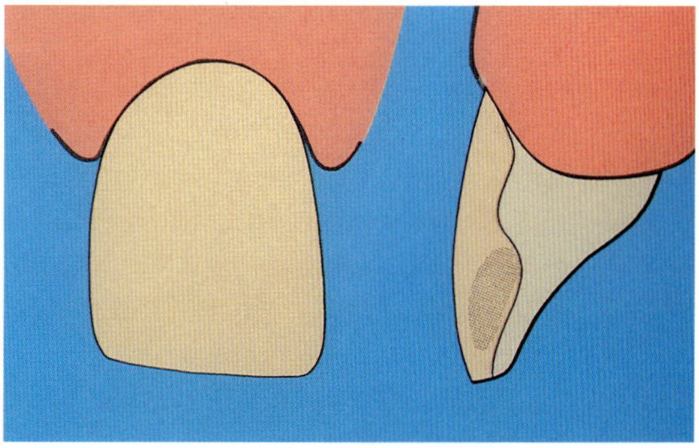

Fig. 6-154 Preparing through proximal contacts requires more circumferential tooth reduction.

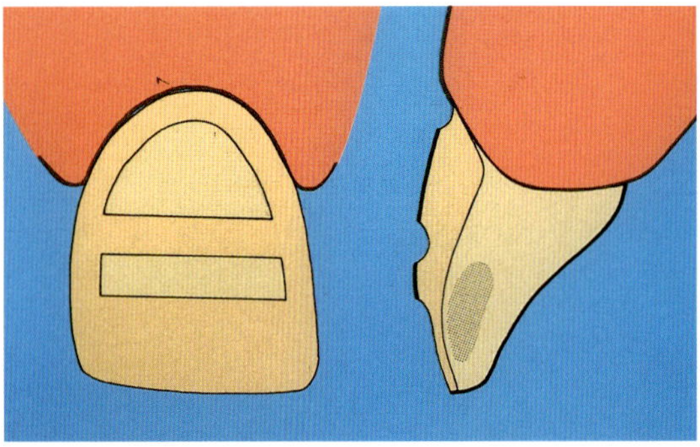

Figs. 6-155a

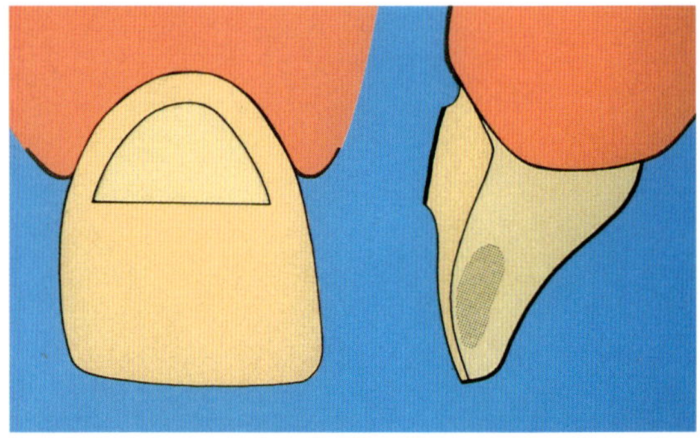

Figs. 6-155b

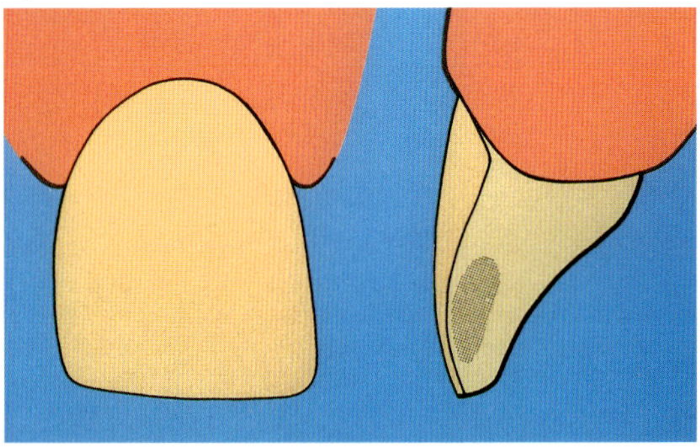

Figs. 6-155c

Figs. 6-155a to c The facial surface is now reduced to the predetermined depth.

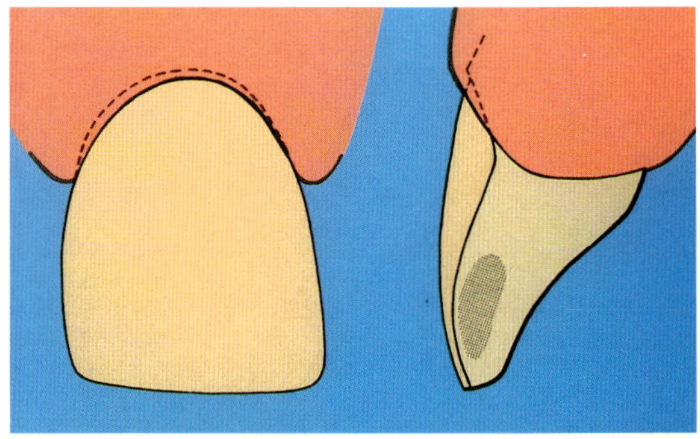

Fig. 6-156 Subgingival margin extension is done only in selected instances.

sion creates a facial three-quarter crown type preparation with more circumferential axial reduction (Fig. 6-154). An incisal line of draw would demand extensive proximal reduction similar to a crown preparation. Thus the contacts would have to be opened even more. When a facial line of draw is possible, proximal taper can be kept more conservative.

4. The facial surface now has three remaining islands of tooth structure that can be removed to the depth of the grooves (Fig. 6-155). At this point, the majority of the preparation is completed and additional design features will be dictated by individual demands. Subgingival extension is occasionally necessary to cover dark teeth with thin gingival tissues or pre-existing defects (Fig. 6-156).
5. Incisal extension on maxillary incisors should be dictated by the necessity to lengthen or reshape the incisal edge of the tooth. When an intact incisal edge exists, the preparation may leave the lingual one half to two thirds of enamel intact (Fig. 6-157) option *(a)*. This will provide a laboratory guide for maintaining existing incisal form. Due to minimal esthetic alteration, the necessity to place a provisional restoration is significantly reduced. Option *(b)* is used to cover slight worn incisal edges and option *(c)* used to totally rebuild incisal edges. When preparing over an intact incisal edge, adequate vertical reduction can be assured using depth grooves (Fig. 6-158). Usually the incisal is already short and preparation consists primarily of placing finish lines. Adequate bulk must be prepared along the lingual and interproximal surfaces to allow for ease of veneer fabrication and placement (Figs. 6-15q and 6-100). Extremely thin incisal bevels are vul

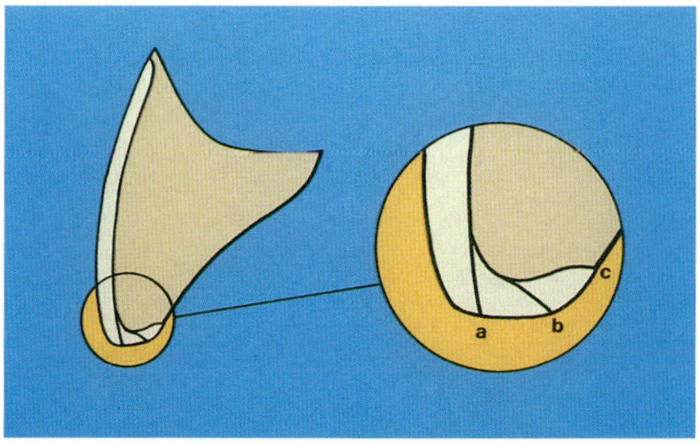

Fig. 6-157 Options for incisal veneer preparation; for intact incisals use *(a)*. When the veneer must modify the incisal edge use *(b)* or *(c)*.

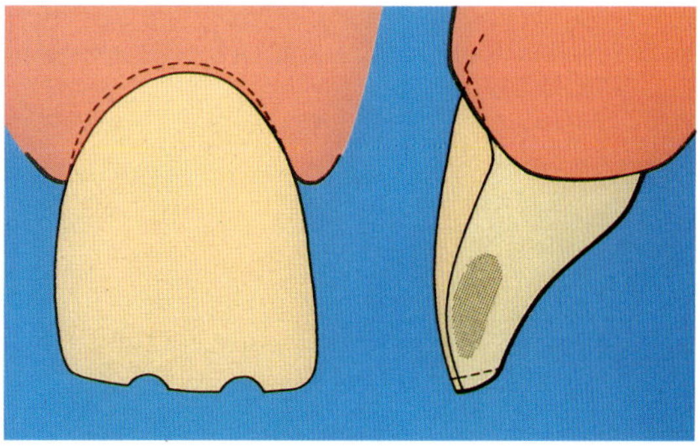

Fig. 6-158 Depth cuts in incisal edge.

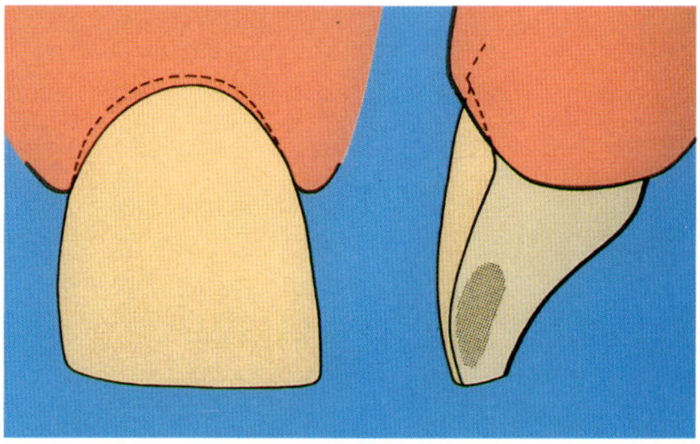

Fig. 6-159 Incisal length reduction.

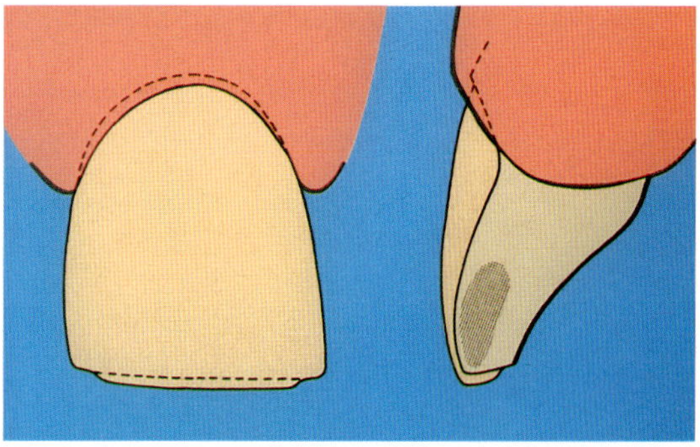

Fig. 6-160 Preparing bulk at margins minimizes fracture potential during fabrication and cementation.

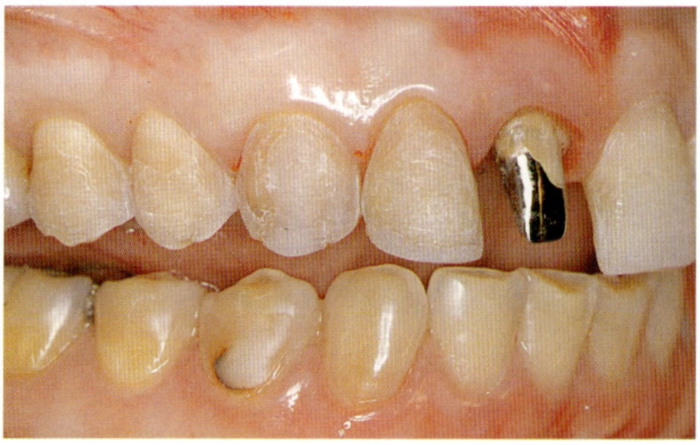

Fig. 6-161a Facial reduction only with occlusal restorations and enamel defects.

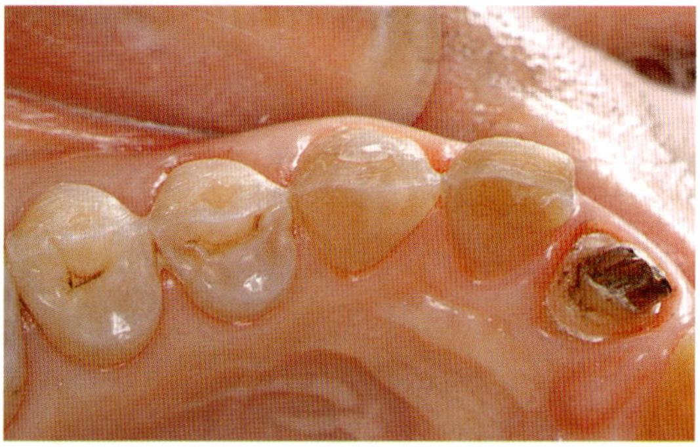

Fig. 6-161b Facial occlusal preparation covering defects in Fig. 6-161a.

nerable to fracture. All internal surfaces of the preparation must be smooth and rounded to minimize die abrasion problems during fabrication and to minimize areas of stress concentration during cementation. Every effort should be made to provide distinct margins and smooth preparation surfaces. This will allow for easier fabrication and minimize irregularities that may prevent the veneers from seating completely.

Incisal or occlusal reduction on maxillary canines or bicuspids is dictated by the necessity to reshape these surfaces for

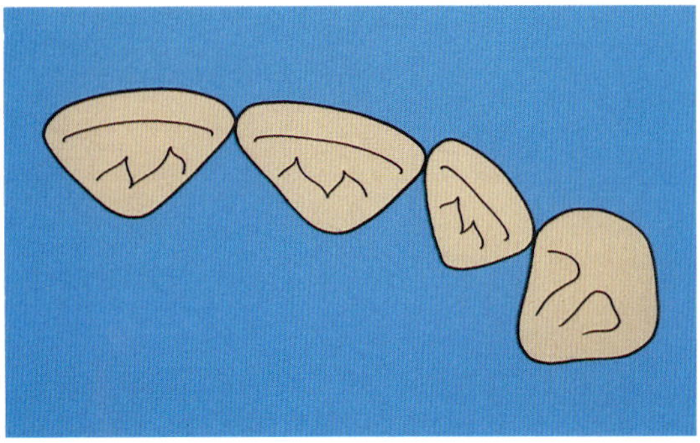

Fig. 6-162a Preoperative diagram of rotated lateral.

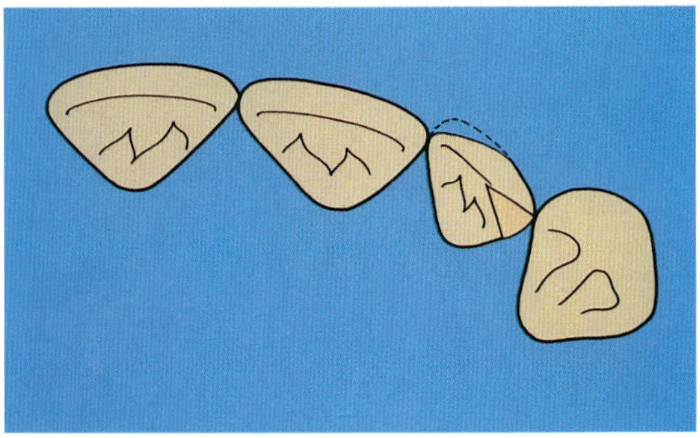

Fig. 6-162b Enameloplasty to remove mesial-buccal and distal-lingual excess.

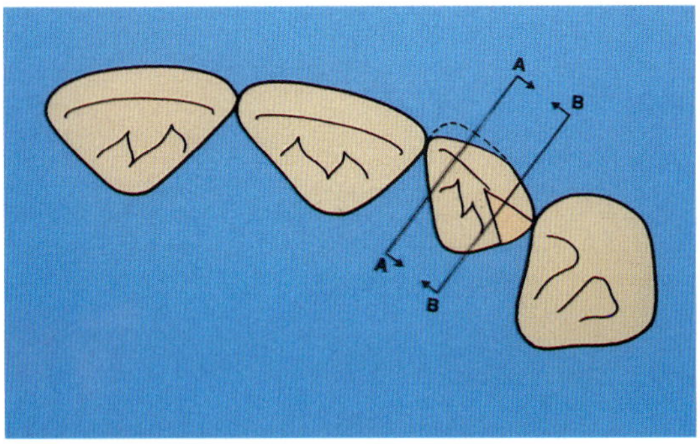

Fig. 6-162c Cross sections "AA" and "BB."

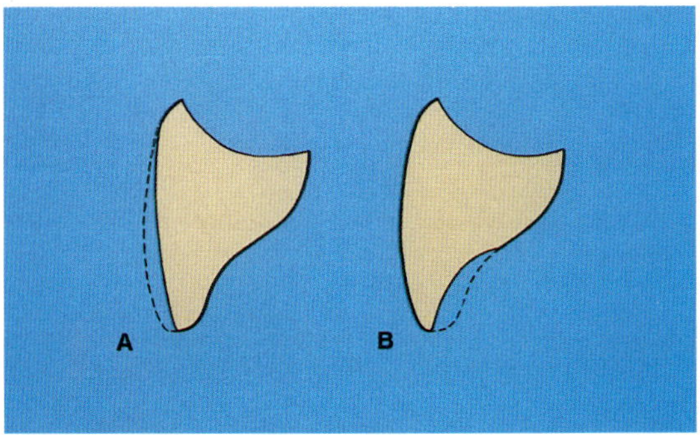

Fig. 6-162d Cross section "AA" showing mesial-buccal contouring; cross section "BB" showing distal-lingual contouring.

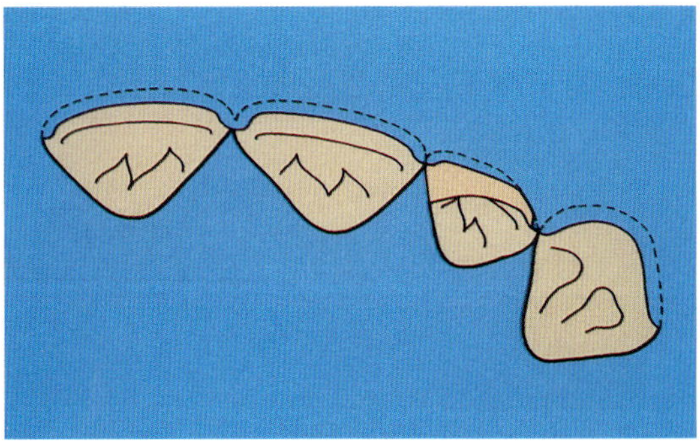

Fig. 6-163 Incisal view of veneer preparations on all teeth.

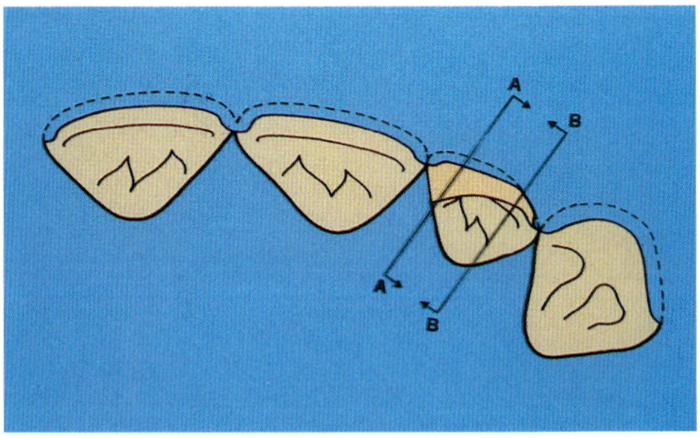

Fig. 6-164a Cross sections "AA" and "BB."

esthetic needs. It is often necessary to extend over the cusp tips to cover mesio-occlusal surfaces that show (Fig. 6-161).

For the majority of ceramic veneer preparations the sequence is now complete. The surface can be left with a medium to fine diamond prepared surface. In some instances, additional preparation modification may be necessary to solve isolated treatment problems.

Preparing Rotated Teeth

The first step in preparing rotated teeth is to contour any surfaces that extend beyond the desired buccal and lingual contours (Fig.

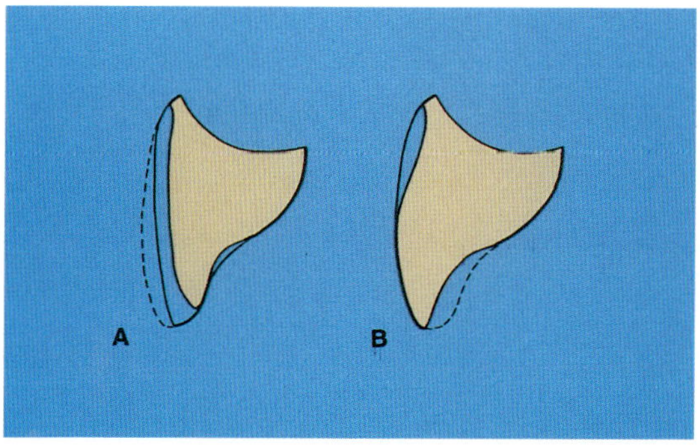

Fig. 6-164b Section "AA" shows additional facial reduction and placement of lingual finish line to build up deficient area. Section "BB" shows only placement of a facial gingival margin because the remaining facial surface is already deficient.

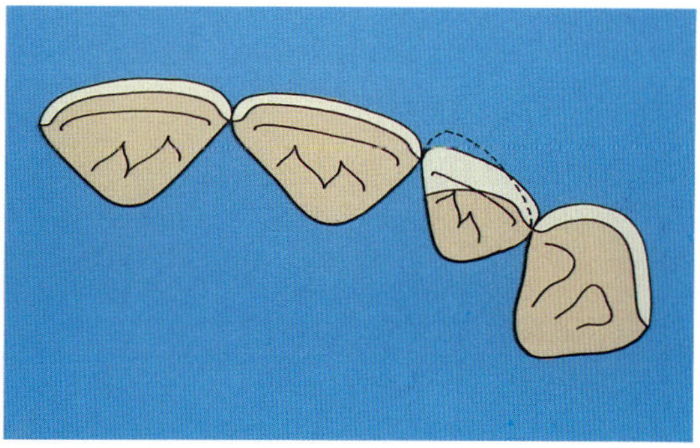

Fig. 6-165 Postoperative incisal view. Dotted line shows previous contour of rotated lateral.

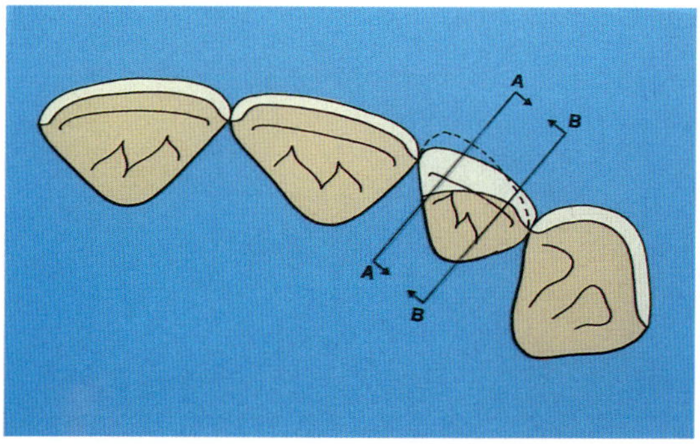

Fig. 6-166a Sections "AA" and "BB" through postoperative veneers.

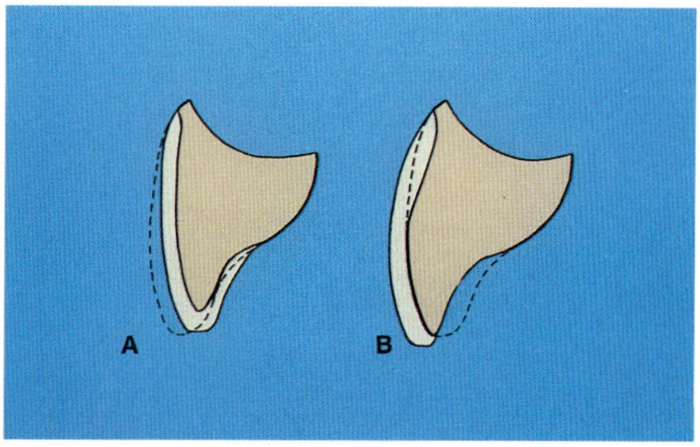

Fig. 6-166b Cross sections show how ceramic veneers have aligned teeth; dotted lines show previous contour.

6-162). Facial reduction now proceeds as described above and when tooth deficiency exists, only margins are prepared. Lingual margins must extend far enough to cover deficient areas and allow for augmentation or replacement of missing tooth structures (Figs. 6-163 and 6-164), and allow for normal tooth recontouring with the veneer (Fig. 6-165). Rotated teeth will generally require significant lingual coverage as well as adequate tooth removal of overextended areas to provide a preparation that is adequate for fabricating a veneer that will restore a rotated tooth to an ideal contour (Fig. 6-166).

Preparing Malpositioned Teeth

A tooth that is protruding facially must first be contoured into proper alignment (Figs. 6-167 and 6-168). Next the facial and incisal surfaces are prepared as if the tooth were in an ideal position. The lingual surface is deficient and so will require little reduction. A lingual finish line must be placed far enough gingivally to allow for proper recontouring of the deficient lingual surface (Figs. 6-169 and 6-170). Inadequate lingual extension gingivally will result in an unnatural abrupt contour change on the lingual surface of the veneer. These contours are undesirable and difficult to finish and polish (Fig. 6-171). Lingually

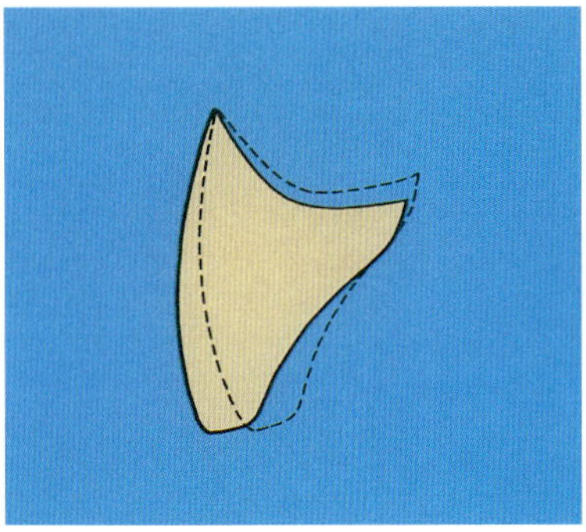

Fig. 6-167 Preoperative view of tooth tipped facially. Dotted line shows desired contour.

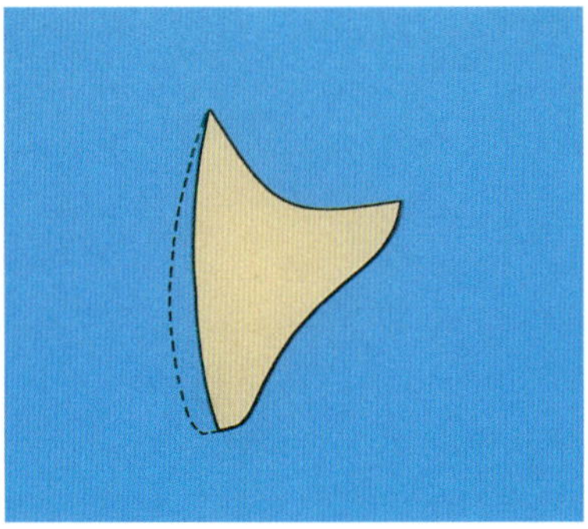

Fig. 6-168 Enameloplasty of facial to ideal contour. Note lingual deficiency.

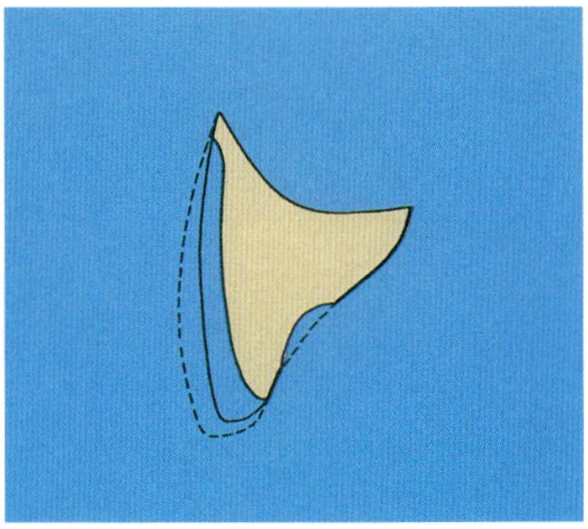

Fig. 6-169 Ceramic veneer preparation requiring additional facial reduction and lingual finish line only.

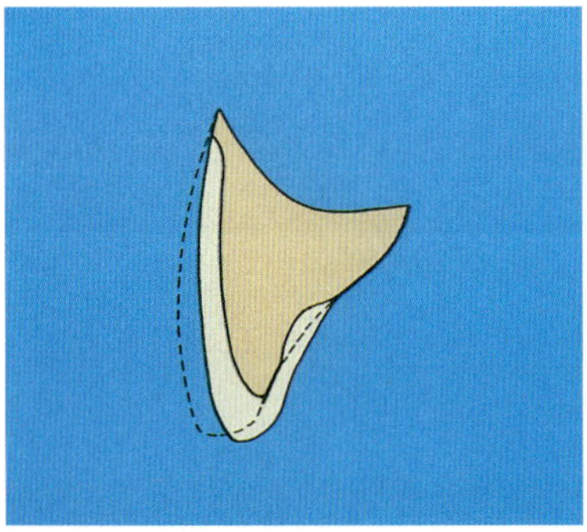

Fig. 6-170 Postoperative view. Dotted lines show original contour.

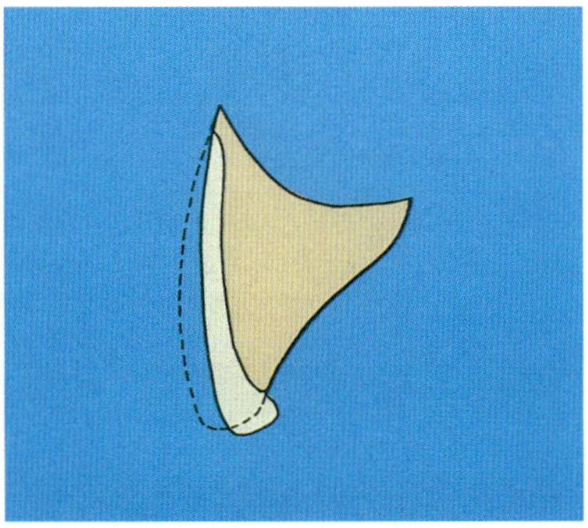

Fig. 6-171 If no lingual finish line is prepared, repositioning the incisal edge without rebuilding the deficient lingual results in an unacceptable incisal contour.

tipped teeth will require an opposite but similar approach.

Preparing for Diastema Closure

The preparation strategy is modified when preparing proximal surfaces to close or reduce diastemas. Underextending the proximal margins lingually will not provide the ceramist sufficient area to overbuild the proximal contact and establish a new lingual contour that blends smoothly with the remaining proximal and lingual tooth structure (Fig. 6-172). It is necessary to extend the preparation through the entire proximal contact to the lingual line angles. Proper extension will allow the ceramist room to fabricate the veneers with new proximal contours that blend smoothly with remaining tooth structures (Fig. 6-173).

Preparing for diastema closure requires a more aggressive preparation and the widening of existing diastemas. These preparations often require provisional restorations to protect prepared teeth from sensitivity and improve compromised esthetics. Greater preparation time should be planned.

Preparing Mandibular Teeth

The preparation sequence is the same as described for maxillary incisors. The design is consistent in that the incisal and/or buccal cusp tips are routinely covered (Fig. 6-174). Because mandibular incisal edges are thin, a flat or slight angular incisal reduction is

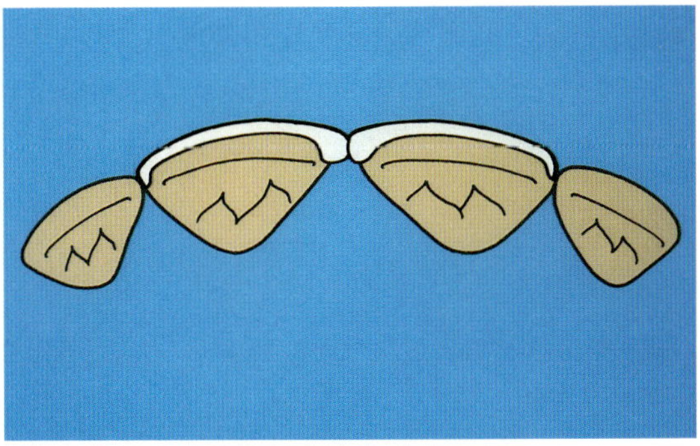

Fig. 6-172 Deficient proximal preparation extension into the diastema between teeth 8 and 9 results in a poor mesiolingual veneer contour.

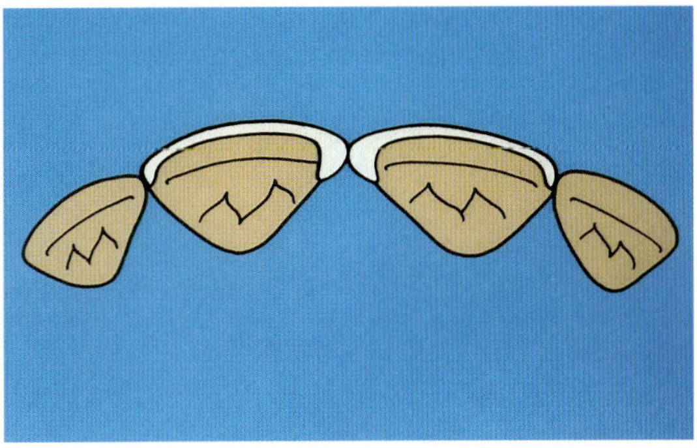

Fig. 6-173 Correct proximal preparation extension results in smoothly contoured veneers adjacent to over contoured mesial contacts used to close the diastema.

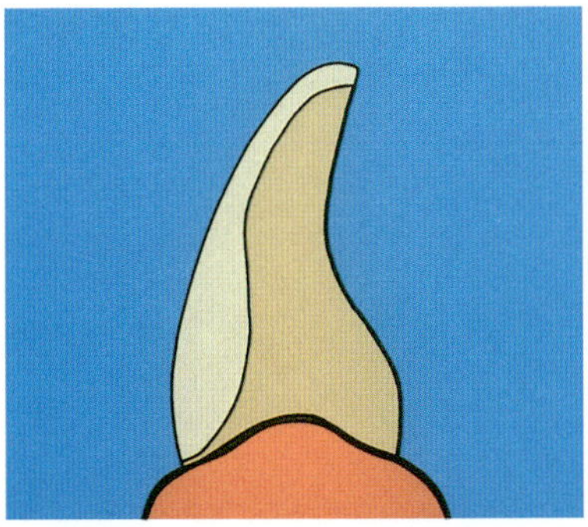

Fig. 6-174 Diagram of typical mandibular ceramic veneer design.

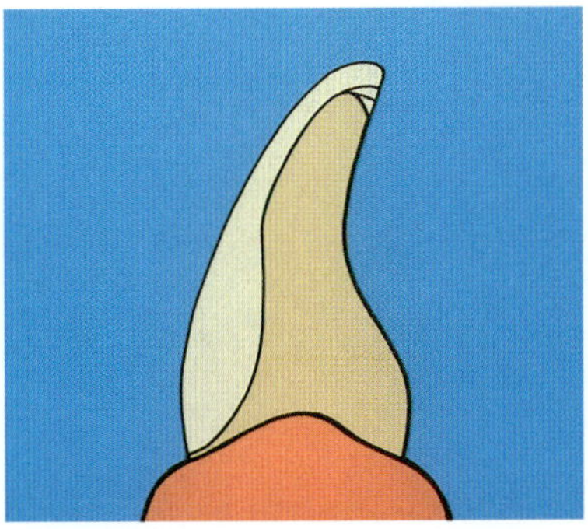

Fig. 6-175 Variations in incisal-lingual margin design depending on incisal edge thickness.

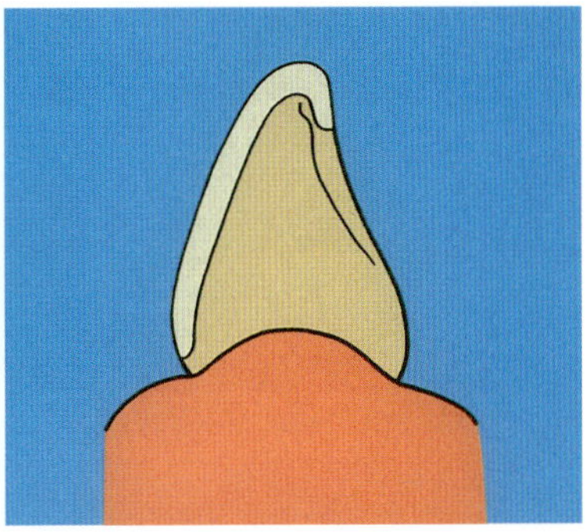

Fig. 6-176 Incisal extension of mandibular canines routinely extends onto the lingual due to increased thickness.

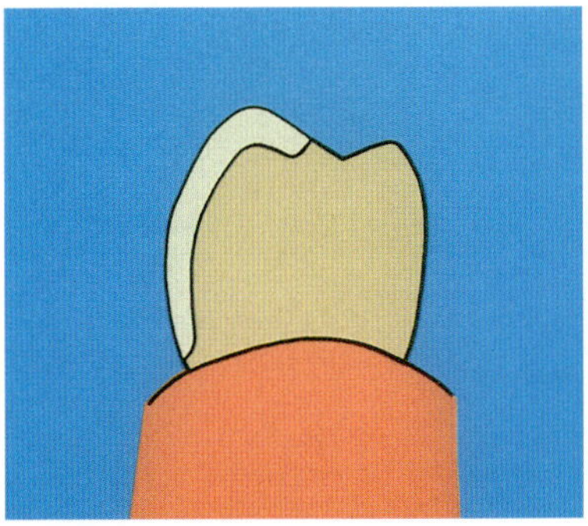

Fig. 6-177 Ceramic veneers should at least cover the buccal cusp on mandibular bicuspids.

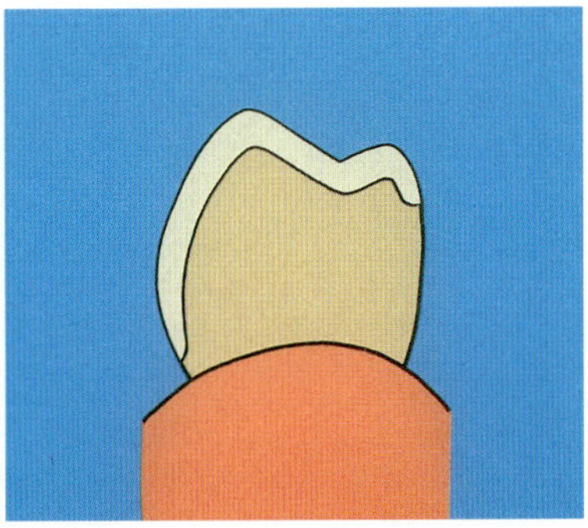

Fig. 6-178 Full occlusal coverage may be necessary for esthetic or functional reasons.

adequate (Fig. 6-175). Routine lingual extension is avoided unless necessary for a special reason such as changing contour. Canines have more incisal bulk and extending onto the lingual surface is more common (Fig. 6-176). The occlusal extension of the mandibular bicuspid should cover the buccal cusp tip and include the functional contacts (Fig. 6-177). When using veneers to make significant color changes, it may be necessary to cover the entire occlusal surface (Fig. 6-178). Occlusal reduction should be

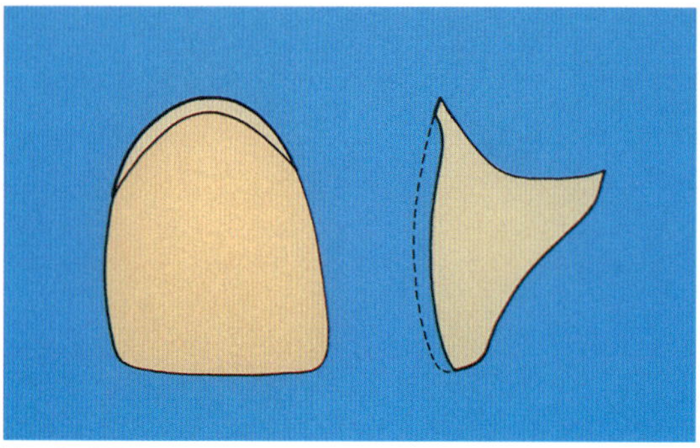

Fig. 6-179

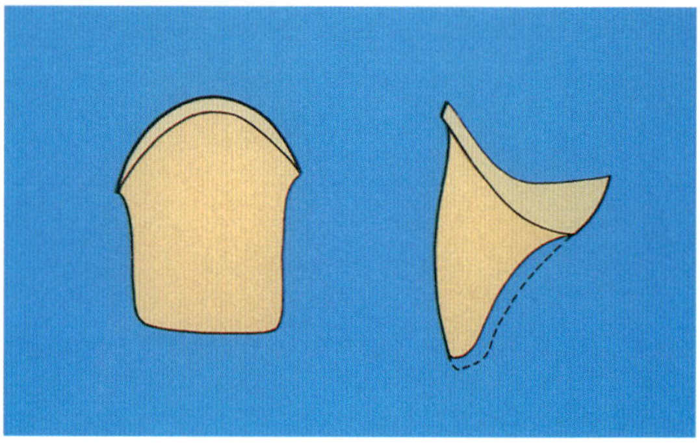

Fig.6-180

Fig. 6-179 Facial reduction of a full veneer similar to a ceramic veneer.

Fig. 6-180 Proximal and lingual reduction will cover faulty tooth structure and be tapered for restoration placement. Note conservative depth compared to all ceramic crowns.

Fig. 6-181 Tooth with only one defective contact.

Fig. 6-182 Facial as ceramic veneers.

Fig. 6-183 Prepare only one proximal surface to cover defect. Incisal reduction is often required to provide structural strength for fabrication and placement.

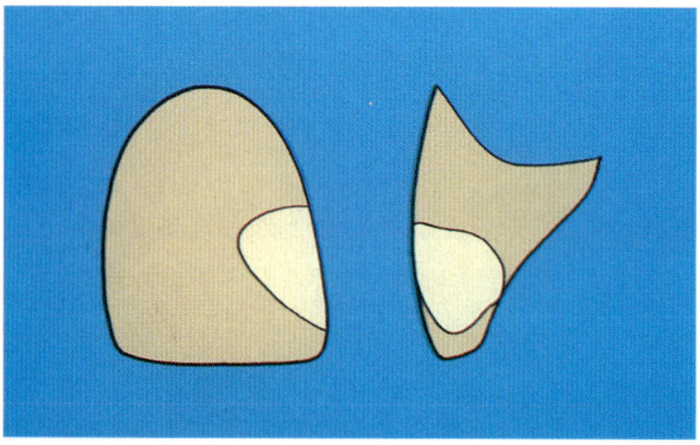

Fig 6-181

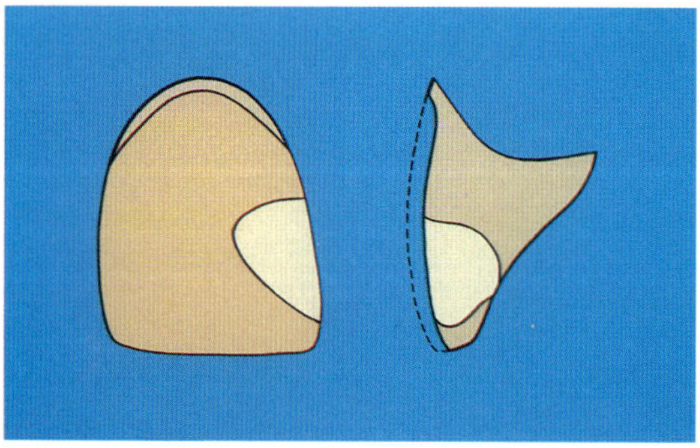

Fig. 6-182

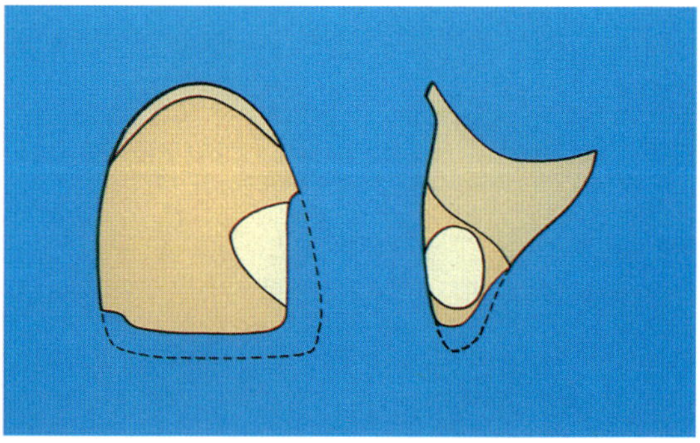

Fig. 6-183

between 0.5 and 1.5 mm in order to maintain occlusal enamel required for maximum bond strengths. This full coverage veneer will be discussed next in greater detail.

Full Coverage Anterior Veneers

When veneers are desired and teeth are intact and unrestored, the decision to do a ceramic veneer is relatively easy. Teeth with large proximal restorations or other defects may not have adequate remaining sound tooth structure and more extensive coverage required. The decision to crown or veneer is often a difficult one, especially when a broken down tooth is to be restored along with several other teeth needing veneers. When teeth are questionable, "full veneers" may provide a good alternative to risking the placement of a facial veneer on a defective tooth. Facial reduction is to the same depth as adjacent veneer preparations. Interproximal and lingual finish lines should be similar in depth to the facial veneer depth but

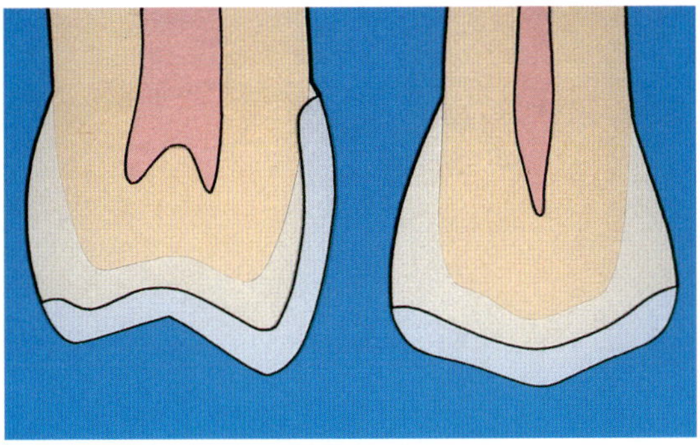

Fig. 6-184 Occlusal-facial full veneer on maxillary bicuspid. Proximal contacts left intact.

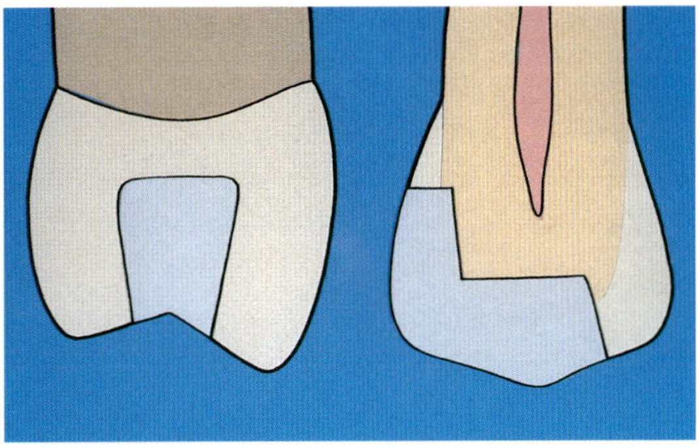

Fig. 6-185 Preoperative view of maxillary bicuspid requiring a ceramic veneer with a preexisting two surface restoration.

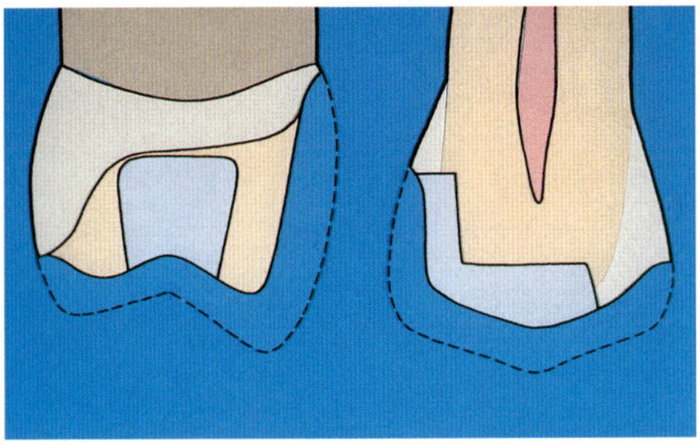

Fig. 6-186 The full veneer covers the facial, occlusal and one proximal surface.

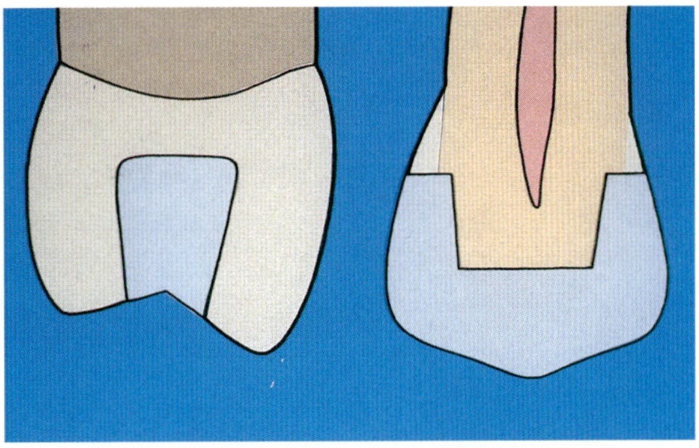

Fig. 6-187 Preoperative view with both proximals restored.

must be deep enough to establish a line of draw. Remaining axial surfaces should be prepared to eliminate undercuts and provide 0.5 to 1.0 mm of occlusal clearance. These superficial crown-like preparations will provide a uniform facial ceramic thickness that will match adjacent facial veneers (Fig. 6-179). Maintenance of enamel and the utilization of ceramic bonding techniques will ensure a maximum prognosis both esthetically and functionally (Fig. 6-180). Full veneers may also provide an alternative to traditional esthetic crowns that require more extensive tooth reduction. The long term prognosis of this restoration has not been established, but the ease of matching adjacent veneers and the conservation of tooth structure make them a desirable alternative.

Placing facial veneers on a tooth with a large interproximal restoration may leave the tooth in a weakened state. Extending the veneer to cover these defective areas is often desirable (Figs. 6-181 and 6-182). Only the defective proximal and lingual surfaces need to be covered. Intact proximal contacts can be maintained as with facial veneers (Fig. 6-183).

Full Coverage Posterior Veneers

The utilization of full veneers on posterior teeth is philosophically the same as with anteriors. The mandibular full veneer has already been indicated as an esthetic possibility and an alternative to a conventional crown. Full occlusal veneers may be indicated on maxillary as well as mandibular teeth, when a facial veneer is to be done and an occlusal or proximal restoration or defect exists. Extending the veneer to cover these

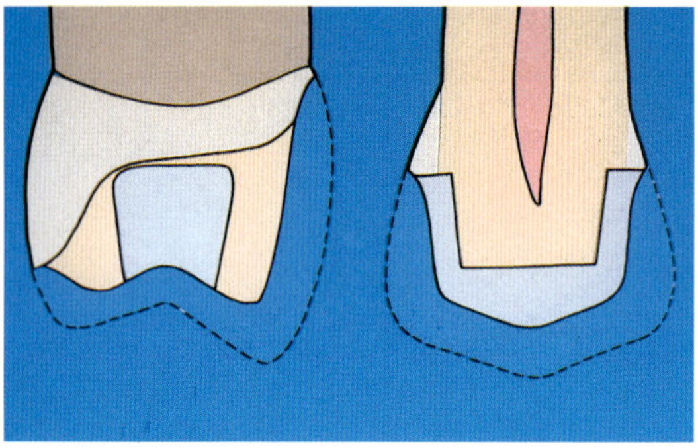

Fig. 6-188 The full veneer covers the facial, occlusal and both proximal surfaces.

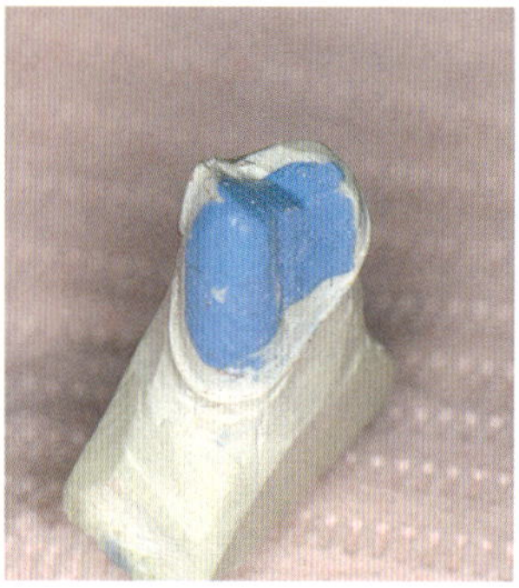

Fig. 6-189 Die of "full veneer" as in Fig. 6-186.

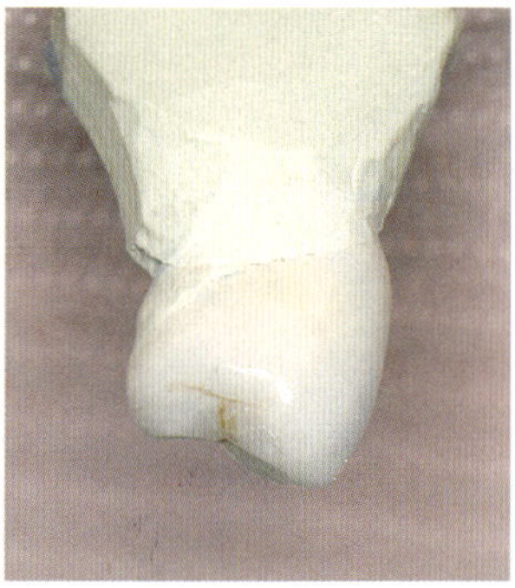

Fig. 6-190 Full veneer seated on the die.

defective areas will completely restore the tooth and eliminate the need for a secondary restoration at a later date. Posterior full veneers may cover the facial and occlusal surfaces and one or both proximal surfaces (Fig. 6-184). Extension is dictated by defective tooth structure and not retentive factors as with crowns. Facial depth is dictated by veneer principles. Occlusal reduction should be between 0.5 and 1.5 mm and kept in enamel where possible. Proximal extension should cover defective tooth structure. Unrestored proximal areas may be left intact (Figs. 6-185 and 6-186). Previous restorations may be incorporated into the full veneer preparation and removed and replaced at the cementation appointment (Figs. 6-187 and 6-188). The defects can also be filled in at the preparation appointment with an appropriate restorative material to which the veneer can be bonded. A fluoride-releasing base is advised, especially for deeper defects. Fixed prosthodontics will be significantly modified in the future as the application of conservative bonded restorations increases and longitudinal success is substantiated by clinical research (Figs. 6-189 and 6-190).

Treating Gingival Margins in Dentin or Gingival Defects

Whenever possible, the margins of the veneer preparations should be kept in enamel to maximize the bond strengths and minimize the possibility of microleakage. Modified procedures should be followed when esthetic or functional demands dictate extension onto gingival dentin.

When preparing onto a root surface and no defect exists, a normal depth of finish line is prepared (Figs. 6-191 and 6-192). During the cementation appointment, meticulous attention to technique detail must be followed and the newest generation of dental bonding agents used. This will minimize potential problems. An alternative approach is to prepare the area deeper in order to place a fluoride-releasing liner. However, this is of reduced benefit with the newer multipurpose bonding agents.

When a gingival defect or previous restoration exists, the preparation margin should include the entire defect (Figs. 6-193 and 6-194). Defects can be blocked out on the die for veneer fabrication. During the cementation appointment, any remaining defective tooth structure or restorative material should be removed. In the deeper portion of the defect, a tooth colored fluoride-releasing liner should be placed. This liner will cover deeper dentin that is closer to pulpal tissues and provide a secondary defense against bacterial migration should microleakage occur (Fig. 6-195). The newer multipurpose bonding agents may prevent microleakage but until long term success is documented, placing a

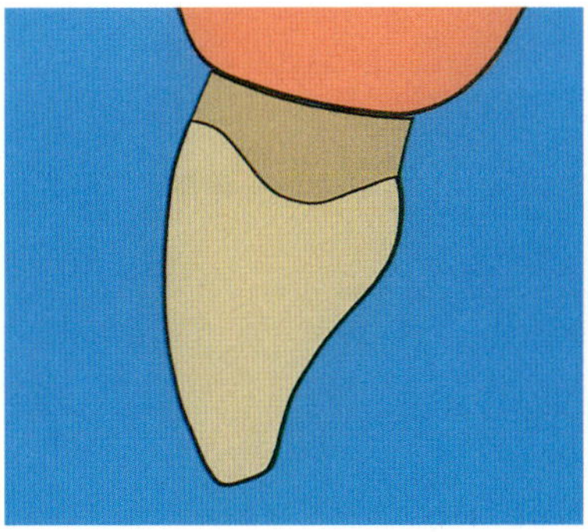

Fig. 6-191 Tooth with cementum exposed.

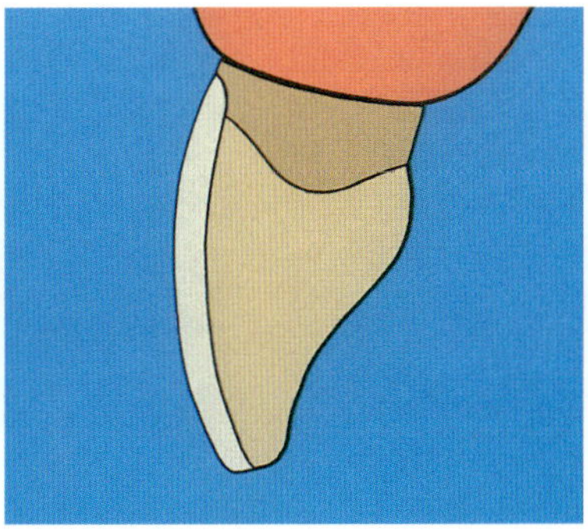

Fig. 6-192 Ceramic veneer extending onto cementum.

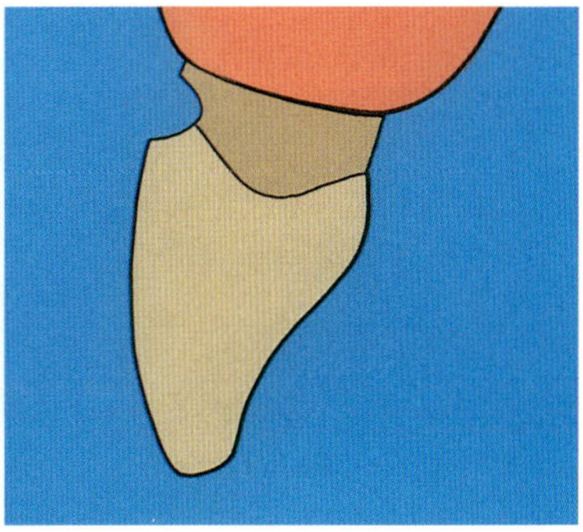

Fig. 6-193 Preexisting gingival defect.

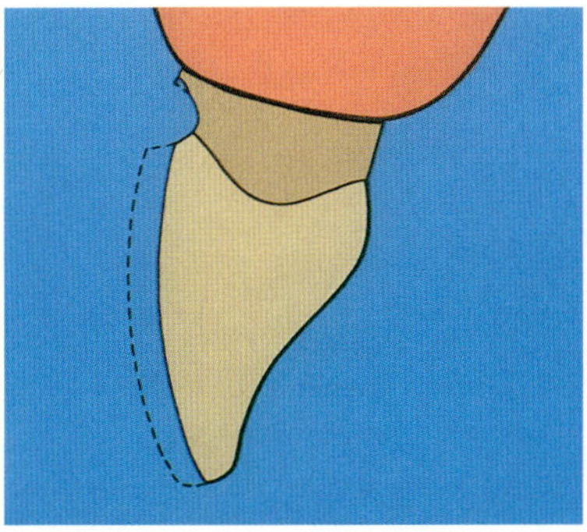

Fig. 6-194 Veneer preparation should cover the defect.

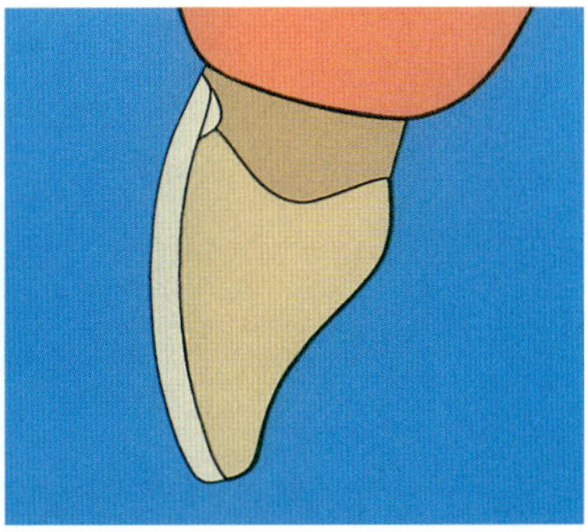

Fig. 6-195 Deep area should have a fluoride-releasing base in case of microleakage.

fluoride-releasing liner in such circumstances is advisable. The newer light cured fluoride-releasing restorative materials provide improved bonds over older chemically cured materials. When predictable long term fluoride-releasing composite cements are developed, this procedure may become redundant.

Large defects should be filled prior to final veneer cementation. An appropriate composite may be placed over the fluoride-releasing liner or a light cured fluoride-releasing restoration may be used to fill most of the defect. This will minimize the amount of composite veneer cement needed to fill this defect, which reduces volumetric contraction during polymerization of the cement.

Impression Technique

The same principals used for fixed prosthodontic impressions should be applied to impressions for veneers. There are some unique modifications that may be required for consistent success. An accurate impression of all prepared surfaces is mandatory. Fragile veneers fabricated on inaccurate dies will have a significantly increased possibility of fracture during delivery procedures.

Gingival Retraction

In most instances the gingival preparation margins are positioned at the free gingival margin or only slightly subgingivally. By placing one long, small diameter, chemical free retraction cord subgingivally, adequate

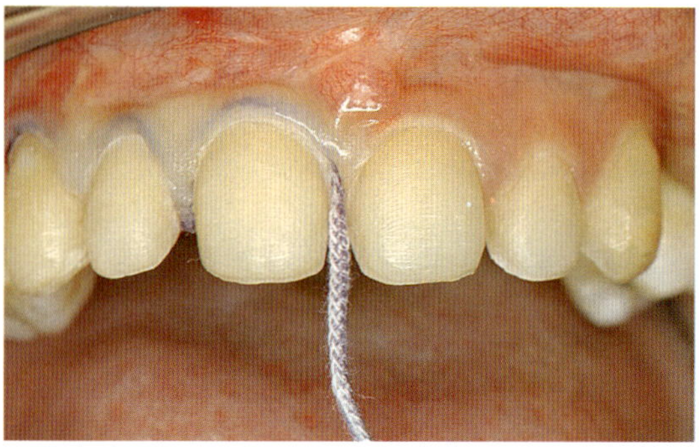

Fig. 6-196 Placing a continuous chemical free retraction cord usually provides retraction for conservative veneer preparations.

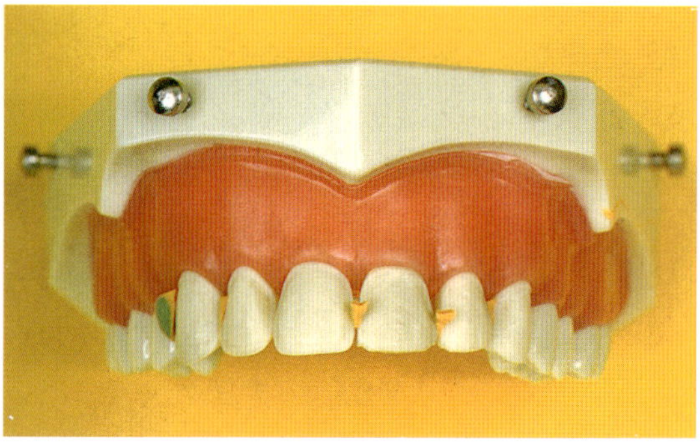

Fig. 6-197a Model demonstrating interproximal impression tear.

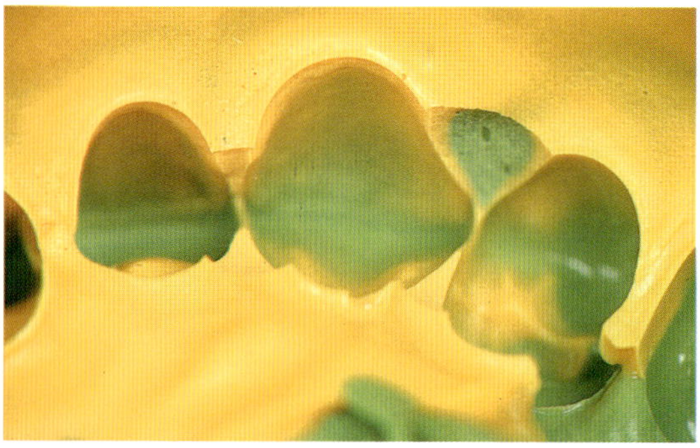

Fig. 6-197b Impression with interproximal tear through margin.

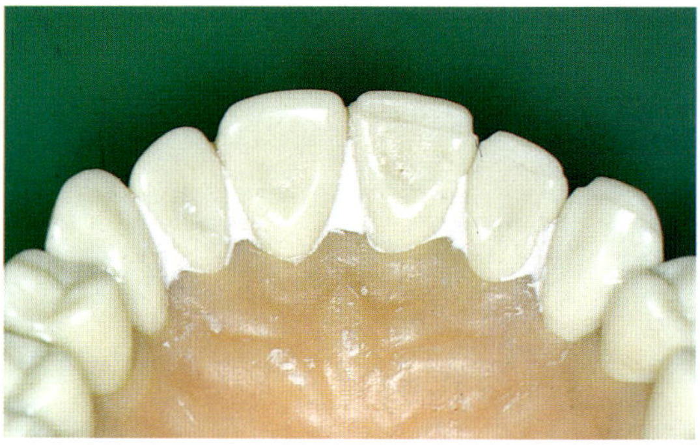

Fig. 6-198 Block out lingual interproximal areas under contacts.

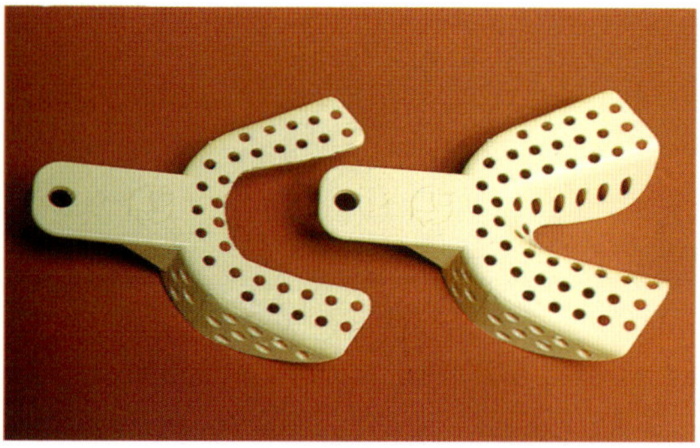

Fig. 6-199 Tray with lingual flange removed (left).

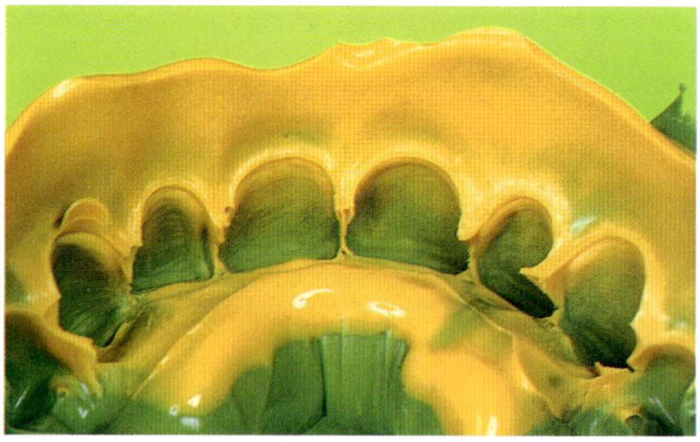

Fig. 6-200 Acceptable impression with intact interproximal extension.

retraction can be achieved (Fig. 6-196). Chemicals can be applied to localized areas of bleeding. The nonchemical string provides sufficient mechanical retraction with minimal to no chemical irritation. The cord can be left in place until an acceptable impression is achieved.

Embrasure Blockout

Because proximal tooth contacts remain in many instances, open gingival embrasures will allow impression material to flow through and tear upon removal (Fig. 6-197). To prevent this, open embrasures with proximal contacts should be sealed from the lingual with rubber dam sealing putty or soft wax (Fig. 6-198). This will prevent the facial impression material from fusing with the lingual and facilitate removal without tearing.

Impression Tray Modification

Rigid mandibular plastic trays, which localize the material and minimize waste, are useful for most veneer impressions. By cutting back the lingual flange, the impression can be removed in a more facial direction and the potential for interproximal tear is reduced (Fig. 6-199). When dual bite trays are used, the opposing teeth should be withdrawn first and the veneer impression pulled facially upon removal (Fig. 6-200).

Provisional Restoration or Stabilization

Because of the conservative preparations used for most veneers, it is often unnecessary to place a provisional restoration. The decision to place an interim restoration should be made prior to the preparation appointment. A provisional restoration should be fabricated when tooth reduction is sufficient to create unacceptable interim esthetics or sensitivity is not tolerable. In addition, a provisional restoration can be used to help determine esthetic and functional contours. The disadvantages of fabricating provisional restorations are that they may result in gingival irritation, they may come loose and they require time and material. Thus the fee must be adjusted if provisionals are used. Some dentists routinely provide and charge for provisional restorations. In contrast, many patients can easily tolerate the interim period without provisional restorations and prefer to save a fee if given the choice. These decisions must be finalized at the consultation appointment so that the appropriate materials can be prepared and sufficient appointment time is scheduled.

Vacuum Formed Provisional Coverage

One of the quickest and easiest ways to protect prepared teeth is to fabricate a vacuum formed vinyl mouthguard or stent. An alginate impression should be made prior to the final impression and poured in quick setting stone. A 0.020- to 0.035-inch flexible clear vinyl stent is vacuum formed and ready before the patient is dismissed (Fig. 6-201) (see Home Bleaching). This stent is cut so it extends just onto the soft tissue and provides excellent protection against thermal changes. These clear stents are esthetic and do not interfere with phonetics. Routine fabrication of this type of provisional is inexpensive and can be provided as a service to patients to

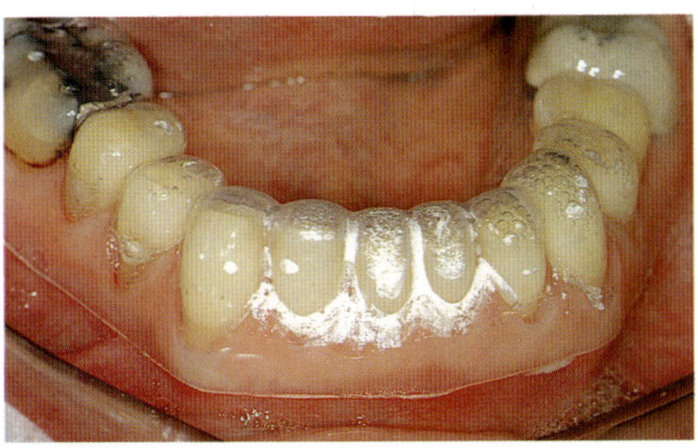

Fig. 6-201 Vacuum formed vinyl provisional.

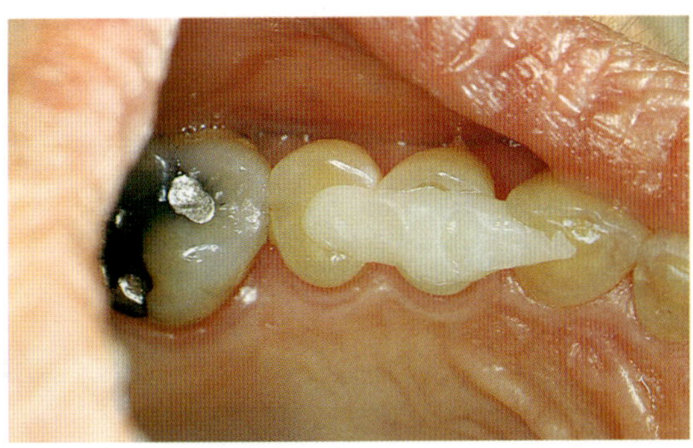

Fig. 6-202 Composite temporarily bonded to opposing teeth to prevent hypereruption of prepared mandibular teeth.

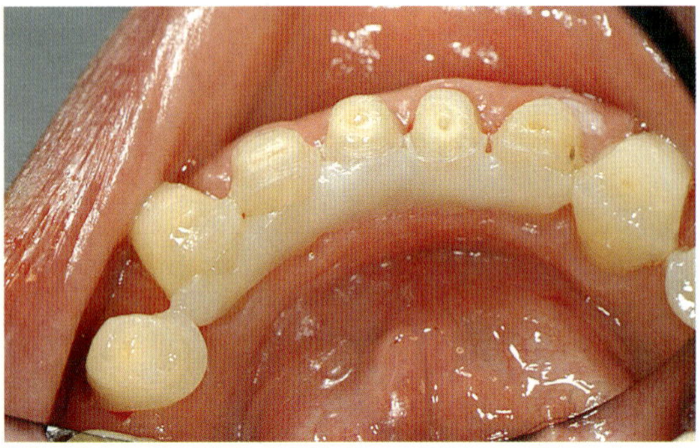
Fig. 6-203 Mandibular teeth temporarily splinted with a lingual bar of composite.

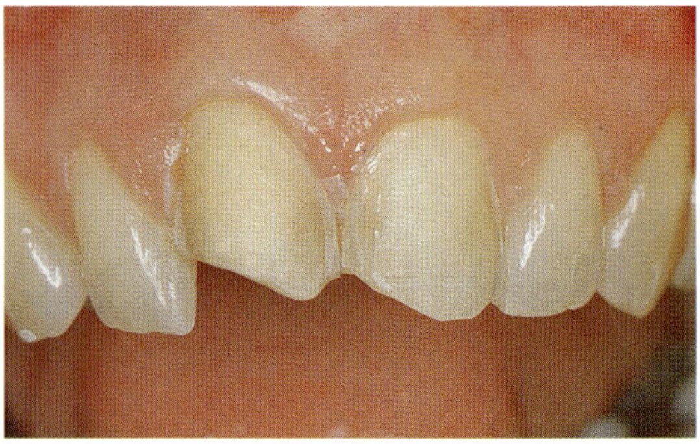
Fig. 6-204a Prepared teeth requiring provisional restorations.

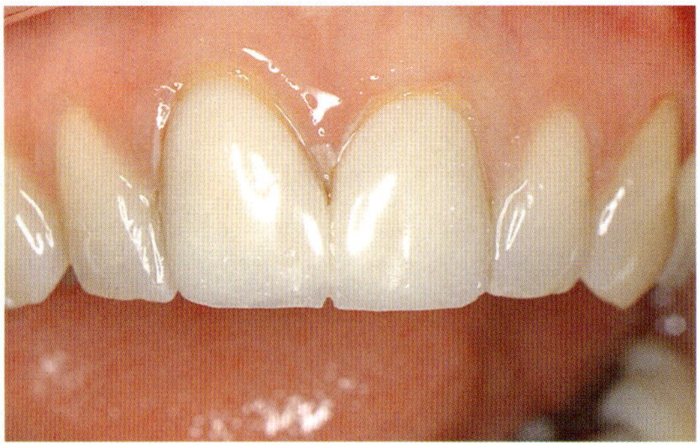
Fig. 6-204b Provisional veneers in place.

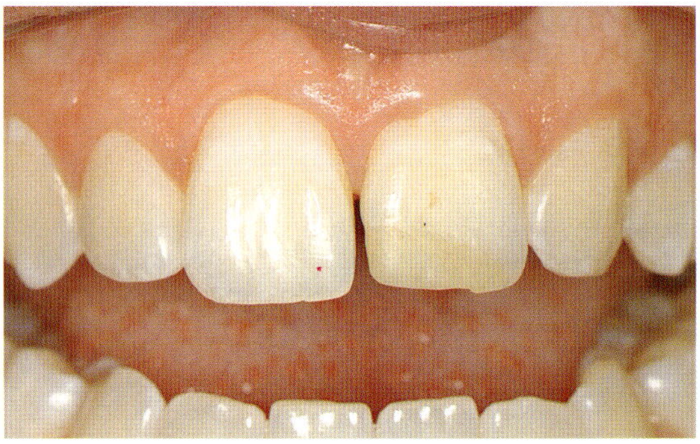
Fig. 6-205a Preoperative view.

use if needed. They will also save a trip back to your office should teeth become overly sensitive after the anesthesia dissipates.

Position Stabilization Using Composite Resin

Mandibular teeth that have been prepared for veneers will normally have the incisal or occlusal contacts reduced to provide room for the veneer. The possibility of hypereruption must be minimized. When a provisional splint is not indicated, a simple and easy way to prevent hypereruption is to simply temporarily bond composite resin occlusal stops on the opposing teeth (Fig. 6-202). These should be formed in a nonmatching shade of composite so they can easily be seen and removed at the delivery appointment.

Composite can also be used to fill open interproximal contacts to prevent proximal migration (Fig. 6-203). Any tooth movement will result in the need for proximal corrections and addition of porcelain, resulting in a wasted delivery appointment. Positional stabilization is important. Teeth that have had diastemas or open contacts for many years are less apt to migrate but still may be splinted to avoid potential problems.

Direct Composite Provisional Restorations

When provisional veneers are required, prepared teeth can be spot etched and composite veneers fabricated directly. Care must be taken not to leave bulky cervical margins that may irritate the gingival tissues (Figs. 6-204a and b). This type of provisional restoration will take time to fabricate and bond properly. Because very little, if any mechanical retention exists, determining the amount of area to etch and bond to is a

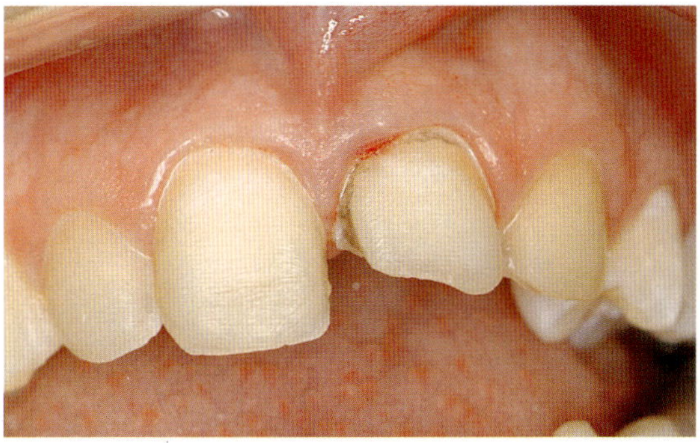

Fig. 6-205b Prepared teeth; provisional required on tooth 9 only.

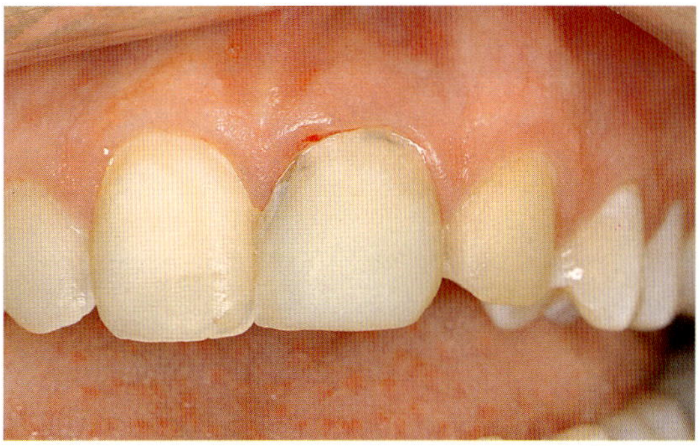

Fig. 6-205c Composite temporarily bonded to tooth 9 (spot etched). Note gingival leakage and irritation after 1 week.

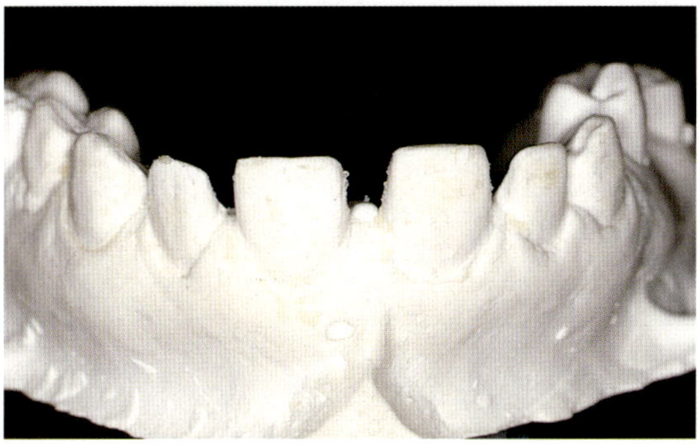

Fig. 6-206 Indirect model of prepared teeth.

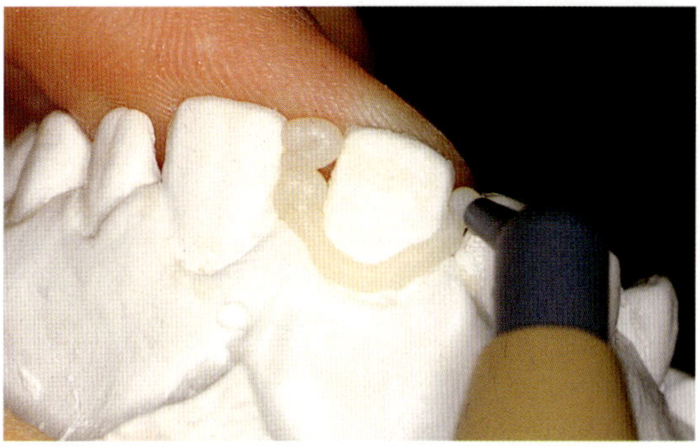

Fig. 6-207 Adding composite to form provisional veneers.

subjective decision. Locking composite into proximal undercuts will improve retention. This type of provisional will also require additional time to remove the composite completely at the delivery appointment. All areas where the provisionals were bonded should be lightly prepared to regain a fresh surface for bonding the veneers.

An additional problem is microleakage around the unbonded margins (Figs. 6-205a to c). This may present an esthetic problem or lead to tissue irritation. Provisional veneers should not be used for extended periods of time. Directly fabricated composite provisional veneers are useful when indicated and convenient and they provide an excellent use for outdated composite.

Indirect Provisional Restorations

The use of an indirect model fabrication technique increases the ease with which an excellent provisional restoration may be fabricated. Preliminary impressions should be made prior to the final impression and poured in a quick-setting plaster or stone (Fig. 6-206). Accurate detailed models provide the basis for many indirect fabrication approaches. Composite may be adapted in layers similar to the direct provisional veneer techniques (Fig. 6-207). Any crown and bridge provisional material may also be used. Indirect models allow the use of clear matrix techniques. A hard vinyl matrix or stent can be vacuum fabricated, as outlined in the section on vital bleaching, from preoperative study models or diagnostic mock-ups of proposed contours (Fig. 6-208). The matrix should be trimmed to retain sufficient soft and hard tissue stops to ensure positional accuracy. Almost any matrix material may be

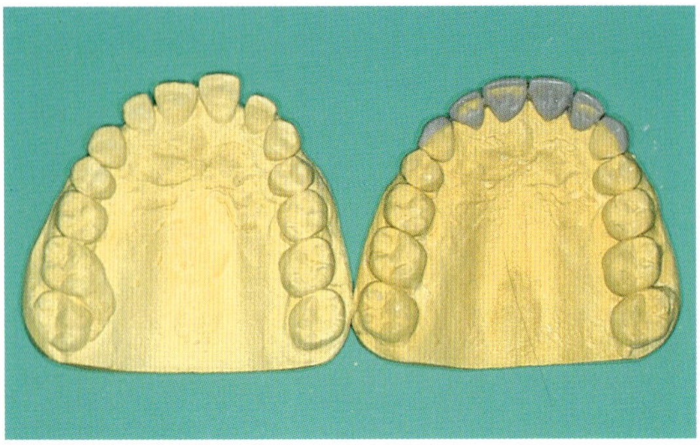

Fig. 6-208

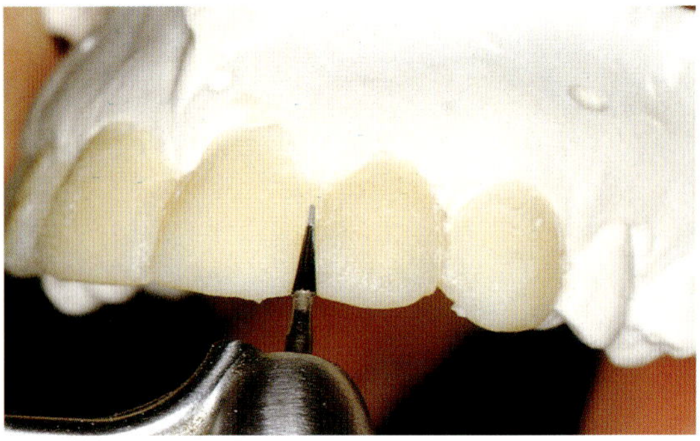

Fig. 6-209

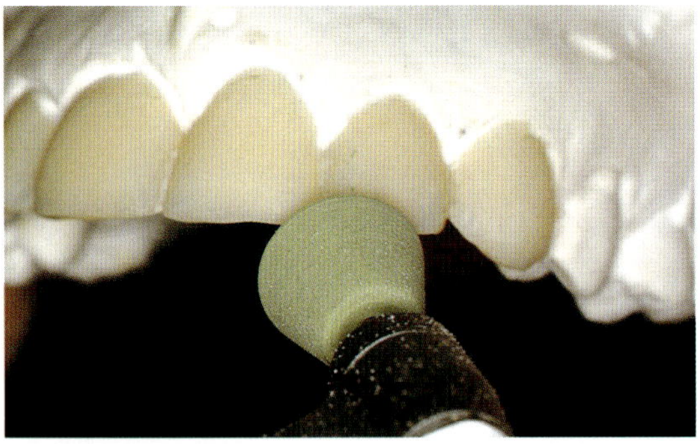

Fig. 6-210

Fig. 6-208 Diagnostic waxup can be used to form a vinyl stent that may be used with other provisional materials when using an indirect model.

Fig. 6-209 Contouring the provisionals on the model.

Fig. 6-210 Final polishing.

Fig. 6-211 A set of completed indirect provisional veneers.

Fig. 6-212 Excess polycarboxylate cement is easily seen.

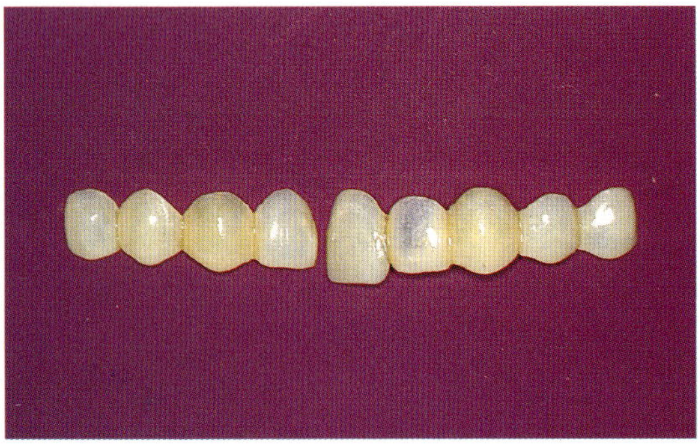

Fig. 6-211

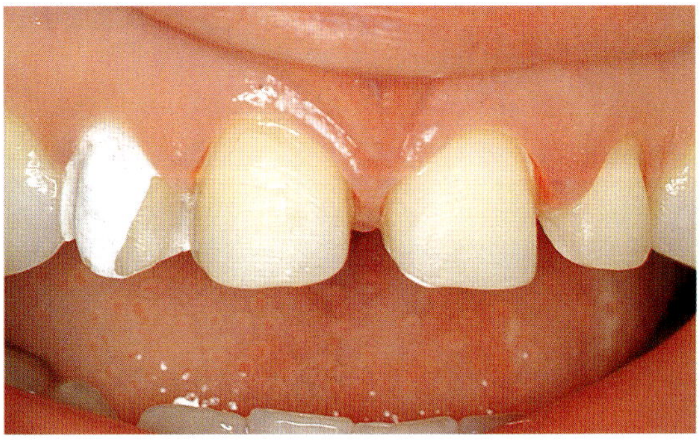

Fig. 6-212

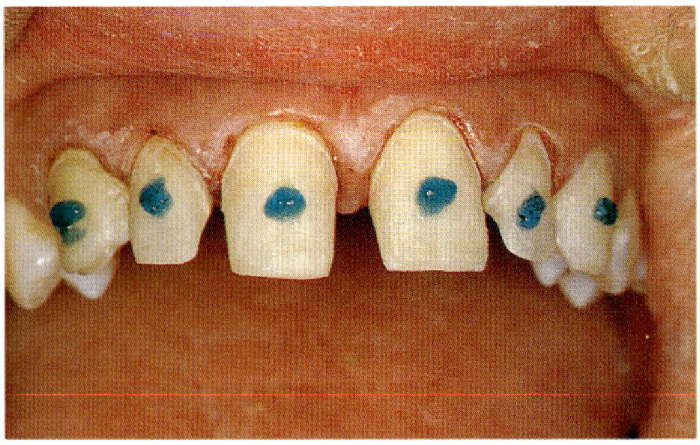

Fig. 6-213 Spot etching prepared teeth so composite cement may be used.

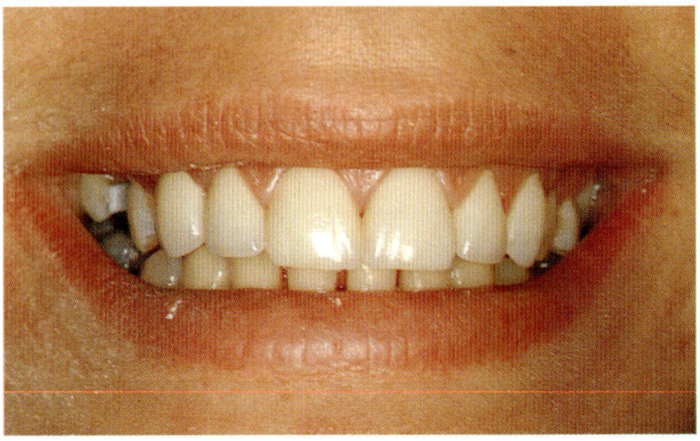

Fig. 6-214 Healthy tissues at cementation appointment.

used. The clear matrix is also useful during tooth preparation to ensure adequate tooth reduction. The indirect model, if fabricated while making the final impression, requires little additional time than direct bonding. It also allows for greater material control by individuals not as experienced in direct bonding or delegation of fabrication to auxiliaries. The indirect provisional restoration can be accurately trimmed on the model and polished (Figs. 6-209 and 6-210). Whenever possible, multiple unit provisional veneer restorations should be splinted (Fig. 6-211). This will provide greater retention and resistance to dislodging. Polycarboxylate cement can be used for cementation and is easily visualized and removed at the delivery appointment (Fig. 6-212). For thin provisional veneers, polycarboxylate cements may be opaque. If more translucent resin cements are desirable, use spot etching techniques (Fig. 6-213). Veneer provisionals must provide good interim esthetic results, but more importantly they should ensure healthy tissues at the delivery appointment (Fig. 6-214).

LABORATORY COMMUNICATION

The usual procedures for shade determination, color perception and correct lighting used for ceramic crowns are also used for ceramic veneers. The purpose of this section is to focus on unique techniques for shade control and success with veneer restorations.

Selection of Shade

Multiple ceramic veneers allow for a shade change that may be the primary reason for treatment. A preoperative shade consultation using various visualization techniques should be performed. Computer imaging provides an excellent way for patients to visualize themselves and analyze proposed changes (Fig. 6-215). Photographs of other cases and shade guides have limited value and may lead to patient expectations that are not communicated to the dentist. A final desired shade should be selected and recorded in the patient chart.

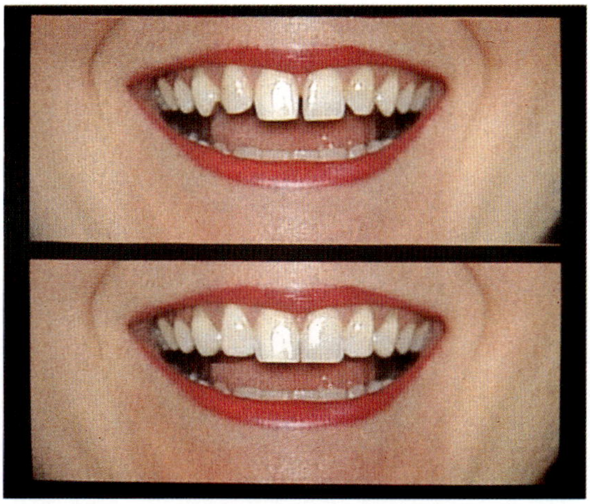

Fig. 6-215 Computer imaged simulation.

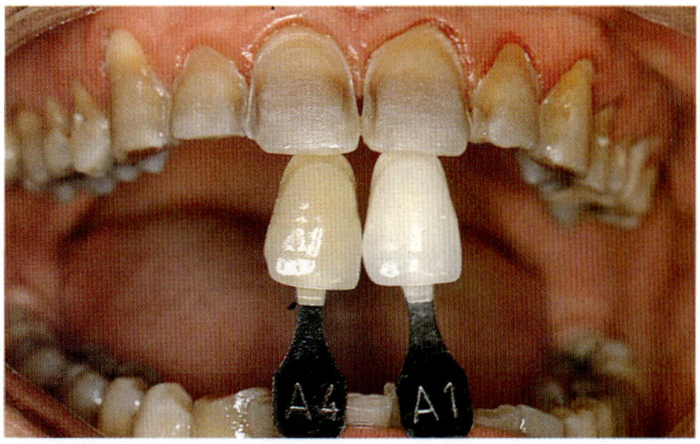

Fig. 6-216 Photograph of prepared teeth with shade guides simulating prepared and desired shades.

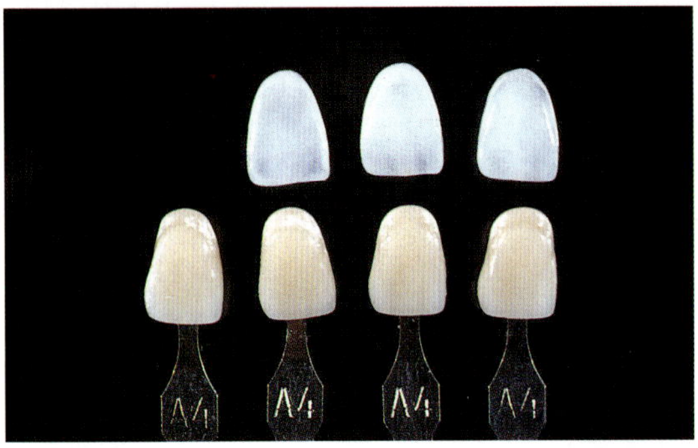

Fig. 6-217

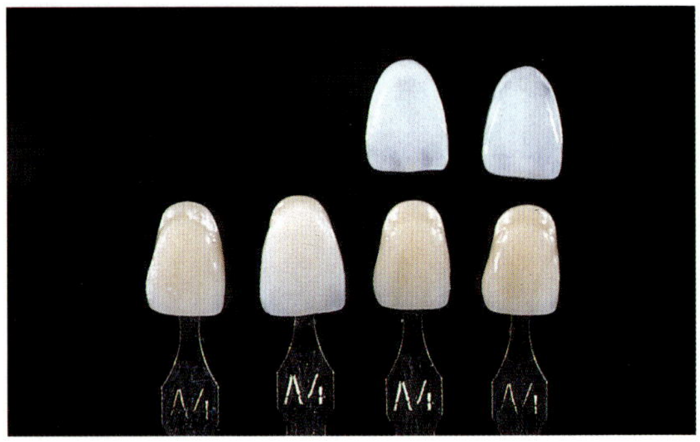

Fig. 6-218

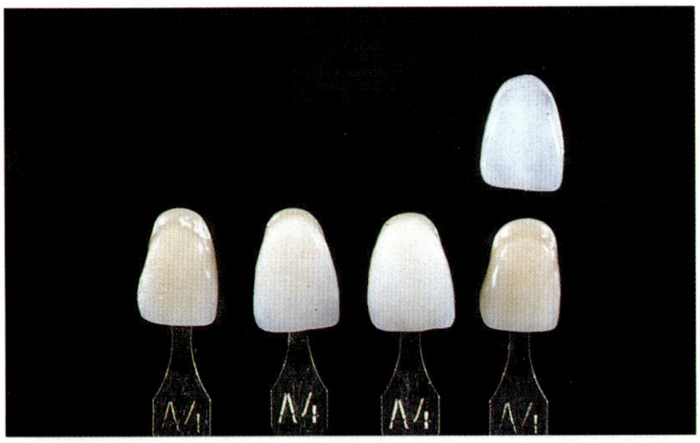

Fig. 6-219

Fig. 6-217 Three ceramic veneers above, four identical shade tabs below. Top left 50% opacification, middle 100% opacification; top right veneer is an opalescent ceramic. Note different translucencies.

Fig. 6-218 Fifty percent opacification veneer seated with clear gel.

Fig. 6-219 Fifty percent and 100% opacification veneers seated with clear gel.

Fig. 6-220 All veneers seated with clear gel. Note variations in lightening and vitality.

Fig. 6-221 Ceramic discs (0.5 mm thick) with varying opacities.

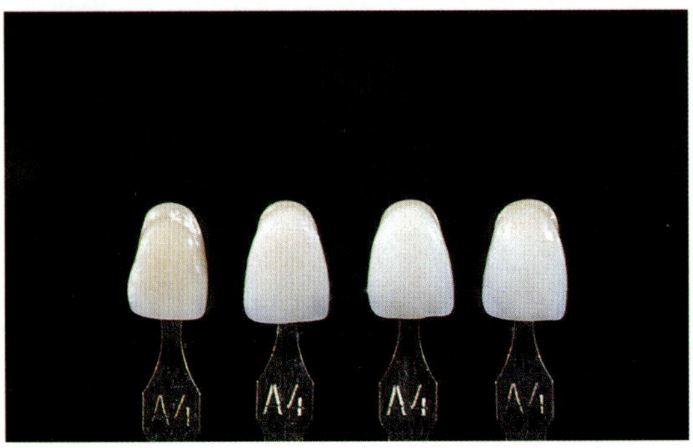

Fig. 6-220

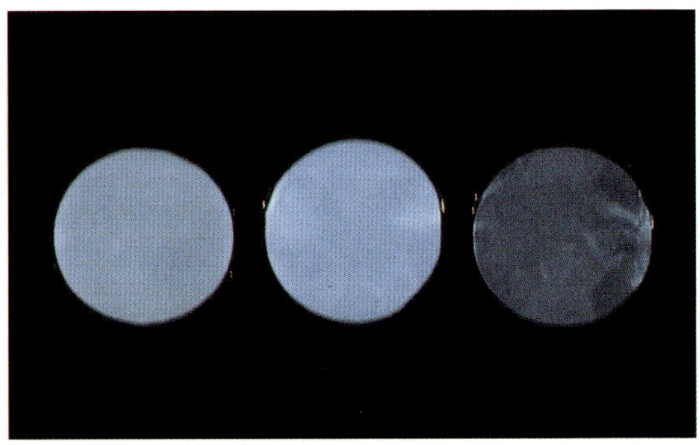

Fig. 6-221

Shade of Existing Teeth

Because ceramic veneers are thin, color from the underlying tooth may alter the final veneer shade. Thus it is of critical importance that the ceramist know the shade of the prepared tooth. Any color irregularities on the tooth should be noted. A computer imaged print is ideal or an instant photograph can be used to show the prepared teeth with reference shade guides of both the actual and desired shades. This visual data provides the ceramist with important information (Fig. 6-216). Depending upon the amount of shade change requested, the ceramist will modify several factors to provide greater opacity. The two main techniques utilized to increase opacity are (1) providing greater die relief and space for opaque resin cements and (2) opacifying the ceramic veneer (Figs. 6-217 to 6-220). Different ceramic systems opacify the veneers in different ways.

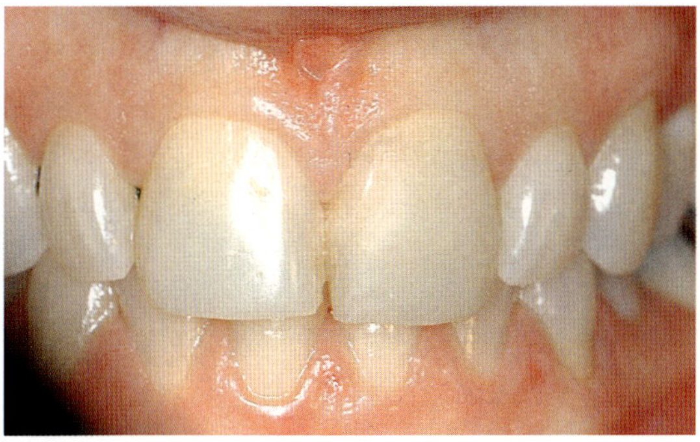

Fig. 6-222a Preoperative view.

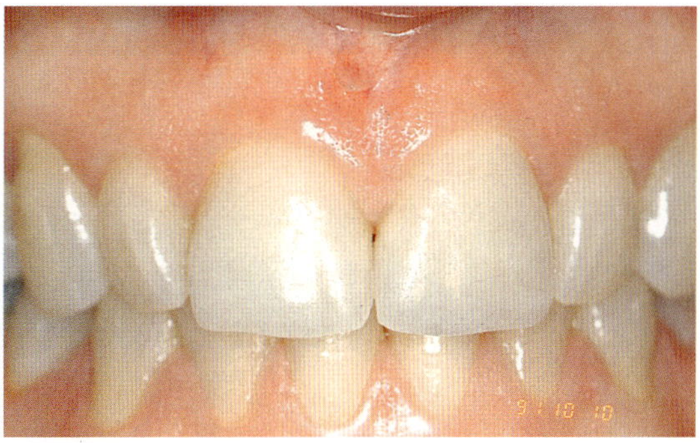

Fig. 6-222b Postoperative view with maximum translucency.

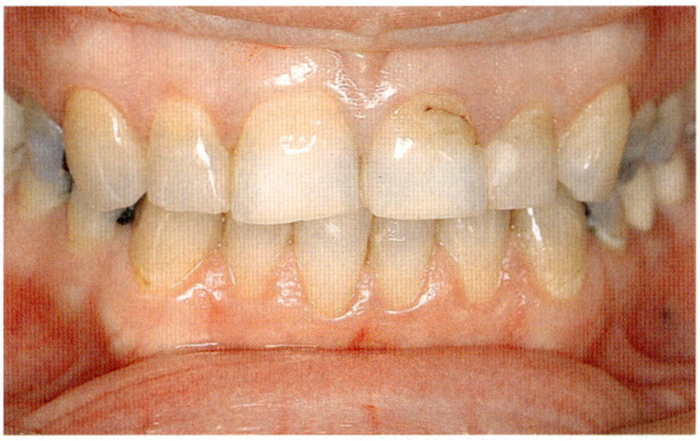

Fig. 6-223a Preoperative view.

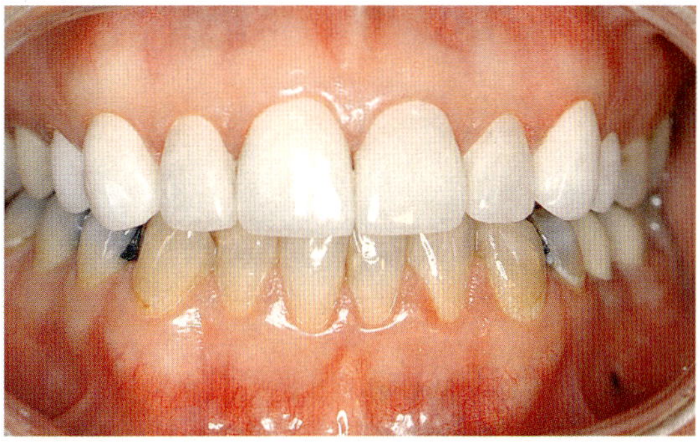

Fig. 6-223b Postoperative view with maximum lightening required and resultant maximum opacity.

Opacity or translucency control is a major factor in optimizing esthetic results (Fig. 6-221). When minimal color change is desired, a more translucent veneer will allow actual tooth color to show through, providing a more natural appearance (Fig. 6-222). In contrast, when blocking out discolored teeth and very white veneers are desired, maximum opacity will be required and a less natural appearing veneer may be the result (Fig. 6-223). There are limitations on how much underlying color a thin ceramic veneer and opaque resin can block out and still be esthetically acceptable to the patient. Increased veneer depth or full crowns may be required when patients are unwilling to compromise. Expectations and reality must be made clear to the patient to avoid disappointment and failure. Usually the educated patient with severely discolored teeth will happily accept a compromise that is a significant esthetic improvement but avoids the amount of tooth removal necessary for full crown preparations.

Good communication between the dentist and ceramist is mandatory in order to control opacity and translucency, for optimal results. The dentist should have a general understanding of the techniques used to modify opacity. There is little or no standardization of veneer ceramic systems and a variety of methods may be used. Understanding how an individual ceramist controls opacity is a must for good communications. A visit to the laboratory to meet your technician and to observe materials and techniques used will help the dentist to improve communication. A ceramist who does not understand these principles should be avoided.

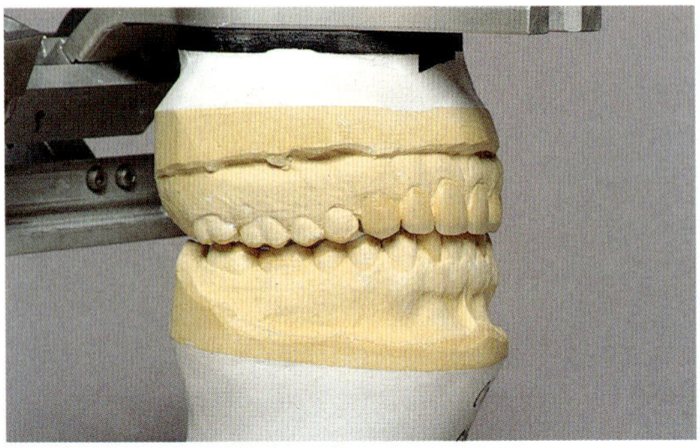

Fig. 6-224a Right lateral view of diagnostic waxup.

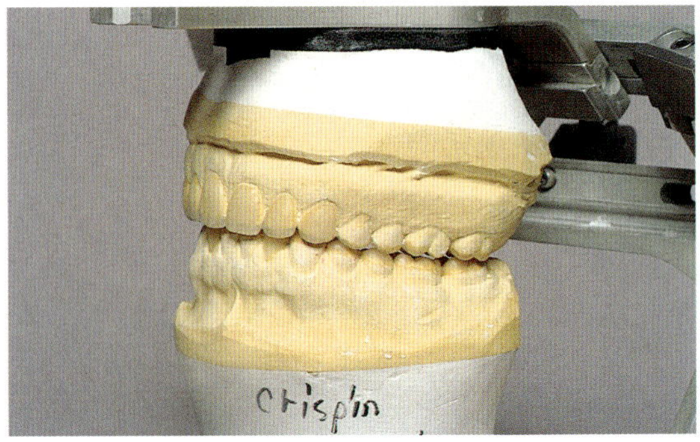

Fig. 6-224b Left lateral view of diagnostic waxup.

Communication of Desired Contour

Photographic prints only provide two-dimensional images for the ceramist. Preoperative models and models of the proposed final contour provide more accurate information on three-dimensional contours. Desired contours may be presented as diagnostic waxups. It is advisable to do these in tooth colored waxes to avoid color distraction during patient consultations (Fig. 6-224). Models may be taken of provisional restorations that have been placed and contoured to satisfy the patient's esthetic treatment goals and provided to the ceramist.

Patient Visit to the Laboratory

For difficult or demanding esthetic cases, it is advisable to have the patient visit the laboratory for direct visualization by the ceramist. This may demand a small laboratory fee but clearly gives the ceramist information that will provide more optimal results. This also places a greater responsibility for the esthetic result in the hands of the laboratory.

CLINICAL PROCEDURES (PLACEMENT)

Preappointment Veneer Inspection

The ceramic veneers should be inspected prior to the clinical delivery appointment. The veneers should individually be placed on the dies to verify accuracy. The veneers should all be seated together to ensure that contour and contact criteria have been met (Fig. 6-225). Finally, the internal surfaces of each veneer must be examined to ensure a complete and uniform etch. A uniform frosty appearance should be seen (Fig. 6-226). A small drop of water should spread quickly over the etched surface upon contact. Any shiny or nonuniform surfaces should be re-etched. Gel etching solutions sometimes underetch borders if not agitated (Fig. 6-227).

Failure to preinspect the veneers may lead to a wasted appointment or accepting compromise that could have been avoided. Place the veneers back into the laboratory storage container until the delivery appointment.

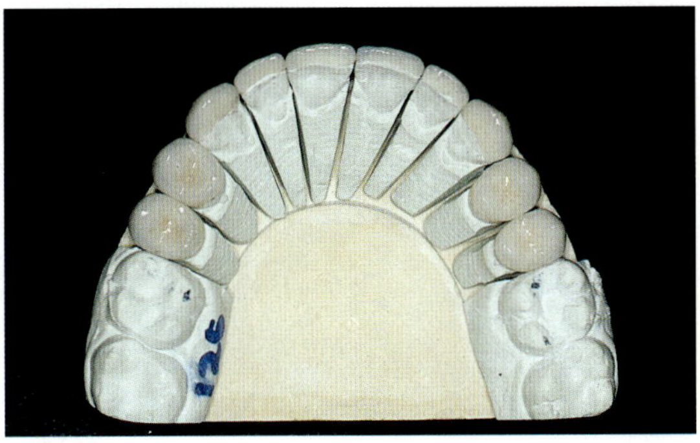

Fig. 6-225a All veneers seated on working model (occlusal view).

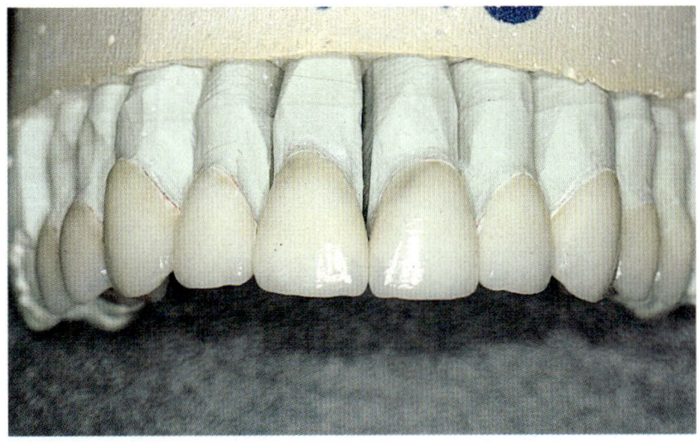

Fig. 6-225b All veneers seated on working model (facial view).

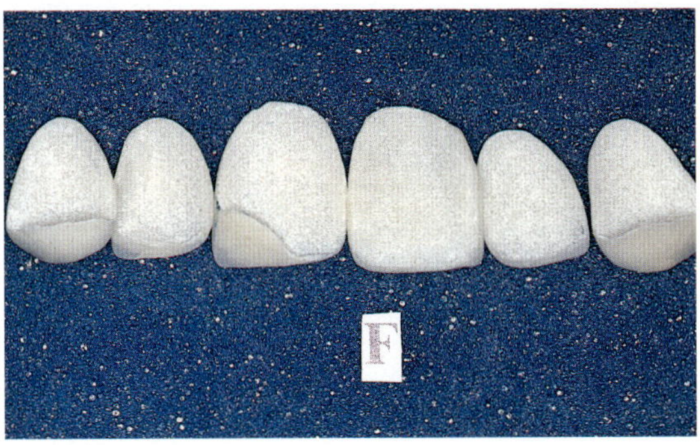

Fig. 6-226 Properly etched veneers.

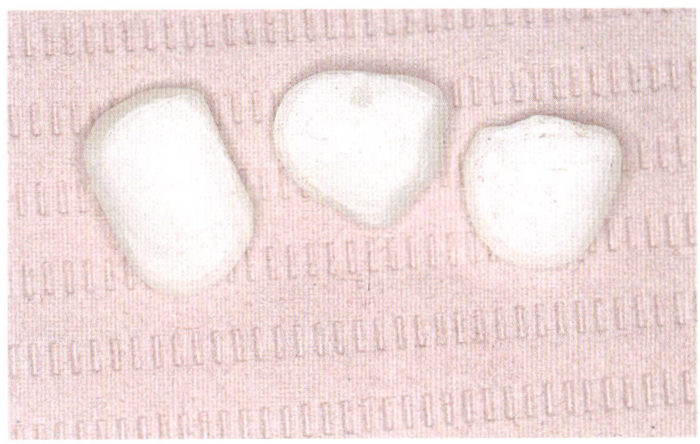

Fig. 6-227 Improperly etched veneers. Note spots and shiny margins.

Preparing for the Clinical Appointment

The veneers should be placed on a clearly labeled surface and a strict policy established (Fig. 6-228). No instruments or other materials should come near this isolated area. This will minimize needless accidents. The veneer must either be in position on its corresponding tooth or on its numbered area at all times. Attention to these simple procedures will eliminate most problems in handling the fragile veneers.

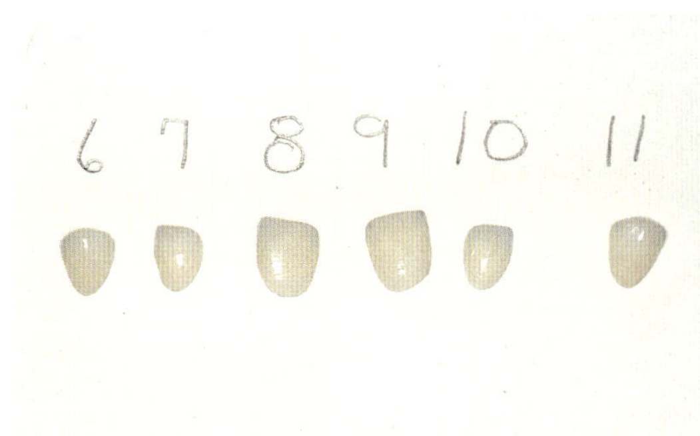

Fig. 6-228 Place veneers in safe, clearly labeled area during cementation appointment.

Tooth and Tissue Preparation

1. Remove any remaining defective tooth structure or old restorations that will be covered by the veneers.

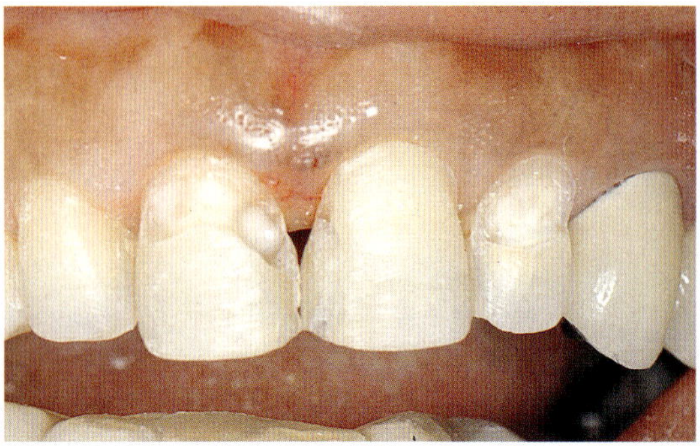

Fig. 6-229

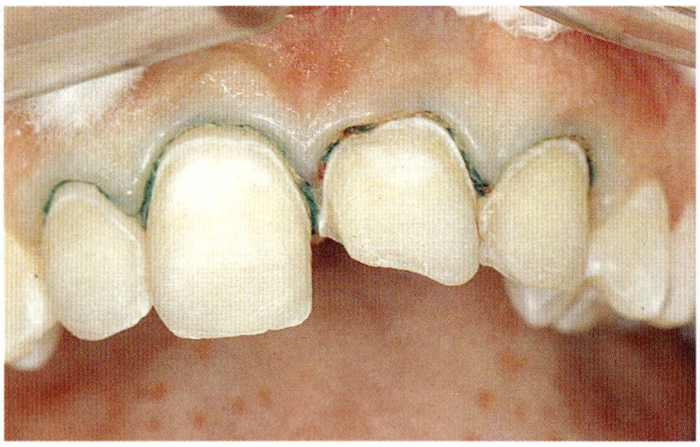

Fig. 6-230

Fig. 6-229 Placement of fluoride liner in deep areas.

Fig. 6-230 Retract tissues with chemical free retraction cord.

Fig. 6-231 Postcementation marginal stains due to inadequate removal of iron containing chemicals.

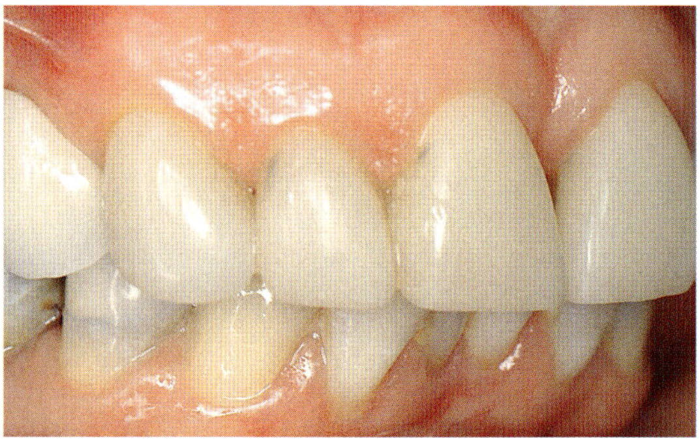

Fig. 6-231

2. Place fluoride-releasing liners in vulnerable or deep areas (Fig. 6-229).
3. Partially fill large voids with an appropriate restorative to minimize cement thickness and unnecessary volumetric contraction in these areas.
4. Carefully clean all prepared surfaces with nonfluoridated pumice to minimize veneer contamination.
5. If soft tissues interfere with veneer seating, pack a chemical-free string for mechanical retraction as done during impression procedures (Fig. 6-230). String retraction is advisable in many instances to minimize gingival fluid contamination and to help contain excess cement. If necessary, chemicals may be used. Chemicals containing iron must be carefully washed away or margin discoloration after cementation can occur (Fig. 6-231).

Veneer Try-in Procedures

1. Veneers should be tried in individually to verify accuracy consistent with the accuracy on the die. Veneers not seating completely may require adjustment. Check for overextended margins that may prevent seating and adjust if necessary with fine high speed diamonds and water spray. If inaccuracy appears to be internal, inspect the die for abraded areas or differences from the prepared tooth. Check for a fulcrum of movement that might localize a high spot. The prepared tooth should always be adjusted first when an internal inaccuracy prevents seating. This will eliminate the need to re-etch the inner surface of the veneer. Silicone fit-checking materials should be avoided because they remain in microetched areas. If used, coat the etched veneer surface with unfilled resin to fill etched areas and minimize silicone penetration.

Fig. 6-232 Use fine diamond and water to adjust proximal contacts.

Fig. 6-233 The veneer on tooth 8 is optically connected; the veneer on tooth 9 is not. Note tooth 9 is lighter due to air space between tooth and veneer.

Fig. 6-234 Six veneers held in place with water-soluble clear gel.

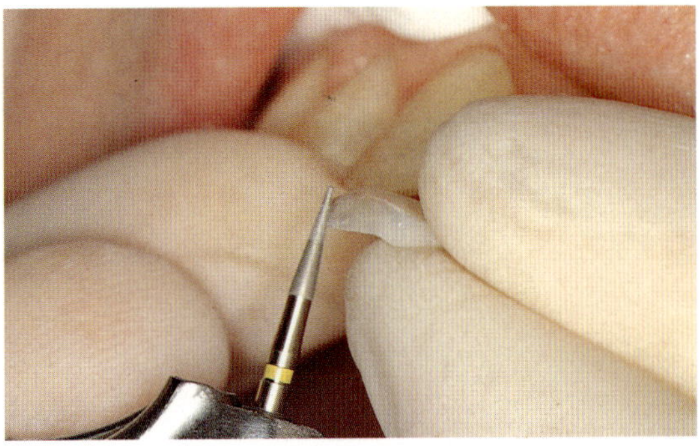

Fig. 6-232

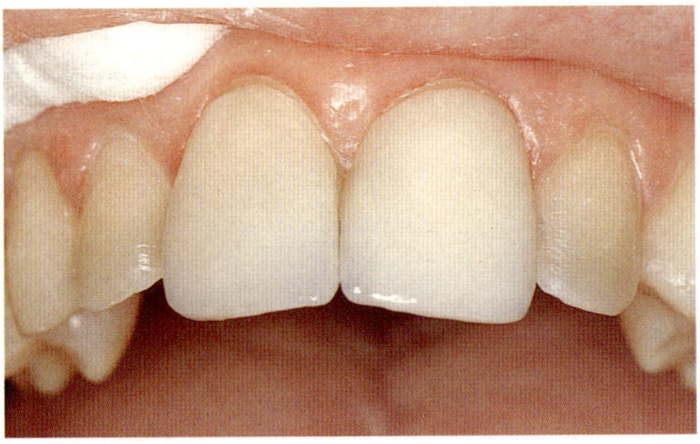

Fig. 6-233

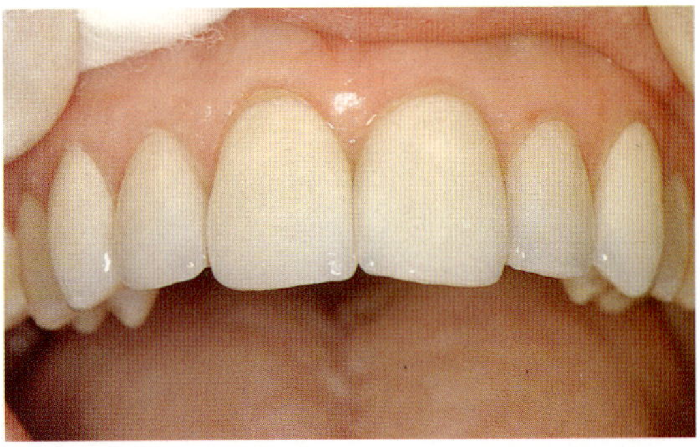

Fig. 6-234

2. Once seated individually, veneers are tried in two at a time to evaluate interproximal contacts. Push on each individual veneer from the facial and the adjacent veneer should not move laterally. Deflecting or heavy contact must be adjusted using fine high speed diamonds and water or fine ceramic adjusting stones on low speed (Fig. 6-232). All adjusted contacts should be polished with rubber porcelain polishing wheels prior to cementation. Care must be exercised to avoid excessive heat and vibration, the two main causes of ceramic chipping.
3. The veneers are now ready to try in all at once and to evaluate contour and color. They must be placed with a material that optically connects the veneer to the tooth for correct color evaluation (Fig. 6-233). In most instances the use of a clear water-soluble gel will optically connect the veneers to the tooth for esthetic evaluation and provide an increased viscosity medium that will hold the veneers in place for patient evaluation (Fig. 6-234). At this point the **patient must verify that the color of the veneers is acceptable and they are not too small.** Often the veneers are perceived as being too large compared to prepared teeth. This is acceptable, for the contour of the cemented veneers can easily be reduced. If the veneers are too small they must be returned to the laboratory for ceramic additions. If the color is acceptable, cementation using a clear or translucent cement can be initiated. If shade modifications are necessary, various materials and techniques must be tried until the colors are acceptable. When a subtle generalized shade modification is desired, the use of a colored cement may provide the solution. When more complicated color alterations are required, several alternatives are available, and these will be described next.
4. **Generalized polychromatic shade modifi-**

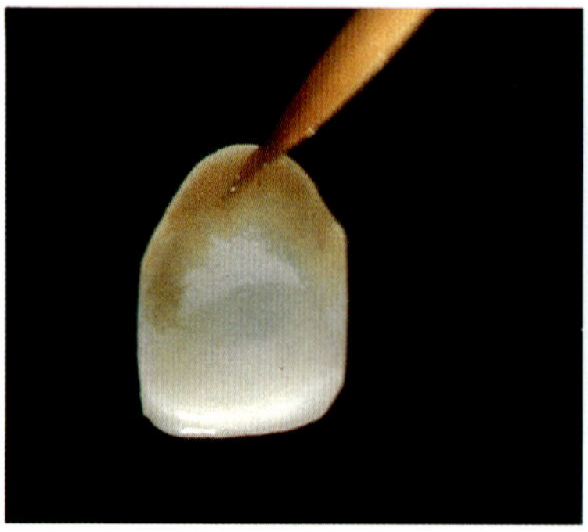

Fig. 6-235 Paint high chroma composite tint on the inner gingival surface of the veneer.

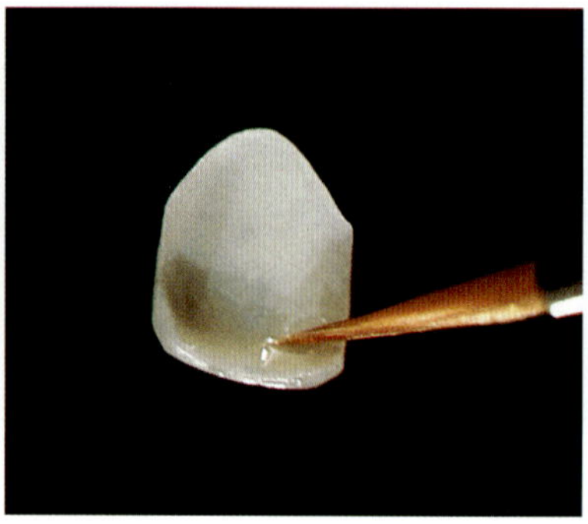

Fig. 6-236 Place grey tint on inner incisal third.

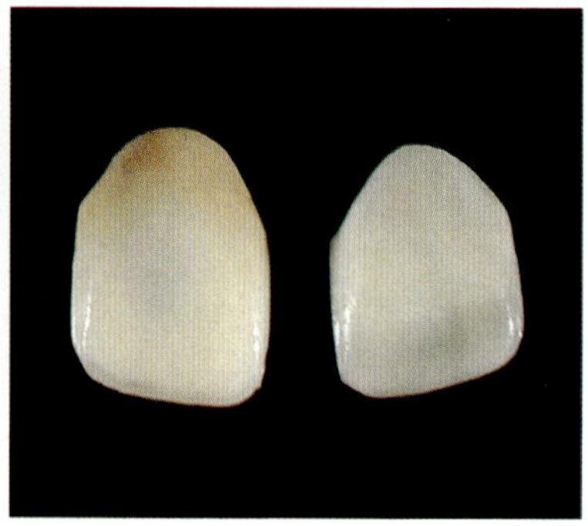

Fig. 6-237 Note how tints can be seen through the veneer and modify color.

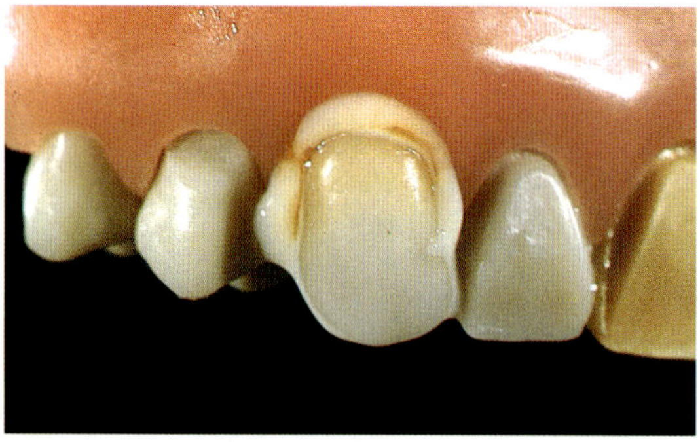

Fig. 6-238 Seat veneer with right and left rocking motion to extrude cement evenly.

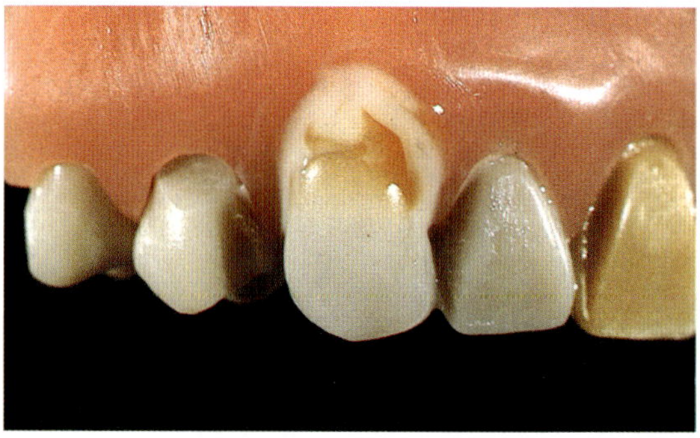

Fig. 6-239 Seating the veneer from incisal to gingival forces all tints gingivally (incorrect).

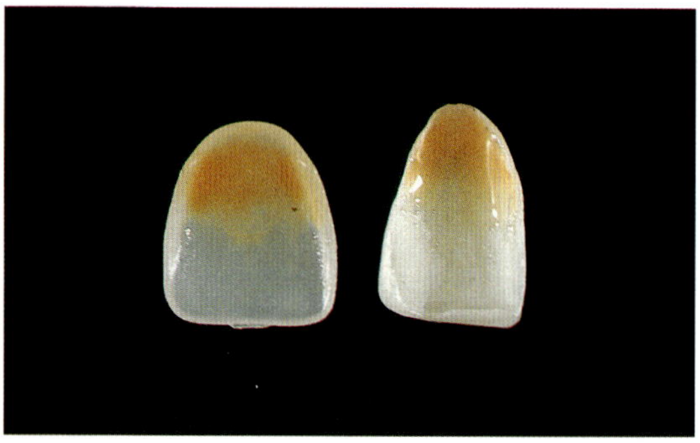

Fig. 6-240a Gingival tint placed on translucent veneer (**left**) and opaque veneer (**right**).

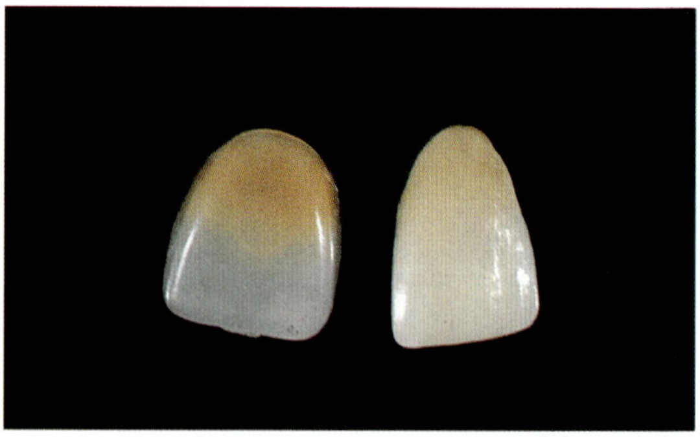

Fig. 6-240b Note how opaque veneer blocks more of the color from the lingual.

cation. When a generalized shade modification is necessary for only a portion of the veneer, composite tints (high chroma, lower viscosity composites) may be used. For example, when chroma enhancement of a particular hue is desired in the gingival one third, a thin layer of the appropriate colored composite tint is painted on the inside of the veneer (Fig. 6-235). The selected cement or try-in paste is placed over the tint and the veneer seated as if cementing. Another common technique is to use a slight amount of blue or grey composite tint in the incisal region to

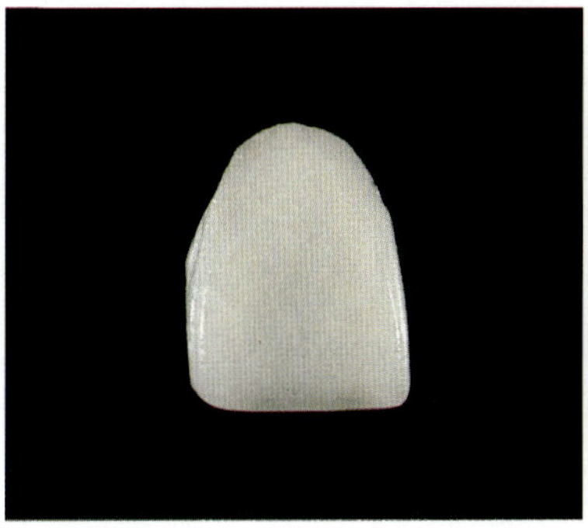

Fig. 6-241a

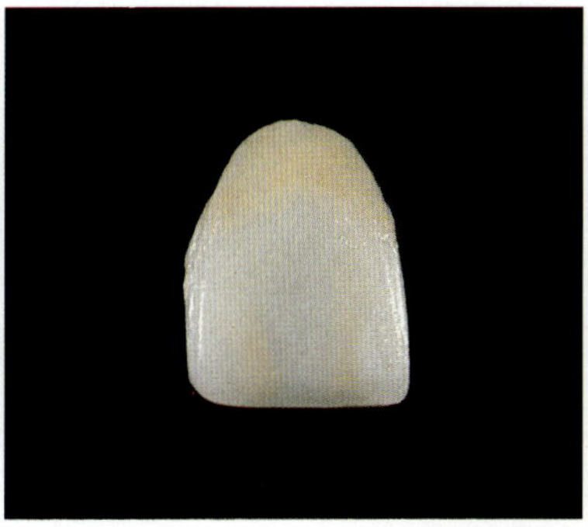

Fig. 6-241b

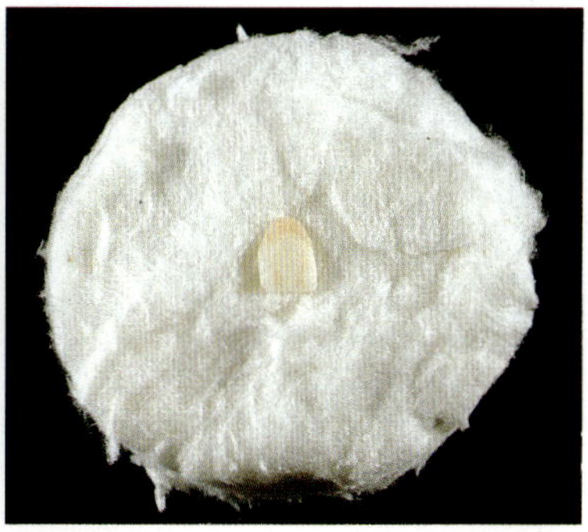

Fig. 6-242

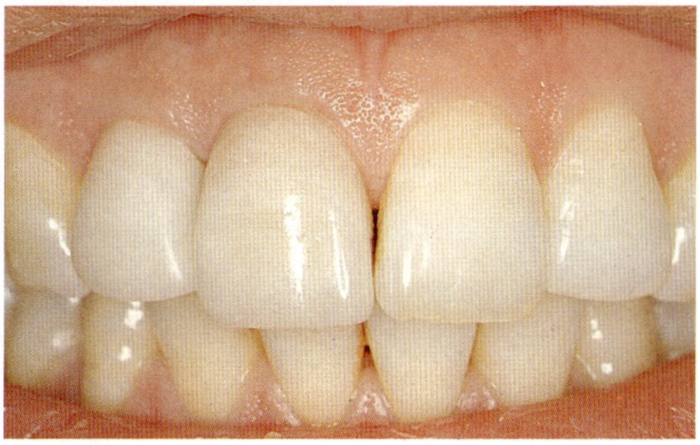

Fig. 6-243

Fig. 6-241a Uncolored veneer.

Fig. 6-241b Application of extrinsic low fusing ceramic stains.

Fig. 6-242 Veneer on sagar pillow ready to go into ceramic oven to fuse stain.

Fig. 6-243 Porcelain veneer on tooth 8 with extrinsic ceramic stain placed to mimic tooth 9.

increase the appearance of translucency (Fig. 6-236). Subtle shade alterations make veneers look less monochromatic and are useful when slight shade modifications are necessary to match veneers to non-veneered teeth (Fig. 6-237).

Limitations exist for shade modification with composite tints. They can be used only to make generalized shade alterations and it takes practice to control the flow of the tint when cementing. Horizontal bands of color are most common. When seating the veneer, a side to side seating force, with consistent pressure incisal to gingival, will force the excess cement to extrude laterally (Fig. 6-238). This will maintain the tint in the correct horizontal position. Asymmetric facial seating pressure, forcing the excess cement incisally or gingivally, will allow the cement and tint to flow vertically thus disrupting the horizontal orientation of the tint (Fig. 6-239).

Another limitation of this technique is the opacity of the veneer itself. The color of thicker or more opaque veneers will be less modified by tints (Fig. 6-240).

Care should be taken to document exactly the materials and techniques used to achieve these desired esthetic results, for these procedures must be repeated during cementation. Complicated mixtures of colored tints should be prepared in sufficient quantities for use during final cementation.

Finally, localized characterizations, such as opacities and cracks, cannot be added using this approach.

5. **Localized polychromatic shade modification.** Specific localized characterizations like opacities, cracks, color spots, etc. cannot be achieved using composite tints. With excellent laboratory communication techniques, acceptable results may be achieved during fabrication. Generally, these characterizations will require chairside color modification for best results.

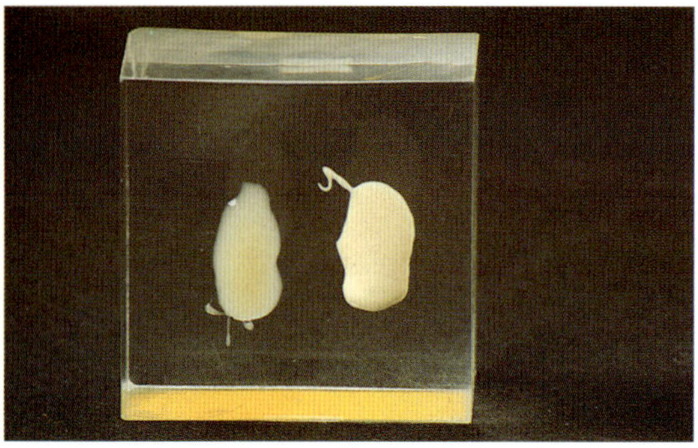

Fig. 6-244 Translucent cement (left); opaque cements (right).

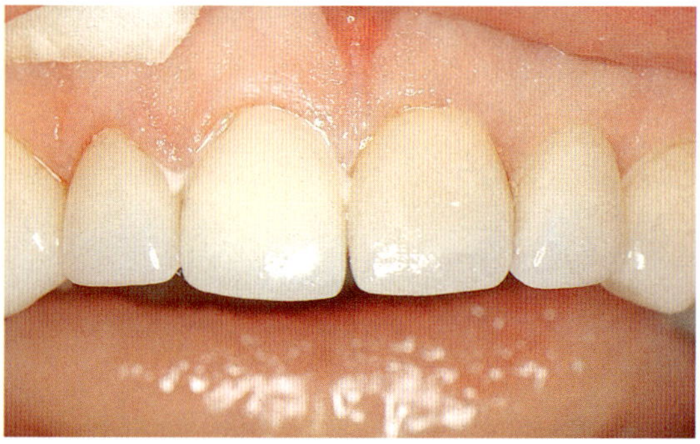

Fig. 6-245 Veneers tried-in with translucent cement (left) and opaque cement (right).

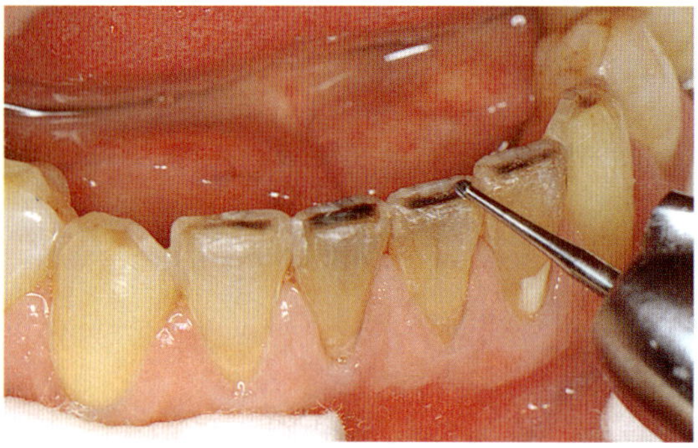

Fig. 6-246a Removing additional tooth structure to create a greater cement thickness in the localized area.

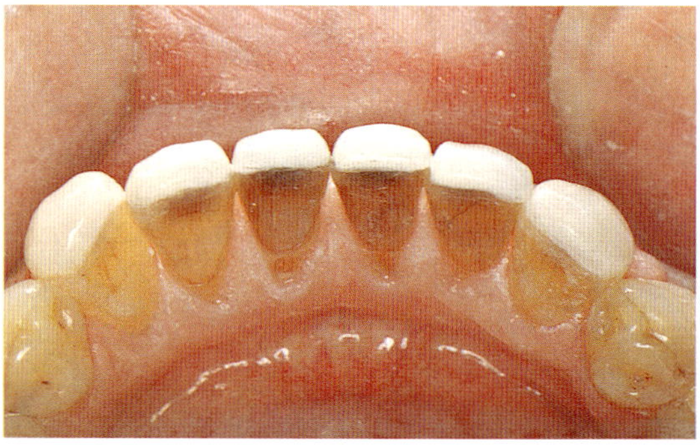

Fig. 6-246b Postoperative incisal view.

This is particularly true for matching veneers to natural teeth. The use of low fusing (lower temperature) ceramic stains is mandatory for optimal ceramic veneer esthetics in these situations. The stains are simply painted on the external veneer surface until the desired esthetic results are achieved (Fig. 6-241). The veneer is positioned on a refractory pillow and placed in a glazing oven to fuse the ceramic stain to the surface of the veneer (Fig. 6-242). The procedure is very similar to that discussed for finalizing conventional ceramic crowns and can be repeated until the desired esthetic results are achieved (Fig. 6-243). Low fusing stains may also be used for generalized shade modifications in opaque veneers when composite tints are not effective.

0. **Value modification (opacity control).** Value, or the achromatic measure of the degree of greyness in a restoration, is one of the most critical and necessary esthetic factors to control in ceramic veneers. Often a primary reason for placing veneers is to lighten teeth while covering unwanted colors. Blocking out dark areas with a relatively thin piece of ceramic will require a knowledge of various techniques used to modify veneer opacity.

Initially the appropriate amount of intrinsic opacity must be prescribed from and provided by the laboratory as described in the laboratory communications section. Translucent to maximally opaqued veneers can be fabricated to meet the specific esthetic demands of each situation.

During the try-in procedures, relative opacity can be further enhanced or modified through the use of opaque composite

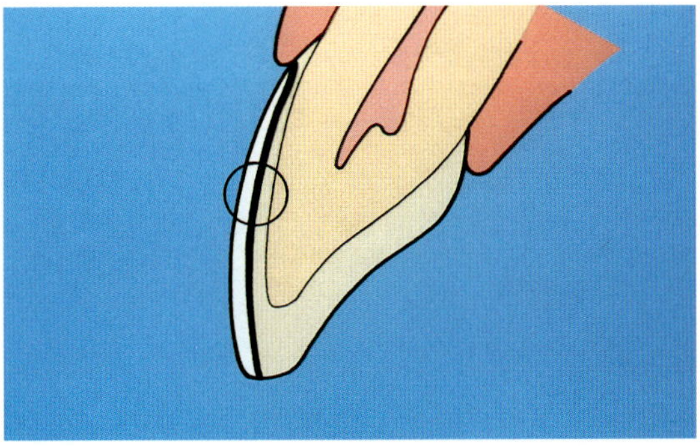

Fig. 6-247a Cross section diagram of cemented veneer.

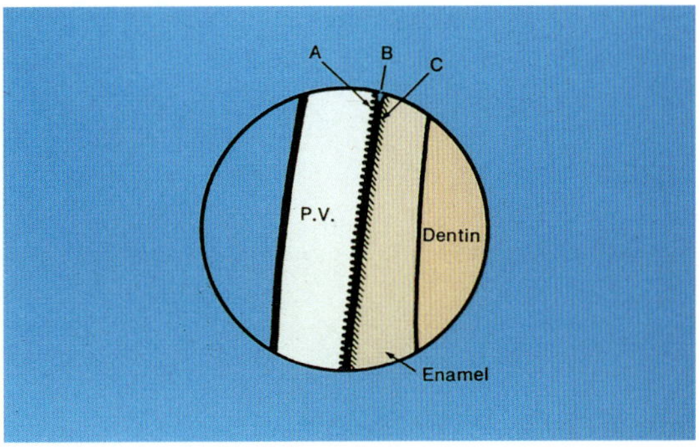

Fig. 6-247b Close up of circled area in Fig. 6-247a. Going from *(PV)* veneer to tooth the layer would be as follows: etched ceramic, *(A)* bonding agent, *(B)* composing cement (tints), *(C)* bonding agent, and enamel.

resin cements (Figs. 6-244 and 6-245). Generalized opacity enhancement and a resultant lightening of the veneers can easily be achieved by using opaque cements by themselves for maximum opacification or in conjunction with more translucent composite resin cements. Multiple trials using various ratios of translucent cements, opaque cements and color modifiers are attempted until the desired results are achieved.

If dark areas are still visible through portions of the veneer, and a maximum opacity cement is already being used, additional opacity can be achieved by removing additional tooth structure in specific areas. This will create a thicker film thickness of cement and greater opacity (Fig. 6-246). The negative aspect of blocking out dark teeth using maximum opacity techniques with thin veneers is the loss of depth and a nonvital appearance. This still may be preferable to placement of crowns on dark teeth. This opaque look can be minimized by preparing deeper veneers. With improved dentin bonding techniques, this alternative is becoming more acceptable.

Once the proper materials have been selected, ample amounts of tints, cements and opaques should be placed in a light protective box. Enough material should be dispensed for the cementation of all the veneers.

Cementation and Finishing Procedures

Figure 6-247 demonstrates the interfaces and materials used.

1. Veneer preparation
   - Ultrasonically clean veneer in acetone for 5 minutes.
   - Dry thoroughly.
   - Apply a silane coupling agent.
   - Apply a multipurpose bonding agent to the etched surfaces simultaneously with tooth application. (Do not cure.)
   - Place in a safe area until ready to cement.
2. Tooth preparation
   - Retract tissues if necessary.
   - When the ceramic veneer will form the majority of the contact, use diamond strips or discs to lighten adjacent natural tooth contacts until thin mylar strips easily pass through (Fig. 6-248a).
   - Clean all bonding surfaces with non-fluoridated pumice and rinse thoroughly (Fig. 6-248b).
   - Use cotton roll isolation and adequate

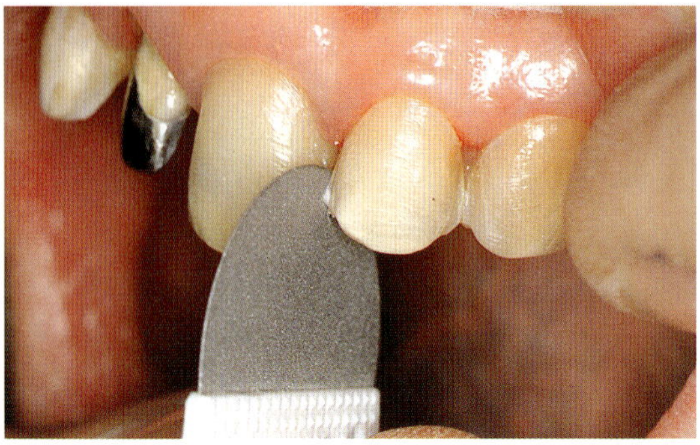
Fig. 6-248a

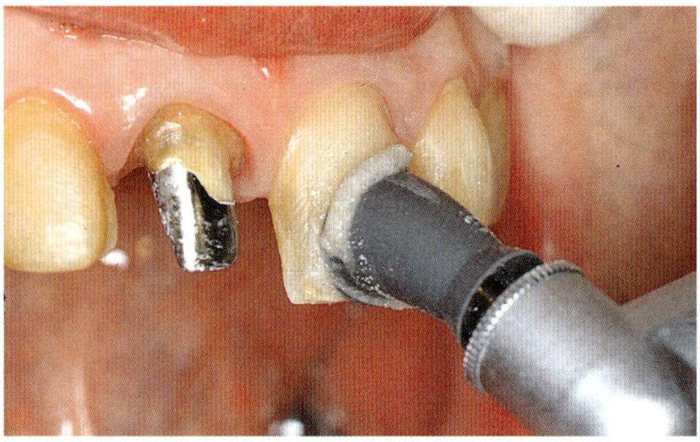
Fig. 6-248b

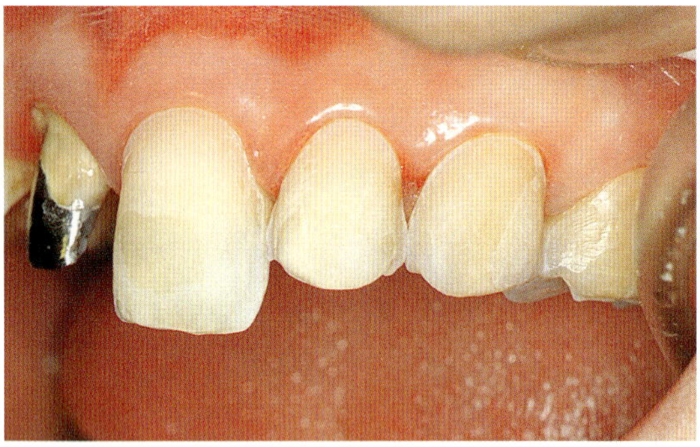
Fig. 6-248c

Fig. 6-248a Use a diamond disc or strip to break the remaining natural tooth contacts when the veneers provide a majority of the contact.

Fig. 6-248b Thoroughly clean all bonding surfaces of teeth.

Fig. 6-248c Etch all surfaces with 37% phosphoric acid.

Fig. 6-248d Apply multipurpose dental bonding agents to all surfaces if dentin is exposed.

Fig. 6-248e Use dry air source.

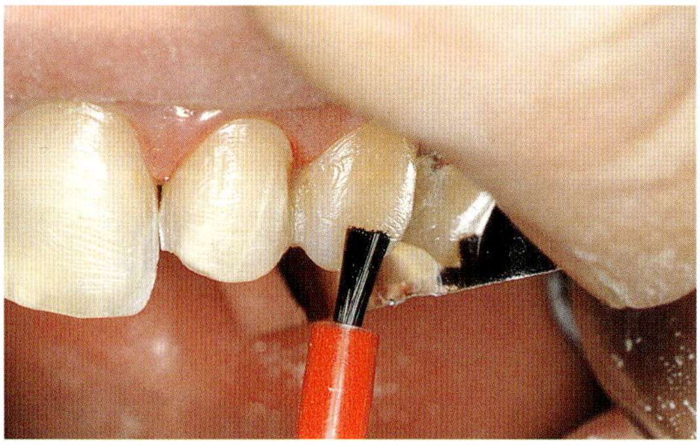
Fig. 6-248d

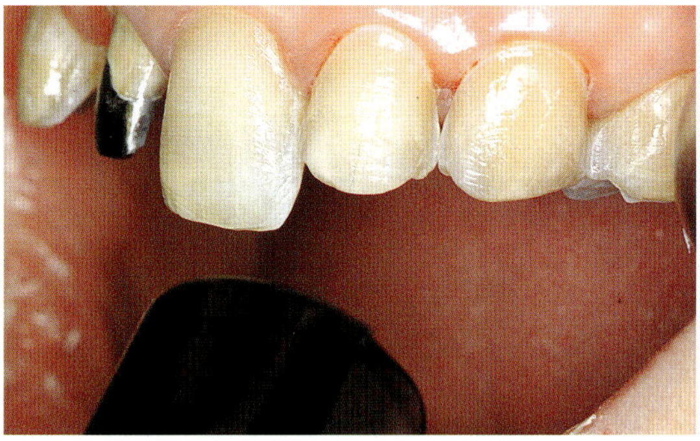
Fig. 6-248e

saliva evacuation.
- Retract checks with one-piece retractor.
- Etch for 15 to 20 seconds with 37% phosphoric acid. For multiple veneers use a liquid etchant to accelerate the speed of application. Place a matrix between prepared and adjacent teeth (Fig. 6-248c).
- Apply multipurpose bonding agents when margins are in dentin or more than one third of the surface area is dentin. Use on all bonding surfaces including the veneers (Fig. 6-248d).
- When preparations are only in enamel, an enamel bonding agent (unfilled resin) may be used to simplify the process. Use on all bonding surfaces.
- A warm air electric dryer should be used after the application of bonding agents. On these shiny surfaces it is not possible to visually detect any water or oil contamination from an operatory air source (Fig. 6-248e).

3. Veneer placement:

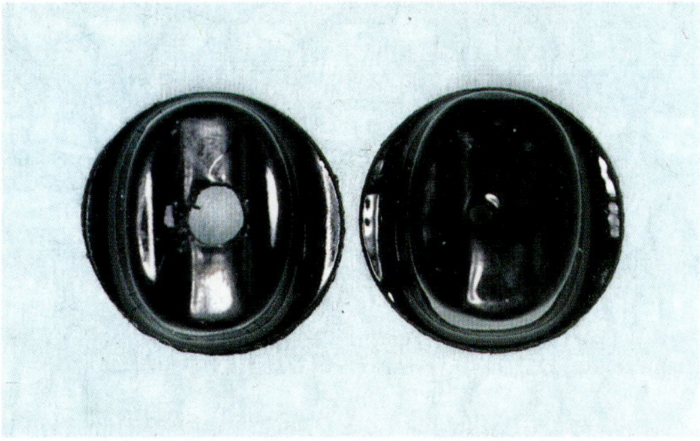

Fig. 6-249 Shield placed over large curing tip to make 2- to 3-mm beam.

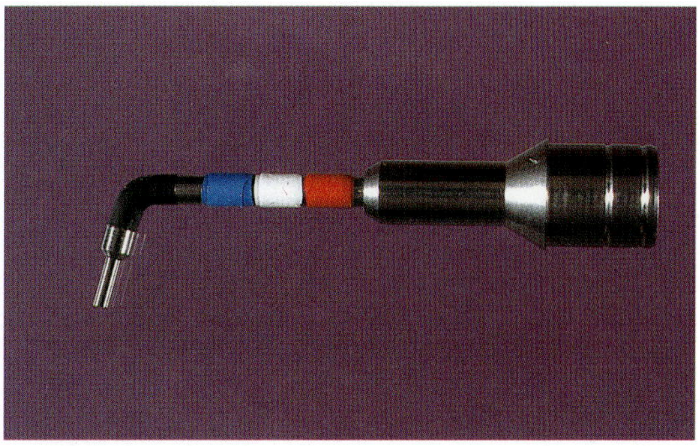

Fig. 6-250 Use of 2- to 3-mm curing tip is recommended.

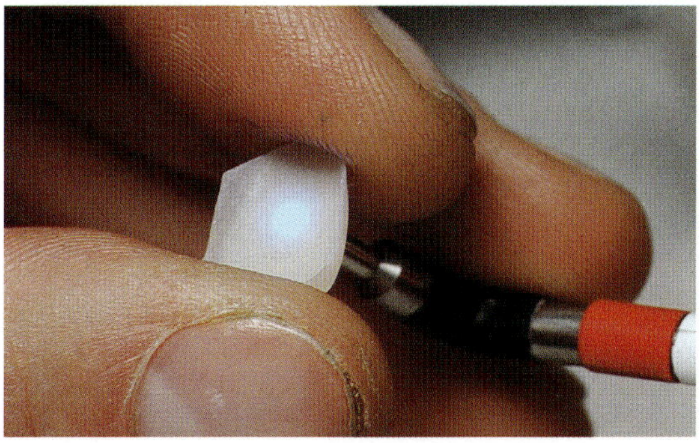

Fig. 6-251 Small tip will cure central portion of veneer only.

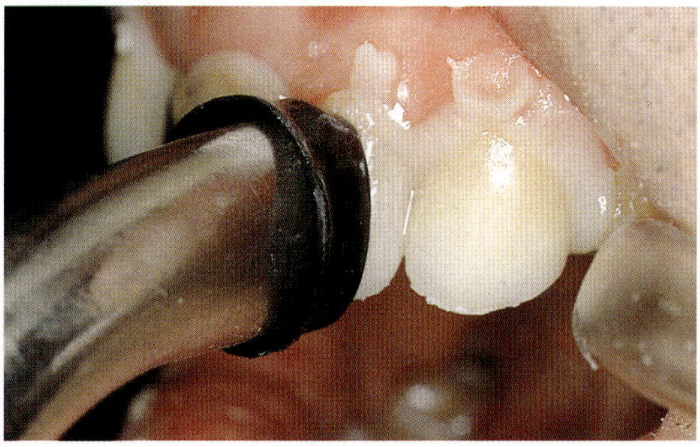

Fig. 6-252 Tacking in all veneers at once.

- Apply tints, opaques and cements as predetermined during the try-in procedures.
- Seat all the veneers and leave excess cement at this time. (Do not shine the operatory light directly on the veneers to avoid premature cement polymerization.)
- Starting at the midline, completely seat one veneer and tack in place with a 2- or 3-mm-diameter curing light tip for 10 seconds (Figs. 6-249 to 6-252).
- Tack all veneers in place moving distally in both directions.
- With a fine brush and rubber tip remove excess cement (Figs. 6-253a and b). Leave some excess cement at the margin to compensate for polymerization shrinkage.
- Pull thin mylar or very thin metal strips through the interproximals in a facial to lingual direction. If they do not easily pass through, do not force them and omit this step (Fig. 6-253c).
- With an 8- to 13-mm-diameter curing tip, cure all veneers for 1 minute from the facial and 1 minute from the lingual (Fig. 6-253d).
- Multiple lights will expedite this process.

4. Delivery appointment finishing procedures:

At the delivery appointment, it is not advisable to attempt final contour and polishing procedures. It is difficult for patients to make final contouring decisions at this point because of the newness of the esthetic results. It is best to postpone final contouring for 1 to 3 weeks. Also, the composite cement will not reach its maximum strength during the delivery

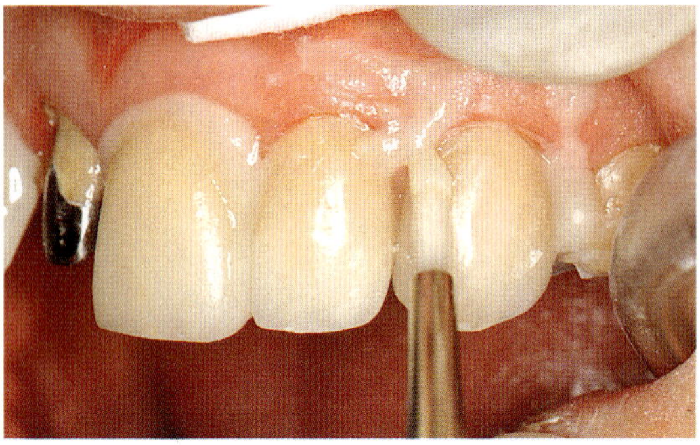

Fig. 6-253a Remove most of excess with a fine brush.

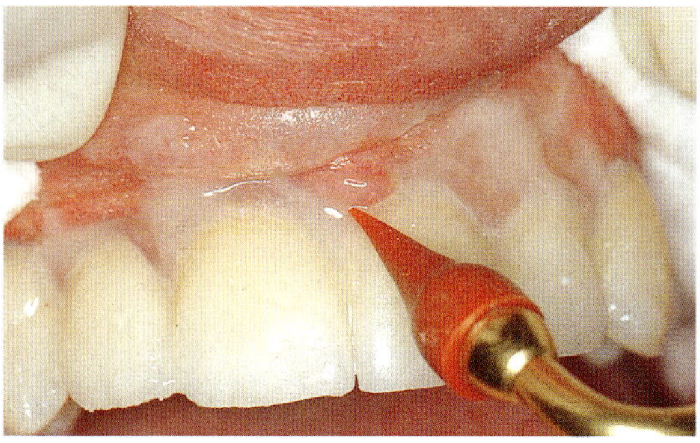

Fig. 6-253b A rubber tip works well for cement removal.

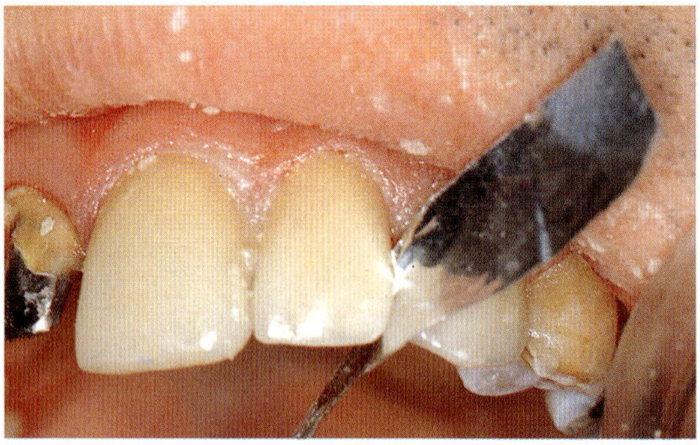

Fig. 6-253c Pull 0.0005-inch mylar strips from buccal to lingual. Ultrathin metal bands may work better.

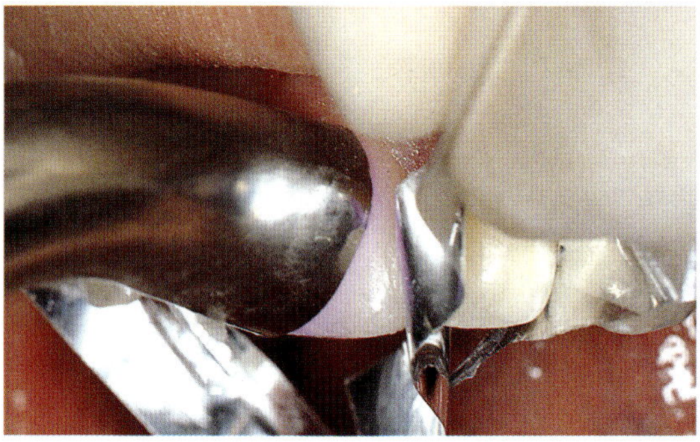

Fig. 6-253d Thoroughly cure veneer with a large (8- to 13-mm) curing tip from the buccal and lingual.

appointment. Finally, the finishing and polishing procedures are time-consuming and premature polishing might only have to be repeated if contour changes are required at a later time.

The goals of the delivery appointment should include (1) removal of excess cement, (2) contouring all gingival margins to maintain and promote gingival heath, (3) adjustment of occlusal and functional contacts and (4) making only obvious contour adjustments.

The marginal fit of ceramic restorations may not be routinely as good as that of conventional crowns and chipping away excess cement may create a void at a margin. Excess cement should be amputated or ground flush with a 30-fluted carbide finishing bur. A 30-fluted finishing bur will cleanly cut away cement flush to the margins with little effect on the glazed ceramic or tooth surface (Fig. 6-253e). A long, pointed 30-fluted carbide works effectively for both gingival and proximal margins (Fig. 6-253f). In most areas where margins are flush, cement is easily removed using this bur as an explorer without grinding. Further finishing may not be necessary. Lingual margins can be smoothed and occlusion adjusted using a fine flame finishing diamond (Figs. 6-253g and h). At this point ceramic overhangs or obvious contour problems may be adjusted using fine diamonds (Fig. 6-253i). Remaining interproximal composite cement excess should be removed with a #12 scalpel blade (Fig. 6-253j). Finally, interproximal contacts not kept open by proximal strips may be opened by the use of a fine proximal saw (Fig. 6-253k). These

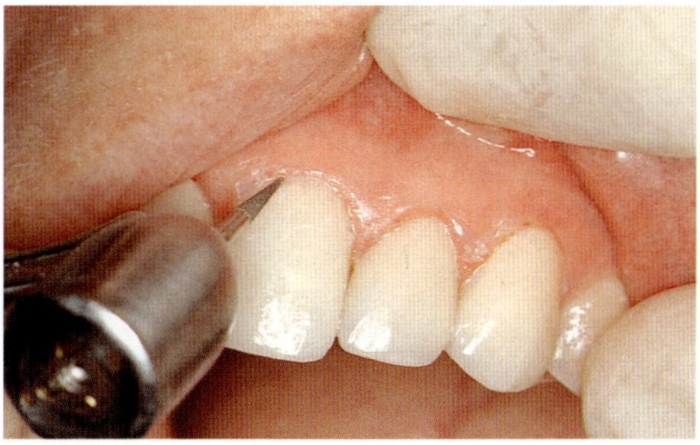

Fig. 6-253e Initial excess removal should be with a long pointed 30-fluted carbide.

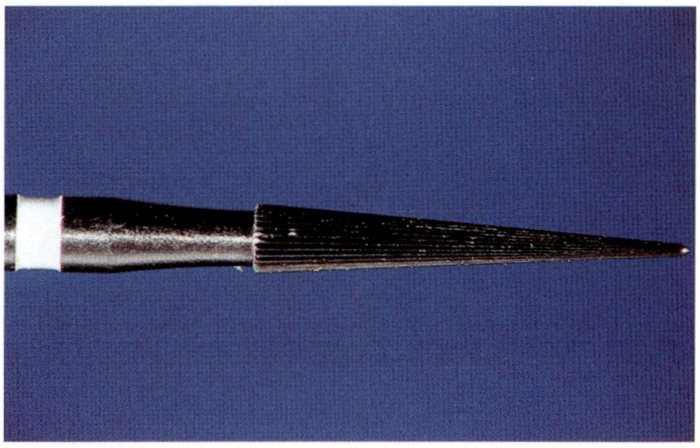

Fig. 6-253f Close up of 30-fluted carbide.

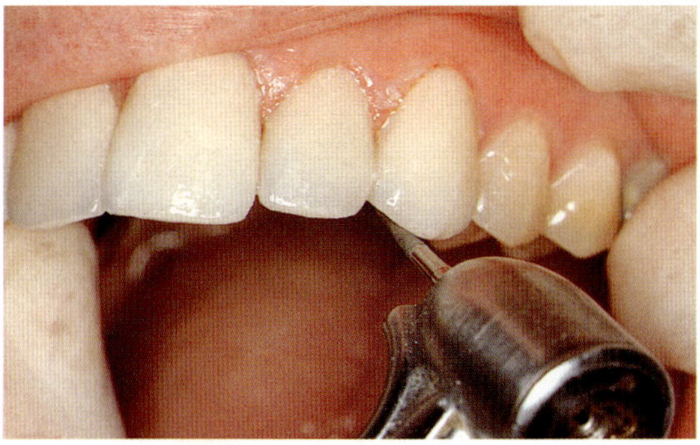

Fig. 6-253g Adjust occlusal contacts.

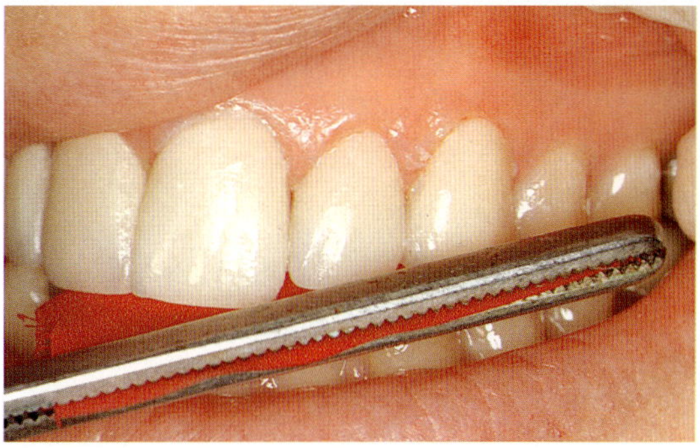

Fig. 6-253h Mark and check occlusal contacts.

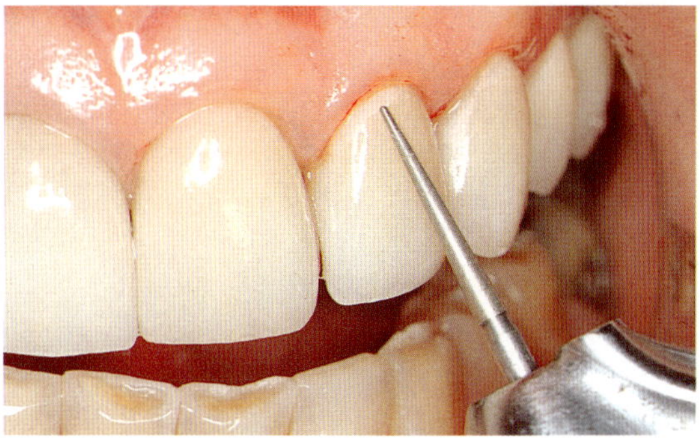

Fig. 6-253i

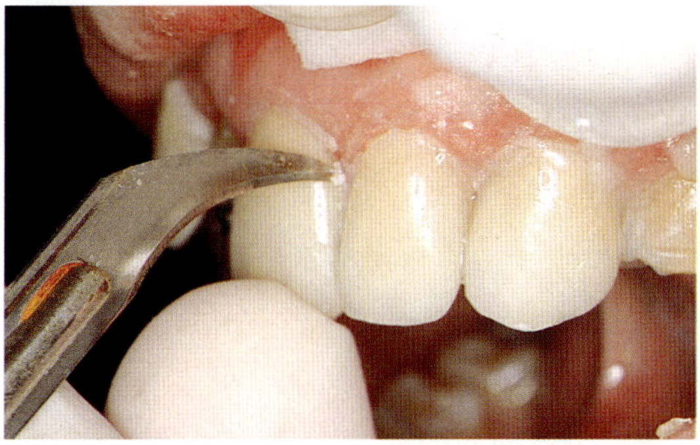

Fig. 6-253j

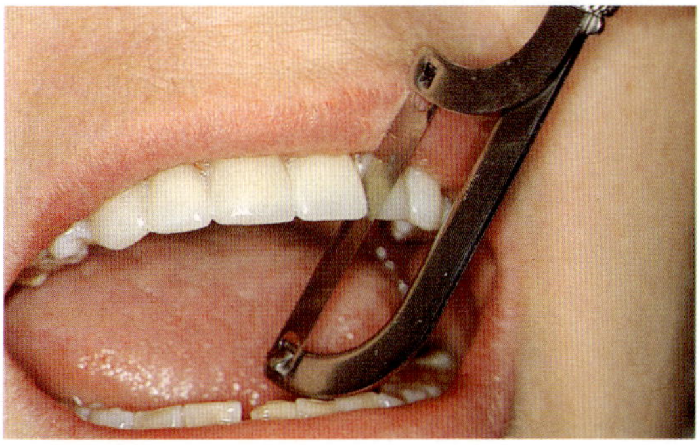

Fig. 6-253k

Fig. 6-253i Remove any ceramic excess with fine diamond burs and water.

Fig. 6-253j A #12 scalpel blade is useful for deep interproximal cement removal.

Fig. 6-253k Use interproximal saws to open any remaining bonded contacts.

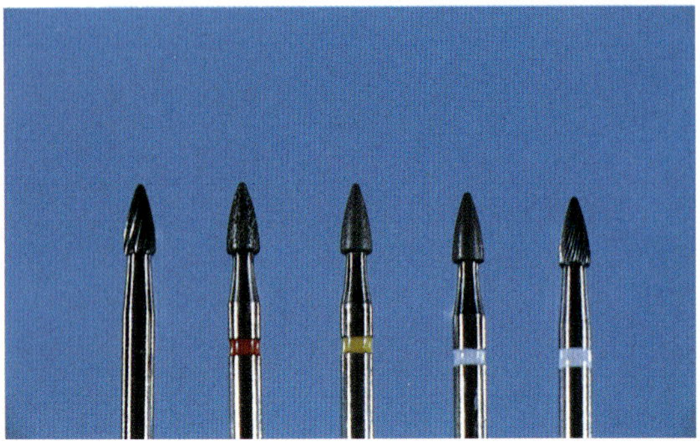

Figs. 6-254a

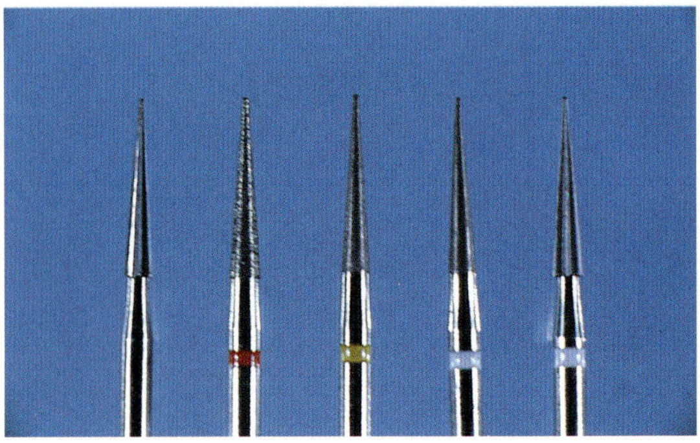

Figs. 6-254 b

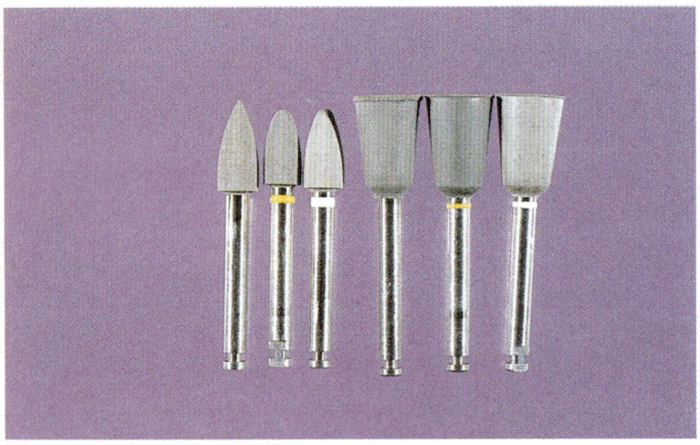

Fig. 6-255

Figs. 6-254a and b The high speed finishing sequence includes the red strip fine diamond to contour and the yellow and white extrafine diamonds to smooth. Finally the 30-fluted carbide (**far right**) is used for additional smoothness.

Fig. 6-255 The low speed polishing sequence includes abrasive rubber polishing points and cups of different grits.

work extremely well as long as the majority of cement is removed first. Gross contouring of interproximal ceramic excess may be done with fine finishing pointed diamonds or diamond impregnated strips as necessary.

The patient is now dismissed and instructed to keep the veneers meticulously clean and to start evaluating for possible contour modification after about a week to avoid premature decisions. Sometimes patients have concerns about size, unusual contacts in excursion, etc. Assure the patient a period of adaptation is essential and necessary adjustments will be done in 2 or 3 weeks.

5. Final finishing and polishing:

   After 2 or 3 weeks the patient may have valid contouring suggestions based upon actual experience. A telephone call should be made to get feedback prior to making the final polishing appointment so the appropriate length of time can be reserved.

- Finalize all contours using fine high speed diamonds and water.
- Check functional contacts and contours.
- Evaluate periodontal response, contour any questionable areas and reinforce oral hygiene procedures.
- Using fine diamonds (rotary and strips) to complete all adjustments.
- Polishing sequence (Fig. 6-254).
  (a) Fine to extrafine high speed diamonds (about 30- to 8-μm particles per size) with water and abrasive discs
  (b) Appropriately shaped 30-fluted carbide finishing burs at high speed with water
  (c) Ceramic polishing rubber cup and point sequence using slow speed and water (Figs. 6-255 and 6-256a and b)
  (d) Diamond polishing paste(s) using cups, pads and/or felt wheels (Figs.

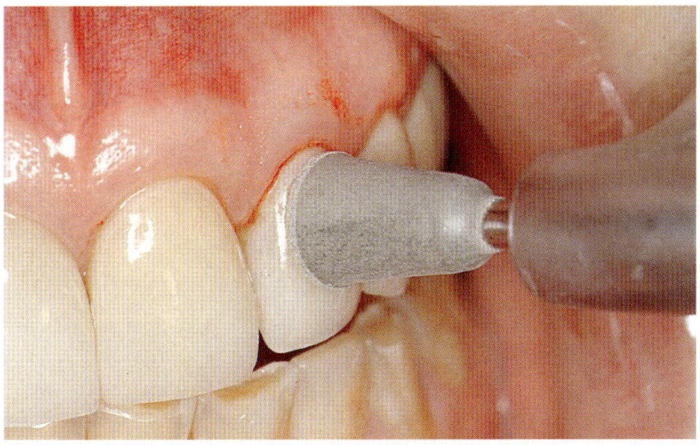

Fig. 6-256a Abrasive cups work well for gingival areas.

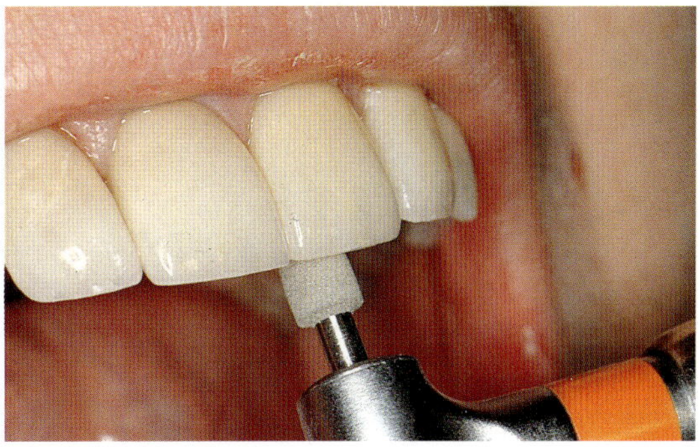

Fig. 6-256b Abrasive cups work well for lingual contours.

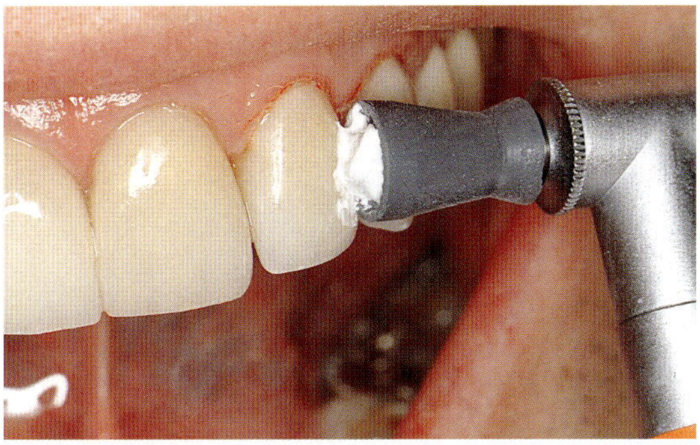

Fig. 6-256c Final polish with diamond polishing paste.

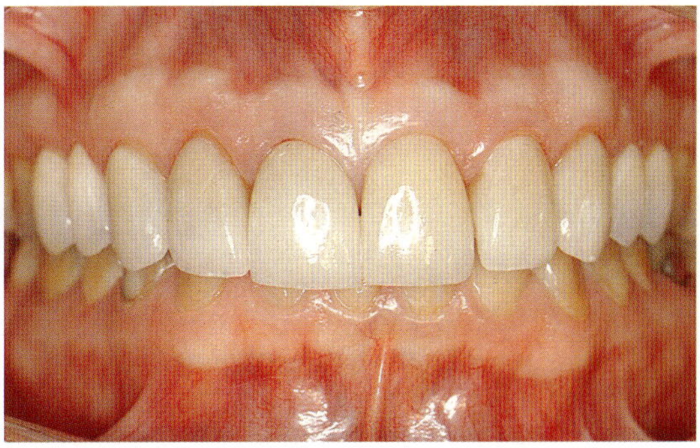

Fig. 6-256d Postoperative close up view.

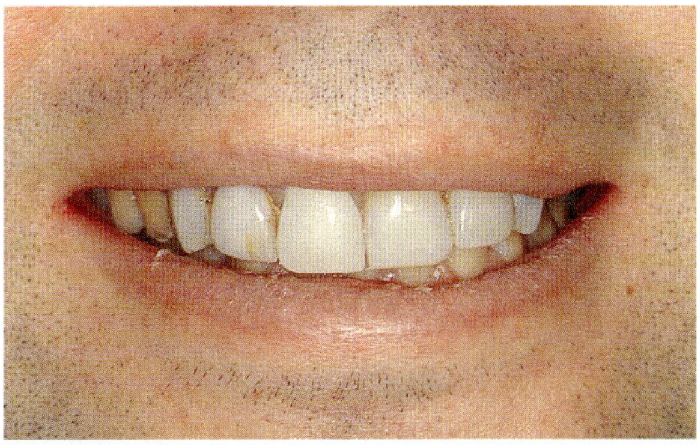

Fig. 6-257a Preoperative smile.

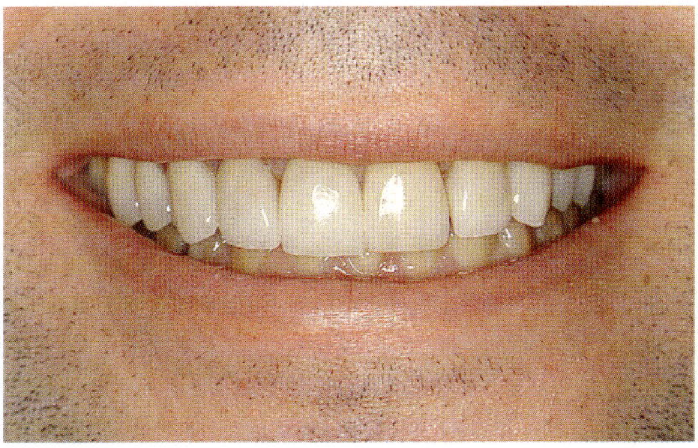

Fig. 6-257b Postoperative smile.

6-256c and d).

- Final patient home care instructions should be given.
- Set recall for 1 to 3 months.
- Figure 6-257 shows the pretreatment and posttreatment views. (Note that the all ceramic crown on tooth 8 was fabricated out of the same conventional ceramic as the veneers and was shaded with low fusing ceramic stains to match.)

LABORATORY PROCEDURES

Introduction

There are two methods of fabrication for ceramic veneers. They are the "refractory die" and "platinum foil" techniques. A basic understanding of each technique is helpful. Ultimately it is the end product that is most important and this is largely dependent upon the ceramist.

Advantages of the platinum foil technique:
1. Fabricate and use standard stone removable dies.
2. Can die space as usual.
3. A platinum foil matrix can quickly be adapted to a die and fabrication started.
4. Easy to measure thickness of the veneer during fabrication.
5. Veneers can be tried on the prepared tooth prior to final glazing.

Disadvantages of the platinum foil technique:
1. Foil distortion possible.
2. Difficult to assess actual color.
3. Cost of foil (can recycle).

Advantages of refractory die techniques:
1. Overall accuracy and fit generally better.
2. Easier technique for a less experienced technician to master.

Disadvantages of refractory die technique:
1. Requires duplication of stone dies or double pouring an impression. Generally the former is preferred because refractory die spacing is eliminated as well as refractory model margin trimming.
2. Divestment is required.
3. Fit must be verified on stone dies.
4. More difficult to control veneer thickness.

Refractory Die Technique

1. The appropriate ceramic refractory die material must be matched with each ceramic used so that they have a similar coefficient of thermal expansion. Also the refractory die must be hard enough so margin adjustments can be made and the die does not deteriorate during fabrication, thermal cycles and handling. In contrast the material must be soft enough to allow for easy divestment after fabrication.
2. The refractory die model is formed by pouring a correctly vacuum mixed refractory die material into the original impression or a duplicate impression of the trimmed and die spaced master stone

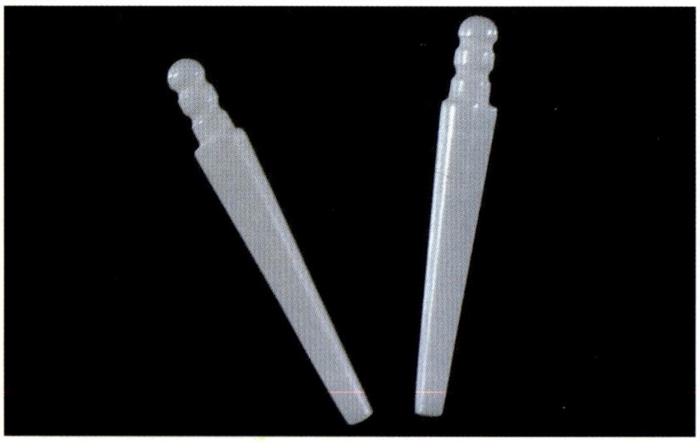

Fig. 6-258 Ceramic dowel pins.

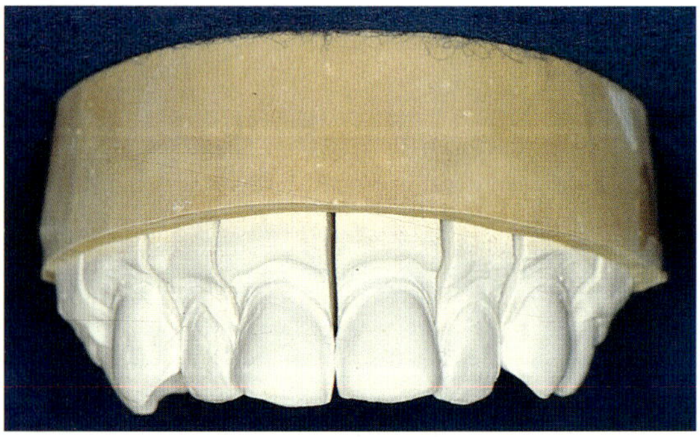

Fig. 6-259a Refractory dies trimmed with stone base.

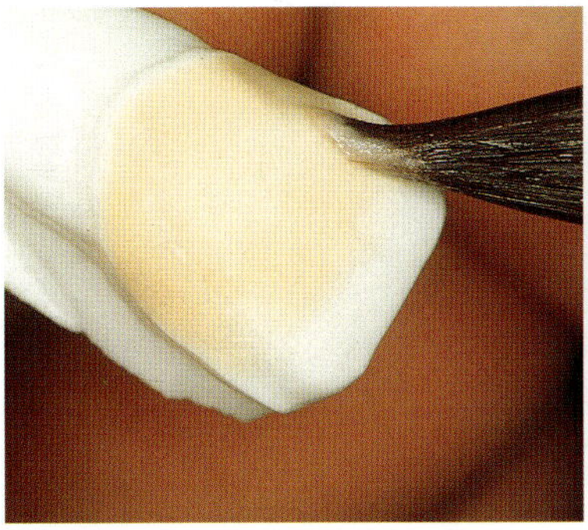

Fig. 6-259b Application of a thin internal layer of opaque ceramic.

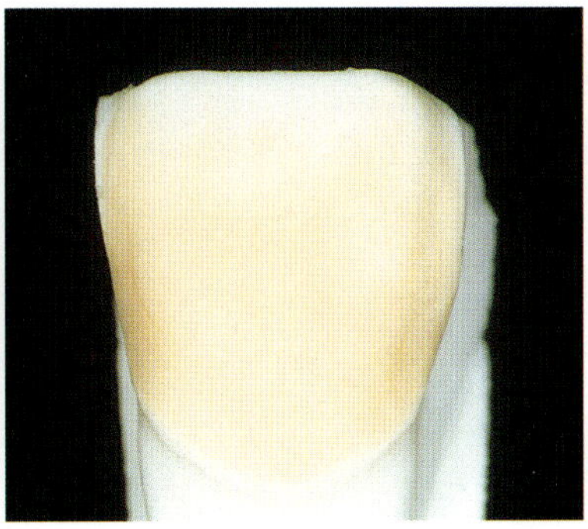

Fig. 6-259c Initial layer of opaque ceramic.

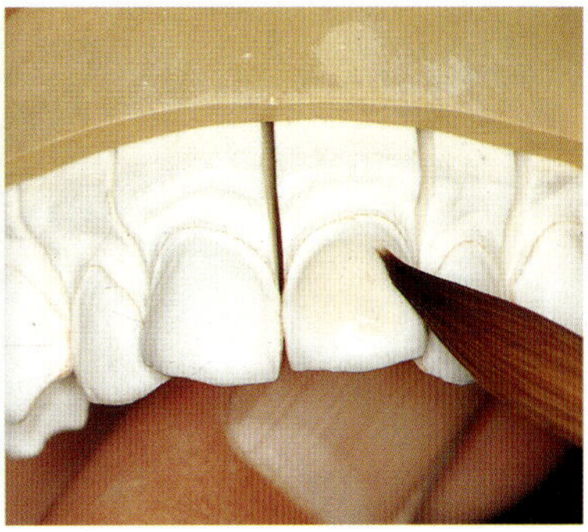

Fig. 6-259d Ceramic application to refractory die.

model. After setting, the refractory model is trimmed so that only a horseshoe base remains. This is tapered apically and "V" shaped vertical positioning grooves are ground into the lateral surfaces of each die with a rotary instrument. This base is coated with a gypsum separating medium and inserted into a base of model stone. Refractory ceramic dowel pins have been developed which may improve this removable die system (Fig. 6-258). Remove the refractory model and separate the individual dies and trim as needed (Fig. 6-259a).

3. The refractory die is first run through the recommended thermal cycle. The ammonia gas released will contaminate the ceramic oven baffle so it is desirable to place the dies in a burnout oven first and then transfer to the ceramic oven. Once cooled to room temperature, the dies are soaked in distilled water until air bubbles stop surfacing.
4. Ceramic addition may now begin. There are many ceramic systems available for the fabrication of veneers. Generally they are slightly higher chroma ceramics that allow for more color saturation in a ceramic restoration that is thinner than conventional ceramic crowns. The most critical requirement of a veneer system is the ability to modify opacity or the ability to selectively mask a variety of tooth colors. When little color change is desired, a more translucent veneer will allow natural tooth color to enhance the final color match. In contrast when more extreme color changes are desired, greater opacity or optical scattering is desired to prevent the color from the underlying tooth from effecting the color of the final veneer. This is accomplished in three ways. First, opacifiers can be added to the veneer ceramic in varying amounts to enhance or reduce the veneer opacity. Second, a layering approach can be used similar to that for ceramometal crowns. A thin opaque masking dentin layer can be applied first and covered with outer layers of more translucent ceramic material (Figs. 6-259b and c). The third and newest technique is to use what is commonly called an opalescent ceramic that more effectively scatters light and gives the illusion of brightness without the dead opaque look. While this last method may not provide the level of tooth color coverage of the first two methods provided, it results in extremely vital-looking veneers when mild to moderate color modification is desired. For maximum color masking, other supportive opacity enhancement techniques may be required during cementation as previously described. All of these ceramic techniques may require the use of opaque cements

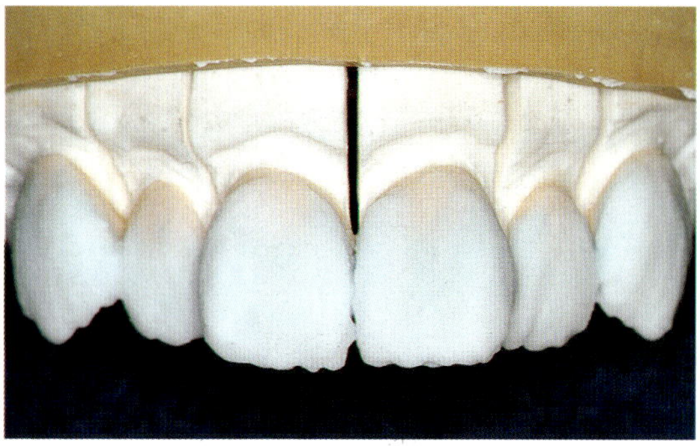

Fig. 6-259e Full contour ceramic buildup.

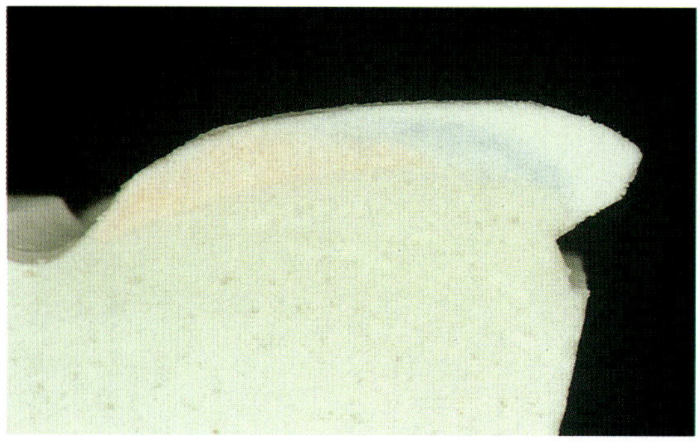

Fig. 6-259f Cross section showing layers of different ceramic materials.

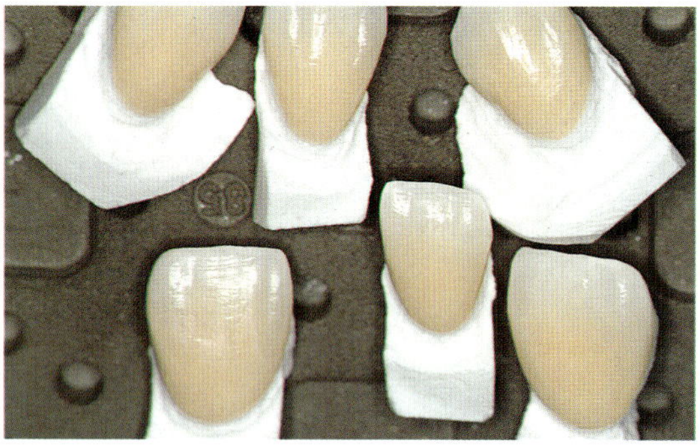

Fig. 6-259g Sintered veneers.

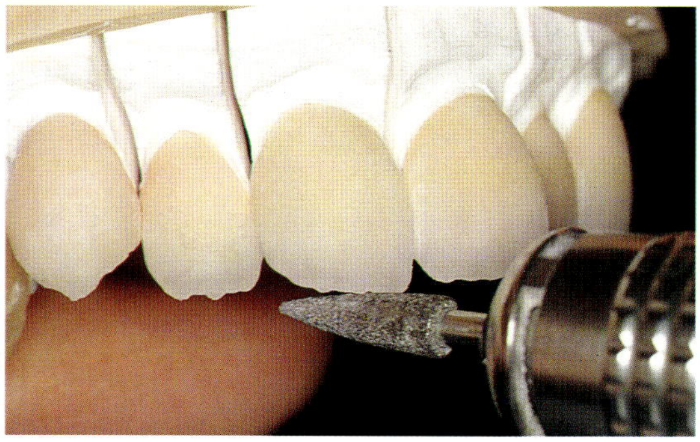

Fig. 6-259h Contouring the veneers on the dies.

or more extensive preparation for extreme hue or value changes.

5. The initial applications of opaque or dentin ceramic is critical to the fit, therefore a thin well condensed layer is applied first. Ultrasonic vibration is advisable (Fig. 6-259d).
6. The ceramic veneer is now built to full contour using dentin and enamel type ceramic blends. A transparent exterior surface may be applied if room permits (Figs. 6-259e and f).
7. The die is removed from the model and the ceramic sintered using the recommended thermal cycle under vacuum (Fig. 6-259g).
8. Once cooled the die and veneers are returned to the master model for final contouring and ceramic additions as needed (Fig. 6-259h). Fine diamonds with water should be used for contouring and the adjusted surface should be steam cleaned before further ceramic additions or glazing. Margins should be finalized and when the veneer is complete and cleaned, it can be glazed at atmospheric pressure.
9. The completed veneer must now be divested. Cut away the majority of the refractory die using a separating disc (Fig. 6-259i). A rotary stone can be used to remove most of the remaining refractory material (Fig. 6-259j). Finally, the remaining refractory material is carefully air abraded away using aluminous oxide (Fig. 6-259k).
10. The veneers are now carefully seated back on the stone dies and examined for marginal accuracy and proximal contacts. Adjustments can be made using fine diamonds and water. Adjusted surfaces should be polished with rubber ceramic polishing wheels (Fig. 6-259l).
11. The inner bonding surfaces of the ceramic

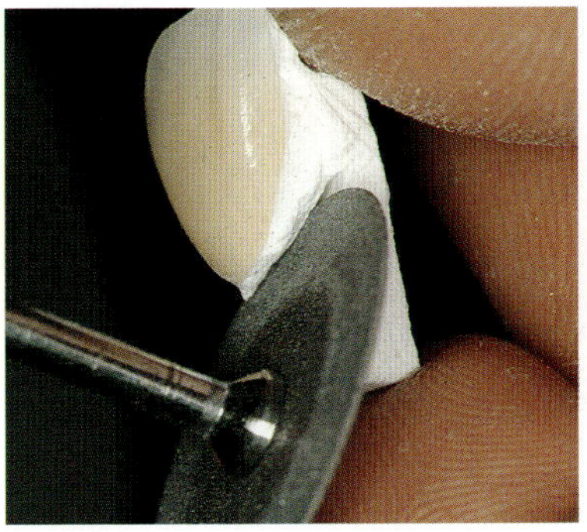

Fig. 6-259i Use a disc to cut the veneer away from the die.

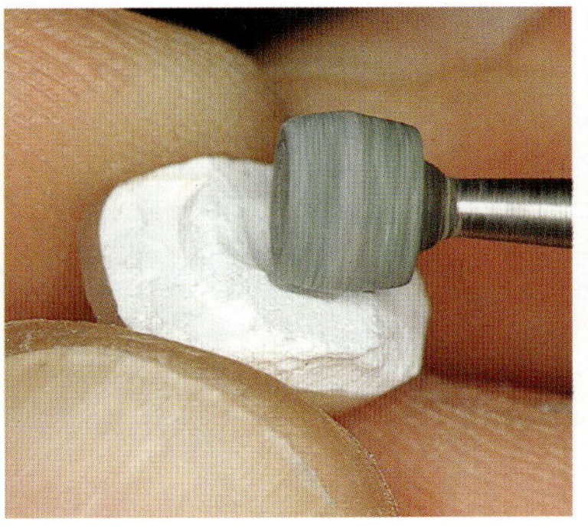

Fig. 6-259j Remove refractory excess with a stone.

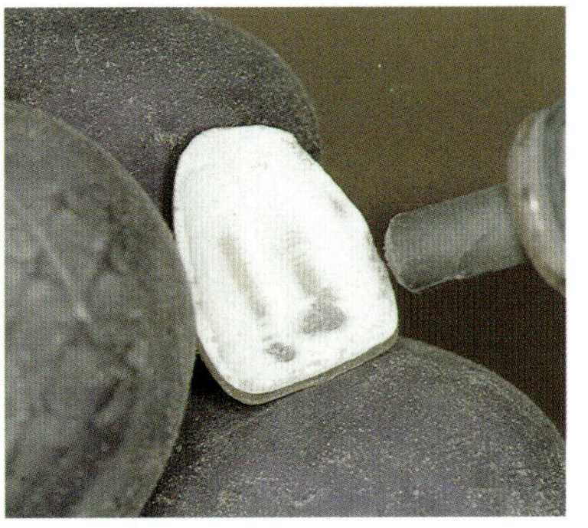

Fig. 6-259k Air abrade remaining refractory off veneer.

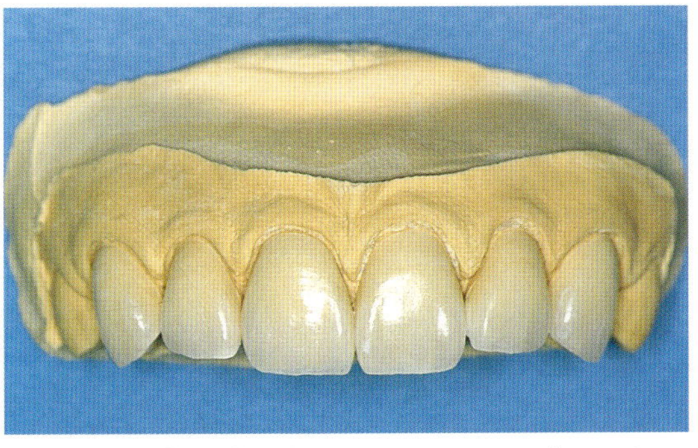

Fig. 6-259l Completed veneers on one piece stone model.

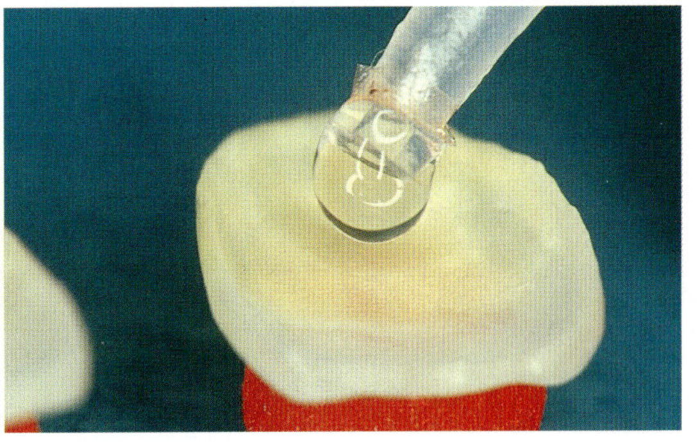

Fig. 6-259m Etch internal bonding surfaces with hydrofluoric acid.

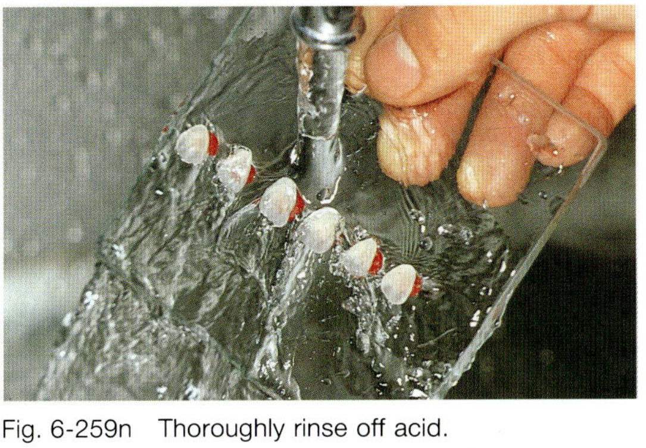

Fig. 6-259n Thoroughly rinse off acid.

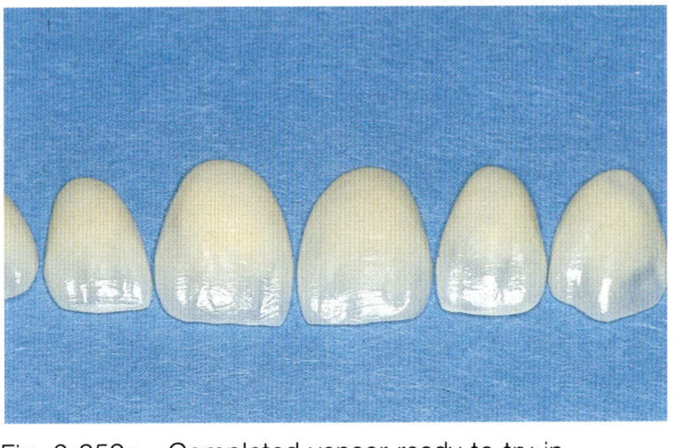

Fig. 6-259o Completed veneer ready to try-in.

veneer are now etched with hydrofluoric acid to create micromechanical retention and enhanced bond strengths to the composite cement. Hydrofluoric acid is dangerous so wear glasses and gloves and follow manufacturer's directions meticulously (Figs. 6-259m and n).

12. The finished veneers are rinsed and ultrasonically cleaned and placed in a safe container until the delivery appointment (Fig. 6-259o).

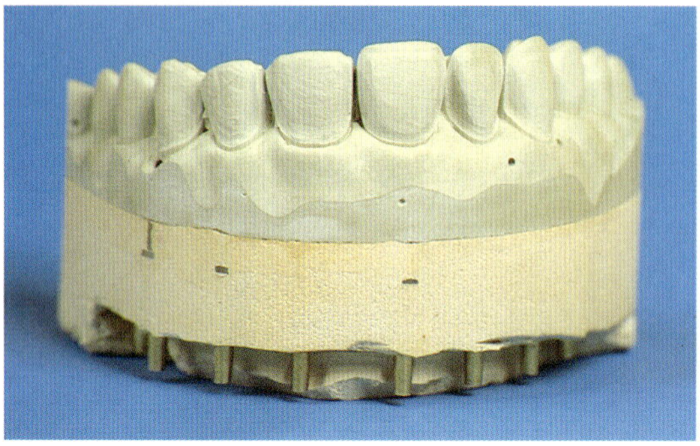

Fig. 6-260a Stone working model as poured.

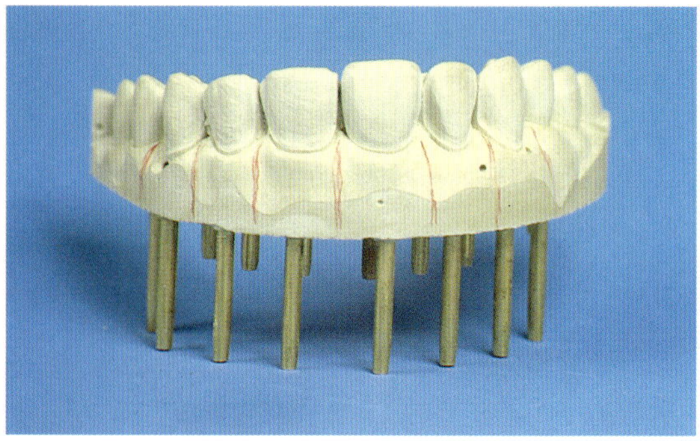

Fig. 6-260b Stone working model as poured, pinned and removed from base.

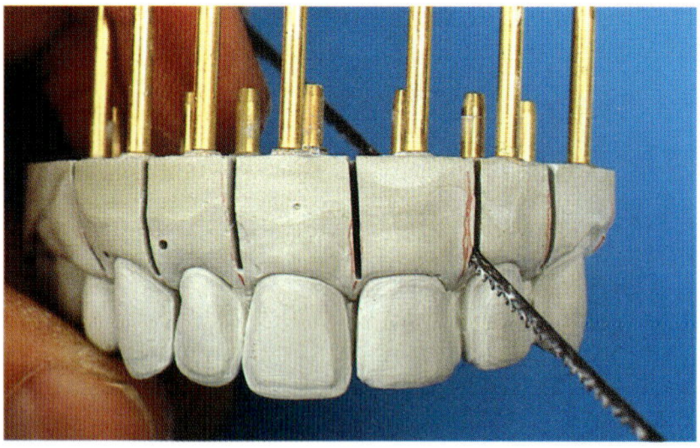

Fig. 6-260c Sectioning dies from a gingival direction.

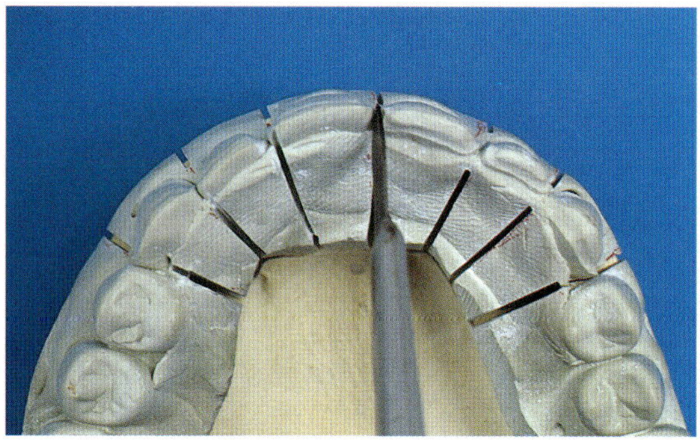

Fig. 6-260d Use scalpel to score a cleavage line near preparation margins.

Platinum Foil Technique

1. Fabricating a ceramic veneer using the platinum foil technique requires the fabrication of a standard removable die working model (Figs. 6-260a and b). The dies are sectioned from the gingival to incisal direction (Figs. 6-260c to e). The use of epoxy or hardened stone dies is advised. Depending upon the amount of color change required, a variable thickness of die spacer is used (Fig. 6-260f). An increased thickness will increase the thickness of cement and its effect upon veneer esthetics.
2. A platinum foil matrix is adapted, burnished and swaged over the prepared surface (Figs. 6-260g to i). It is cut back to 1 or 2 mm beyond the margins.
3. Begin ceramic fabrication by adapting the ceramic to the gingival portion first (Fig. 6-260j). The remaining veneer is built up with body modifiers and incisal ceramic materials (Figs. 6-260k and l). The ceramic veneers are sintered and contoured, and correction additions are made as with ceramic crowns (Fig. 6-260m). The veneers should be colored and glazed prior to foil removal (Fig. 6-260n).
4. The completed veneers are soaked in water and the foil is peeled out (Fig. 6-261).
5. The veneer can now be coated with wax leaving only the surface to be etched exposed (Fig. 6-262). The veneer is now immersed in hydrofluoric acid for the appropriate recommended time. A proper etched surface will appear frosty and even (Fig. 6-263). Underetched areas will appear shiny (Fig. 6-264). Overetched surfaces

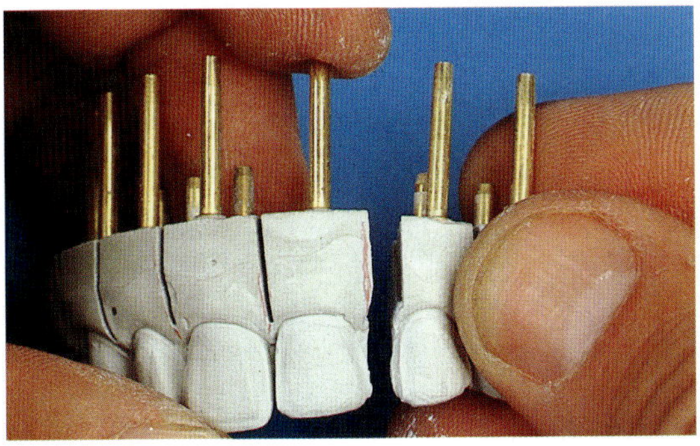
Fig. 6-260e Carefully separating dies.

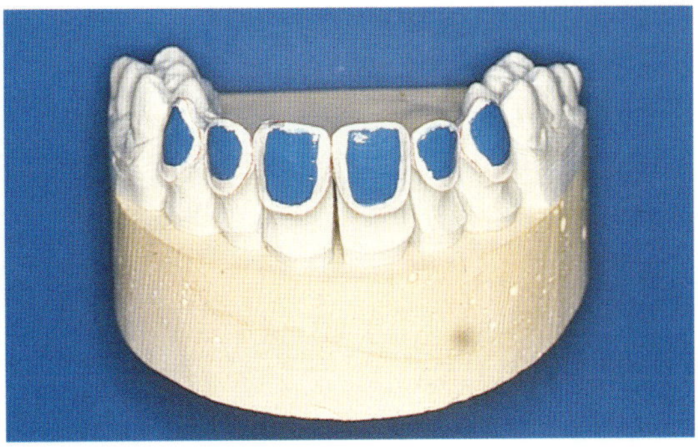
Fig. 6-260f Final trimmed and die spaced working model.

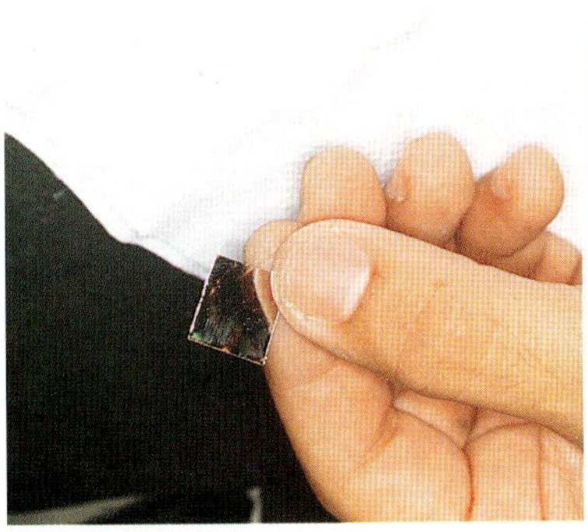
Fig. 6-260g Platinum foil matrix.

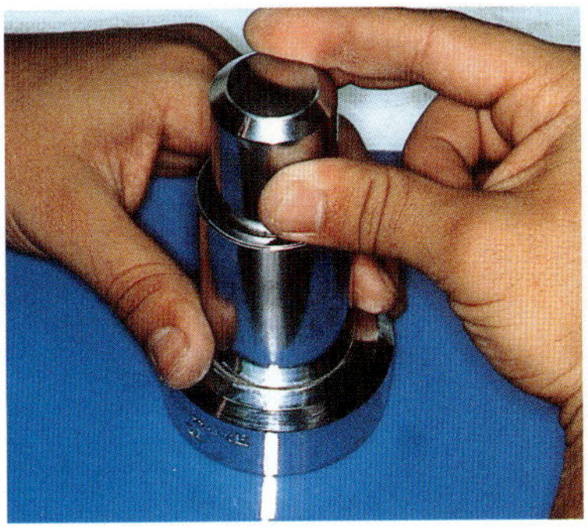
Fig. 6-260h Swagger to adapt foil.

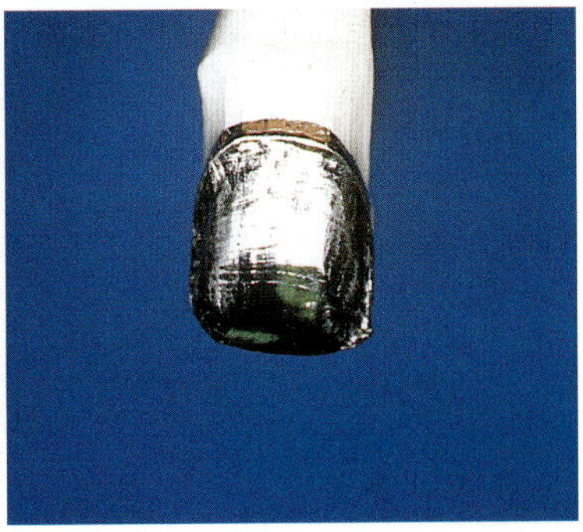
Fig. 6-260i Final adapted platinum foil on die.

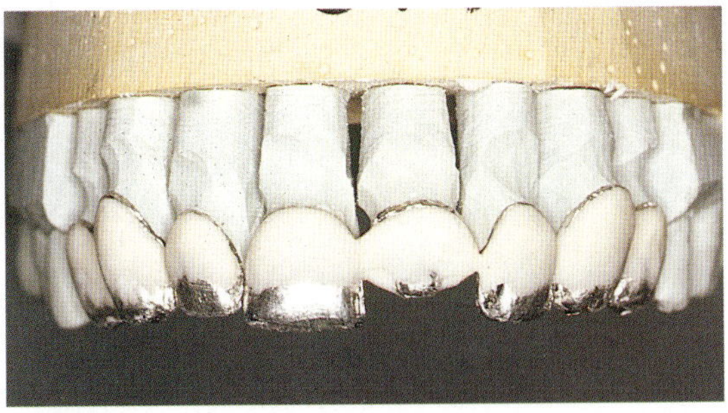
Fig. 6-260j Apply gingival ceramic first.

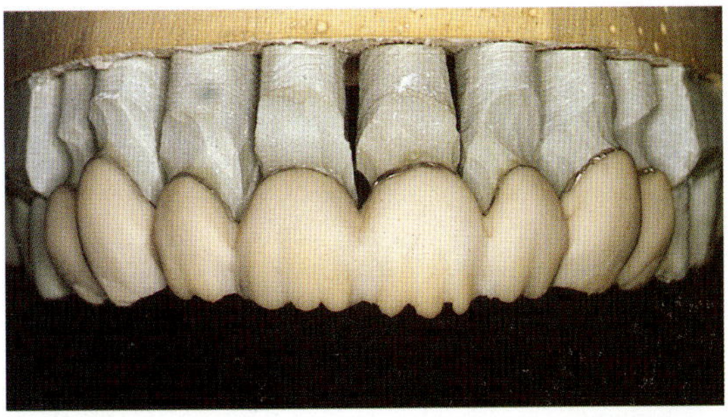
Fig. 6-260k Apply dentin and ceramic modifiers next.

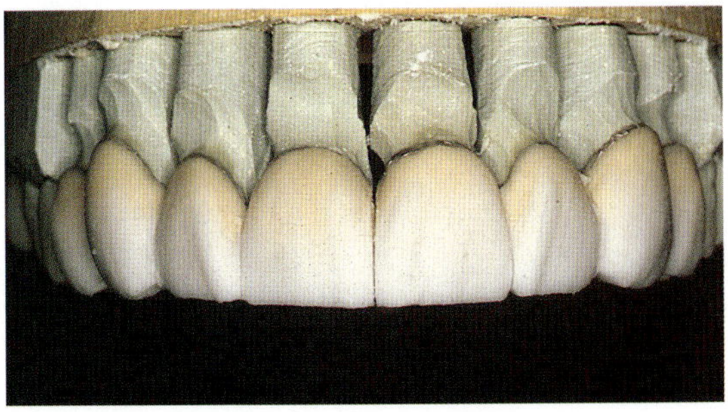
Fig. 6-260l Apply enamel ceramic last.

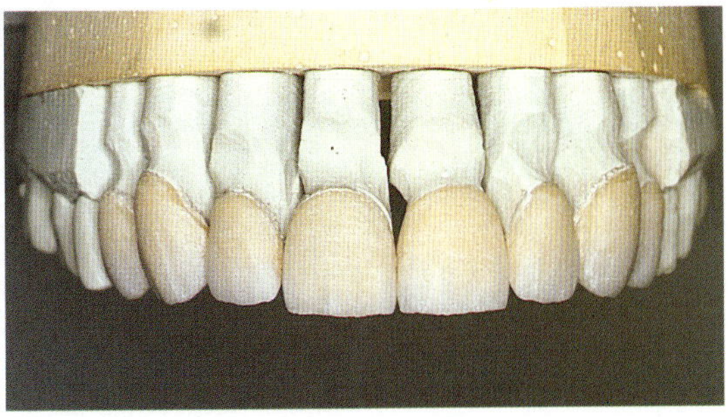
Fig. 6-260m Sintered and contoured ceramic veneers.

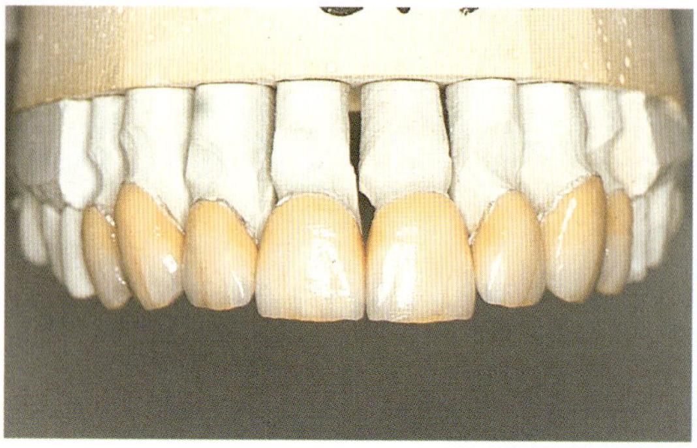

Fig. 6-260n Final stained and glazed ceramic veneers.

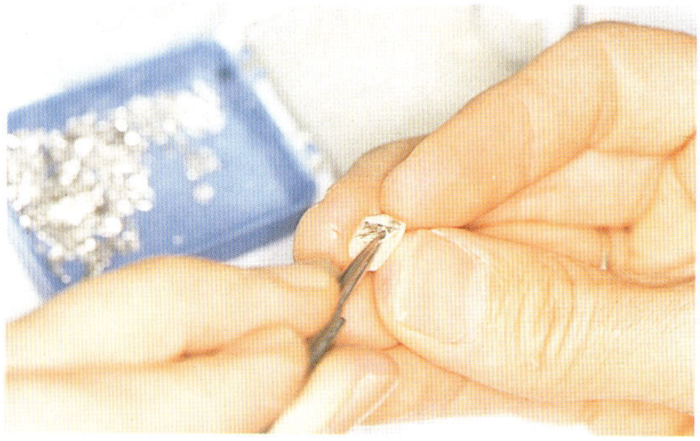

Fig. 6-261 Removing platinum foil matrix

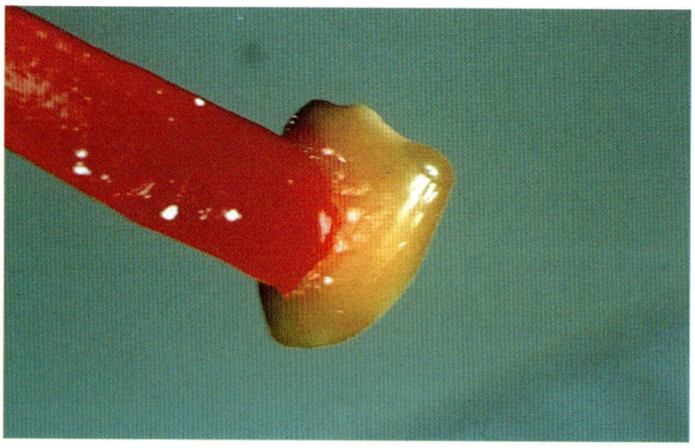

Fig. 6-262a Apply wax to all areas that are not to be etched.

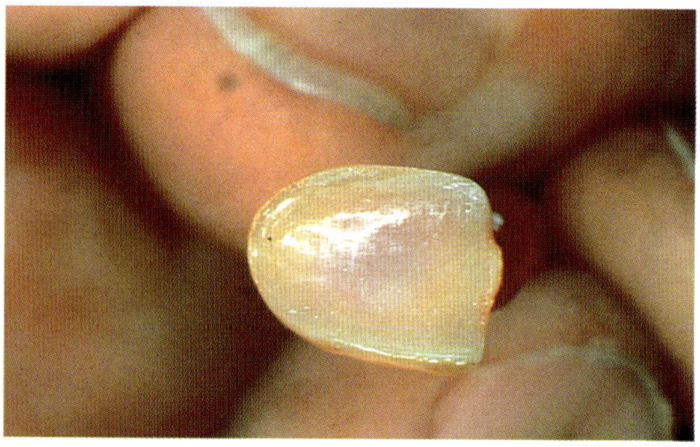

Fig. 6-262b Leave only the surfaces to be etched exposed.

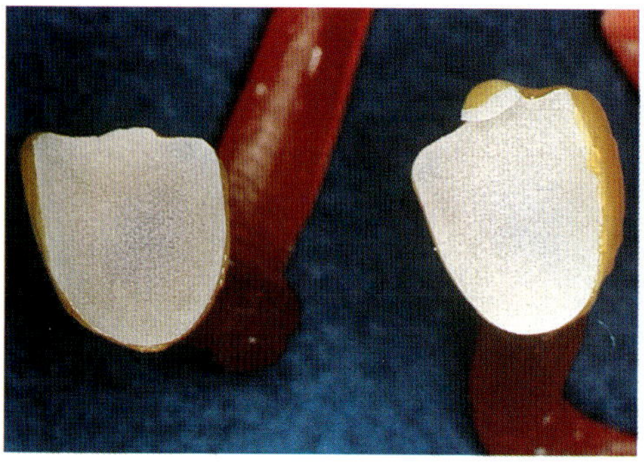

Fig. 6-263 Properly etched ceramic veneers.

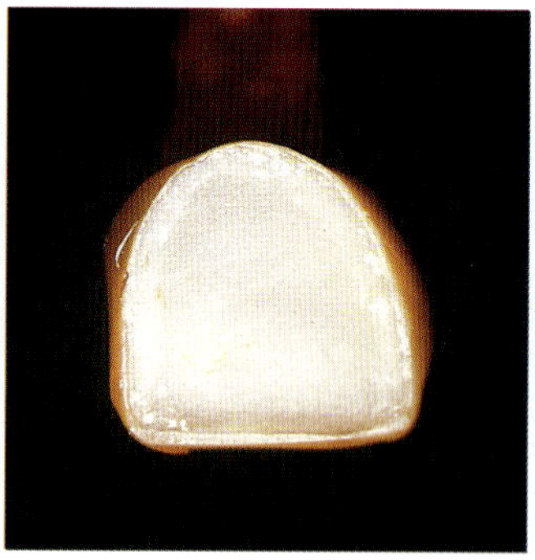

Fig. 6-264 Underetched ceramic veneers.

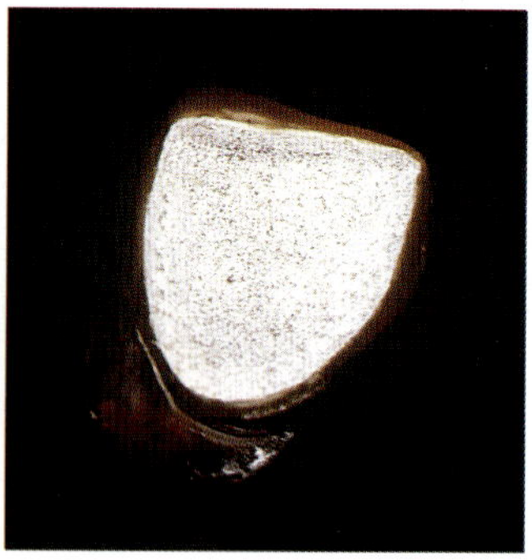

Fig. 6-265 Overetched ceramic veneers.

appear as if coated with talcum powder (Fig. 6-265).

6. The waxed veneer can now be sprayed with an aerosol spray coolant and the wax will easily fall off the veneer.
7. The completed veneers should be placed in a safe storage container until the delivery appointment.

(Figs. 6-260f to 6-265 courtesy of Daniel Materdomini)

INTRODUCTION TO CONTEMPORARY ESTHETIC FIXED PARTIAL DENTURES

BACKGROUND AND LIMITATIONS

Esthetic fixed partial dentures (FPDs) have evolved significantly in the last few decades. In only 25 to 30 years dentistry has gone from the use of conservative partial coverage metal retainers with cemented ceramic pontic facings to full coverage ceramometal restorations with ceramic margins. The excellent level of esthetics achievable with ceramometal FPDs combined with their predictable strength and proven longevity makes them the primary choice for most esthetic FPDs.

Currently there is no nonmetallic fixed partial denture that can match this predictability. All the FPDs described in this chapter must be viewed as esthetic alternatives that lack the predictable long term prognosis of ceramometal alternatives. Until long term clinical studies (8 to 10 years) prove that a system has a longevity similar to ceramometal, placing such restorations in one's practice must be regarded as somewhat experimental and this should be made clear to the patient during the treatment planning consultation. A clear understanding of the prognosis and responsibilities of the dentist and the patient must be established before starting. Otherwise, if failures of these untested systems occur, a difficult situation could develop leading to some very strained patient-dentist relationships.

The purpose of this section is to provide an introduction to a few proposed contemporary esthetic FPD designs. Most of the clinical procedures are covered in other sections.

TRADITIONALLY DESIGNED ALL CERAMIC FIXED PARTIAL DENTURES

A traditionally designed all ceramic FPD is one that has full coverage retainer design and a pontic suspended between the retainers. Preparation design is essentially that of a full ceramic crown. Increased bulk is recommended adjacent to the connectors using a box design or a deeper shoulder. Conventional ceramic systems are not strong enough for FPDs. Some method of strengthening is required.

Indications

The decision to use an all ceramic traditional FPD should be based primarily upon esthetic goals. The elimination of the metallic substructure, as discussed in the section on all ceramic crowns may enhance the translucency of the final restoration and make esthetic goals easier to attain. More conservative preparations are sometimes possible. When used adjacent to all ceramic crowns of the same material, it eliminates a potential esthetic mismatch that often occurs when trying to match dissimilar materials. Other indications may include the desire to eliminate metal for physiologic or even psychological reasons. Metal phobias are becoming more common and some patients are willing to accept restorations with diminished strength in order to eliminate metal in their mouth. All ceramic traditional FPDs should not be considered as a replacement for ceramometal FPDs at this time but as a selected esthetic alternative that is done for a specific reason.

Contraindications

The main contraindication should be a situation where the patient is not willing to accept a FPD with reduced strength for any reason. When maximum strength is a priority, use a ceramometal FPD. Other contraindications might include (1) inadequate space for adequate ceramic bulk, (2) parafunctional activity such as bruxism, (3) matching existing ceramometal restorations and finally (4) an unwillingness by the treating dentist to place a restoration with a more guarded prognosis than clinically proven ceramometal FPDs.

Materials

Two materials, at least, market the use of their material for anterior all ceramic traditional FPDs. The first is the strengthened sintered glass ceramic Optec (Jeneric/Pentron, Wallingford, CT). This material has about twice the strength of conventional ceramics but is significantly weaker than a ceramometal FPD. It has been advocated for use in anterior fixed partial dentures. This material should be used for short span anterior fixed partial dentures where adequate space exists to develop bulk in the lingual and connector regions. Limited space leading to thin retainers or the presence of greater than normal functional stresses may contraindicate the use of this material. Some authors have claimed reasonable success with this material while others have described surveys that are not as successful. Other totally strengthened ceramic materials may be used in a similar application but their manufacturers have marketed this application less aggressively.

Fabrication of Optec FPDs requires a refractory die and is similar to the technique described in the section on laboratory procedures for all ceramic crowns. Because of the bulk of ceramic in the pontic area, this portion must be built incrementally in separate sections and connected later after bulk contraction has taken place (Fig. 6-266).

This material has been shown to have a slightly higher abrasion potential than conventional ceramic materials so meticulous attention should be given to functional contact surface quality. Because of its limited strength, the use of composite resin cements and optimal all purpose bonding techniques is required to further support and strengthen this all ceramic FPD alternative.

The second and newest ceramic material that is advocated for use in the fabrication of anterior traditional FPDs is the aluminous oxide, core strengthening material In-ceram

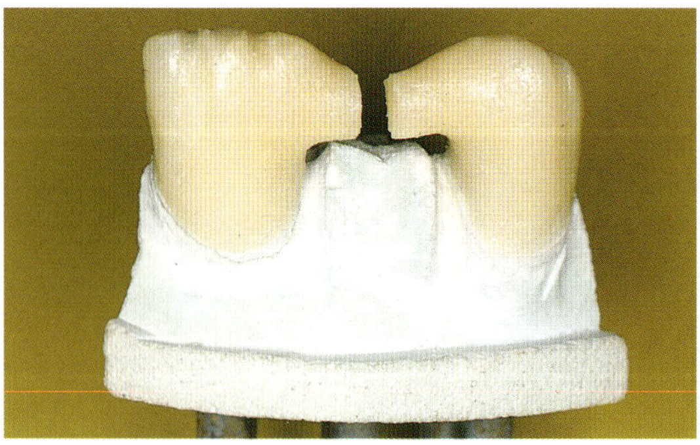

Fig. 6-266a Initial two part buildup on refractory die.

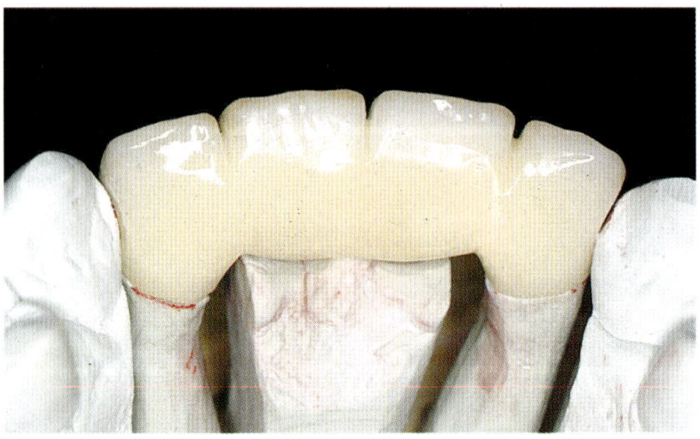

Fig. 6-266b Completed all ceramic FPD, showing bulk in lingual connector region.

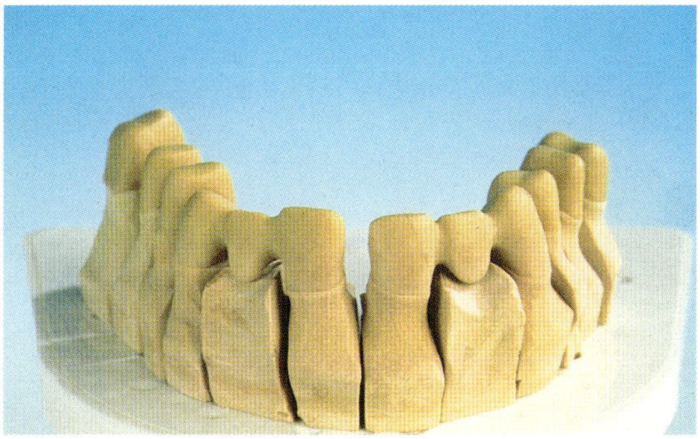

Fig. 6-267a In-Ceram FPD substructures on dies (courtesy of Vident, Baldwin Park, CA).

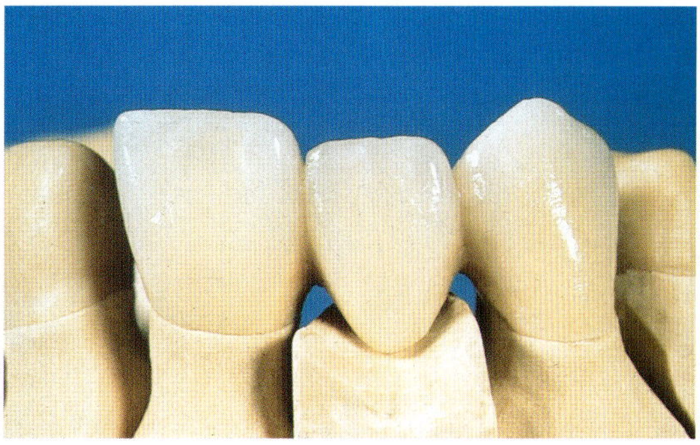

Fig. 6-267b Completed In-Ceram FPD (courtesy of Vident, Baldwin Park, CA).

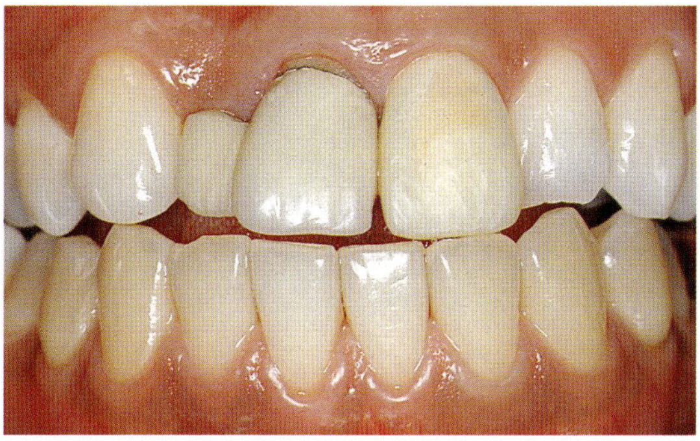

Fig. 6-268a

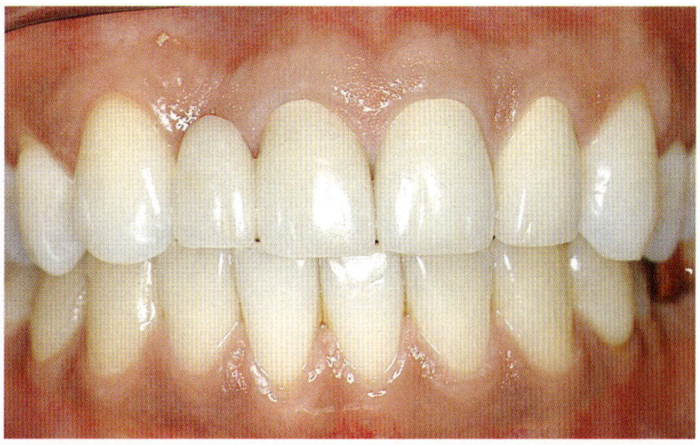

Fig. 6-268b

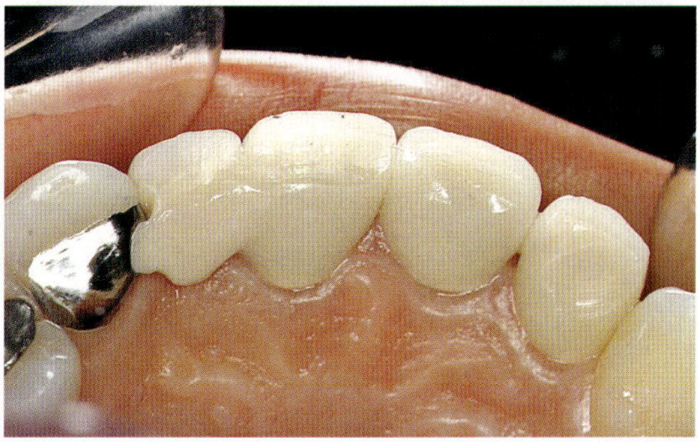

Fig. 6-268c

Fig. 6-268a Preoperative view.

Fig. 6-268b Postoperative facial view. In-Ceram FPD to replace teeth 7 and 8.

Fig. 6-268c Postoperative lingual view showing ceramic bulk between tooth 7 cantilever pontic and tooth 8 retainer.

(Vident, Baldwin Park, CA). In-Ceram, described previously in this chapter, is currently the strongest ceramic material available for use in fabricating FPDs. One advantage of In-Ceram is that it appears to be strong enough that composite resin cements are not mandatory for success. The option to use fluoride-releasing glass ionomer luting cements is still possible. However, the use of composite resin cements and all purpose bonding techniques should be strongly considered for any all ceramic FPD. As with single units, a core of In-Ceram is formed, much like a metal substructure for a ceramometal FPD, and veneered with more esthetic conventional ceramic (Fig. 6-267). In-Ceram bulk should be maximum in nonesthetic lingual, proximal and connector regions and minimal in the more esthetic facial areas where adequate room is needed for the veneering ceramic (Fig. 6-268). In-Ceram is claimed to be more translucent than previous aluminous oxide core materials. Using the newer opalescent veneering ceramic materials, highly esthetic restorations can be provided.

Currently In-Ceram is being advocated for short span anterior FPDs with one or two pontics. Research is currently in progress analyzing more extensive anterior designs as well as posterior designs. Initial success has led to some optimism but is there a demand for such FPDs? More extensive anterior FPDs include a greater area and the need to closely match adjacent natural teeth is diminished. Many posterior FPDs are less esthetically demanding and the alternative of a weaker material may be less desirable. If the clinical success rate is shown to be high, then reasons other than esthetic demands may provide a stimulus to place these later In-Ceram FPDs. Currently all ceramic FPDs should be limited to short span anterior situations. Venturing beyond that point should be considered experimental at this time.

CERAMIC VENEER FIXED PARTIAL DENTURES

A ceramic veneer FPD is designed to have a pontic suspended between porcelain veneer retainers. This all ceramic alternative to the previously described traditionally designed all ceramic FPD provides an alternative requiring much less tooth reduction.

Indications

Ceramic veneer FPDs are indicated for the replacement of a single anterior tooth when intact abutment teeth exist. The retainers may be used on either the buccal or lingual surfaces depending upon space present and esthetic goals.

The lingual approach would replace the more predictable ceramometal bonded FPD (Maryland bridge) and may selectively be used when the use of metal is not desired.

The facial veneer approach has more distinct indications. When an edentulous space exists and ceramic veneers are treatment planned for the adjacent teeth, this approach is useful in matching adjacent restorations. Another esthetic advantage of this approach is that tooth size adjustments can be made when asymmetries exist between abutment teeth and the edentulous space. For in-

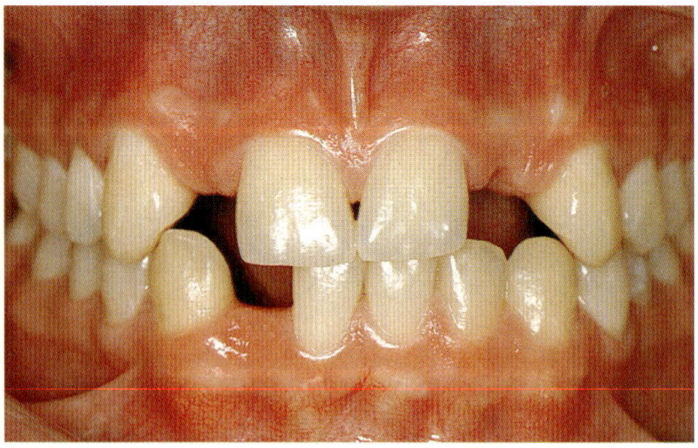

Fig. 6-269a Preoperative view.

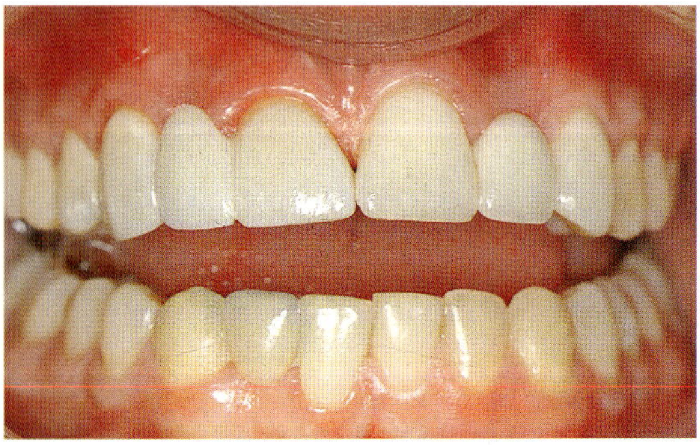

Fig. 6-269b Postoperative view of porcelain veneer FPDs

stance, when an edentulous space is too large, facial veneers can be used to widen retainers and narrow the pontic making a more acceptable tooth size relationship (Fig. 6-269). This would not be possible using a lingual approach.

Contraindications

The main deterrent to using this type of FPD is an unwillingness to accept a guarded prognosis in spite of the potential esthetic advantages. A second contraindication is a lack of adequate buccal-lingual width in the connector region. Bulk in the connectors is mandatory for maximum predictability (Fig. 6-270). Thin connectors are vulnerable to fracture and the prognosis is significantly reduced. In addition, any above normal strength requirements resulting from habits, patient activities or occupational duties should be viewed as potential deterrents to the use of this type of restoration. Some form of postoperative orthotic or mouth protection is required when a veneer FPD is used under these circumstances.

Design

The preparation adjacent the pontic is extended to the lingual line angle as described in the section on porcelain veneer preparation for diastemas. This will allow for maximum buccal-lingual connector width and maximum potential strength.

The materials used must be totally strengthened ceramics that allow for maximum strength and esthetics in the thinnest possible space. Conventional and core strengthened ceramic materials might be successful but have not been advocated by the manufacturers or restorative dentists so they cannot be recommended.

CERAMIC VENEER/ COMPOSITE SUBSTRUCTURE FIXED PARTIAL DENTURES

An innovative and esthetic FPD was designed to combine the stability, versatility and esthetics of a ceramic veneer with a strong yet more flexible high strength composite substructure (Fig. 6-271). Failures with nonmetallic all ceramic FPDs often occur in the connector region due to stress induced strain that exceeds the material's ability to resist or compensate. This combination design is an attempt to provide a more flexible yet strong substructure made of composite. A ceramic veneer is cemented over the pontic substructure and provides all the advantages of a ceramic veneer.

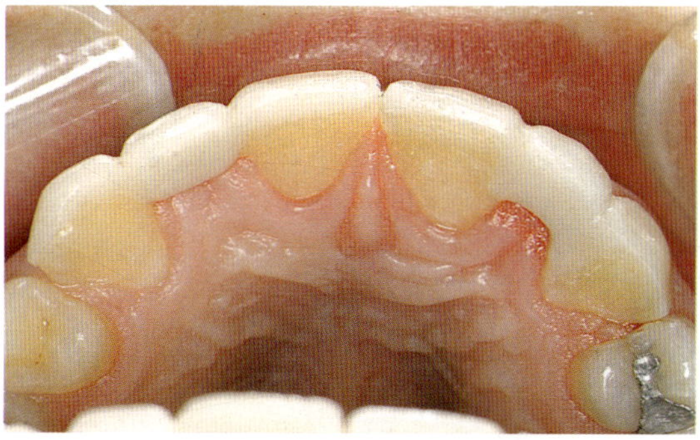

Fig. 6-270 Lingual view showing adequate connector bulk (teeth 9 to 11) and inadequate connector bulk (teeth 6 to 8).

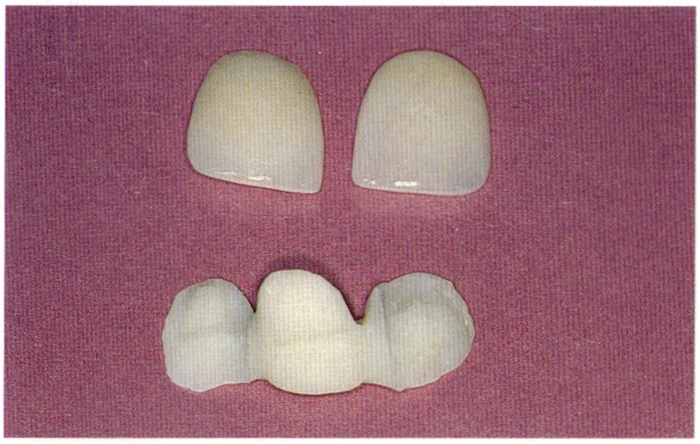

Fig. 6-271 (**top**) Porcelain veneers; (**bottom**) composite substructure.

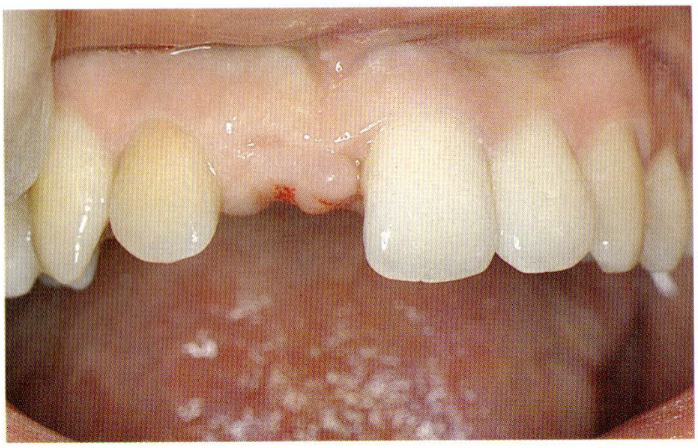

Fig. 6-272a

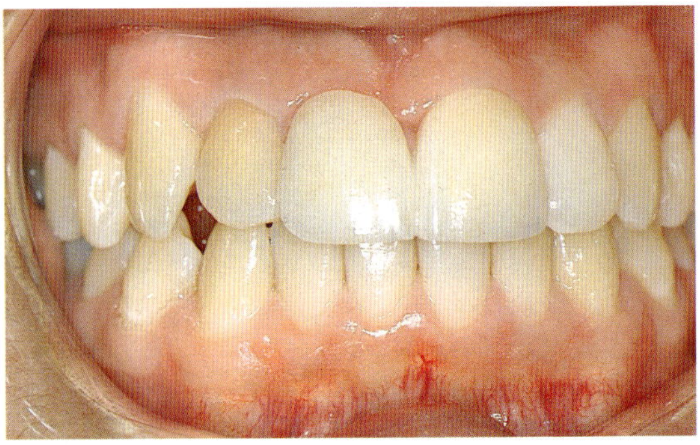

Fig. 6-272b

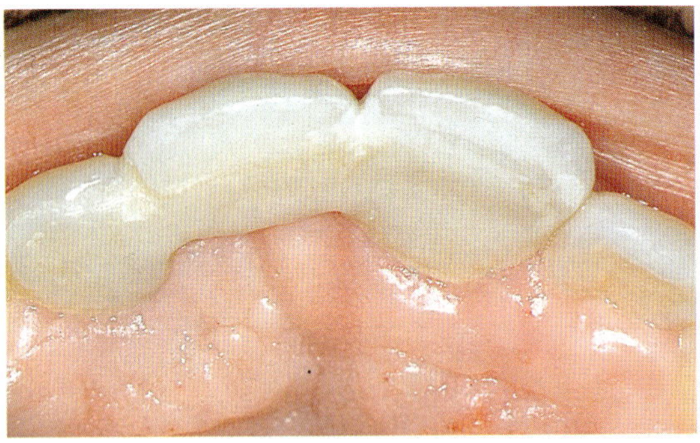

Fig. 6-272c

Fig. 6-272a Preoperative view.

Fig. 6-272b Facial postoperative view.

Fig. 6-272c Lingual postoperative view; note lingual composite substructure (teeth 7 to 9) and porcelain veneers (teeth 8 and 9).

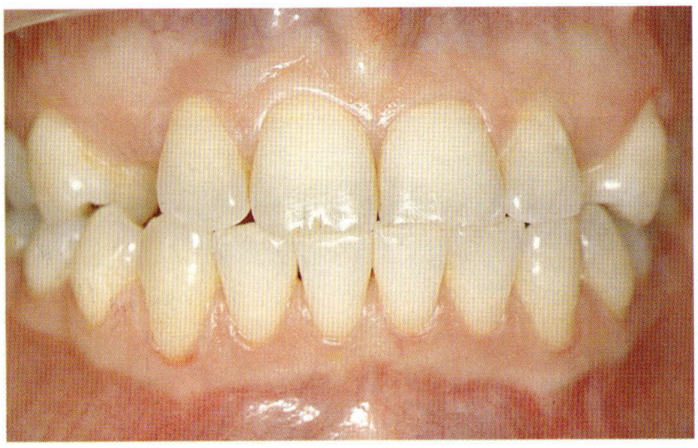

Fig. 6-273a

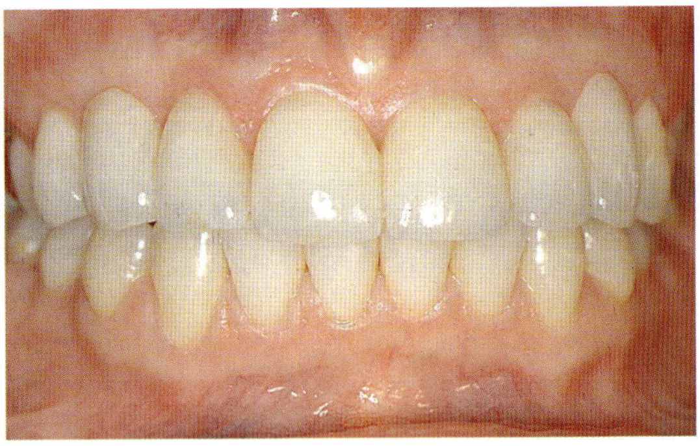

Fig. 6-273b

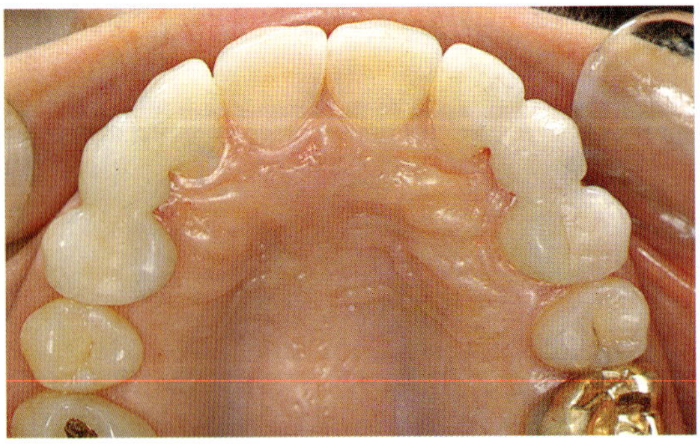

Fig. 6-273c

Fig. 6-273a Preoperative view.

Fig. 6-273b Postoperative view (teeth 5 to 12 porcelain veneers).

Fig. 6-273c Postoperative view. Note composite FPD substructure in teeth 5 to 7 and 10 to 12.

Indications

This FPD design is used as a potentially more esthetic alternative to a ceramometal bonded FPD (Maryland FPD). It is an extremely esthetic and conservative alternative to conventionally designed FPDs (Fig. 6-272). It is a useful adjunctive technique when adjacent ceramic veneers are used and an esthetic match of an edentulous space is mandatory (Fig. 6-273).

Contraindications

Low strength and lack of long term clinical research are the main deterrents to their use. This type of FPD, while showing good preliminary success, must be placed only with the patient's clear understanding that it is an attempt to provide maximum esthetics and strength is significantly less than conventional or bonded ceramometal FPD designs.

Design

The preparation is similar to a ceramometal bonded FPD but due to the reduced strength of the composite substructure, additional room must be provided lingually and especially in the connector region. Maximum lingual enamel coverage, as demonstrated when using metallic retainers, appears to be slightly less important and the need for bulk in the connector region and adjacent areas more significant. Maximum lingual coverage should still be utilized in areas where room exists (between 0.5 and 1.0 mm).

The composite substructure should be designed for maximum lingual bulk and strength. The "Encore FPD" technique (da Vinci Dental Studio, Woodland Hills, CA) uses a high strength larger particle size composite and reinforcing mesh veneered with a more polishable composite. This is fabricated in a nitrogen atmosphere under pressure. This innovative technique has been used extensively with good success.

The ceramic veneer is fabricated out of a conventional ceramic material for maximum esthetics. A vertical strut is cut in the pontic's facial composite substructure to provide increased ceramic bulk and resistance to cracks resulting from substructure flexure.

Cementation procedures are similar to the procedures used for ceramic veneers. The FPD components are tried in for esthetic evaluation. The substructure is generally cemented first using previously described techniques. Care must be taken to eliminate any composite resin cement excess from the surface on which the veneer will be cemented. Finally, the ceramic veneer is cemented and finalized as a conventional veneer. Finishing and polishing is done as with ceramic veneers or composites as discussed in previous chapters. The composite substructure and ceramic veneer may also be cemented simultaneously. This is especially useful when a single veneer is used. When used in conjunction with adjacent veneers, a veneer should be cemented separately from the substructure to minimize any chance of veneer displacement.

CERAMIC INLAY/ METAL REINFORCED FIXED PARTIAL DENTURES

Inlay retainers with rigid connectors have never been a predictable design in traditional fixed prosthodontics using luting cements. Newer bonding techniques that have increased the retention of this minimal retainer have renewed interest and utilization. All ceramic, inlay retained FPD designs lack the bulk and subsequent strength to have predictable success. Consequently a metallic substructure is advocated. This substructure

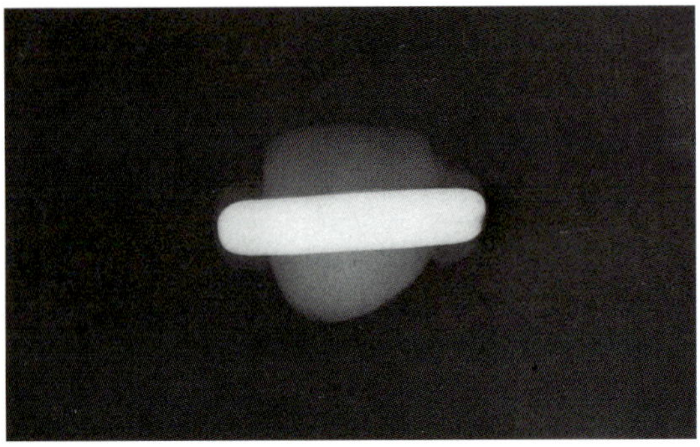

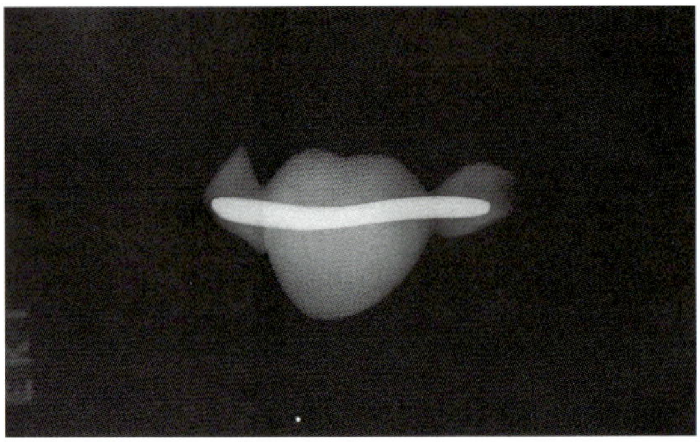

Figs. 6-274a and b Radiographs of posterior and anterior inlay FPDs showing reinforcement bars.

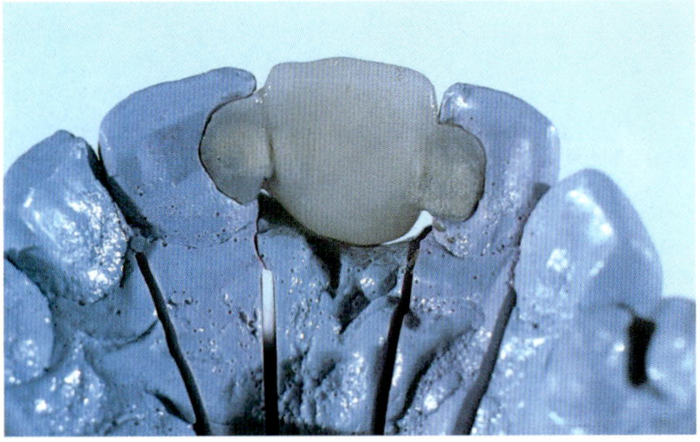

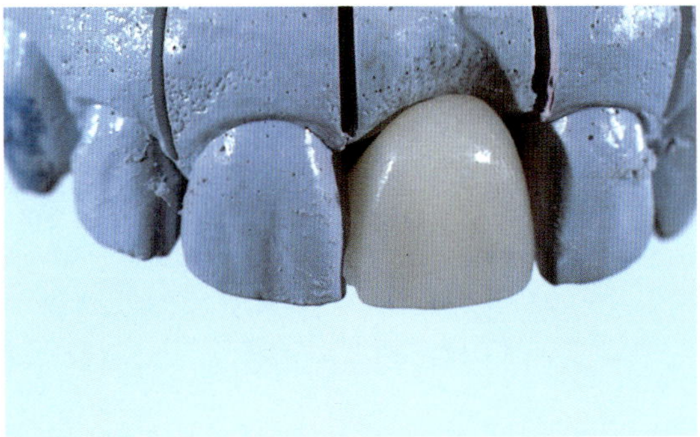

Figs. 6-275a and b Anterior inlay FPD, bar reinforced.

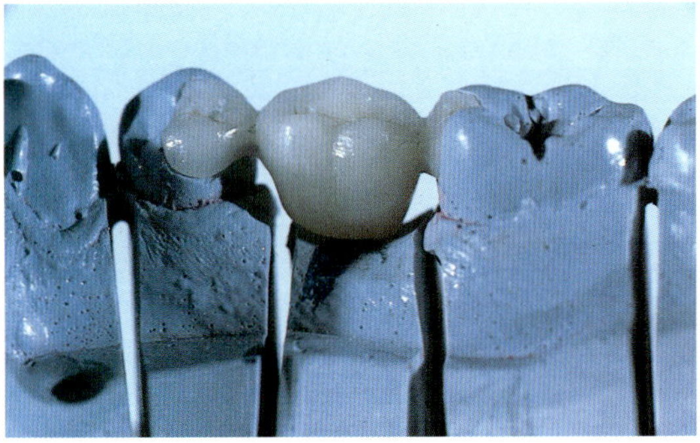

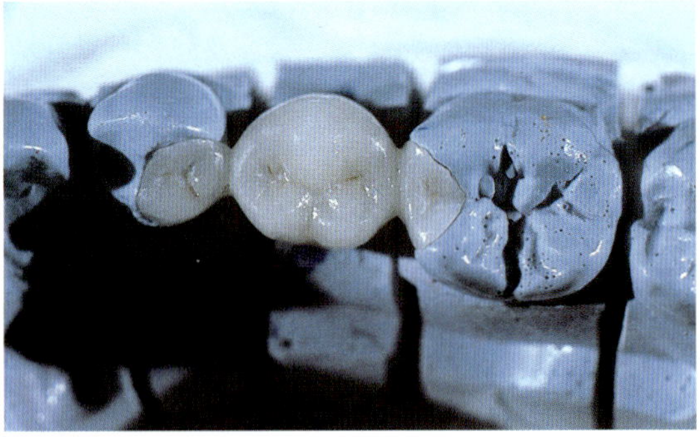

Figs. 6-276a and b Posterior inlay FPD, bar reinforced.

(Note: Fixed partial dentures courtesy of Tetra Dynamics.)

ranges from a custom cast type to a prefabricated bar (Fig. 6-274). While these FPD designs are metal reinforced, they have been included in this chapter because they are a contemporary design that is reasonably esthetic and very conservative.

Indications

Utilization of this type of FPD might include situations where adjacent retainers are intact or have existing intracoronal restorations and insufficient external enamel for utilization of other bonded FPD designs (Figs. 6-275 and 6-276). Patient esthetic demands should be maximum and a desire for a conservative approach a priority. This FPD design may also be utilized when intact retainers exist and esthetic demands eliminate the use of other less esthetic ceramometal bonded FPD designs. Utilization of this FPD design follows the basic principals outlined in the section on ceramic inlays. The preparations must be large enough to attain adequate bulk for FPD strength and space for the metal substructure. The design must also have adequate surface area for sufficient bond strengths. Initial reports on this type of FPD appear to be positive. Long term results are not available.

Many new esthetic FPD designs have been and will continue to be developed as the desire for esthetic yet conservative restorations continue to increase as a priority. Good clinical research is necessary and mandatory before any of these designs can be recommended for routine use. Until that time, all these FPD designs, as with many other techniques described in this textbook, must be used with guarded optimism.

REFERENCES

DENTAL CERAMIC MATERIALS

Barghi, N., McKechan-Whitmer, M., and Aranda, R.: Comparison of Fracture Strength of Porcelain-Veneered-to-High Noble and Base Metal Alloys. (1987). J. Prosth. Dent. Vol. 57 (1), p. 23.

Barreiro, M.M., Riesgo, O., and Vicente, E.E.: Phase Identification in Dental Porcelains for Ceramo-Metallic Restorations. (1989). Dent. Mat., Vol. 5, p. 51.

Broadbent, R.H.W., O'Brien, W.J., and Fan, P.L.: Translucency in Dental Porcelains. (1980). J. Dent. Res. Vol. 59 (1), p. 70.

Calamia, J.R.: High Strength Porcelain Bonded Restorations: Anterior and Posterior. (1989). Quint. Int. Vol. 20 (10), p. 717.

Campbell, S.D.: A Comparative Study of Metal Ceramic and All-Ceramic Esthetic Materials: Modulus of Rupture. (1989). J. Prosth. Dent. Vol. 62(4), p. 476.

Cochran, M.A., Carlson, T.J., Moore, B.K., Richmond, N.L., and Brackett, W.W.: Tensil Bond Strengths of Five Porcelain Repair Systems. (1988). Oper. Dent. Vol. 13, p. 162.

Claus, H.: The Structure and Microstructure of Dental Porcelain in Relationship to the Firing Conditions. (1989). Int. J. Prosth. Vol. 2 (4), p. 376.

Claus, H.: The Structural Basis of Dental Porcelain. (1980). Vita Zahnfabrik, Bad Säckingen, Germany.

DeGroot, K., Tencer, A., Waite, P., Nichols, J., and Kay, J.: Significance of the Porosity and Physical Chemistry of Calcium Phosphate Ceramics. (1988). Annals N.Y. Acad. Sci. Vol. 523, p. 272.

Drummond, J.L., Novickas, D., and Lenke, J.W.: Physiological Aging of an All-Ceramic Restorative Material. (1991). Dent. Mat. Vol. 7, p. 133.

Fan, P.L. and Stanford, J.W.: Ceramics: Their Place in Dentistry. (1987). Int. Dent. J. Vol. 37, p. 197.

Grossman, D.G.: Cast Glass Ceramics. (1985). Dent. Clin. N.A., Vol. 2, p. 725.

Kelly, J.R., Giordano, R., Pober, R., and Cima, M.J.: Fracture Surface Analysis of Dental Ceramics: Clinically Failed Restorations. (1990). Int. J. Prosthodont. Vol. 3 (5), p. 430.

Kelly, J.R., Cambell, S.D., and Bowen, H.K.: Fracture-Surface Analysis of Dental Ceramics. (1989). J. Prosthet. Dent. Vol. 62 (5), p. 536.

Lumo, P.S., Goodkind, R.J., and Swanson, S.: Residual Stress in Several Ceramo Metal Systems. (1989). J. Prosth. Dent. Vol. 62 (3), p. 278.

Mackert, J.R., and Evans, A.L.: Effect of Cooling Rate on Leucite Volume Fraction in Dental Porcelains. (1991). J. Dent. Res. Vol. 70 (2), p. 137.

Malhotra, M.C. and Maickel, L.B.: Shear Bond Strength in Porcelain Metal Restorations. (1980). J. Prosth. Dent. Vol. 43 (4), p. 397.

McCrory, P.V., Tinston, S., Piddock, V., Kelly, P., Combe, E.C., and Arnell, R.D.: Tin Oxide Coating of Aluminous Porcelain by Reactive Ion Plating. (1991). J. Dent. Vol. 19 (3), p. 171.

McLean, J.W.: Ceramics in Clinical Dentistry. (1988). Br. Dent. J. Vol. 164, p. 187.

McLean, J.W.: The Science and Art of Dental Ceramics. (1991). Oper. Dent. Vol. 16, p. 149.

Messer, P.F., Piddock, V., and Lloyd, C.H.: The Strength of Dental Ceramics. (1991). J. Dent. Vol. 19 (1), p. 51.

Miller, A., Long, J., Miller B., and Cole, J.: Comparison of the Fracture Strength of Ceramometal Crowns Versus Several All-Ceramic Crowns. (1992). J. Prosth. Dent. Vol. 68 (1), p. 38.

O'Brien, W.J., Kay K.S., Boenke, K.M., and Groh, C.L.: Sources of Color Variation on Firing Porcelain. (1991). Dent. Mat. Vol. 7, p. 170.

Piddock, V.: Effect of Alumina Concentration on the Thermal Diffusivity of Dental Porcelain. (1989). J. Dent. Vol. 17 (16), p. 290.

Piddock, V., Marquis, P.M., and Wilson, H.J.: The Mechanical Strength and Microstructure of All-Ceramic Crowns. (1987). J. Dent. Vol. 15, p. 153.

Piddock, V., Qualthrough, A.J.E.: Dental Ceramics — An Update. (1990). J. Dent. Vol. 18, p. 227.

Piddock, V., Qualthrough, A.J.E., and Brough, I.: An Investigation of an Ion Strengthening Paste for Dental Porcelains. (1991). Int. J. Prosthodont. Vol. 4 (2), p. 132.

Rosenstein, S.F. and Porter, S.S.: Apparent Fracture Toughness of All-Ceramic Crown Systems. (1989). J. Prosth. Dent. Vol. 62 (5), p. 529.

Seghi, R.R., Crispin, B.J., and Mito, W.: The Effect of Ion Exchange on the Flexural Strength of Feldspathic Porcelains. (1990). Int. J. Prosthodont. Vol. 3 (2), p. 130.

Seghi, R.R., Daher, T., and Caputo, A.: Relative Flexural Strength of Dental Restorative Ceramics. (1990). Dent. Mat. Vol. 6, p. 181.

Seghi, R.R., Rosenstein, S.F., and Bauer, P.: Abrasion of Human Enamel by Different Dental Ceramics in Vitro. (1991). J. Dent. Res. Vol. 70 (3), p. 221.

Sproull, R.C.: History of Porcelain, in Dental Porcelain: The State of the Art (1977). (Yamada ed.). Univ. of S. Cal., Los Angeles, CA. USA.

Sumithra, N., Waknine, S., and Schulman, A.: Bond Strength of Etched Porcelain Denture Teeth to PMMA. (1986). Quint. Int. Vol. 17 (11), p. 745.

Taira, M., Nomura, Y., Wakasa, K., Yamaki, M., and Matsui, A.: Studies on Fracture Toughness of Dental Ceramics. (1990). J. Oral. Rehab. Vol. 17, p. 551.

Tjan, A.H.L. and Nemetz, H.: A Comparison of the Shear Bond Strength Between Two Composite Resins and Two Etched Ceramic Materials. (1988). Int. J. Prosthodont. Vol. 1 (1), p. 73.

Wassenaar, P.: G-C Ceramicoat: An Ion Exchange Hardener for Ceramics. (1990). Aust. Dent. J. Vol. 35 (5), p. 474.

Yamamoto, M.: A Newly Developed "Opal" Ceramic and its Clinical Use, with Special Attention to its Relative Refractive Index. (1989). QDT Yearbook. Vol. 9.

ALL CERAMIC CROWNS

Abbatie, M.P., Tjan, A.H.L., and Fox, W.M.: Comparison of the Marginal Fit of Various Ceramic Crown Systems. (1989). J. Prosth. Dent. Vol. 61, p. 527.

Adair, P.J. and Grossman, D.G.: The Castable Ceramic Crown. (1984). Int. J. Perio. Rest. Dent. Vol. 23, p. 33.

Bruke, C.E. and Phillip, G.E.: The Fit of Molded All-Ceramic, Twin Foil and Conventional Ceramic Crowns. (1987). J. Prosth. Dent. Vol. 58, p. 408.

Campbell, S.D.: Esthetic Modification of Cast Dental-Ceramic Restorations. (1990). Int. J. Prosthodont. Vol. 3 (2), p. 123.

Campbell, S.D.: A Comparative Strength Study of Metal Ceramic and All-Ceramic Esthetic Materials: Modulus of Rupture. (1989). J. Prosth. Dent. Vol. 62(4) p. 476.

Castellani, D.: Differential Treatment Planning for Single Anterior Crowns. (1990). Int. J. Perio. Rest. Dent. Vol. 10 (3), p. 231.

Claus, H.: Vita In-Ceram, A New System for Producing Aluminum Oxide Crown and Bridge Substructures. (1990). Quint. Zahntech. Vol. 16, p.35.

Crispin, B.J. and Watson, J.F.: Margin placement of esthetic veneer crowns: Part I, anterior tooth show. (1981). J. Prosth. Dent. 45(3) p. 278. (Research article).

Crispin, B.J. and Watson, J.F.: Margin placement of esthetic veneer crowns: Part II, anterior tooth show. (1981). J. Prosth. Dent. 45(4) p. 389. (Research article).

Crispin, B.J. and Watson, J.F., and Shay, K.: Margin placement of esthetic veneer crowns: Part IV, patient acceptance of supragingival margins. (1985). J. Prosth. Dent. Vol. 53, No. 2, p. 165.

Crispin, B.J., Hewlett, E., and Seghi, R.R.: Color stability of Porcelain Stains Subjected to Glazing Temperatures. (1991). J. Prosth. Dent. 66, p. 20.

Davis, D.R.: Comparison of Fit of Two Types of All Ceramic Crowns. (1988). J. Prosth. Dent. Vol. 59 (1), p. 12.

Day, G.P. and Devlin, R.: Optec HSP: An Integrated System for All-Ceramic Restorations. (1987). Trends Tech. Cont. Dent. Lab. Nat. Assoc. Dent. Labor.

Derand, T.: Reinforcement of Porcelain Crowns with Silicon Carbide Fibers. (1980). J. Prosth. Dent. Vol. 43 (1), p. 40.

Dickinson, A.J.G., Moore, B.K., Harris, R.K., and Dykema, R.W.: A Comparative Study of the Strength of Aluminous Porcelain and All-Ceramic Crowns. (1989). J. Prosth. Dent. Vol. 61 (3), p. 297.

Doyle, M.G., Munoz, C.A., Goodacre, C.J., Friedlander, L.D., and Moore, B.K.: The Effect of Tooth Preparation Design on the Breaking Strength of Dicor Crowns: Part 2. (1990). Int. J. Prosthodont. Vol. 3 (3), p. 241.

Doyle, M.G., Goodacre, C.J., Munoz, C.A., and Andres, C.J.: The Effect of Tooth Preparation Design on the Breaking Strength of Dicor Crowns: Part 3. (1990). Int. J. Prosthodont. Vol. 3 (4), p. 327.

Eden, G.T. and Kacicz, J.M.: Dicor Crown Strength Improvement Due to Bonding. (1987). J. Dent. Res. Vol. 66, p. 207.

El Sherif, M.H., Jacobi, R., and Lindke, L.: The Ceramic Reverse Three-Quarter Crown for Anterior Teeth: Laboratory Procedures. (1990). J. Prosth. Dent. Vol. 64 (2), p. 127.

Fall, T.W., Hesby, R.A., Pelleu, G.B., and Eastwood, G.W.: Marginal Opening of Single and Twin Platinum Full-Bonded Aluminous Porcelain Crown. (1985). J. Prosth. Dent. Vol. 53, p. 29.

Friedlander, L.D., Munoz, C.A., Goodacre, C.J., Doyle, M.G., and Moore, B.K.: The Effect of Tooth Preparation Design on the Breaking Strength of Dicor Crowns: Part I. (1990). Int. J. Prosthodont. Vol. 3 (2), p. 159.

Hensel, W., Sato, T., Wohlwend, A., and Schärer, P.: A Clinical Case Report Utilizing a Castable Ceramic Crown System. (1987). Quint. Int. Vol. 18 (5), p. 323.

Hojjatie, B. and Anusavich, K.J.: Three-Dimensional Finite Element Analysis of Glass-Ceramic Dental Crowns. (1990). J. Biomechan. Vol. 23 (11), p. 1157.

Holmes, R. and Sneed, W.D.: Treatment of Severe Chemo-mechanical Erosion Using Castable Ceramic Restorations and a New Dentin/Enamel Bonding System: A Case Report. (1990). Quint. Int. Vol. 21 (11), p. 863.

Hondrum, S.O.: The Strength of Cemented Alumina Core and Magnesia Core Crowns. (1988). Int. J. Prosthdont. Vol. 1 (2), p. 190.

Hummert, T., Barghi, N., and Berry, T.: Effect of Fitting Adjustments on Compressive Strength of a New Foil Crown System. (1991). J. Prosth. Dent. Vol., 66 (2), p. 172.

Hung, S.H., Hung, K., Eick, J.D., and Chappell, R.P.: Marginal Fit of Porcelain-Fused-To-Metal and Two Types of Ceramic Crowns. (1990). J. Prosth. Dent. Vol. 63 (1), p. 26.

Hunt, P.R. and Rafetto, R.F.: Full Circle in Ceramics: The Development of a New Porcelain Fused to Metal Restoration. (1980). Compend. Cont. Ed. Vol. 1 (1), p. 7

Jacobi, R., Schillingburg, H.T., and Duncanson, M.G.: A Comparison of the Abrasiveness of Six Ceramic Surfaces and Gold. (1991). J. Prosth. Dent. Vol. 66 (3), p. 303.

Jensen, E., Schultes, A.M., Handelman, S.L., and Proskin, H.M.: Plaque Retention on Dicor Crowns and Gingival Health Evaluated Over a 4-Year Period. (1990). Int. J. Perio. Rest. Dent. Vol. 10 (6), p. 455.

Josephson, B.A., Schulman, A., Dunn, Z.A., and Hurwitz, W.: A Compressive Strength Study of All-Ceramic Crown. (1985). J. Prosth. Dent. Vol. 53 (3), p. 301.

Josephson, B.A., Schulman, A., Dunn, Z.A., and Hurwitz, W.: A Compressive Strength Study of All-Ceramic Crown. Part II. (1991). J. Prosth. Dent. Vol. 65 (3), p. 388.

Latta, M.A.: The Continuing Ceramic Evolution: Dicor Plus and Dicor Castable Ceramic. (1990). Esth. Dent. Update. Vol. 2.

Lugassy, A.A., Moffa, J.P., and Elison, J.A.: Cast Glass Ceramic Crowns: A One-Year Clinical Study. (1986). Cal. Dent. Assoc. J. Vol. 14, p. 72.

Mater, H.J.: Willi Glass Crowns Eliminate the "Blue Gums" Phenomenon. (1989). Can. Dent. Assn. J. Vol. 55 (8), p. 612.

Malament, K.A., and Grossman, D.G.: The Cast Glass-Ceramic Restoration. (1987). J. Prosth. Dent. Vol. 57 (6), p. 674.

McLean, J.W., Jeansonne, E.E., Bruggers, H., and Lynn D.B.: A New Metal-Ceramic Crown. (1978). J. Prosth. Dent. Vol. 40 (3) p. 273.

O'Brien, W.J.: Magnesia Ceramic Jacket Crowns. (1985). Dent. Clin. N.A. Vol. 29 (4), p. 719.

Philip, G.K. and Bruke, C.E.: Compressive Strengths of Conventional, Twin Foil, and All Ceramic Crowns. (1984). J. Prosth. Dent. Vol. 52 (2), p. 215.

Savitt, E.D., Malament, K.A., Socransky, S.S., Melcer, A.J., and Backman, K.J.: Effects on Colonization of Oral Microbiota by a Cast Glass-Ceramic Restoration. (1987). Int. J. Perio. Prosthodont. Vol. 7 (2), p. 22.

Schössow, D.: The Kera-Platinum Technique Porcelain Crown: "Renaissance of the Jacket Crown." (1984). Quint of Dent. Tec. Vol. 8 (4), p. 231.

Sorensen, J.A. and Okamoto, S.K.: Comparison of Marginal Fit of All-Ceramic Crown Systems. (1987). J. Dent. Res. (Abstract). Vol. 49 (2), p. 283.

Sozio, R.B. and Riley, E.J.: The Shrink-Free Ceramic Crown. (1983). J. Prosth. Dent. Vol. 49 (2), p. 182.

Vahidi, F., Egloff, E.T., and Panno, F.V.: Evaluation of Marginal Adaptation of All-Ceramic Crowns and Metal Ceramic Crowns. (1991). J. Prosth. Dent. Vol. 66 (4), p. 426.

Watson, J.F. and Crispin, B.J.: Margin placement of esthetic veneer crowns: Part III, attitudes of dentists and patients. (1981). J. Prosth. Dent 45(5) p. 499.

Weaver, J.D., Johnson, G.H. and Bales, D.J.: Marginal Adaptation of Castable Ceramic Crowns. (1991). J. Prosth. Dent. Vol. 66 (6), p. 747.

Wohlwend, A., Strub, J.R., and Schärer, P.: Metal Ceramic and All-Porcelain Restorations: Current Considerations. (1989). Int. J. Prosthodont. Vol. 2 (1), p. 13.

CERAMIC INLAYS AND ONLAYS

Albers, H.F.: Tooth Colored Restoratives. 7th ed. (1985). Alto Books, Cotati, CA. U.S.A.

Banks, R.G.: Conservative Posterior Ceramic Restorations: A Literature Review. (1990). J. Prosth. Dent. Vol. 63 (6), p. 619.

Bessing, C., and Molin, M.: An in Vivo Study of Glass Ceramic (Dicor®) Inlays. Preliminary Report. (1990). Acta Odontol. Scand. Vol. 48, p. 351.

Bowen, R.L., Eighmiller, F.G., and Marjenhoff, W.R.: Glass-Ceramic Inserts Anticipated for "Megafilled" Composite Restorations. (1991). J.A.D.A. Vol. 122, p. 71.

Cavel, W.T., Kelsey, W.P., III, and Barkmeier, W.W.: Pilot Study of the Clinical Evaluation of Castable Ceramic Inlays and a Dual-cure Resin Cement. (1988). Quint. Int. Vol. 19, p. 257.

Christensen, G.T.: Tooth-Colored Inlays and Onlays. (1988). J.A.D.A. Special Issue, p. 12E.

Christensen, G.T.: A Look at State of the Art Tooth-Colored Inlays and Onlays. (1992). J.A.D.A. Vol. 123, p. 66.

Crispin, B.J.: Computerized Design and Manufacturing of Esthetic Dental Restorations. (1992). Dent. Clin. N.A. Vol. 36 (3), p. 797.

Derand, T.: Stress Analysis of Cemented or Resin-Bonded Loaded Porcelain Inlays. (1991). Dent. Mat. Vol. 7, p. 21.

Douglas, W.H., Morin, D., and Delong, R.: Stiffness of Teeth as a Function of Cavity preparation and Restorative Materials. (1983). J. Dent. Res. (Abstract 450). Vol. 62, p. 219.

El-Mowafy, O.M., Brown, J.W., and McComb, D.: Radiopacity of Direct Ceramic Inlay Restoratives. (1991). J. Dent. Vol. 19, p. 366.

Hasegawa, E.A., Boyer, D.B., Daniel, C.N., and Chan: Hardening of Dual-Cured Cements Under Composite Resin Inlays. (1991). J. Prosth. Dent. Vol. 66(2), p. 187.

Hirato, K., Nakashima, M., Sekine, I., Mukouyama, Y., and Kimura, K.: Dentinal Fluid Movement Associated with Loading of Restorations. (1991). J. Dent. Res. Vol. 70 (6), p. 975.

Hornbrook, D.S., and Pai, M.D.: Silane-Coupling Agents: The Missing Link in Porcelain-Resin Bonding. (1992). Esth. Dent. Update. Vol. 3 (1), p.13.

James, D.F.: An Esthetic Inlay Technique for Posterior Teeth. (1983). Quint. Int. Vol. 14, p. 1.

Jensen, M.E.: Preliminary Research Report, Etched-Porcelain Resin Bonded Restorations: A Study of Cuspal Flexure, Strength and Microleakage. Dow Institute for Dental Research, Iowa City, IA., U.S.A.

Jensen, M.E., Redford, D.A., Williams, B.T., and Gardner, F.: Posterior Etched-Porcelain Restorations: An In Vitro Study. (1987). Compend. Cont. Ed. Dent. Vol. 8, p. 615.

Joynt, R.B., Wieczkowski, G., Klockowski, R., and Davis, E.I.: Effects of Composite Restorations on Resistance to Cuspal Fracture in Posterior Teeth. (1987). J. Prosth. Dent. Vol. 57, p. 431.

Lacy, A.M., Zhang, K., Koh, A., Wilshire, W.A., and Watanabe, L.: Marginal Microleakage Around Class II Resin and Dicor Inlays (1988). J. Dent. Res. (Abstract 669). Vol. 67, p. 196.

Leinfelder, K.F., Isenberg, B.P., and Essig, M.E.: New Method for Generating Ceramic Restorations: CAD-CAM System. (1989). J.A.D.A. Vol. 118, p. 703.

Leung, R.L. and Confortes, I.: Porcelain Inlays and Onlays. (1988) Cal. Dent. Assn. J. Sept., p. 38.

Mörman, W.H., Brandestini, M., Lutz, F., Barbakow, F., and Gutsch, T.: CAD-CAM Ceramic Inlays and Onlays: A Case Report After 3 Years in Place. (1990). J.A.D.A. Vol. 120, p. 517.

Qualtrough, A.J.E., Wilson, N.H.E., and Smith, G.A.: The Porcelain Inlay: A Historical View. (1990). Oper. Dent. Vol. 15, p. 61.

Reality. Miller, M.B. (Ed). Houston, TX. U.S.A.

Rekow, E.D.: Computer Aided Design and Manufacturing in Dentistry. A Review of the State of the Art. (1987). J. Prosth. Dent. Vol. 58, p. 512.

Rekow, E.D.: Dental Cad-Cam Systems: What is the State of the Art? (1991). J.A.D.A. Vol. 122, p. 43.

Rees, J.S. and Jacobsen, P.H.: Stresses Generated by Luting Resins During Cementation of Composite and Ceramic Inlay. (1992). J. Oral Rehabil. Vol. 19, p. 115.

Shaffer, H. and Zobler, C.: Complete Restoration with Resin-Bonded Porcelain Inlay. (1991). Quint. Int. Vol. 22 (2) p. 87.

Shortall, A.C., Baylis, R.L., Baylis, M.A., and Grundy, J.R.: Marginal Seal Comparisons Between Resin-Bonded Class II Porcelain Inlays, Posterior Composite Restorations and Direct Composite Resin Inlays. (1989). Int. J. Prosthdont. Vol. 2, p. 217.

Sorensen, J.A.: Improved Seating of Ceramic Inlays with a Silicone Fit-Checking Medium. (1991). J. Prosth. Dent. Vol. 65, p. 646.

Sorensen, J.A., Engleman, M.S., Torres, T.J., and Avera, S.P.: Shearbond Strength of Composite to Various Porcelain Surface Treatments. (1991)..Int. J. Prosthodont. Vol. 4 (1), p. 17.

Sorensen, J.A., Kang, S.K., and Avera, S.P.: Porcelain-Composite Interface Microleakage with Various Porcelain Surface Treatments. (1991). J. Dent. Mater. Vol. 7, p. 118.

Stampalia, L.L., Nicholls, J.I., Brudvik, J.S., and Jones, D.W.: Fracture Resistance of Teeth With Resin-Bonded Restorations. (1986). J. Prosth. Dent. Vol. 55, p. 694.

CERAMIC VENEERS

Albers, H.F.: Tooth Colored Restorations, 7th ed. (1985). Alto Books. Cotati, CA, U.S.A.

Albers, H.F.: Porcelain Veneers. (1990). Adept Report, Vol. 1 (3).

Barham, T.P., Mayhew, R.B., Cowan, R.D., Lubow, R.M., Pierson, W.P., and Voss, J.E.: Gingival Response to Laminate Veneer Restorations. (1983). Oper. Dent. Vol. 8 p. 122.

Barnes, D.M. and Strassler, H.E.: Veneers: A Comparison of Three Techniques. (1990). Esth. Dent. Update, Vol. 1 (5), p. 74.

Barreto, M.T., Shiu, A., and Renner, R.P.: Anterior Porcelain Laminate Veneers: Clinical and Laboratory Procedures. (1986). Quint. Dent. Tech. Sept., p. 493.

Bertolotti, R.L.: Laboratory Laminate Veneers: A Viable Alternative. (1989). Oral Health, p. 11.

Blackman, R., Barghi, N., and Duke, E.: Influence of Ceramic Thickness on Polymerization of Light-Cured Resin Cement. (1990). J. Prosth. Dent. Vol. 63 (3), p. 295.

Boksman, L., Jordan, R.E., Suzuki, M., Galii, K.A., and Burgoyne, A.R.: Etched Porcelain Labial Veneers. (1985). Ontario Dent. Vol. 62, (1).

Calamia, J.R.: Etched Porcelain Veneers: A New Treatment Modality Based on Scientific and Clinical Evidence. (1983). N.Y.J. Dent. Vol. 53 (6), p. 255.

Calamia, J.R. and Simonsen, R.J.: Effect of Coupling Agents on Bond Strength of Etched Porcelain. (1984). J. Dent. Res. (Abstract 79). Vol. 63, p. 179.

Calamia, J.R.: Etched Porcelain Veneers: The Current State of the Art. (1985). Quint. Int. Vol. 16 (1), p. 5.

Christensen, G.: Veneering of Teeth: State of the Art. (1985). Dent. Clin. N.A. Vol. 29 (2), p.373.

Clyde, J.S. and Gilmour, A.: Porcelain Veneers: A Preliminary Review. (1988). Br. Dent. J. Vol. 164, p. 9.

Crispin, B.J., Hewlett, G.R., and Dayan, S.: Evaluation of Enamel Thickness and Instrumentation as it Relates to Porcelain Veneer Preparations. (in press).

El-Sherif, M. and Jacobi, R.: The Ceramic Reverse Three-Quarter Crown for Anterior Teeth: Preparation Design. (1989). J. Prosth. Dent. Vol. 61 (1), p. 4.

Exner, H.V.: Predictability of Color Matching and the Possibilities for Enhancement of Ceramic Laminate Veneers. (1991). J. Prosth. Dent. Vol. 65 (5), p. 619.

Faunce, F.G. and Myers, D.R.: Laminate Veneer Restoration of Permanent Incisions. (1976). J.A.D.A. Vol. 93, p. 790.

Faunce, F.G.: Management of Discolored Teeth. (1983). Dent. Clin. N. Am. Vol. 27, p. 657.

Feinman, R.A.: Mandibular Laminate Provisionalization. (1984). Quint. Int. Vol. 20 (10), p. 771.

Friedman, M.J.: Potentials and Controversies of Etched Porcelain Veneer Techniques. (1987). Esth. Dent. Update. Vol. 2 (4), p. 62.

Friedman, M.J.: Multiple Potential of Etched Porcelain Laminate Veneers. (1987). J.A.D.A. (Special Issue). December, p. 82-E.

Friedman, M.J.: Augmenting Restorative Dentistry with Porcelain Veneers. (1991). J.A.D.A. Vol. 122, p. 29.

Garber, D.A., Goldstein, R.E., and Feinman, R.: Porcelain Laminate Veneers. (1988). Quint. Pub. Co., Chicago, IL USA.

Highton, R., Caputo, A.A., and Matyas, J.: A Photoelastic Study of Stresses on Porcelain Laminate Preparations (1987). J. Prosth. Dent. Vol. 58 (2), p. 157.

Horn, H.R.: A New lamination: Porcelain Bonded to Enamel. (1983). N.Y.S. Dent. J. Vol. 49, p. 401.

Horn, H.R.: Porcelain Laminate Veneers Bonded to Etched Enamel. (1983). Dent. Clin. N.A. Vol. 27, p. 671.

Hornbrook, D.S. and Pai, N.D.: Silane-Coupling Agents: The Missing Link in Porcelain-Resin Bonding. (1992). Esth. Dent. Update. Vol. 3 (1), p.13.

Hsu, C.S., Stangel, I., and Nathanson, D.: Shear Bond Strength of Resin to Etched Porcelain. (1985). J. Dent. Res. (Special Issue). (Abstract 1095).

Ibsen, R.L.: Establishing Cuspid-Guided Occlusion with Bonded Porcelain. (1989). J. Esth. Dent. Vol. 1 (3).

Lacy, A.M., Wada, C., Du, W., and Watanabe, L.: In Vitro Microleakage at the Gingival Margin of Porcelain and Resin Veneers. (1992). J. Prosth. Dent. Vol. 67 (1).

Lang, S.A. and Starr, C.R.: Castable Glass Ceramics for Veneer Restorations. (1992). J. Prosth. Dent. Vol. 67 (5), p. 590.

Liu, P., Isenberg, B.P., and Leinfelder, K.F.: Evaluating CAD-CAM Generated Ceramic Veneers. (1993). J.A.D.A. Vol. 124, p. 59.

Linden, J.J., Swift, E.J., Boyer, D.B., and Davis, B.K.: Photo-Activation of Resin Cements Through Porcelain Veneers. (1991). J. Dent. Res. Vol. (70) 2, p. 154.

Miller, B.J. and Nesbit, M.: Etched Porcelain Restorations for Patients with Microdontia. (1989). Quint. Int. Vol. 20 (9), p. 621.

Minato, K.S.: Esthetic Porcelain Veneers, Part I. (1986). Hawaii Dent. J. Vol. 17 (7).

Minato, K.S.: Esthetic Porcelain Veneers, Part II. (1987). Hawaii Dent. J. Vol. 17 (7).

Nash, R.W.: A Veneering Porcelain with High Color Saturation. (1990). Dent. Today. Vol. 9 (4).

Nash, R.W.: A Temporization Technique for Multiple Indirect Veneers. (1991). Esth. Dent. Update. Vol. 2 (4), p. 60.

Nicholls, J.I.: Tensil Bond of Resin Cements to Porcelain Veneers. (1988). J. Prosth. Dent. Vol. 60, p. 443.

Nixon, R.: Use of Porcelain Laminate Veneers Enhances Foreshortened, Worn Teeth. (1984). Dent. Today. (Oct.) p. 27.

O'Keefe, K.L., Pease, P.L, and Herrin, H.K.: Variables Affecting the Spectral Transmittance of Light Through Porcelain Veneer Samples. (1991). J. Prosth. Dent. Vol. 66 (4), p. 434.

Pincus, C.: Building Mouth Personality. (1948). Alpha Omegan, Vol. 42, p. 163.

Reality: Reality Publishing Company, Houston TX, U.S.A.

Rucker, L.M., Richter, W., Macentee, M., and Richardson, A.: Porcelain and Resin Veneers Clinically Evaluated: 1-Year Results. (1990). J.A.D.A. Vol. (121), p. 594.

Schaffer, H. and Kulmer, S.: Functional Reconstruction of Abraded Canines by Resin-Bonded All-Ceramic Guiding Elements. (1990). Int. J. of Prosthodont. Vol. 3 (6), p.538.

Sheets, C.G. and Taniguchi, T.: Advantages and Limitations in the Use of Porcelain Veneer Restorations (1990). J. Prosth. Dent. Vol. 64 (4), p. 406.

Sorensen, J.P., Strutz, J.M., Avera, S.P., and Materdomini, D.: Marginal Fidelity and Microleakage of Porcelain Veneers Made by two Techniques. (1992). J. Prosth. Dent. Vol. 67 91), p. 16.

Sorensen, J.A., Kang, S.K., and Avera, S.P.: Microleakage of Porcelain-Composite Interface with Various Porcelain Surface Treatments. (1991). Dent. Mat. Vol. 7, p. 118.

Sorensen, J.A., Engelman, M.J., Torres, T.J., and Avera, S.P.: Shear Bond Strength of Composite to Porcelain. (1991). J. Prosth. Dent. Vol. 4 (1).

Strassler, H.E. and Buchness, G.F.: Etched Porcelain Laminate Veneers: Our Newest Cosmetic Bonding Treatment Modality. (1985). B.C.D.S. Forum. Vol. 5(2), p.7.

Strassler, H.E., and Nathanson, D.: Clinical Evaluation of Etched Porcelain Veneers Over a Period of 18 to 42 Months. (1989). Esth. Dent., p. 21.

Sumithra, N., Waknine, S., and Schulman, A.: Bond Strength of Etched Porcelain Denture Teeth to PMMA. (1986). Quint. Int. Vol. 17 (11), p. 745.

Tjan, A.H.L. and Nemetz, H.: A Comparison of the Shear Bond Strength Between Two Composite Resins and Two Etched Ceramic Materials. (1988). Int. J. Prosthodont. Vol. 1 (1), p. 74.

Ton, C.G., Setcos, J.C., and Weinstein, A.R.: Indirect Dental Laminate Veneers — An Overview. (1987). J. Dent. Vol. 15 (3), p. 117.

INTRODUCTION TO CONTEMPORARY ESTHETIC FIXED PARTIAL DENTURES

Calamia, J.R.: High-Strength Porcelain Bonded Restorations: Anterior and Posterior. (1989). Quint. Int. Vol. 20 (10), p. 717.

Campbell, S.D. and Sozio, R.B.: Evaluation of the Fit and Strength of an All-Ceramic Fixed Partial Denture. J. Prosth. Dent. Vol. 59 (3), p. 301.

Claus, H.: Vita In-Ceram, A New System for Producting Aluminum Oxide Crown and Bridge Substructures. (1990). Quint. Zahntec. Vol. 16, p. 35.

Christensen, G.: Personal Communication. American Academy of Esthetic Dentistry, Santa Barbara, (1991).

Crocker, W.P.: The Cementation of Porcelain Jacket Crowns with Adhesive Resins. (Jan. 1992). Brit. Dent. J. p. 64.

Hornbrook, D.S.: Anterior Tooth Replacement Using a Two-Component Resin-Bonded Bridge. (1993). Compend. Contin. Educ. Dent. Vol. 14 (1), p. 52.

Ibsen, R.L. and Strassler, H.E.: An Innovative Method for Fixed Anterior Tooth Replacement Utilizing Porcelain Veneers. (1986). Quint. Int. Vol. 17 (8), p. 455.